Henke's
Med-Math

Dosage Calculation, Preparation & Administration

Sixth Edition

Susan Buchholz, RN, MSN

Associate Professor
Georgia Perimeter College
Lawrenceville, Georgia

Sister Grace Henke, SC, RN, MSN, EdD

Integrated Scientific and Ethics Review Board
St. Vincent Catholic Medical Centers
New York City, New York

 Wolters Kluwer | Lippincott Williams & Wilkins
Health
Philadelphia · Baltimore · New York · London
Buenos Aires · Hong Kong · Sydney · Tokyo

Acquisitions Editor: Hilarie Surrena
Development Editors: Helen Kogut, Laura Scott
Director of Nursing Production: Helen Ewan
Senior Managing Editor/Production: Erika Kors
Production Editor: Mary Kinsella
Design: Holly Reid McLaughlin
Cover/Interior design: Karen Quigley
Art Director, Illustration: Brett MacNaughton
Manufacturing Coordinator: Karin Duffield
Compositor: Circle Graphics

Sixth Edition

9 8 7 6 5 4 3 2

Printed in China

Library of Congress Cataloging-in-Publication Data

Buchholz, Susan, RN.
 Henke's med-math : dosage calculation, preparation, and administration / Susan Buchholz, Grace Henke. — 6th ed.
  p. ; cm.
 Includes index.
 ISBN 978-0-7817-7628-8
 1. Pharmaceutical arithmetic. I. Henke, Grace. II. Henke, Grace. Med-math. III. Title. IV. Title: Med-math.
 [DNLM: 1. Pharmaceutical Preparations—administration & dosage—Nurses' Instruction. 2. Pharmaceutical Preparations—administration & dosage—Programmed Instruction. 3. Drug Dosage Calculations—Nurses' Instruction. 4. Drug Dosage Calculations—Programmed Instruction. QV 18.2 B919h 2009]
 RS57.H46 2009
 615'.1401513—dc22

                        2008024079

CCS0309

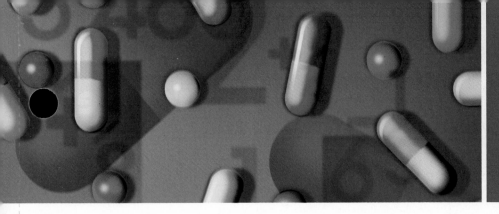

Reviewers

Christine Boyle, RN, BScN, MA
Nursing Faculty and Coordinator Bridge to
Canadian Nursing Program
Mount Royal College
Calgary, Alberta, Canada

Peggy Irene Bozarth, RN, MSN
Professor
Hopkinsville Community College
Hopkinsville, Kentucky

Julie A. Calvery, MS, RN
Instructor
University of Arkansas—Fort Smith
Fort Smith, Arkansas

Michelle Carr, AAS, BSN, MSN, CHPN
Assistant Professor
Brevard Community College
Cocoa, Florida

Charlene B. Gagliardi, RN, BSN, MSN
Instructor
Mount St. Mary's College
Los Angeles, California

Karin Freas Gapper, EdD, RN
Associate Professor
Queensborough Community College
Bayside, New York

Jacqueline Guhde, MSN, RN, CNS
Instructor
The University of Akron
Akron, Ohio

Lucy Hampton, BSN, RN, CNOR
Director Medical Programs
Tennessee Technology Center at
Chattanooga State Technical Community College
Chattanooga, Tennessee

Beverly Anne Lansiquot, BSN, MSN, RN
Coordinator
Sir Arthur Lewis Community College
Morne Fortune, Castries, St. Lucia

Jane Mighton, RN, BSN, MSN
Nursing Instructor
Langara College
Vancouver, British Columbia, Canada

Lori L. Neubauer, RN, BSN, BC
Vocational Nursing Director, Instructor
Angelina College, Crockett Campus
Crockett, Texas

Mandi Newton, PhD, RN
Research Fellow
University of Alberta
Edmonton, Alberta, Canada

Lynda G. Nicol, RN, BScN
Sessional Instructor
University of Alberta
Edmonton, Alberta, Canada

Wanda Pierson, RN, BSN, MSN, MA, PhD
Nursing Department Chair
Langara College
Vancouver, British Columbia, Canada

Colleen M. Quinn, RN, MSN
Associate Dean, Nursing
Broward Community College, South Campus
Fort Lauderdale, Florida

Christy L. Raymond, RN, BScN, Med
Faculty, Clinical Coordinator
Grant MacEwan College
Edmonton, Alberta, Canada

Elaine Ridgeway, MSN, CRNP
Nursing Instructor
Bowie State University
Bowie, Maryland

Tami J. Rogers, DVM, MSN, BSN
Professor of Nursing
Valencia Community College
Orlando, Florida

Sharon Tighe, EdD, MN, RN-C, ARNP
Professor
Daytona Beach Community College
Daytona Beach, Florida

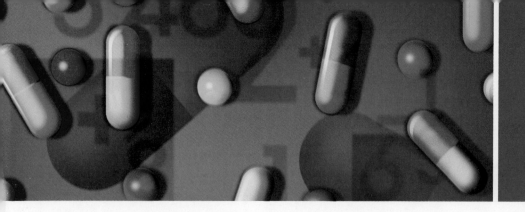

New!! Up to date!! Relevant!!

Even though it sounds like an advertisement for something other than a textbook, the sixth edition of Henke's Med-Math: Dosage Calculation, Preparation and Administration can be summarized with the above heading. The sixth edition, which presents up-to-date information about drugs, medication administration, and safe practices; new material including illustrations, pictures, and tables; and more relevant drugs, also emphasizes the basics of dosage calculation. The more you practice and solve problems, the better, more accurate, and more safe you become!

The text is designed to be used by nursing students in various types of nursing programs. Other healthcare professionals who administer drugs will also find it useful. It is a good review book for practicing nurses or nurses returning to practice.

Beginning nursing students can start at the beginning and work through each chapter. Students who are confident of their math abilities can take the proficiency tests in each chapter and work forward. Experienced nurses can also take the proficiency tests and then concentrate on chapters that address their learning needs.

Text Organization

The first five chapters present the basics:

Chapter 1 concentrates on the arithmetic needed to calculate doses.

Chapter 2 identifies abbreviations used in prescriptions and explains how to interpret them.

Chapter 3 explains dosage measurement systems (metric, apothecary, household) and teaches students how to convert among systems.

Chapter 4 clarifies information printed on drug labels and types of drug packaging.

Chapter 5 defines the forms in which drugs are manufactured and the equipment used in administration.

Chapters 6 to 10 concentrate on calculating doses for

- oral solid and liquid problems
- injections from liquids and powders
- intravenous medications and pediatric doses

Chapter 11 explains the dimensional analysis method of drug calculation.

Chapters 12 and 13 present information and techniques for safe administration, including universal precautions, pregnancy categories, and legal and ethical considerations. Also included is information on how to administer drugs orally, parenterally, and topically.

Key Elements of the Text

- Dosage problems simulate actual clinical experience
- Easy-to-learn formulas and a step-by-step approach in solving problems
- Shows three methods of calculation (formula, proportion expressed as two ratios, proportion expressed as two fractions)
- Chapter 11 fully explains the Dimensional Analysis Method
- Proficiency Test Answer key shows how to set up and solve problems using all four methods of calculation (formula, proportion expressed as two ratios, proportion expressed as two fractions, dimensional analysis)
- Self-tests and proficiency tests offer varied opportunities to translate text into clinical application material
- Simple to complex organization of the text
- Abbreviations approved by The Joint Commission

Key Features

- Self-tests in the chapter include answers at the end of each chapter
- Proficiency tests at the end of each chapter with answers in Appendix A
- *Test your Clinical Savvy*—"what if" situations that stimulate critical thinking
- Glossary with definitions and common abbreviations
- Enclosed CD-ROM contains math problems for students to practice calculations
- Handy quick-reference plastic card with common conversions and formulas

New to This Edition

- *Putting It Together*—case studies with application of dosage calculations and critical thinking questions with suggested answers in Appendix B
- Update of drug labels and drug names including common trade names and generic names
- Reorganization of the chapters to present a better flow to learning
- More information in Chapters 12 and 13 relevant to medication administration, including use of computerized charting and safety information

Aids for Students and Faculty

- Free CD-ROM
  Includes over 15 minutes of video clips on safe medication administration, a dosage calculation tool, and access to free additional dosage calculation quizzes
- Instructor's Resource CD-ROM
  Includes a Testbank and Power Point presentations corresponding to each chapter, and is available for teachers to help to optimize the teaching of dosage calculations and medication administration

- thePoint

  Go online! Students and instructors can access this information at http://thepoint.lww.com/Buchholz6e

I welcome comments and suggestions via e-mail, and I hope the book helps all who are involved with calculating correct medication dosages.

Susan Buchholz, RN, MSN
sbuchhol@gpc.edu

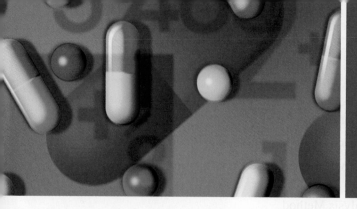

Acknowledgments and Dedication

This edition is dedicated to my friends, family, church community at Oakhurst Baptist Church, neighbors, nursing students, colleagues at Georgia Perimeter College and DeKalb Medical, my Creator and Christ and everyone who helped me through the bad karma year of 2007!

Special thanks to:

Ginger Pyron: editing, spiritual support, theme support

Laura Lacey-Bordeaux: photography and spiritual support

Mary Logan: emotional and spiritual support

Amy Williams, Edy Burel, Kerri Bond, MyAnh Nguyen, Barbara MacLaren, Jamilla Fontenot, Lindsey Combs, Moshena Harris, Sarah Harrington, Heather Hoagland, Lauren Cartee, Jacob Bailey, Rebecca Sharma, Erica Wells: obtaining drug labels and helping me through the craziness of last year

Sister Grace Henke: original text and format

Mr. Wok: hunger support

Laura Scott, Liz Harris, Helen Kogut, Margaret Zuccarini, Hilarie Surrena (and others at Lippincott Williams and Wilkins): for your editorial assistance, expertise, and support

Pharmaceutical companies: providing medication labels

DeKalb Medical: providing medication labels and protocols

Andrew and Chelsea: I am so proud of how you are growing up. You are the main reason I keep going each day.

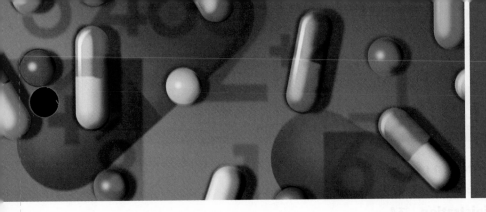

Contents

CHAPTER 1

Arithmetic Needed for Dosage   1

Multiplying Whole Numbers   2

Dividing Whole Numbers   3

Fractions   4

Types of Fractions   4
Reducing Fractions   4
Adding Fractions   6
Subtracting Fractions   6
Multiplying Fractions   7
Dividing Fractions   8
Changing Fractions to Decimals   8

Decimals   10

Reading Decimals and Converting Decimals to Fractions   10
Addition and Subtraction of Decimals   11
Multiplying Decimals   12
Dividing Decimals   12
Clearing the Divisor of Decimal Points   13
Rounding Off Decimals   14
Comparing the Value of Decimals   15

Percents   15

Percents That Are Whole Numbers   16
Percents That Are Decimals   16
Percents That Are Fractions   17
Fractions Converted to Percents   17
Ratios Converted to Percents   17
Decimals Converted to Percents   18

Fractions, Ratio, and Proportion   18

Solving Proportions With an Unknown   19
Proportions Expressed as Two Fractions   19
Proportions Expressed as Two Ratios   19
Ratio and Proportion in Dosage   20

Proficiency Test in Arithmetic   22

Answers to Self-Tests   23

Interpreting the Language of Prescriptions   30

Time of Administration of Drugs   30
Military Time: The 24-hour Clock   33

Routes of Administration   34

Metric and SI Abbreviations   36

Apothecary Abbreviations   37

Household Abbreviations   38

Terms and Abbreviations for Drug Preparations   39

Proficiency Tests   41

Answers to Self-Tests   45

Metric, Apothecary, and Household Systems of Measurement   47

Metric System   47
Measures of Weight   47
Weight Equivalents   47
Converting Solid Equivalents   48

Apothecary System   55
Apothecary Abbreviations   55
Solid Apothecary Measure—The Grain   55
Solid Equivalents—Apothecary and Metric   55

Household System   57
Household Measures   57
Metric Liquid Measures   57
Liquid Apothecary Measures   58
Conversions Among Liquid Measures   58

Other Conversions   59
Temperature Conversions   59
Milliunits and Milliequivalents   59

Proficiency Test   61

Answers to Self-Tests   63

Drug Labels and Packaging   65

Drug Labels   65

Drug Packaging   69

Unit-Dose Packaging   69
Multidose Packaging   73

Proficiency Tests   79

Answers to Self-Tests   83

CHAPTER 5

Drug Preparations and Equipment to Measure Doses   84

Drug Preparations   84

Oral Route   84
Parenteral Route   87
Topical Route   87

Equipment to Measure Doses   89

Medicine Cups   90
Syringes   91
Rounding Off Numbers in Liquid Dosage Answers   93
Needles for Intramuscular and Subcutaneous Injections   95

Proficiency Test   96

Answers to Self-Tests   99

CHAPTER 6

Calculation of Oral Medications— Solids and Liquids   101

Proportions Expressed as Two Fractions   101

Proportions Expressed as Two Ratios   102

Formula Method   103

Oral Solids   103

Application of the Rule for Oral Solids   103
Clearing Decimals When Using the Formula Method   105
Special Types of Oral Solid Orders   113

Oral Liquids   114

Special Types of Oral Liquid Orders   120

Oral Solid and Liquid Problems Without Written Calculations   120

Proficiency Tests   123

Putting It Together   121

Answers to Self-Tests   129

CHAPTER 7

Liquids for Injection   141

Calculating Injection Problems   142

3-mL Syringe   142
1-mL Syringe   142
IV Medications   144

Special Types of Problems in Injections From a Liquid   149

   When Supply Is a Ratio   *149*
   When Supply Is a Percent   *153*

Insulin Injections   156

   Types of Insulin   *156*
   Types of Insulin Syringes   *158*
   Preparing an Injection Using an Insulin Syringe   *158*
   Mixing Two Insulins in One Syringe   *159*
   Sliding-Scale Regular Insulin Dosages   *161*
   Insulin Pens and Prefilled Insulin Devices   *162*

Injections From Powders   163

   Application of the Rule for Injections From Powders   *163*

Distinctive Features of Injections From Powders   167

Where to Find Information About Reconstitution of Powders   169

Critical Thinking: Test Your Clinical Savvy   175

Putting It Together   176

Proficiency Tests   178

Answers to Self-Tests   189

CHAPTER 8

Calculation of Basic IV Drip Rates   203

Types of Intravenous Fluids   203

Kinds of Intravenous Drip Factors   204

   Infusion Pumps   *204*
   Labeling IVs   *205*

Calculating Basic IV Drip Rates   206

   Solving IV Calculations Using an Infusion Pump   *207*
   Applying the Rule   *208*
   Determining Hours an IV Will Run   *210*
   Choosing the Infusion Set   *212*
   Need for Continuous Observation   *212*

Adding Medications to IVs   213

Medications for Intermittent Intravenous Administration   215

   Explanation   *215*

Ambulatory Infusion Device   218

Enteral Nutrition   218

   Calculation of Tube Feedings   *219*
   Recording Intake   *220*

Proficiency Test   225

Answers to Self-Tests   227

CHAPTER
9

Special Types of Intravenous Calculations   237

Amount of Drug in a Solution   237

Medications Ordered in Units/hr or mg/hr   238

Units/hr—Rule and Calculation   238
mg/hr, g/hr—Rule and Calculation   240
mg/min—Rule and Calculation   243

Medications Ordered in mcg/min, mcg/kg/min, or milliunits/min   245

mcg/min—Rule and Calculation   245
mcg/kg/min—Rule and Calculation   247
Milliunits/min—Rule and Calculation   248

Body Surface Nomogram   249

m²—Rule and Calculation   251

Patient-Controlled Analgesia (PCA)   252

Heparin and Insulin Protocols   254

Heparin Protocol   254
Insulin Protocol   256

Critical Thinking: Test Your Clinical Savvy   259

Putting It Together   259

Proficiency Test   261

Answers to Self-Tests   263

CHAPTER
10

Dosage Problems for Infants and Children   280

Dosage Based on mg/kg and Body Surface Area   281

Converting Ounces to Pounds   281
Converting Pounds to Kilograms   282
Steps and Rule—mg/kg Body Weight   283
Determining BSA in m²   290

Administering Intravenous Medications   295

General Guidelines for Continuous IV Medications   303

Critical Thinking: Test Your Clinical Savvy   305

Putting It Together   305

Proficiency Test   307

Answers to Self-Tests   309

CHAPTER
11

Dimensional Analysis   320

Oral Solid Medication Equation and Calculation   320

Oral Liquid Medication Equation and Calculation   322

Parenteral Liquid Medication Equation and Calculation 323

Insulin Equation and Calculation 323

Dimensional Analysis Method With Equivalency Conversions 325

Dimensional Analysis Method With Weight-Based Calculations 328

    Calculation of Medications Based on BSA 329

Dimensional Analysis Method With Reconstitution of Medications 330

Dimensional Analysis Method With Calculation of Intravenous Fluids 332

Dimensional Analysis Method With Advanced Intravenous Calculations 333

    Calculating mL/hr 333
    Calculating mg/hr or units/hr 334
    Calculating mL/hr for Drugs Ordered in mcg or mcg/min 335
    Calculating mL/hr for Drugs Ordered in mcg/kg/min 336

Heparin and Insulin Intravenous Calculations 337

    Heparin Protocol 337
    Insulin Protocol 338

Proficiency Test 340

Answers to Self-Tests 343

CHAPTER 12

Information Basic to Administering Drugs 351

Drug Knowledge 351

    Generic and Trade Names 351
    Drug Classification and Drug Category 352
    Side Effects and Adverse Effects 352
    Pregnancy Category 352
    Dosage and Route 353
    Action 353
    Indications 353
    Contraindications and Precautions 354
    Interactions and Incompatibilities 354
    Nursing Implications 355
    Signs of Effectiveness 355
    Teaching the Patient 355

Pharmacokinetics 355

    Absorption 355
    Distribution 356
    Biotransformation 356
    Excretion 356
    Tolerance 356
    Cumulation 357
    Half-Life 357
    Therapeutic Range 357

Legal Considerations 358

Criminal Law 358
Civil Law 359

Ethical Principles in Drug Administration 361

Autonomy 361
Truthfulness 362
Beneficence 362
Nonmaleficence 362
Confidentiality 362
Justice 362
Fidelity 362

Specific Points That May Be Helpful in Giving Medications 362

Three Checks and Six Rights 362
Medication Orders 363
Medication Orders for Physicians and Healthcare Providers 364
Knowledge Base 364
Medication Safety 364
Oral Medications—Tablets and Capsules 365
Liquid Medications 365
Giving Medications 366
Charting 366
Evaluation 367
Error in Medication 367

Clinical Thinking: Test Your Clinical Savvy 367

Proficiency Test 370

Answers to Self-Tests 373

CHAPTER
13 **Administration Procedures 374**

Standard Precautions Applied to Administration of Medications 374

General Safeguards in Administering Medications 374

Systems of Administration 377

Medication Administration Record 377
Ticket System 378
Mobile Cart System 379
Computer Scanning 380
Computer Order Entry 380

Routes of Administration 380

Oral Route 380
Parenteral Route 382
Administering Injections 391
IV Administration 394
Application to Skin and Mucous Membranes 395

Special Considerations 404

   Neonatal and Pediatric Considerations 404

   Geriatric Considerations 405

Critical Thinking: Test Your Clinical Savvy 405

Proficiency Tests 409

Answers to Self-Tests 415

Appendix A   Proficiency Test Answers 417

Appendix B   Putting It Together Answers 483

Glossary 500

Index 507

Arithmetic Needed for Dosage

LEARNING OBJECTIVES

1. Addition and subtraction of fractions

2. Multiplication and division of whole numbers, fractions, and decimals

3. Converting mixed fractions to improper

4. Reading decimals

5. Clearing and rounding of decimals

6. Addition, subtraction, multiplication, and division of decimals

7. Changing decimals to fractions

8. Percents

9. Solving ratio and proportion

10. Proficiency test in arithmetic

When a medication order differs from the fixed amount at which a drug is supplied, you must calculate the dose needed. Calculation requires knowledge of the systems of dosage measurements (see Chapter 3) and the ability to solve arithmetic. This chapter covers the common arithmetic functions needed for the safe administration of drugs.

Beginning students invariably express anxiety that they will miscalculate a dose and cause harm. Although *everyone* is capable of error, no one has to cause an error. The surest way to prevent a mistake is to exercise care in performing basic arithmetic operations.

For students who believe their arithmetic skills are already satisfactory, this chapter contains self-tests and a proficiency exam. Once you pass the proficiency exam, you can move on to other chapters in the book.

Students with math anxiety and those with deficiencies in performing arithmetic will want to work through this chapter page by page. Examples demonstrate how to perform calculations; the self-tests provide practice and drill. FINE POINTS boxes explain details about the calculation. After you've mastered the content, take the proficiency exam to verify your readiness to move on.

Since calculators are readily available, why go through all the arithmetic? For one thing, using a calculator can actually complicate the process, because you must know what numbers and functions to enter. In clinical situations you may encounter some problems that require a calculator's help, but it's good to know how to make calculations on your own. Solving the arithmetic problems yourself helps you think logically about the amount ordered and the relative dose needed. And when you can mentally calculate dosage, you increase your speed and efficiency in preparing medications. None of the arithmetic problems in this chapter require a calculator.

1	2	3	4	5	6	⑦	8	9	10	11	12
2	4	6	8	10	12	14	16	18	20	22	24
3	6	9	12	15	18	21	24	27	30	33	36
4	8	12	16	20	24	28	32	36	40	44	48
5	10	15	20	25	30	35	40	45	50	55	60
6	12	18	24	30	36	42	48	54	60	66	72
7	14	21	28	35	42	49	56	63	70	77	84
⑧	16	24	32	40	48	㊴56	64	72	80	88	96
9	18	27	36	45	54	63	72	81	90	99	108
10	20	30	40	50	60	70	80	90	100	110	120
11	22	33	44	55	66	77	88	99	110	121	132
12	24	36	48	60	72	84	96	108	120	132	144

FIGURE 1-1

The multiplication table. The numbers going down the left side (from 1 to 12) are the row numbers. The numbers going across the top (from 1 to 12) are the column numbers. To multiply any two numbers from 1 to 12, find the column for one number, find the row for the other number, and read across the row until you intersect the column.

Multiplying Whole Numbers

If you need a review, first study the multiplication table (Fig. 1-1) for the numbers 1 through 12. Then do the problem, aiming for 100% accuracy without referring to the table.

Example	Multiply 8 by 7 (8 × 7).

1. Find row 8.

2. Find column 7.

3. Read across row 8 until you intersect column 7. The answer is 56.

SELF-TEST 1 **Multiplication**

After studying the multiplication table, write the answers to these problems. Answers are given at the end of the chapter; aim for 100%.

1. 2 × 6 = _____

2. 9 × 7 = _____

3. 4 × 8 = _____

4. 5 × 9 = _____

5. 12 × 9 = _____

6. 8 × 3 = _____

7. 11 × 10 = _____

8. 2 × 7 = _____

9. 8 × 6 = _____

10. 8 × 9 = _____

11. 3 × 5 = _____

12. 6 × 7 = _____

13. 4 × 6 = _____

14. 9 × 6 = _____

15. 8 × 8 = _____

16. 7 × 8 = _____

17. 2 × 9 = _____

18. 8 × 11 = _____

19. 4 × 9 = _____

20. 3 × 8 = _____

21. 12 × 11 = _____

22. 9 × 5 = _____

23. 9 × 9 = _____

24. 7 × 5 = _____

1	2	3	4	5	6	7	8	⑨	10	11	12
2	4	6	8	10	12	14	16	18	20	22	24
3	6	9	12	15	18	21	24	27	30	33	36
4	8	12	16	20	24	28	32	36	40	44	48
5	10	15	20	25	30	35	40	45	50	55	60
6	12	18	24	30	36	42	48	54	60	66	72
7	14	21	28	35	42	49	56	63	70	77	84
8	16	24	32	40	48	56	64	72	80	88	96
9	18	27	36	45	54	63	72	81	90	99	108
10	20	30	40	50	60	70	80	90	100	110	120
11	22	33	44	55	66	77	88	99	110	121	132
⑫	24	36	48	60	72	84	96	⑩⑧	120	132	144

FIGURE 1-2

Division table. The numbers going down the left side (from 1 to 12) are the row numbers. The numbers going across the top (from 1 to 12) are the column numbers. To divide, find the divisor (the number performing the division) in the row. Read across the row to the dividend (the number to be divided). The number at the top of that column is the answer.

Dividing Whole Numbers

The division table is helpful when you're dividing large numbers by smaller ones. Study the table (Fig. 1-2) for the division of numbers 2 through 12. Again, aim for 100% accuracy without referring to the table.

Example Divide 108 by 12 (108 ÷ 12).

1. Find 12 (the smaller number) in the left row.

2. Read across that row until you find 108 (the larger number).

3. The number at the top of that column is the answer: 9.

Remember, because $9 \times 12 = 108$, then $108 \div 12 = 9$ (see Fig. 1-2).

SELF-TEST 2 Division

After studying the division of larger numbers by smaller numbers, write the answers to the following problems. Answers are given at the end of the chapter.

1. 63 ÷ 7 = _____	**9.** 49 ÷ 7 = _____	**17.** 81 ÷ 9 = _____
2. 24 ÷ 6 = _____	**10.** 18 ÷ 3 = _____	**18.** 32 ÷ 8 = _____
3. 36 ÷ 12 = _____	**11.** 72 ÷ 8 = _____	**19.** 36 ÷ 6 = _____
4. 42 ÷ 6 = _____	**12.** 48 ÷ 8 = _____	**20.** 18 ÷ 9 = _____
5. 35 ÷ 5 = _____	**13.** 28 ÷ 7 = _____	**21.** 21 ÷ 3 = _____
6. 96 ÷ 12 = _____	**14.** 21 ÷ 7 = _____	**22.** 48 ÷ 4 = _____
7. 12 ÷ 3 = _____	**15.** 24 ÷ 8 = _____	**23.** 144 ÷ 12 = _____
8. 27 ÷ 9 = _____	**16.** 84 ÷ 12 = _____	**24.** 56 ÷ 8 = _____

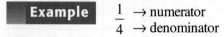 Fractions

A *fraction* is a portion of a whole number. The top number in a fraction is called the *numerator* and the bottom number is called the *denominator*. The line between the numerator and the denominator is a division sign. Therefore, you can read the fraction $\frac{1}{4}$ as "one divided by four."

| **Example** | $\frac{1}{4}$ → numerator |
| | $\phantom{\frac{1}{4}}$ → denominator |

Types of Fractions

In a *proper* fraction, the numerator is smaller than the denominator.

| **Example** | $\frac{2}{5}$ (Read as "two fifths.") |

In an *improper* fraction, the numerator is larger than the denominator.

| **Example** | $\frac{5}{2}$ (Read as "five halves.") |

A *mixed number* has a whole number plus a fraction.

| **Example** | $1\frac{2}{3}$ (Read as "one and two thirds.") |

In a *complex* fraction, both the numerator and the denominator are already fractions.

| **Example** | $\dfrac{\frac{1}{2}}{\frac{1}{4}}$ (Read as "one half divided by one fourth.") |

RULE   **REDUCING FRACTIONS**

Find the largest number that can be divided evenly into the numerator *and* the denominator. ■

| **Example** | *EXAMPLE 1* |

Reduce $\frac{4}{12}$

$$\frac{\overset{1}{\cancel{4}}}{\underset{3}{\cancel{12}}} = \frac{1}{3}$$

EXAMPLE 2

Reduce $\frac{7}{49}$

$$\frac{\overset{1}{\cancel{7}}}{\underset{7}{\cancel{49}}} = \frac{1}{7}$$

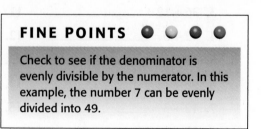

FINE POINTS ● ○ ● ●

Check to see if the denominator is evenly divisible by the numerator. In this example, the number 7 can be evenly divided into 49.

Sometimes fractions are more difficult to reduce because the answer is not obvious.

Example   *EXAMPLE 1*

Reduce $\frac{56}{96}$

$$\frac{56}{96} = \frac{\overset{1}{\cancel{8}} \times 7}{\underset{1}{\cancel{8}} \times 12} = \frac{7}{12}$$

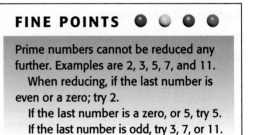

FINE POINTS ● ○ ● ●

Use the multiplication table (Fig. 1-1) to change the numbers to their multiples.

EXAMPLE 2

Reduce $\frac{54}{99}$

$$\frac{54}{99} = \frac{\overset{1}{\cancel{9}} \times 6}{\underset{1}{\cancel{9}} \times 11} = \frac{6}{11}$$

When you need to reduce a very large fraction, it may be difficult to determine the largest number that will divide evenly into both the numerator and the denominator. You may have to reduce the fraction several times.

Example   *EXAMPLE 1*

Reduce $\frac{189}{216}$

Try to divide both by 3 $\dfrac{\overset{63}{\cancel{189}}}{\underset{72}{\cancel{216}}} = \dfrac{63}{72}$

Then use multiples $\dfrac{63}{72} = \dfrac{\overset{1}{\cancel{9}} \times 7}{\underset{1}{\cancel{9}} \times 8} = \dfrac{7}{8}$

FINE POINTS ● ○ ● ●

Prime numbers cannot be reduced any further. Examples are 2, 3, 5, 7, and 11.
   When reducing, if the last number is even or a zero; try 2.
   If the last number is a zero, or 5, try 5.
   If the last number is odd, try 3, 7, or 11.

EXAMPLE 2

Reduce $\frac{27}{135}$

Try to divide both by 3 $\dfrac{\overset{9}{\cancel{27}}}{\underset{45}{\cancel{135}}} = \dfrac{\overset{1}{\cancel{9}}}{\underset{5}{\cancel{45}}} = \dfrac{1}{5}$

Then divide by 9.

SELF-TEST 3   Reducing Fractions

Reduce these fractions to their lowest terms. Answers are given at the end of the chapter.

1. $\frac{16}{24}$

2. $\frac{36}{216}$

3. $\frac{18}{96}$

4. $\frac{70}{490}$

5. $\frac{18}{81}$

6. $\frac{8}{48}$

7. $\frac{12}{30}$

8. $\frac{68}{136}$

9. $\frac{55}{121}$

10. $\frac{15}{60}$

Adding Fractions

If you need to add two fractions that have the *same* denominator, first add the two numerators; write that sum over the denominator and, if necessary, reduce again.

$$\frac{1}{5} + \frac{3}{5} = \frac{4}{5}$$

If the two fractions have *different* denominators, the process takes two steps. First convert each fraction, multiplying both of its numbers by their lowest common denominator. After you've converted both fractions, add their two numerators together. If necessary, reduce again.

$$\frac{3}{5} + \frac{2}{3} =$$

$$\frac{3(\times 3)}{5(\times 3)} = \frac{9}{15}$$

$$\frac{2(\times 5)}{3(\times 5)} = \frac{10}{15}$$

$$\frac{9}{15} + \frac{10}{15} = \frac{19}{15}$$

Subtracting Fractions

To subtract two fractions that have the *same* denominator, first subtract their numerators and then write the difference over the denominator. Reduce if necessary.

$$\frac{27}{32} - \frac{18}{32} = \frac{9}{32}$$

If the two fractions have *different* denominators, first convert each fraction using the lowest common denominator (just as you did in the adding example, above). Then subtract the numerators, and reduce again if necessary.

$$\frac{7}{8} - \frac{2}{3} =$$

$$\frac{7(\times 3)}{8(\times 3)} = \frac{21}{24}$$

$$\frac{2(\times 8)}{3(\times 8)} = \frac{16}{24}$$

$$\frac{21}{24} - \frac{16}{24} = \frac{5}{24}$$

SELF-TEST 4 Adding and Subtracting Fractions

Add and subtract these fractions. Answers are given at the end of the chapter.

1. $\frac{3}{7} + \frac{2}{7} =$

2. $\frac{3}{5} + \frac{1}{5} =$

3. $\frac{2}{4} + \frac{1}{4} =$

4. $\frac{2}{3} + \frac{1}{6} =$

5. $\frac{1}{2} + \frac{1}{3} =$

6. $\frac{15}{16} - \frac{5}{16} =$

7. $\frac{3}{7} - \frac{2}{7} =$

8. $\frac{3}{5} - \frac{2}{15} =$

9. $\frac{11}{15} - \frac{7}{10} =$

10. $\frac{8}{9} - \frac{5}{12} =$

Multiplying Fractions

There are two ways to multiply fractions. Use whichever method is more comfortable for you.

First Way

Multiply the numerators across. Multiply denominators across. Reduce the answer to its lowest terms.

Example $\frac{2}{7} \times \frac{3}{4} = \frac{2 \times 3}{7 \times 4} = \frac{6}{28}$

$$\frac{6}{28} = \frac{3 \times \overset{1}{\cancel{2}}}{14 \times \underset{1}{\cancel{2}}} = \frac{3}{14}$$

Second Way (When You Are Multiplying Several Fractions)

First, reduce each fraction by dividing its numerator evenly into its denominator. Multiply the remaining numerators across. Multiply the remaining denominators across. Check to see if further reductions are possible. In example 1, because of several fractions, you can use any numerator to divide into any of the denominators.

Example *EXAMPLE 1*

$$\frac{3}{14} \times \frac{7}{10} \times \frac{5}{12} = \frac{\overset{1}{\cancel{3}}}{\underset{2}{\cancel{14}}} \times \frac{\overset{1}{\cancel{7}}}{\underset{2}{\cancel{10}}} \times \frac{\overset{1}{\cancel{5}}}{\underset{4}{\cancel{12}}} = \frac{1}{16}$$

FINE POINTS ● ○ ● ●

$14 \div 7 = 2$

$10 \div 5 = 2$

$12 \div 3 = 4$

The denominators are being divided by the numerators to reduce.

If you're multiplying mixed numbers, you first need to change each of them into an improper fraction. The process: For each fraction, multiply the whole number by the denominator; then add that total to the numerator.

EXAMPLE 2

$$1\frac{1}{2} \times \frac{4}{6} = \frac{\overset{1}{\cancel{3}}}{\underset{1}{\cancel{2}}} \times \frac{\overset{2}{\cancel{4}}}{\underset{2}{\cancel{6}}} = \frac{2}{2} = 1$$

EXAMPLE 3

$$\frac{4}{5} \times 6\frac{2}{3} = \frac{4}{\cancel{5}} \times \frac{\overset{4}{\cancel{20}}}{3} = \frac{16}{3}$$

SELF-TEST 5 Multiplying Fractions

Multiply these fractions. Answers are given at the end of the chapter.

1. $\frac{1}{6} \times \frac{4}{5} \times \frac{5}{2} =$

2. $\frac{4}{15} \times \frac{3}{2} =$

3. $1\frac{1}{2} \times 4\frac{2}{3} =$

4. $\frac{1}{5} \times \frac{15}{45} =$

5. $3\frac{3}{4} \times 10\frac{2}{3} =$

6. $\frac{7}{20} \times \frac{2}{14} =$

7. $\frac{9}{2} \times \frac{3}{2} =$

8. $6\frac{1}{4} \times 7\frac{1}{9} \times \frac{9}{5} =$

Dividing Fractions

To divide two fractions, first invert the fraction that is after the division sign, then change the division sign to a multiplication sign.

Example   *EXAMPLE 1*

$$\frac{1}{75} \div \frac{1}{150} = \frac{1}{\underset{1}{\cancel{75}}} \times \frac{\overset{2}{\cancel{150}}}{1} = 2$$

EXAMPLE 2

$$\frac{\frac{1}{4}}{\frac{3}{8}} = \frac{1}{4} \div \frac{3}{8} = \frac{1}{\underset{1}{\cancel{4}}} \times \frac{\overset{2}{\cancel{8}}}{3} = \frac{2}{3}$$

EXAMPLE 3

$$\frac{1\frac{1}{5}}{\frac{2}{3}} = \frac{6}{5} \div \frac{2}{3} = \frac{\overset{3}{\cancel{6}}}{5} \times \frac{3}{\underset{1}{\cancel{2}}} = \frac{9}{5}$$

FINE POINTS ● ○ ● ●

Complex fractions such as

$$\frac{\frac{1}{4}}{\frac{3}{8}}$$ are read as $\frac{1}{4} \div \frac{3}{8}$

The vertical arrangement acts just like a division sign.

SELF-TEST 6 ▸ Dividing Fractions

Divide these fractions. Answers are given at the end of the chapter.

1. $\frac{1}{75} \div \frac{1}{150} =$

2. $\frac{1}{8} \div \frac{1}{4} =$

3. $2\frac{2}{3} \div \frac{1}{2} =$

4. $75 \div 12\frac{1}{2} =$

5. $\frac{7}{25} \div \frac{7}{75} =$

6. $\frac{1}{2} \div \frac{1}{4} =$

7. $\frac{3}{4} \div \frac{8}{3} =$

8. $\frac{1}{60} \div \frac{7}{10} =$

Changing Fractions to Decimals

To change a fraction into a decimal, begin by dividing the numerator by the denominator. Remember that the line between the numerator and the denominator is a division sign; so $\frac{1}{4}$ can be read as $1 \div 4$.

In a division problem, each number has a name. The number that's being divided (your fraction's numerator) is the *dividend;* the one that does the dividing (your fraction's denominator) is the *divisor*; and the answer is the *quotient.*

$$\text{divisor} \rightarrow 16\overline{)640.} \quad \begin{array}{l} \leftarrow \text{quotient} \\ \leftarrow \text{dividend} \end{array}$$
$$\underline{64}$$
$$0$$

1. Look at the fraction $\frac{1}{4}$

$$\frac{1}{4} \quad \begin{array}{l} \leftarrow \text{numerator} = \text{dividend} \\ \leftarrow \text{denominator} = \text{divisor} \end{array}$$

2. Write

$$4\overline{)1}$$

3. Some people find it easier to simply extend the fraction's straight line to the right, and then strike out the numerator and place that same number down into the "box."

$$\frac{1}{4} = \frac{\cancel{1}}{4\overline{)1}}$$

4. Once you've set up the structure for your division problem, place a decimal point immediately after the dividend. Put another decimal point on the quotient line (above), lining up that point exactly with the decimal point below.

By placing your decimal points carefully, you can avoid serious dosage errors.

$$\frac{\cancel{1}}{4}\overline{)1.} \begin{array}{l} \cdot \leftarrow \text{quotient} \\ \\ \leftarrow \text{dividend} \end{array}$$

5. Complete the division.

$$\frac{\cancel{1}}{4}\overline{\begin{array}{r} .25 \\ )1.00 \\ \underline{8} \\ 20 \\ \underline{20} \\ 0 \end{array}} = 0.25$$

> **FINE POINTS** ● ○ ● ●
>
> If the answer does not have a whole number, place a zero before the decimal point. .25 is incorrect; 0.25 is correct.
>
> The number of places to carry out the decimal will vary depending on the drug and equipment used. For these exercises, carry answers to the thousandths place (three decimal places).

Example

EXAMPLE 1

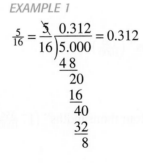

$$\frac{5}{16} = \frac{\cancel{5}}{16\overline{\begin{array}{r} 0.312 \\ )5.000 \\ \underline{4\ 8} \\ 20 \\ \underline{16} \\ 40 \\ \underline{32} \\ 8 \end{array}}} = 0.312$$

EXAMPLE 2

$$\frac{640}{8} = \frac{\cancel{640}}{8}\overline{\begin{array}{r} 80. \\ )640. \end{array}} = 80$$

> **FINE POINTS** ● ○ ● ●
>
> In the answer, note the space between 8 and the decimal point. When such a space occurs, fill it with a zero to complete your answer.

EXAMPLE 3

$$\frac{1}{75} = \frac{\cancel{1}}{75\overline{\begin{array}{r} 0.013 \\ )1.000 \\ \underline{75} \\ 250 \\ \underline{225} \\ 25 \end{array}}} = 0.013$$

SELF-TEST 7   **Converting Fractions to Decimals**

Divide these fractions to produce decimals. Answers are given at the end of the chapter. Carry decimal point to three decimal places if necessary.

1. $\frac{1}{6}$ 4. $\frac{9}{40}$

2. $\frac{6}{8}$ 5. $\frac{1}{8}$

3. $\frac{4}{5}$ 6. $\frac{1}{7}$

Decimals

Most medication orders are written in the metric system, which uses decimals.

Reading Decimals and Converting Decimals to Fractions

Start by counting how many places come after the decimal point. One space after the decimal point is the *tenths* place. Two spaces is the *hundredths* place. Three places is the *thousandths* place; and so on. When you read the decimal aloud, it sounds like you're reading a fraction:

0.1 is read as "one tenth" $\left(\frac{1}{10}\right)$.

0.01 is read as "one hundredth" $\left(\frac{1}{100}\right)$.

0.001 is read as "one thousandth" $\left(\frac{1}{1000}\right)$.

Always read the number by its name first, and then count off the decimal places. If a whole number precedes the decimal, read it just as you normally would.

Since decimals are parts of a whole number, you can write them as fractions:

Example   0.56 = "fifty-six hundredths" $\left(\frac{56}{100}\right)$

0.2 = "two-tenths" $\left(\frac{2}{10}\right)$

0.194 = "one hundred ninety-four thousandths" $\left(\frac{194}{1000}\right)$

0.31 = "thirty-one hundredths" $\left(\frac{31}{100}\right)$

1.6 = "one and six-tenths" $\left(1\frac{6}{10}\right)$

17.354 = "seventeen and three hundred fifty-four thousandths" $\left(17\frac{354}{1000}\right)$.

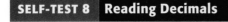

SELF-TEST 8   Reading Decimals

Write these decimals in longhand and as fractions. Answers are given at the end of the chapter.

1. 0.25 _____

2. 0.004 _____

3. 1.7 _____

4. 0.5 _____

5. 0.334 _____

6. 136.75 _____

7. 0.1 _____

8. 0.150 _____

Addition and Subtraction of Decimals

To add decimals, stack them vertically, making sure that all the decimal points line up exactly. Starting at the far right of the stack, add each vertical column of numbers. In your answer, be sure your decimal point lines up exactly with the points above it.

EXAMPLE 1

$$\begin{array}{r} 0.8 \\ + 0.6 \\ \hline 1.4 \end{array}$$

EXAMPLE 2

$$\begin{array}{r} 10.30 \\ + 3.28 \\ \hline 13.58 \end{array}$$

To subtract decimals, stack your two decimals as you did for addition, lining up the decimal points as before. Starting at the far right of the stack, subtract the numbers; and again, make sure that the decimal point in your answer aligns with those above it.

EXAMPLE 1

$$13 - 12.54 = \begin{array}{r} \overset{2\ 9}{1\cancel{3}.\cancel{0}0} \\ - 12.54 \\ \hline 0.46 \end{array}$$

EXAMPLE 2

$$14.56 - 0.47 = \begin{array}{r} \overset{4\ 16}{14.\cancel{5}6} \\ - 0.47 \\ \hline 14.09 \end{array}$$

SELF-TEST 9   Addition and Subtraction of Decimals

Add and subtract these decimals. Answers are given at the end of the chapter.

1. $0.9 + 0.5 =$

2. $5 + 2.999 =$

3. $10.56 + 357.5 =$

4. $2 + 3.05 + 0.06 =$

5. $15 + 0.19 + 21 =$

6. $98.6 - 66.5 =$

7. $0.45 - 0.38 =$

8. $1.724 - 0.684 =$

9. $7.066 - 0.2 =$

10. $78.56 - 5.77 =$

Multiplying Decimals

Line up the numbers on the right. Do not align the decimal points. Starting on the right, multiply each digit in the top number by each digit in the bottom number, just as you would with whole numbers. Add the products. Place the decimal point in the answer by starting at the right and moving the point the same number of places equal to the sum of the decimal places in both numbers multiplied, count the number of places that you totaled earlier. If you end up with any blank spaces, fill each one with a zero.

EXAMPLE 1

$$2.6 \times 0.03 = \quad \begin{array}{r} 2.6 \ \text{(1 decimal place)} \\ \times\, 0.03 \ \text{(2 decimal places)} \\ \hline 0.078 \ \text{(3 decimal places from the right)} \end{array}$$

EXAMPLE 2

$$200 \times 0.03 = \quad \begin{array}{r} 200 \ \text{(no decimal place)} \\ 0.03 \ \text{(2 decimal places)} \\ \hline 6.00 \ \text{(2 decimal places from the right)} \\ \text{or} \\ 6 \end{array}$$

Dividing Decimals

A reminder: The number being divided is called the *dividend;* the number doing the dividing is called the *divisor;* and the answer is called the *quotient.*

$$\text{divisor} \rightarrow 16 \overline{)5.000} \begin{array}{l} \ 0.312 \rightarrow \text{quotient} \\ \rightarrow \text{dividend} \end{array}$$

Note: As soon as you write your dividend, place a decimal point immediately after it. Then place another decimal point directly above it, on the quotient line.

Example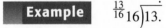

That completes your division.

Example

$$16\overline{)13.000} = 0.812$$

```
    0.812
16)13.000
   12 8
      20
      16
      40
      32
       8
```

Clearing the Divisor of Decimal Points

Before dividing one decimal by another, clear the divisor of decimal points. To do this, move the decimal point to the far right. Move the decimal point in the dividend *the same number of places* and, directly above it, insert another decimal point in the quotient.

Example

EXAMPLE 1

$$0.2\overline{)0.004} = 0.2\overline{)0.004}$$

Hence, $2\overline{)00.04} = 0.02$

EXAMPLE 2

$$4.3\overline{)5.427} \text{ becomes } 43.\overline{)54.270}$$

```
         1.262
43.)54.270
    43
    11 2
     8 6
     2 67
     2 58
        90
        86
         4
```

FINE POINTS ● ○ ● ●

When you're dividing, the answer may not come out even. The dosage calculation problems give directions on how many places to carry out your answer. In example 2, the answer is carried out to three decimal places.

SELF-TEST 10 **Multiplication and Division of Decimals**

Do these problems in division of decimals. The answers are given at the end of this chapter. If necessary, carry the answer to three places.

1. $3.14 \times 0.02 =$

2. $100 \times 0.4 =$

3. $2.76 \times 0.004 =$

4. $7.8\overline{)140}$

5. $6\overline{)140}$

6. $0.025\overline{)10}$

Rounding Off Decimals

How do you determine the number of places to carry out division? The answer depends on the way the drug is dispensed and the equipment needed to administer the drug. Some tablets can be broken into halves or fourths. Some liquids are prepared in units of measurement: tenths, hundredths, or thousandths. Some syringes are marked to the nearest tenth, hundredth, or thousandth place. Intravenous rates are usually rounded to the nearest whole number. As you become familiar with dosage, you'll learn how far to round off your answers. To practice, first review the general rule for rounding off decimals.

RULE	**ROUNDING OFF DECIMALS**
	To round off a decimal, you simply drop the final number. Exception: If the final number is 5 or higher, drop it and then increase the adjacent number by 1. ■

Example	0.864 becomes 0.86
	1.55 becomes 1.6
	0.33 becomes 0.3
	4.562 becomes 4.56
	2.38 becomes 2.4

To obtain an answer that's rounded off to the nearest tenth, look at the number in the hundredth place and follow the above rule for rounding off.

Example	0.12 becomes 0.1
	0.667 becomes 0.7
	1.46 becomes 1.5

If you want an answer that's rounded off to the nearest hundredth, look at the number in the thousandth place and follow the above rule for rounding off.

Example	0.664 becomes 0.66
	0.148 becomes 0.15
	2.375 becomes 2.38

And if you want an answer that's rounded off to the nearest thousandth, look at the number in the ten-thousandths place and follow the same rules.

Example	1.3758 becomes 1.376
	0.0024 becomes 0.002
	4.5555 becomes 4.556

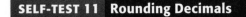

SELF-TEST 11 Rounding Decimals

Round off these decimals as indicated. Answers are given at the end of the chapter.

Nearest Tenth	Nearest Hundredth	Nearest Thousandth
1. 0.25 = _____	**6.** 1.268 = _____	**11.** 1.3254 = _____
2. 1.84 = _____	**7.** 0.750 = _____	**12.** 0.0025 = _____
3. 3.27 = _____	**8.** 0.677 = _____	**13.** 0.4520 = _____
4. 0.05 = _____	**9.** 4.539 = _____	**14.** 0.7259 = _____
5. 0.63 = _____	**10.** 1.222 = _____	**15.** 0.3482 = _____

Comparing the Value of Decimals

Understanding which decimal is larger or smaller can help you solve dosage problems. Example: "Will I need more than one tablet or less than one tablet?"

> **RULE** **DETERMINING THE VALUE OF DECIMALS**
>
> **The decimal with the higher number in the tenth place has the greater value.** ▪

> **Example** Compare 0.25 with 0.5.
>
> Since 5 is higher than 2, the greater of these two decimals is 0.5.

SELF-TEST 12 Value of Decimals

In each pair, underline the decimal with the greater value. Answers are given at the end of the chapter.

1. 0.125 and 0.25

2. 0.04 and 0.1

3. 0.5 and 0.125

4. 0.1 and 0.2

5. 0.825 and 0.44

6. 0.9 and 0.5

7. 0.25 and 0.4

8. 0.7 and 0.350

Percents

Percent means "parts per hundred." Percent is a fraction, containing a variable numerator and a denominator that's always 100. You can write a percent as a fraction, a ratio, or a decimal. (To write a ratio, use two numbers separated by a colon. Example: 1:100. Read this ratio as "one is to a hundred.")

Percent written as a fraction: $5\% = \frac{5}{100}$

Percent written as a ratio: $5\% = 5{:}100$

Percent written as a decimal: $5\% = 0.05$

Whole numbers, fractions, and decimals may all be written as percents.

Example   Whole number: 4% (four percent)

Decimal: 0.2% (two-tenths percent)

Fraction: $\frac{1}{4}$% (one-fourth percent)

Percents That Are Whole Numbers

Example   *EXAMPLE 1*

Change to a fraction.

$4\% = \frac{4}{100} = \frac{1}{25}$

EXAMPLE 2

Change to a decimal.

$4\% = \frac{4}{100} \quad 100\overline{)4.00}^{.04} = 0.04$

Percents That Are Decimals

These may be changed in three ways:

1. By moving the decimal point two places to the left

$0.2\% = 00.2 = 0.002$

2. By keeping the decimal, placing the number over 100, and then dividing

$0.2\% = \frac{0.2}{100} \quad 100\overline{)0.200}^{0.002} = 0.002$

3. By turning it into a complex fraction. If you're using this method, remember to invert the number after the division sign and then multiply. A whole number always has a denominator of 1.

$0.2\% = \frac{\frac{2}{10}}{100} =$

$\frac{2}{10} \div \frac{100}{1} =$

$\frac{2}{10} \times \frac{1}{100} = \frac{2}{1000}$

$\frac{\frac{1}{2}}{\frac{1000}{500}} = \frac{1}{500}$

Solving Proportions With an Unknown

When one of the numbers in a proportion is unknown, the letter x substitutes for that missing number. By following three steps you can determine the value of x in a proportion.

Step 1. Cross-multiply.

Step 2. Clear x.

Step 3. Reduce.

Here's how the three steps work.

Proportions Expressed as Two Fractions

Suppose you want to solve this proportion:

$$\frac{1}{0.125} = \frac{x}{0.25}$$

Step 1. Cross-multiply the numerators and denominators.

$$\frac{1}{0.125} \diagdown \frac{x}{0.25}$$

$$0.125x = 0.25$$

Step 2. Clear x by dividing both sides of the equation with the number that precedes x.

$$x = \frac{0.25}{0.125}$$

Step 3. Reduce the number.

$$0.125\overline{)0.250.}^{\,2.}$$

$$x = 2$$

Example	$\frac{45}{180} = \frac{3}{x}$
	$45x = 540$
	$x = \frac{540}{45}$
	$x = 12$

Proportions Expressed as Two Ratios

Suppose you start with this proportion:

$$4 : 3.2 :: 7 : x$$

Step 1. Cross-multiply the two outside numbers (called *extremes*) and the two inside numbers (called *means*).

$$4 : 3.2 :: 7 : x$$

$$4x = 22.4$$

Step 2.   Clear x by dividing both sides of the equation with the number that precedes x.

$$x = \frac{22.4}{4}$$

Step 3.   Reduce the number.

$$\begin{array}{r} 5.6 \\ 4\overline{)22.4} \end{array}$$

$$x = 5.6$$

Example $11 : 121 :: 3 : x$

$11x = 363$

$$\begin{array}{r} 33. \\ 11\overline{)363.} \\ \underline{33} \\ 33 \\ \underline{33} \\ \underline{33} \end{array}$$

$$x = 33$$

SELF-TEST 15 | Solving Proportions

Solve these proportions. Answers are given at the end of the chapter.

1. $\frac{120}{4.2} = \frac{16}{x}$

2. $750 : 250 :: x : 5$

3. $\frac{14}{140} = \frac{22}{x}$

4. $2 : 5 :: x : 10$

5. $\frac{81}{3} = \frac{x}{15}$

6. $0.125 : 0.5 :: x : 10$

Ratio and Proportion in Dosage

When the amount of drug ordered by a physician or healthcare provider differs from the supply, you can solve the dosage problem with proportion, using either two ratios or two fractions.

Example   Order: 0.5 mg of a drug

Supply: A liquid labeled 0.125 mg per 4 mL

You know that the liquid comes as 0.125 mg in 4 mL. And you know that the amount you want is 0.5 mg. You don't know, however, what amount of liquid is needed to equal 0.5 mg. So, you need one more piece of information: the unknown, or x.

You can set up and solve this arithmetic operation as a proportion, using either two fractions or two ratios separated by colons. Notice that both methods eventually become the same calculation.

Two Fractions   *Two Ratios Using Colons*

$$\frac{0.5}{0.125} \diagtimes \frac{x}{4}$$

$$0.125x = 2$$

$$\downarrow$$

$$0.5 : 0.125 :: x : 4$$

$$0.125x = 2$$

$$\frac{0.125x}{0.125} = \frac{2}{0.125}$$

$$\downarrow$$

$$\downarrow$$

$$\frac{0.125x}{0.125} = \frac{2.0}{0.125}$$

$$\downarrow$$

$$x = \frac{2}{0.125}$$

$$x = \frac{2}{0.125}$$

$$\downarrow$$

$$\downarrow$$

$$x = \frac{2}{0.125}\ \ \overset{16.}{0.125\,)\overline{2.000.}}$$
$$\underline{1\ 25}$$
$$750$$
$$\underline{750}$$

$$x = \frac{2}{0.125}\ \ \overset{16.}{0.125\,)\overline{2.000.}}$$
$$\underline{1\ 25}$$
$$750$$
$$\underline{750}$$

$$x = 16$$

So far, you've learned two ways to solve dosage calculation problems: the *ratio method* (i.e., the proportion of two ratios); and the *proportion method* (i.e., the proportion of two fractions). Chapter 6 introduces the simpler *formula method,* which is derived from ratio and proportion. And Chapter 11 explains another less complicated way: the *dimensional analysis method.* Throughout the book, proficiency test problems illustrate solutions reached by all four methods of calculation.

Name: _____

These arithmetic operations are needed to calculate doses. See Appendix A for answers. Your instructor can provide other practice tests if necessary.

A. Multiply

     a) $\begin{array}{r} 647 \\ \times 38 \\ \hline \end{array}$ **b)** $\frac{8}{9} \times \frac{12}{32}$ **c)** $\begin{array}{r} 0.56 \\ \times 0.17 \\ \hline \end{array}$

B. Divide. If necessary, report to two decimal places.

     a) $82\overline{)793}$ **b)** $5\frac{1}{4} \div \frac{7}{4}$ **c)** $0.015\overline{)0.3}$

C. Add and reduce

     a) $\frac{7}{15} + \frac{8}{15}$ **b)** $\frac{3}{8} + \frac{2}{5}$ **c)** $0.825 + 0.1$

D. Subtract and reduce

     a) $\frac{11}{15} - \frac{7}{10}$ **b)** $\frac{8}{15} - \frac{4}{15}$ **c)** $1.56 - 0.2$

E. Change to a decimal. If necessary, report to two decimal places.

     a) $\frac{1}{18}$ **b)** $\frac{3}{8}$

F. Change to a fraction and reduce to lowest terms.

     a) 0.35 $\frac{35}{100}$ **b)** 0.08 $\frac{8}{100}$

G. In each set, which number has the greater value?

     a) _____ 0.4 and 0.162

     b) _____ 0.76 and 0.8

     c) _____ 0.5 and 0.83

     d) _____ 0.3 and 0.25

H. Reduce these fractions to their lowest terms as decimals. Report to two decimal places.

     a) $\frac{20}{12}$ **b)** $\frac{7}{84}$ **c)** $\frac{6}{13}$

I. Round off these decimals as indicated.

     a) nearest tenth   5.349 _____

     b) nearest hundredth   0.6284 _____

     c) nearest thousandth   0.9244 _____

J. Change these percents to a fraction, ratio and decimal.

     a) $\frac{1}{3}\%$ **b)** 0.8%

K. Change these fractions, ratios and decimals to a percent.

     a) $\frac{7}{100}$ **b)** $1:10$ **c)** 0.008

L. Solve these proportions.

     a) $\frac{32}{128} = \frac{4}{x}$

     b) $8:72 :: 5:x$

     c) $\frac{0.4}{0.12} = \frac{x}{8}$ (nearest whole number)

Answers

Self-Test 1 Multiplication

1. 12	**5.** 108	**9.** 48	**13.** 24	**17.** 18	**21.** 132
2. 63	**6.** 24	**10.** 72	**14.** 54	**18.** 88	**22.** 45
3. 32	**7.** 110	**11.** 15	**15.** 64	**19.** 36	**23.** 81
4. 45	**8.** 14	**12.** 42	**16.** 56	**20.** 24	**24.** 35

Self-Test 2 Division

1. 9	**5.** 7	**9.** 7	**13.** 4	**17.** 9	**21.** 7
2. 4	**6.** 8	**10.** 6	**14.** 3	**18.** 4	**22.** 12
3. 3	**7.** 4	**11.** 9	**15.** 3	**19.** 6	**23.** 12
4. 7	**8.** 3	**12.** 6	**16.** 7	**20.** 2	**24.** 7

Self-Test 3 Reducing Fractions

1. $\frac{16}{24} = \frac{4}{6} = \frac{2}{3}$ (Divide by 4, then 2.)

Alternatively: $\frac{16}{24} = \frac{2}{3}$ (Divide by 8.)

2. $\frac{36}{216} = \frac{6}{36} = \frac{1}{6}$ (Divide by 6, then 6.)

3. $\frac{18}{96} = \frac{9}{48} = \frac{3}{16}$ (Divide by 2, then 3.)

4. $\frac{70}{490} = \frac{7}{49} = \frac{1}{7}$ (Divide by 10, then 7.)

5. $\frac{18}{81} = \frac{2}{9}$ (Divide by 9.)

6. $\frac{8}{48} = \frac{1}{6}$ (Divide by 8.)

7. $\frac{12}{30} = \frac{6}{15} = \frac{2}{5}$ (Divide by 2, then 3.)

Alternatively: $\frac{12}{30} = \frac{2}{5}$ (Divide by 6.)

8. $\frac{68}{136} = \frac{34}{68} = \frac{1}{2}$ (Divide by 2, then 34.)

9. $\frac{55}{121} = \frac{5}{11}$ (Divide by 11.)

10. $\frac{15}{60} = \frac{1}{4}$ (Divide by 15.)

Alternatively: $\frac{15}{60} = \frac{3}{12} = \frac{1}{4}$ (Divide by 5, then 3.)

Self-Test 4 Adding and Subtracting Fractions

1. $\frac{5}{7}$

2. $\frac{4}{5}$

3. $\frac{3}{4}$

4. $\frac{(2 \times 2)}{\frac{3}{6}} + \frac{1}{6} = \frac{4}{6} + \frac{1}{6} = \frac{5}{6}$

5. $\frac{1}{2} + \frac{1}{3} = \frac{3}{6} + \frac{2}{6} = \frac{5}{6}$

6. $\frac{10}{16}$ or $\frac{5}{8}$

7. $\frac{1}{7}$

8. $\frac{(3 \times 3)}{\frac{5}{15}} - \frac{2}{15} = \frac{9}{15} - \frac{2}{15} = \frac{7}{15}$

9. $\frac{11}{15} - \frac{7}{10} = \frac{22}{30} - \frac{21}{30} = \frac{1}{30}$

10. $\frac{8}{9} - \frac{5}{12} = \frac{32}{36} - \frac{15}{36} = \frac{17}{36}$

Self-Test 5 Multiplying Fractions (Two Ways to Solve)

First Way   *Second Way*

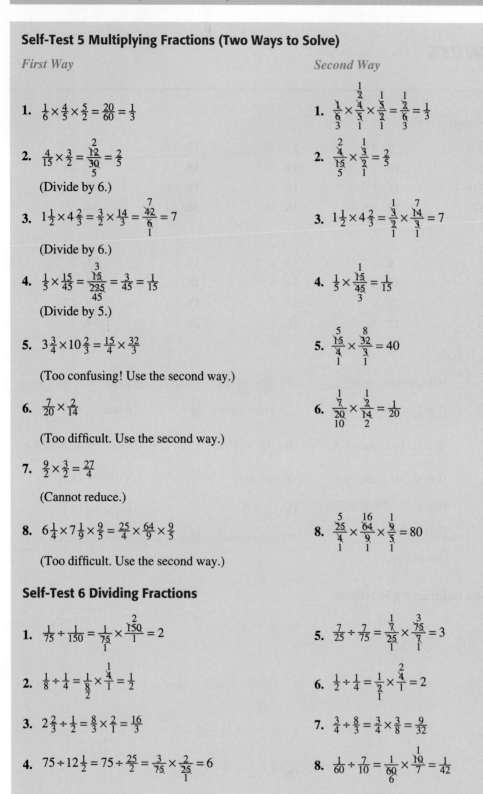

1. $\frac{1}{6} \times \frac{4}{5} \times \frac{5}{2} = \frac{20}{60} = \frac{1}{3}$

2. $\frac{4}{15} \times \frac{3}{2} = \frac{\overset{2}{12}}{\underset{5}{30}} = \frac{2}{5}$

   (Divide by 6.)

3. $1\frac{1}{2} \times 4\frac{2}{3} = \frac{3}{2} \times \frac{14}{3} = \frac{\overset{7}{42}}{\underset{1}{6}} = 7$

   (Divide by 6.)

4. $\frac{1}{5} \times \frac{15}{45} = \frac{\overset{3}{15}}{\underset{45}{225}} = \frac{3}{45} = \frac{1}{15}$

   (Divide by 5.)

5. $3\frac{3}{4} \times 10\frac{2}{3} = \frac{15}{4} \times \frac{32}{3}$

   (Too confusing! Use the second way.)

6. $\frac{7}{20} \times \frac{2}{14}$

   (Too difficult. Use the second way.)

7. $\frac{9}{2} \times \frac{3}{2} = \frac{27}{4}$

   (Cannot reduce.)

8. $6\frac{1}{4} \times 7\frac{1}{9} \times \frac{9}{5} = \frac{25}{4} \times \frac{64}{9} \times \frac{9}{5}$

   (Too difficult. Use the second way.)

1. $\frac{1}{\underset{3}{6}} \times \frac{4}{5} \times \frac{\overset{1}{5}}{\underset{1}{2}} = \frac{\overset{1}{2}}{\underset{3}{6}} = \frac{1}{3}$

2. $\frac{\overset{2}{4}}{\underset{5}{15}} \times \frac{3}{\underset{1}{2}} = \frac{2}{5}$

3. $1\frac{1}{2} \times 4\frac{2}{3} = \frac{\overset{1}{3}}{\underset{1}{2}} \times \frac{\overset{7}{14}}{\underset{1}{3}} = 7$

4. $\frac{1}{5} \times \frac{\overset{1}{15}}{\underset{3}{45}} = \frac{1}{15}$

5. $\frac{\overset{5}{15}}{\underset{1}{4}} \times \frac{\overset{8}{32}}{\underset{1}{3}} = 40$

6. $\frac{\overset{1}{7}}{\underset{10}{20}} \times \frac{\overset{1}{2}}{\underset{2}{14}} = \frac{1}{20}$

8. $\frac{\overset{5}{25}}{\underset{1}{4}} \times \frac{\overset{16}{64}}{\underset{1}{9}} \times \frac{\overset{1}{9}}{\underset{1}{5}} = 80$

Self-Test 6 Dividing Fractions

1. $\frac{1}{75} \div \frac{1}{150} = \frac{1}{\underset{1}{75}} \times \frac{\overset{2}{150}}{1} = 2$

2. $\frac{1}{8} \div \frac{1}{4} = \frac{1}{\underset{2}{8}} \times \frac{\overset{1}{4}}{1} = \frac{1}{2}$

3. $2\frac{2}{3} \div \frac{1}{2} = \frac{8}{3} \times \frac{2}{1} = \frac{16}{3}$

4. $75 \div 12\frac{1}{2} = 75 \div \frac{25}{2} = \frac{\overset{3}{75}}{1} \times \frac{2}{\underset{1}{25}} = 6$

5. $\frac{7}{25} \div \frac{7}{75} = \frac{\overset{1}{7}}{\underset{1}{25}} \times \frac{\overset{3}{75}}{\underset{1}{7}} = 3$

6. $\frac{1}{2} \div \frac{1}{4} = \frac{1}{\underset{1}{2}} \times \frac{\overset{2}{4}}{1} = 2$

7. $\frac{3}{4} \div \frac{8}{3} = \frac{3}{4} \times \frac{3}{8} = \frac{9}{32}$

8. $\frac{1}{60} \div \frac{7}{10} = \frac{1}{\underset{6}{60}} \times \frac{\overset{1}{10}}{7} = \frac{1}{42}$

Self-Test 7 Converting Fractions to Decimals

1.
$$\frac{1}{6} \overline{)1.000}^{.166} = 0.166$$
$$\underline{6}$$
$$40$$
$$\underline{36}$$
$$40$$
$$\underline{36}$$
$$4$$

2.
$$\frac{\overset{3}{\cancel{6}}}{\underset{4}{\cancel{8}}} = \frac{3}{4} \overline{)3.00}^{.75} = 0.75$$
$$\underline{2\ 8}$$
$$20$$
$$\underline{20}$$
$$0$$

3.
$$\frac{4}{5} \overline{)4.0}^{.8} = 0.8$$
$$\underline{4\ 0}$$
$$0$$

4.
$$\frac{9}{40} \overline{)9.000}^{.225} = 0.225$$
$$\underline{8\ 0}$$
$$1\ 00$$
$$\underline{80}$$
$$200$$
$$\underline{200}$$
$$0$$

5.
$$\frac{1}{8} \overline{)1.000}^{.125} = 0.125$$
$$\underline{8}$$
$$20$$
$$\underline{16}$$
$$40$$
$$\underline{40}$$
$$0$$

6.
$$\frac{1}{7} \overline{)1.000}^{.145} = 0.142$$
$$\underline{7}$$
$$30$$
$$\underline{28}$$
$$20$$
$$\underline{14}$$
$$6$$

Self-Test 8 Reading Decimals

1. Twenty-five hundredths $\left(\frac{25}{100}\right)$
2. Four thousandths $\left(\frac{4}{1000}\right)$
3. One and seven tenths $\left(1\frac{7}{10}\right)$
4. Five tenths $\left(\frac{5}{10}\right)$
5. Three hundred thirty-four thousandths $\left(\frac{334}{1000}\right)$

6. One hundred thirty-six and seventy-five hundredths $\left(136\frac{75}{100}\right)$
7. One tenth $\left(\frac{1}{10}\right)$
8. One hundred fifty thousandths $\left(\frac{150}{1000}\right)$. The zero at the end of 0.150 is not necessary. The number could be read as fifteen hundredths $\left(\frac{15}{100}\right)$.

Self-Test 9 Addition and Subtraction of Decimals

1.
$$\begin{array}{r} 0.9 \\ + 0.5 \\ \hline 1.4 \end{array}$$

2.
$$\begin{array}{r} 5.000 \\ + 2.999 \\ \hline 7.999 \end{array}$$

3.
$$\begin{array}{r} 10.56 \\ + 357.50 \\ \hline 368.06 \end{array}$$

4.
$$\begin{array}{r} 2.00 \\ 3.05 \\ + 0.06 \\ \hline 5.11 \end{array}$$

5.
$$\begin{array}{r} 15.00 \\ 0.19 \\ + 21.00 \\ \hline 36.19 \end{array}$$

6.
$$\begin{array}{r} 98.6 \\ - 66.5 \\ \hline 32.1 \end{array}$$

7.
$$\begin{array}{r} 0.\overset{3}{\cancel{4}}5 \\ - 0.38 \\ \hline 0.07 \end{array}$$

8.
$$\begin{array}{r} 1.\overset{6}{\cancel{7}}24 \\ - 0.684 \\ \hline 1.040 \ \text{or} \ 1.04 \end{array}$$

9.
$$\begin{array}{r} \overset{6}{\cancel{7}}.066 \\ - 0.200 \\ \hline 6.866 \end{array}$$

10.
$$\begin{array}{r} 7\overset{7}{\cancel{8}}.\overset{4}{\cancel{5}}6 \\ - \quad 5.77 \\ \hline 72.79 \end{array}$$

Self-Test 10 Multiplication and Division of Decimals

1.
$$\begin{array}{r} 3.14 \\ \times\,0.02 \\ \hline 0.0628 \end{array}$$

2.
$$\begin{array}{r} 100 \\ \times\,0.4 \\ \hline 40.0 \end{array}\ \text{or } 40$$

3.
$$\begin{array}{r} 2.76 \\ \times\,0.004 \\ \hline 0.01104 \end{array}$$

4. $7.8\,\overline{)140.0}$ Now it is
$$\begin{array}{r} 17.948 \\ 78\,\overline{)1400.000} \\ \underline{78}\ \ \ \ \ \ \\ 620\ \ \ \ \ \\ \underline{546}\ \ \ \ \ \\ 74\,0\ \ \ \\ \underline{70\,2}\ \ \ \\ 3\,80\ \ \\ \underline{3\,12}\ \ \\ 680 \\ \underline{624} \\ 56 \end{array}$$

5.
$$\begin{array}{r} 23.333 \\ 6\,\overline{)140.000} \\ \underline{12}\ \ \ \ \ \ \ \\ 20\ \ \ \ \ \\ \underline{18}\ \ \ \ \ \\ 20\ \ \ \ \\ \underline{18}\ \ \ \ \\ 20\ \ \ \\ \underline{18}\ \ \ \\ 20\ \ \\ \underline{18}\ \ \\ 2 \end{array}$$

6. $0.025\,\overline{)10.000}$ Now it is $25\,\overline{)10000.}^{\,400.}$

Note that because there are two places between the 4 and the decimal, you had to add two zeros.

Self-Test 11 Rounding Decimals

Nearest Tenth
1. 0.3
2. 1.8
3. 3.3
4. 0.1
5. 0.6

Nearest Hundredth
6. 1.27
7. 0.75
8. 0.68
9. 4.54
10. 1.22

Nearest Thousandth
11. 1.325
12. 0.003
13. 0.452
14. 0.726
15. 0.348

Self-Test 12 Value of Decimals

1. 0.25
2. 0.1
3. 0.5
4. 0.2
5. 0.825
6. 0.9
7. 0.4
8. 0.7

Self-Test 13 Conversion of Percents

1. Fraction $10\% = \dfrac{\frac{1}{\cancel{10}}}{\frac{\cancel{100}}{10}} = \dfrac{1}{10}$

Decimal $10\% = \dfrac{10}{100}\,\overline{)10.0}^{\,.1} = 0.1$

Quick-rule decimal $10.\% = 0.1$

2. Fraction $0.9\% = \dfrac{\frac{9}{10}}{100} = \dfrac{9}{10} \div 100 = \dfrac{9}{10} \times \dfrac{1}{100} = \dfrac{9}{1000}$

Decimal $0.9\% = \dfrac{0.9}{100} \overset{.009}{\overline{\smash{)}0.900}} = 0.009$

Quick-rule decimal $00.9\% = 0.009$

3. Fraction $\dfrac{1}{5}\% = \dfrac{\frac{1}{5}}{100} = \dfrac{1}{5} \div 100 = \dfrac{1}{5} \times \dfrac{1}{100} = \dfrac{1}{500}$

Decimal $\dfrac{1}{5}\% = \dfrac{1}{5} \div 100 = \dfrac{1}{500} \overset{.002}{\overline{\smash{)}1.000}} = 0.002$

Quick-rule decimal $\dfrac{1}{5}\% = \dfrac{1}{5} \overset{.2}{\overline{\smash{)}1.0}} = 0.2\%$

$00.2 = 0.002$

4. Fraction $0.01\% = \dfrac{\frac{1}{100}}{100} = \dfrac{1}{100} \div \dfrac{100}{1} = \dfrac{1}{100} \times \dfrac{1}{100} = \dfrac{1}{10000}$

Decimal $0.1\% = \dfrac{0.01}{100} \overset{0.0001}{\overline{\smash{)}.0100}} = 0.0001$

Quick-rule decimal $00.01 = 0.0001$

5. Fraction $\dfrac{2}{3}\% = \dfrac{\frac{2}{3}}{100} = \dfrac{2}{3} \div \dfrac{100}{1} = \dfrac{2}{3} \times \dfrac{1}{100} = \dfrac{2}{300} = \dfrac{1}{150}$

Decimal $\dfrac{2}{3}\% = \dfrac{2}{3} \div \dfrac{100}{1} = \dfrac{2}{3} \times \dfrac{1}{100} = \dfrac{2}{300} \overset{.0066}{\overline{\smash{)}2.000}} = 0.0066$

Quick-rule decimal $\dfrac{2}{3}\% = \dfrac{2}{3} \overset{.66}{\overline{\smash{)}2.00}} = 0.66\% = 00.66 = 0.0066$

6. Fraction $0.45\% = \dfrac{\frac{45}{100}}{100} = \dfrac{45}{100} \div \dfrac{100}{1} = \dfrac{45}{100} \times \dfrac{1}{100} = \dfrac{45}{10000} = \dfrac{9}{2000}$

Decimal $0.45\% = \dfrac{.45}{100} \overset{.0045}{\overline{\smash{)}0.4500}} = 0.0045$

Quick-rule decimal $00.45\% = 0.0045$

7. Fraction $\dfrac{\frac{1}{20}}{\frac{100}{5}} = \dfrac{1}{5}$

Decimal $20\% = \dfrac{20}{100} \overset{0.2}{\overline{\smash{)}20.0}}$

Quick-rule decimal $20.\% = 0.2$

8. Fraction $\quad 0.4\% = \dfrac{\frac{4}{10}}{100} = \dfrac{4}{10} \div \dfrac{100}{1} = \dfrac{\overset{1}{\cancel{4}}}{10} \times \dfrac{1}{\underset{25}{\cancel{100}}} = \dfrac{1}{250}$

Decimal $\quad 0.4\% = \dfrac{0.4}{100} \quad 100\overline{)0.400}^{\,0.004} = 0.004$

Quick-rule decimal $\quad 00.4\% = 0.004$

9. Fraction $\quad \dfrac{1}{10}\% = \dfrac{\frac{1}{10}}{100} = \dfrac{1}{10} \div \dfrac{100}{1} = \dfrac{1}{10} \times \dfrac{1}{100} = \dfrac{1}{1000}$

Decimal $\quad \dfrac{1}{10}\% = \dfrac{1}{10} \div \dfrac{100}{1} = \dfrac{1}{10} \times \dfrac{1}{100} = \dfrac{1}{1000} \quad 1000\overline{)1.000}^{\,0.001} = 0.001$

Quick-rule decimal $\quad \dfrac{1}{10}\% = \dfrac{1}{10} \quad 10\overline{)1.0}^{\,0.1} = 0.1\% = 00.1 = 0.001$

10. Fraction $\quad 2\frac{1}{2}\% = 2.5\% = \dfrac{\frac{25}{10}}{100} = \dfrac{25}{10} \div \dfrac{100}{1} = \dfrac{25}{10} \times \dfrac{1}{100} = \dfrac{25}{1000} = \dfrac{1}{40}$

Decimal $\quad 2.5\% = \dfrac{2.5}{100} \quad 100\overline{)2.50}^{\,0.025} = 0.025$

Quick-rule decimal $\quad 000.2.5\% = 0.025$

11. Fraction $\quad 33\% = \dfrac{33}{100}$

Decimal $\quad 33\% = \dfrac{33}{100} \quad 100\overline{)33.00}^{\,.33} = 0.33$

Quick-rule decimal $\quad 33.\% = 0.33$

12. Fraction $\quad 50\% = \dfrac{50}{100} = \dfrac{1}{2}$

Decimal $\quad 50\% = \dfrac{50}{100} \quad 100\overline{)50.0}^{\,.5} = 0.5$

Quick-rule decimal $\quad 50.\% = 0.5$

Self-Test 14 Fractions, Ratios and Decimals

	Fraction	*Ratio*	*Decimal*
1. 32% =	$\dfrac{32}{100}$	32:100	32% = 0.32
2. 8.5% =	$\dfrac{8.5}{100}$ or $\dfrac{85}{1000}$	8.5:100	08.5% = 0.085
3. 125% =	$\dfrac{125}{100}$	125:100	125% = 1.25

4. $64\% = \dfrac{64}{100}$ $64:100$ $64\% = 0.64$

5. $11.25\% = \dfrac{11.25}{100}$ or $\dfrac{1125}{10000}$ $11.25:100$ $11.25\% = 0.1125$

6. $\dfrac{7}{10} = \dfrac{70}{100} = 70\%$

7. $2:5 = 40:100 = 40\%$

8. $0.08 = 8\%$

9. $0.56 = 56\%$

10. $3.00 = 300\%$

Self-Test 15 Solving Proportions

1. $\dfrac{120}{4.2} = \dfrac{16}{x}$
$120x = 67.2$
$x = 0.56$

$$
\begin{array}{r}
0.56 \\
120\overline{)67.20} \\
\underline{60\ 0} \\
7\ 20 \\
\underline{7\ 20}
\end{array}
$$

2. $750:250::x:5$
$250x = 750 \times 5$
$x = 15$

$\dfrac{\overset{3}{750 \times 5}}{\underset{1}{250}} = 15$

3. $\dfrac{14}{140} = \dfrac{22}{x}$
$14x = 22 \times 140$
$x = 220$

$\dfrac{22 \times \overset{10}{140}}{\underset{1}{14}} = 220$

4. $2:5::x:10$
$5x = 20$
$x = 4$

5. $\dfrac{81}{3} = \dfrac{x}{15}$
$3x = 81 \times 15$
$x = 405$

$\dfrac{81 \times \overset{5}{15}}{\underset{1}{3}} = 405$

6. $0.125:0.5::x:10$
$0.5x = 0.125 \times 10 = \dfrac{\overset{1}{0.125}}{\underset{4}{0.500}} \times 10 = \dfrac{10}{4}\overline{)10.0}^{\,2.5}$
$x = 2.5$

Interpreting the Language of Prescriptions

LEARNING OBJECTIVES

1. Abbreviating times and routes of administration

2. Understanding military time: the 24-hour clock

3. Abbreviating metric, household, and apothecary measures

4. Understanding SI units

5. Reading prescriptions

6. Terms and abbreviations for drug preparations

When you're calculating drug dosages, it's important to understand medical abbreviations. Misunderstanding them can lead to medication errors. If you're unsure about what a medical abbreviation stands for, if the handwriting is illegible, or if you have any question about the medication order, *do not prepare the dose.* Clarify the order or abbreviation with the healthcare provider who prescribed the medication.

Below are three sample medication orders. They may look confusing now, but after you've worked your way through this chapter, they'll make perfect sense:

Morphine sulfate 15 mg sub Q stat and 10 mg q4h prn

Chloromycetin 0.01% Ophth Oint left eye bid

Ampicillin 1 g IVPB q6h

In 2004, The Joint Commission issued a list of "Do Not Use" abbreviations: the ones that were often misread and thus led to medication errors. Some of them (clearly labeled "Do Not Use") appear in this book, either because they are from the minimal required list on the Joint Commission's web site or because they supplement that list. To see a complete roster of abbreviations designated "Do Not Use," go to www.jointcommission.org or search "prohibited abbreviations." Each institution may also have its own "Do Not Use" list. As a nurse, you need to make careful note of abbreviations that are prohibited or dangerous.

Time of Administration of Drugs

The abbreviations for the times of drug administration, which come from Latin words, appear in the following table. Memorize the abbreviations, their meanings, and the sample times that indicate how the abbreviations are interpreted. However, follow your institutional policy for administration times.

Time Abbreviation	Meaning	Explanation		Do Not Use
ac	Before meals	Latin, *ante cibum*		
		Sample Time 7:30 AM, 11:30 AM, 4:30 PM		
pc	After meals	Latin, *post cibum*		
		Sample Time 10 AM, 2 PM, 6 PM		
daily	Every day, daily	Latin, *quaque die*		q.d.
		Sample Time 10 AM		qd
bid	Twice a day	Latin, *bis in die*		
		Sample Time 10 AM, 6 PM		
tid	Three times a day	Latin, *ter in die*		
		Sample Time 10 AM, 2 PM, 6 PM		
qid	Four times a day	Latin, *quater in die*		
		Sample Time 10 AM, 2 PM, 6 PM, 10 PM		
qh	Every hour	Latin, *quaque hora* Because the drug is given every hour, it will be given 24 times in one day.		
at bedtime	At bedtime, hour of sleep	Latin, *hora somni*.		hs
		Sample Time 10 PM		h.s.
qn	Every night	Latin, *quaque nocte*		
		Sample Time 10 PM		
stat	Immediately	Latin, *statim*		
		Sample Time Now!		

The time abbreviations in the following table are based on a 24-hour day. To determine the number of times a medication is given in a day, divide 24 by the number given in the abbreviation.

Time Abbreviation	Meaning	Explanation
q2h or q2°	Every 2 hours	The drug will be given 12 times in a 24-hour period (24 ÷ 2). **Sample Times** even hours at 2 AM, 4 AM, 6 AM, 8 AM, 10 AM, 12 noon, 2 PM, 4 PM, 6 PM, 8 PM, 10 PM, 12 midnight
q4h or q4°	Every 4 hours	The drug will be given six times in a 24-hour period (24 ÷ 4) **Sample Times** 2 AM, 6 AM, 10 AM, 2 PM, 6 PM, 10 PM
q6h or q6°	Every 6 hours	The drug will be given four times in a 24-hour period (24 ÷ 6) **Sample Times** 6 AM, 12 noon, 6 PM, 12 midnight
q8h or q8°	Every 8 hours	The drug will be given three times in a 24-hour period (24 ÷ 8) **Sample Times** 6 AM, 2 PM, 10 PM
q12h or q12°	Every 12 hours	The drug will be given twice in a 24-hour period (24 ÷ 12) **Sample Times** 6 AM, 6 PM

There are four additional time abbreviations that require explanation. They are as follows:

Time Abbreviation	Meaning	Explanation	Do Not Use
every other day	Every other day	Latin, *quaque otra die* This abbreviation is interpreted by the days of the **month:** the nurse writes on the medication record: odd days of the month **Sample Time** 10 AM on the first, third, fifth day, and so on The nurse might write: even days of the month **Sample Time** 10 AM on the second, fourth, sixth day, and so on	qod q.o.d.
prn	As needed	Latin, *pro re nata* **This abbreviation is usually combined with a time abbreviation.** **Example** q4h prn (every 4 hours as needed) This permits the nurse to assess the patient and make a nursing judgment about whether to administer the medication. **Sample** acetaminophen 650 mg po q4h prn (650 milligrams acetaminophen by mouth, every 4 hours as needed for pain) The nurse assesses the patient for pain every 4 hours. If the patient has pain, the nurse may administer the drug. This abbreviation has three administration implications: 1. The nurse **must wait** 4 hours before giving the next dose. 2. Once 4 hours have elapsed, the dose may be given any time thereafter. 3. Sample times are not given because the nurse does not know when the patient will need the drug.	
3 times weekly	Three times per week	Latin, *ter in vicis* Time relates to days of the **week.** **Sample Time** 10 AM on Monday, Wednesday, Friday Do not confuse with tid (three times per **day**).	tiw t.i.w.
biw	Twice per week	Latin, *bis in vicis* Time relates to days of the **week.** **Sample Time** 10 AM on Monday, Thursday Do not confuse with bid (twice per **day**).	

SELF-TEST 1	Abbreviations

After studying the abbreviations for times of administration, give the meaning of the following terms. Include sample times. Indicate if the abbreviation is "Do Not Use" and which words to substitute for it. The correct answers are given at the end of the chapter.

1. tid_____

2. qn_____

3. pc_____

4. qod_____

5. bid_____

6. hs_____

7. stat_____

8. qid_____

9. q4h_____

10. ac_____

11. qd_____

12. q8h_____

13. qh_____

14. prn_____

15. q4h prn_____

Military Time: The 24-Hour Clock

If a handwritten prescription does not clearly distinguish "AM" from "PM" confusion about times of administration can arise. To prevent error, many institutions have converted from the traditional 12-hour clock to a 24-hour clock, referred to as *military time.*

The 24-hour clock begins at midnight as 0000. The hours from 1 AM to 12 noon are the same as traditional time; colons and the terms AM and PM are omitted (Fig. 2-1). Examples:

Traditional	*Military*
12 midnight	0000
1 AM	0100
5 AM	0500
7:30 AM	0730
11:45 AM	1145
12:00 noon	1200

The hours from 1 PM continue numerically; 1 PM becomes 1300. To change traditional time to military time from 1 PM on, add 12. To change military time to traditional time from 1300 on, subtract 12. Examples:

Traditional	*Military*
1 PM	1300
2:30 PM	1430
5 PM	1700
7:15 PM	1915
10:45 PM	2245
11:59 PM	2359

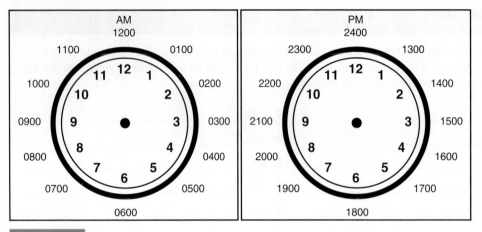

FIGURE 2-1

Example of a military, or 24-hour, clock.

SELF-TEST 2 | Military Time

A. *Change these traditional times to military time. Answers are given at the end of the chapter.*

1. 2 PM _____

2. 9 AM _____

3. 4 PM _____

4. 12 noon _____

5. 1:30 AM _____

6. 9:15 PM _____

7. 4:50 AM _____

8. 6:20 PM _____

B. *Change these military times to traditional times. Answers are given at the end of the chapter.*

1. 0130 _____

2. 1745 _____

3. 1100 _____

4. 2015 _____

5. 1910 _____

6. 0600 _____

7. 0050 _____

8. 1000 _____

Routes of Administration

Of the following abbreviations, some are based on Latin words and some are not. Note the Latin words and also the alternative abbreviations, which are given in parentheses. Figure 2-2 shows the use of several abbreviations for routes of administration.

Route Abbreviation	Meaning	Origin and Explanation	Do Not Use
Write out	Right ear	Latin, *aures dextra*	AD
Write out	Left ear	Latin, *aures laeva*	AL
Write out	Each ear	Latin, *aures utrae*	AU
HHN	Hand-held nebulizer	Medication is placed in a device that produces a fine spray for inhalation.	
IM	Intramuscularly	The injection is given at a 90° angle into a muscle.	
IV	Intravenously	The injection is given into a vein.	
IVP	Intravenous push	Medication is injected directly in a vein.	

(continued)

Route Abbreviation	Meaning	Origin and Explanation	Do Not Use
IVPB	Intravenous piggyback	Medication prepared in a small volume of fluid is attached to an IV (which is already infusing fluid into a patient's vein) at specified times.	
MDI	Metered-dose inhaler	An aerosol device delivers medication by inhalation.	
NEB	Nebulizer	Medication is placed in a device that produces a fine spray for inhalations.	
NGT (ng)	Nasogastric tube	Medication is placed in the stomach through a tube in the nose.	
Write out	In the right eye	Latin, *oculus dextra*	OD
Write out	In the left eye	Latin, *oculus sinister*	OS
Write out	In both eyes	Latin, *oculi utrique*	OU
po (PO)	By mouth	Latin, *per os*	
pr (PR)	In the rectum	Latin, *per rectum*	
Sub-Q or Sub Q	Subcutaneously	The injection is usually given at a 45° angle into subcutaneous tissue.	sc sq s.c. s.q.
SL	Sublingual, under the tongue	Latin, *sub lingua*	
S & S	Swish and swallow	By using tongue and cheek muscles, the patient coats his/her mouth with a liquid medication.	

SELF-TEST 3   Abbreviations (Routes)

After studying the abbreviations for routes of administration, give the meaning of the following terms. Indicate if the abbreviation is "Do Not Use" and which words substitute for it. The correct answers are given at the end of the chapter.

1. SL _____
2. OU _____
3. NGT _____
4. IV _____
5. po _____

6. OD _____
7. IVPB _____
8. OS _____
9. IM _____
10. pr _____

11. S&S _____
12. SC _____
13. AU _____
14. AL _____

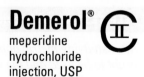

□ 1 mL   **Carpuject®**
                with Luer Lock

Demerol® ℂⅡ

meperidine
hydrochloride
injection, USP

Warning: May be habit forming.

75 mg/mL

For IM, SC or Slow IV Use

Sterile Aqueous Injection 7.5%
pH adjusted with NaOH or HCl.
For usual dosage and route of administration, see package insert.
Store at room temperature up to 25°C (77°F).
Caution: Federal (USA) law prohibits dispensing without prescription.
Demerol® is a registered trademark of Sanofi Pharmaceuticals, Inc.

©Abbott 1997   08-8409-2/R1-11/97   Printed in USA
Abbott Laboratories, North Chicago, IL 60064, USA

FIGURE 2-2

Label states the routes of administration. Meperidine HCL may be administered intramuscularly (IM), subcutaneously, or slowly intravenous (IV). (Courtesy of Abbott Laboratories)

Metric and SI Abbreviations

Metric abbreviations in dosage relate to a drug's weight or volume and are the most common measures in dosage. The International System of Units (Système International d'Unités; SI) was adapted from the metric system in 1960. Most developed countries except the United States have adopted SI nomenclature to provide a standard language of measurement.

Differences between metric and SI systems do not occur in dosage. The meaning and abbreviations for weight and volume are the same. Weight measures are based on the gram; volume measures are based on the liter.

Study the meaning of the abbreviations listed in the following table. Under "Explanation," you'll see one equivalent for each abbreviation, to help you understand what kinds of quantities are involved. Equivalents (metric, household, apothecary) are discussed in Chapter 3. The preferred abbreviation is listed first; variations appear in parentheses.

Metric Abbreviation	Meaning	Explanation	Do Not Use
cc	Cubic centimeter	This is a measure of volume usually reserved for measuring gases. However, you may still find it used as a liquid measure. (One cubic centimeter is approximately equal to 16 drops from a medicine dropper.)	Substitute mL.
g (gm, Gm)	Gram	This is a solid measure of weight. (One gram is approximately equal to the weight of two paper clips.)	
kg (Kg)	Kilogram	This is a weight measure. (One kilogram equals 2.2 pounds.)	
L	Liter	This is a liquid measure. (One liter is a little more than a quart.)	
mcg	Microgram	This is a measure of weight. (One thousand micrograms make up 1 milligram: 1000 mcg = 1 mg.)	μg
mEq	Milliequivalent	No equivalent necessary. Drugs are prepared and ordered in this weight measure.	
mg	Milligram	This is a measure of weight. (One thousand milligrams make up 1 gram: 1000 mg = 1 g.)	
mL (ml)	Milliliter	This is a liquid measure. The terms *cubic centimeter* (cc) and *milliliter* (mL) are interchangeable in dosage (1 cc = 1 mL).	
unit	Unit	This is a measure of biologic activity. Nurses do not calculate this measure.	U

Example penicillin potassium 300,000 units

Important: It is considered safer to write the word *unit* rather than use the abbreviation, because the *U* could be read as a zero and a medication error might result.

SELF-TEST 4 Abbreviations (Metric)

After studying metric abbreviations, write the meaning of the following terms. Indicate if the abbreviation is not to be used and the words to substitute for it. The correct answers are given at the end of the chapter.

1. 0.3 g _____

2. 150 mcg _____

3. 80 U _____

4. 0.5 mL _____

5. 1.7 cc _____

6. 0.25 mg _____

7. 14 kg _____

8. 20 mEq _____

9. 1.5 L _____

10. 50 μg _____

Apothecary Abbreviations

Apothecary measures were common in the United States as far back as colonial times. Today apothecary measures are discouraged, for several reasons: 1) Equivalency with the metric system is not exact. 2) The system requires Roman numerals and fractions. 3) Apothecary symbols can easily be misinterpreted. These apothecary terms are in minimal use:

Minim   Abbreviated m, it is about the size of one drop. The term is found on some syringes. In Figure 2-3, note two sets of marks. The upper lines indicate doses to 3 cubic centimeters. The lower lines indicate minims. On this syringe, 1 cubic centimeter = 16 minims. Substitute "mL" for "cc," although many syringes are marked "cc."

Dram   Abbreviated dr, this is a liquid measure slightly less than a household teaspoon. 1 dr = 4 mL. In Figure 2-4, note that the medication cup has measures in metric, household, and apothecary systems. If the answer to a dosage calculation was 12 mL, one can pour 3 drams.

Grain   Abbreviated "gr" and derived from the Latin word *granum.* In medieval times this solid measure was based on the weight of a grain of wheat. There is no commonly accepted equivalent to the grain in the metric system. Generally, 60 mg = 1 gr, except with acetaminophen (Tylenol) and aspirin: 65 mg = 1 gr. See Figure 2-5. In written prescriptions, the metric gram (g; gm; Gm) can be confused with the apothecary grain (gr). Therefore, it is advisable to write out "grain."

Drop   Abbreviated "gtt" and derived from the Latin word *guttae.* It indicates a liquid measure that was based on a drop of water: 1 gtt = 1 m. The term gtt is used in ordering eye medications. Example: Timoptic 0.25% Ophth Sol 1 gtt left eye bid.

i   This letter indicates "one" in Roman numerals, which are conveyed by letters of the alphabet. Roman numerals never have more than three of the same digit in a row.

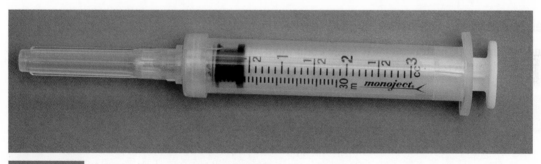

FIGURE 2-3

A 3-mL syringe calibrated in tenths of a milliliter and in minims. (Copyright © Lacey-Bordeaux Photography.)

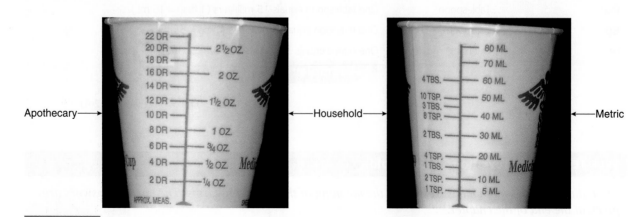

FIGURE 2-4

A medicine cup with metric, household, and apothecary equivalents. Two sides of the cup are shown. (© 2004 Lacey-Bordeaux Photography.)

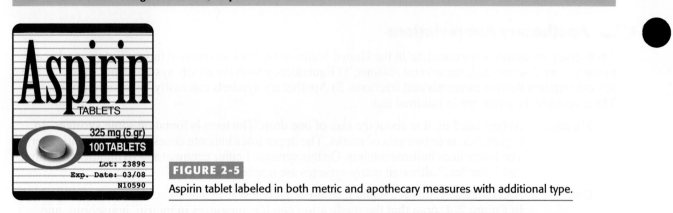

FIGURE 2-5

Aspirin tablet labeled in both metric and apothecary measures with additional type.

SELF-TEST 5   **Abbreviations (Apothecary)**

After studying apothecary abbreviations that are still used in prescriptions, write the meaning of the following terms. The correct answers are given at the end of the chapter.

1. m x _____   6. gr i _____

2. ii dr _____   7. 2 gtt _____

3. 5 gr _____   8. 10 gr _____

4. gtt iii _____   9. m v _____

5. dr i _____

Household Abbreviations

Physicians and healthcare providers may use these common household measures to order drugs, especially if the drug is to be administered at home. The "explanation" column shows metric equivalents.

Household Abbreviation	Meaning	Explanation
pt	Pint	One pint is approximately equal to 500 milliliters (1 pt ≅ 500 mL). One quart is approximately equal to 1 liter, which is equal to 1000 milliliters (1 qt ≅ 1 L = 1000 mL).
qt	Quart	One half of a quart is approximately equal to 1 pint ($\frac{1}{2}$ qt ≅ 1 pt = 500 mL).
tbsp	Tablespoon	One tablespoon equals 15 milliliters (1 tbsp = 15 mL).
tsp	Teaspoon	One teaspoon equals 5 milliliters (1 tsp = 5 mL).
oz	Ounce	One ounce equals 30 milliliters (1 oz = 30 mL).

> **Example**   6 tsp = 1 oz = 30 mL
> 3 tsp = $\frac{1}{2}$ oz = 15 mL
> 2 tbsp = 1 oz = 30 mL = 6 tsp (see Fig. 2-4)

SELF-TEST 6   **Abbreviations (Household)**

After studying household measures, write the meaning of the following terms. The correct answers are given at the end of the chapter.

1. 3 tsp _____   3. $\frac{1}{2}$ qt _____   5. 1 pt _____

2. 1 oz _____   4. 1 tsp _____   6. 2 tbsp _____

Terms and Abbreviations for Drug Preparations

The following abbreviations and terms are used to describe selected drug preparations. Some of these abbreviations are rarely used, yet are included here for reference.

Term Abbreviation	Meaning	Explanation
cap, caps	Capsule	Medication is encased in a gelatin shell.
CR	Controlled release	These abbreviations indicate that the drug has been prepared in a form that allows extended action. Therefore, the drug is given less frequently.
LA	Long acting	
SA	Sustained action	
SR	Slow release	
DS	Double strength	
EC	Enteric coated	The tablet is coated with a substance that will not dissolve in the acid secretions of the stomach; instead, it dissolves in the more alkaline secretions of the intestines.
el, elix	Elixir	A drug is dissolved in a hydroalcoholic sweetened base.
sol	Solution	The drug is contained in a clear liquid preparation.
sp	Spirit	This is an alcoholic solution of a volatile substance (eg, spirit of ammonia).
sup, supp	Suppository	This is a solid, cylindrically shaped drug that can be inserted into a body opening (eg, the rectum or vagina).
susp	Suspension	Small particles of drug are dispersed in a liquid base and must be shaken before being poured; gels and magmas are also suspensions.
syr	Syrup	A sugar is dissolved in a liquid medication and flavored to disguise the taste.
tab, tabs	Tablet	Medication is compressed or molded into a solid form; additional ingredients are used to shape and color the tablet.
tr, tinct.	Tincture	This is a liquid alcoholic or hydroalcoholic solution of a drug.
ung, oint.	Ointment	This is a semisolid drug preparation that is applied to the skin (for external use only).
KVO	Keep vein open	**Example Order** 1000 mL dextrose 5% in water IV KVO. The nurse is to continue infusing this fluid.
TKO	To keep open	
Discontinue	Discontinue	**Example Order** Discontinue ampicillin (do not use D/C)
NKA	No known allergies	This is an important assessment that is noted on the medication record of a patient.
NKDA	No known drug allergies	This is an important assessment that is noted on the medication record of a patient.

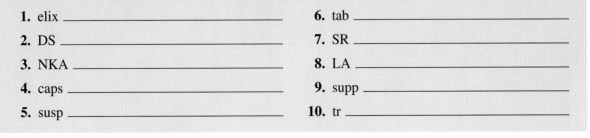

SELF-TEST 7 **Abbreviations (Drug Preparations)**

After studying the abbreviations for drug preparations, write out the meaning of the following terms. The correct answers are given at the end of the chapter.

1. elix _____

2. DS _____

3. NKA _____

4. caps _____

5. susp _____

6. tab _____

7. SR _____

8. LA _____

9. supp _____

10. tr _____

Now consider the formerly confusing orders that appeared at the beginning of this chapter.

Original: Morphine sulfate 15 mg Sub Q stat and 10 mg q4h prn

Interpretation: Morphine sulfate 15 mg subcutaneously immediately and 10 mg every 4 hours as needed.

Original: Chloromycetin 0.01% Opth Oint left eye bid

Interpretation: Chloromycetin 0.01% ophthalmic ointment left eye twice a day.

Original: Ampicillin 1 g IVPB q6h

Interpretation: Ampicillin 1 gram intravenous piggyback every 6 hours.

PROFICIENCY TEST 1   Abbreviations

Name: _____

There are 50 items and each is worth 2 points. Indicate if the abbreviation is "Do Not Use" and which words to substitute for it. See Appendix A for answers.

1. bid _____
2. hs _____
3. prn _____
4. OU _____
5. po _____
6. pr _____
7. SL _____
8. S&S _____
9. tiw _____
10. mL _____
11. q4h _____
12. cc _____
13. SC _____
14. AU _____
15. g _____
16. PC _____
17. qd _____

18. stat _____
19. q12h _____
20. tid _____
21. OS _____
22. kg _____
23. qn _____
24. qh _____
25. OD _____
26. mEq _____
27. AC _____
28. qid _____
29. mg _____
30. IM _____
31. qod _____
32. biw _____
33. NGT _____
34. q8h _____

35. L _____
36. mcg _____
37. q6h _____
38. µg _____
39. U _____
40. tsp _____
41. AD _____
42. gr _____
43. IV _____
44. susp _____
45. tbsp _____
46. IVPB _____
47. m _____
48. Gm _____
49. q2h _____
50. q3h _____

PROFICIENCY TEST 2   **Reading Prescriptions**

Name: _____

Now that you have studied the language of prescriptions, you are ready to interpret medication orders. Write the following orders in longhand. Give sample times. The correct answers are given in Appendix A.

1. Nembutal 100 mg at bedtime prn po _____

2. Propranolol hydrochloride 40 mg po bid _____

_____

3. Ampicillin 1 g IVPB q6h _____

_____

4. Demerol 50 mg IM q4h prn for pain _____

_____

5. Tylenol 325 mg tabs ii po stat _____

_____

6. Pilocarpine gtt ii OU q3h _____

_____

7. Scopolamine 0.8 mg subcutaneously stat _____

_____

8. Digoxin el 0.25 mg po qd _____

_____

9. Kaochlor 30 mEq po bid _____

_____

10. Liquaemin sodium 6000 units subcutaneously q4h _____

_____

11. Tobramycin 70 mg IM q8h _____

_____

12. Prednisone 10 mg po every other day _____

_____

13. Milk of magnesia 1 tbsp po at bedtime qn _____

_____

14. Septra DS tab i every day po _____

_____

15. Morphine sulfate 15 mg subcutaneously stat and 10 mg q4h prn _____

_____

PROFICIENCY TEST 3   Interpreting Written Prescription Orders

Name: _____

Below are actual prescriptions written by physicians and other healthcare providers. Interpret each in longhand. In a real life situation, if the order is not clear, check with the person who wrote the order. Note any "Do Not Use" abbreviations. The correct answers are given in Appendix A.

1. Colace 100 mg po HD	1.
2. Ativan 1mg IVP x 1 now	2.
3. 10 meq KCl in 100cc NS over 1h x 1	3.
4. Tylenol #3 II tabs po q4° pRN Pain	4.
5. Heparin 25,000 IU in 250ª D5W @ 500 u/Hr.	5.
6. Ticlid 250mg I PO BID.	6.
7. lopressor 25mg po BID.	7.
8. Benadryl 25mg po qhs	8.

Answers

Self-Test 1 Abbreviations

1. Three times a day (**sample times:** 10 AM, 2 PM, 6 PM)

2. Every night (**sample time:** 10 PM)

3. After meals (**sample times:** 10 AM, 2 PM, 6 PM)

4. Every other day (**sample times:** odd days of month at 10 AM). Do not use "qod" (write out "every other day").

5. Twice a day (**sample times:** 10 AM, 6 PM)

6. Do not use hs. Use "at bedtime." (**sample time:** 10 PM)

7. Immediately (**sample time:** whatever the time is now)

8. Four times a day (**sample times:** 10 AM, 2 PM, 6 PM, 10 PM)

9. Every 4 hours (**sample times:** 2 AM, 6 AM, 10 AM, 2 PM, 6 PM, 10 PM)

10. Before meals (**sample times:** 7:30 AM, 11:30 AM, 4:30 PM)

11. Do not use qd; use "every day." (**sample time:** 10 AM)

12. Every 8 hours (**sample times:** 6 AM, 2 PM, 10 PM)

13. Every hour

14. Whenever necessary (**sample times:** No time routine can be written.)

15. Every 4 hours as needed (**sample times:** No time routine is written because we do not know when the drug will be needed.)

Self-Test 2 Military Time

A. 1. 1400
2. 0900
3. 1600
4. 1200
5. 0130
6. 2115
7. 0450
8. 1820

B. 1. 1:30 AM
2. 5:45 PM
3. 11 AM
4. 8:15 PM
5. 7:10 PM
6. 6 AM
7. 12:50 AM
8. 10 AM

Self-Test 3 Abbreviations (Routes)

1. Sublingual; under the tongue

2. Do not use OU; use "both eyes"

3. Nasogastric tube

4. Intravenously

5. By mouth

6. Do not use OD; use "right eye"

7. Intravenous piggyback

8. Do not use OS; use "left eye"

9. Intramuscularly

10. Rectally

11. Swish and swallow

12. Do not use SC; use "subcutaneously."

13. Do not use au; use "both ears."

14. Do not use al; use "left ear."

Self-Test 4 Abbreviations (Metric)

1. Three tenths of a gram

2. One hundred fifty micrograms

3. Eighty units. Do not use U; use "unit."

4. Five tenths of a milliliter

5. One and seven tenths of a milliliter. Do not use cc; use "milliliter."

6. Twenty-five hundredths of a milligram

7. Fourteen kilograms

8. Twenty milliequivalents

9. One and five tenths of a liter

10. Fifty micrograms. Do not use μg; use "microgram."

Self-Test 5 Abbreviations (Apothecary)

1. 10 minims
2. 2 drams
3. 5 grains

4. 3 drops
5. 1 dram
6. 1 grain

7. 2 drops
8. 10 grains
9. 5 minims

Self-Test 6 Abbreviations (Household)

1. Three teaspoons
2. One ounce

3. One-half quart
4. One teaspoon

5. One pint
6. Two tablespoons

Self-Test 7 Abbreviations (Drug Preparations)

1. Elixir
2. Double strength
3. No known allergies
4. Capsules

5. Suspension
6. Tablet
7. Slow release
8. Long acting

9. Suppository
10. Tincture

Metric, Apothecary, and Household Systems of Measurement

Medication orders are written in metric terms. In this chapter you will learn solid and liquid measures in the metric system and their equivalents.

When you're preparing liquid doses, a knowledge of apothecary and household equivalents will help you pour exact amounts. Medicine cups are marked in metric, apothecary, and household measures; syringes are marked in metric and apothecary lines.

Metric System

Measures of Weight

These are the solid measures in the metric system and their abbreviations:

Gram: g or gm

Milligram: mg

Microgram: mcg (µg, which uses the Greek letter mu [µ], is no longer accepted by The Joint Commission for its approved abbreviation list)

Kilogram: kg

Weight Equivalents

These are the basic weight equivalents in the metric system:

1 g = 1000 mg

1 mg = 1000 mcg

As you can see, the gram is the largest of these.

To equal the weight of a single gram, you need 1000 mg.

To equal the weight of a single milligram, you need 1000 mcg.

The symbol >, which means "greater than," indicates these relationships:

g > mg > mcg

Read this notation as "A gram is greater than a milligram, which is greater than a microgram."

Converting Solid Equivalents

If the available supply is not in the same weight measure as the medication order, you will have to calculate how much of a drug to give.

| Example | Order: 0.25 g |

Supply: tablets labeled 125 mg

Since 1 g = 1000 mg, you change 0.25 g to milligrams by multiplying the number of grams by 1000.

$$\begin{array}{r} 0.25 \\ \times\, 1000 \\ \hline 250.00 \end{array}$$

To convert the order, you use 0.25 g = 250 mg.

Here's an easy rule to help you remember this type of conversion:

Large to small—multiply by 1000

Small to large—divide by 1000

Following this rule, if you are converting grams to milligrams (a larger measurement to a smaller one), multiply the original number by 1000. If you are converting from micrograms to milligrams (a smaller measurement to a larger one), divide the original number by 1000.

There's another method of conversion as well. In decimals, the thousandth place is three numbers after the decimal point. You can change grams to milligrams by moving the decimal point three places to the *right*, which produces the same answer as multiplying by 1000. You can also change milligrams to grams by moving the decimal point three places to the *left*, which is the same as dividing by 1000. You'll be using this method in some of the calculations to come.

| RULE | **CHANGING GRAMS TO MILLIGRAMS** |

To multiply by 1000, move the decimal point three places to the right. ■

| Example | *EXAMPLE 1* |

0.25 g = _____ mg

0.250 = 250

0.25 g = 250 mg

EXAMPLE 2

0.1 g = _____ mg

0.100 = 100

0.1 g = 100 mg

Grams to Milligrams Quick Method: Should you move the decimal point to the left or to the right? This Quick Method can help you decide.

1. First, write the order.

2. Write the equivalent measure you need.

3. Show which way the decimal point should move by drawing an *arrow*.

4. Make sure the open part of your arrow always faces the larger measure.

5. Remember that in the equivalent 1 g = 1000 mg, the gram is the larger measure, with 1000 mg equaling the weight of 1 gram.

Example

EXAMPLE 1

Order: 0.25 g

Supply: 125 mg

You want to convert grams to milligrams.

0.25 g > _____ mg

The arrow tells you to move the decimal point three places to the *right*.

0.250 = 250

Therefore, 0.25 g = 250 mg

EXAMPLE 2

Order: 1.5 g

Supply: 500 mg

You want to convert grams to milligrams.

1.5 g > _____ mg

1.500 = 1500

Therefore, 1.5 g = 1500 mg

SELF-TEST 1   Grams to Milligrams

Convert from grams to milligrams. For correct answers, see the end of the chapter.

1. 0.3 g = 300 mg	**7.** 0.08 g = 80 mg
2. 0.001 g = 1 mg	**8.** 0.275 g = 275 mg
3. 0.02 g = 20 mg	**9.** 0.04 g = 40 mg
4. 1.2 g = 1200 mg	**10.** 0.325 g = 325 mg
5. 5 g = 5000 mg	**11.** 2 g = 2000 mg
6. 0.4 g = 400 mg	**12.** 0.0004 g = .4 mg

RULE **CHANGING MILLIGRAMS TO GRAMS**

To divide by 1000, move the decimal point three places to the left. ■

Example *EXAMPLE 1*

100 mg = _____ g

100. = 0.1

100 mg = 0.1 g

EXAMPLE 2

8 mg = _____ g

008. = 0.008

8 mg = 0.008 g

Milligrams to Grams Quick Method: The arrow method also works to convert milligrams to grams.

1. First, write the order.

2. Write the equivalent measure you need.

3. Show which way the decimal point should move by drawing an *arrow*.

4. Make sure the open part of your arrow always faces the larger measure.

5. Remember that in the equivalent 1 g = 1000 mg, the gram is the larger measure.

Example *EXAMPLE 1*

Order: 15 mg

Supply: 0.03 g

You want to convert milligrams to grams.

15 mg < g

The arrow tells you to move the decimal point three places to the *left*.

015. = 0.015

15 mg = 0.015 g

EXAMPLE 2

Order: 500 mg

Supply: 1 g

You want to convert milligrams to grams.

500 mg = _____ g

500 mg < g

The arrow tells you to move the decimal point three places to the *left*.

500. = 0.5

500 mg = 0.5 g

SELF-TEST 2 Milligrams to Grams

Convert from milligrams to grams. For correct answers, see the end of the chapter.

1. 4 mg = _____·004_____ g
2. 120 mg = _____·120_____ g
3. 40 mg = _____·040_____ g
4. 75 mg = _____·075_____ g
5. 250 mg = _____·25_____ g
6. 1 mg = _____·001_____ g
7. 50 mg = _____·05_____ g
8. 600 mg = _____·6_____ g
9. 5 mg = _____·005_____ g
10. 360 mg = _____·36_____ g
11. 10 mg = _____·1_____ g
12. 0.1 mg = _____·0001_____ g

RULE   CHANGING MILLIGRAMS TO MICROGRAMS

The second major weight equivalent in the metric system is

1 mg = 1000 mcg.

Some medications are so powerful that smaller microgram doses are sufficient to produce a therapeutic effect. Rather than using milligrams written as decimals, it's easier to write orders in micrograms as whole numbers.

To multiply by 1000, move the decimal point three places to the right. ■

Example

EXAMPLE 1

0.1 mg = _____ mcg

0.100 = 100

0.1 mg = 100 mcg

EXAMPLE 2

0.25 mg = _____ mcg

0.250 = 250

0.25 mg = 250 mcg

Milligrams to Micrograms Quick Method: Should you move the decimal point to the left or to the right? Here are the steps:

1. First, write the order.

2. Write the equivalent measure you need.

3. Show which way the decimal point should move by drawing an *arrow*.

4. Make sure the open part of your arrow faces the larger measure.

5. Remember that in the equivalent 1 mg = 1000 mcg, the milligram is the larger measure, with 1000 mcg equaling the weight of 1 mg.

Example

EXAMPLE 1

Order: 0.1 mg

Supply: 200 mcg

You want to convert milligrams to micrograms.

0.1 mg > _____ mcg

The arrow is telling you to move the decimal point three places to the *right*.

0.100 = 100

Therefore, 0.1 mg = 100 mcg

EXAMPLE 2

Order: 0.3 mg

Supply: 600 mcg

You want to convert milligrams to micrograms.

0.3 mg > _____ mcg

0.300 = 300

Therefore, 0.3 mg = 300 mcg

SELF-TEST 3   Milligrams to Micrograms

Convert from milligrams to micrograms. For correct answers, see the end of the chapter.

1. 0.3 mg = _____ 300 _____ mcg
2. 0.001 mg = _____ 1 _____ mcg
3. 0.02 mg = _____ 20 _____ mcg
4. 0.08 mg = _____ 80 _____ mcg
5. 1.2 mg = _____ 1200 _____ mcg
6. 0.4 mg = _____ 400 _____ mcg
7. 5 mg = _____ 5,000 _____ mcg
8. 0.7 mg = _____ 700 _____ mcg
9. 0.04 mg = _____ 40 _____ mcg
10. 10 mg = _____ 10,000 _____ mcg
11. 0.9 mg = _____ 900 _____ mcg
12. 0.01 mg = _____ 10 _____ mcg

RULE   **CHANGING MICROGRAMS TO MILLIGRAMS**

To divide by 1000, move the decimal point three places to the left. ■

Example

EXAMPLE 1

300 mcg = _____ mg

300. = 0.3

300 mcg = 0.3 mg

EXAMPLE 2

50 mcg = _____ mg

050. = 0.05

50 mcg = 0.05 mg

Micrograms to Milligrams Quick Method: The arrow method also converts micrograms to milligrams.

1. First, write the order.

2. Write the equivalent measure you need.

3. Show which way the decimal point should move by drawing an *arrow*.

4. Make sure the open part of your arrow faces the larger measure.

5. Remember that in the equivalent 1 mg = 1000 mcg, the milligram is the larger measure.

Example

EXAMPLE 1

Order: 100 mcg

Supply: 0.1 mg

You want to convert micrograms to milligrams.

100 mcg < mg

The arrow tells you to move the decimal point three places to the *left*.

100. = 0.1

100 mcg = 0.1 mg

EXAMPLE 2

Order: 50 mcg

Supply: 0.1 mg

You want to convert micrograms to milligrams.

50 mcg = _____ mg

mcg < mg

The arrow tells you to move the decimal point three places to the *left*.

050. = 0.05

50 mcg = 0.05 mg

SELF-TEST 4   Micrograms to Milligrams

Convert from micrograms to milligrams. For correct answers, see the end of the chapter.

1. 800 mcg = _____ .8 _____ mg

2. 4 mcg = _____ .004 _____ mg

3. 14 mcg = _____ .014 _____ mg

4. 25 mcg = _____ .025 _____ mg

5. 1 mcg = _____ .001 _____ mg

6. 200 mcg = _____ .2 _____ mg

7. 50 mcg = _____ .05 _____ mg

8. 750 mcg = _____ .75 _____ mg

9. 325 mcg = _____ .325 _____ mg

10. 75 mcg = _____ .075 _____ mg

11. 0.1 mcg = _____ .001 _____ mg

12. 150 mcg = _____ .150 _____ mg

SELF-TEST 5   Mixed Conversions

Convert mixed metric weight measures. For correct answers, see the end of the chapter.

1. 0.3 mg = _____.003_____ g
2. 0.03 g = _____30_____ mg
3. 15 mcg = _____15,000_____ mg
4. 0.1 g = _____100_____ mg
5. 100 mcg = ___(~~100,000~~) .1___ mg

6. 50 mg = _____.05_____ g
7. 0.014 g = _____14_____ mg
8. 200 mg = _____.2_____ g
9. 0.2 mg = _____200_____ mcg
10. 0.65 mg = _____650_____ mcg

SELF-TEST 6   Common Equivalents

Fill in the blanks to convert mg to g or to mcg.

1. 1000 mg = _____1_____ g
2. 600 mg = _____.6_____ g
3. 500 mg = _____.5_____ g
4. 300 mg = _____.3_____ g
5. 200 mg = _____.2_____ g
6. 100 mg = _____.1_____ g
7. 60 mg = _____.06_____ g

8. 30 mg = _____.03_____ g
9. 15 mg = _____.015_____ g
10. 10 mg = _____.01_____ g
11. 0.6 mg = _____600_____ mcg
12. 0.4 mg = _____400_____ mcg
13. 0.3 mg = _____300_____ mcg
14. 0.25 mg = _____250_____ mcg

SELF-TEST 7   Review of Grams to Milligrams

1. What are the methods for converting grams to milligrams? _____

_____

_____

2. 1 g = _____1000_____ mg
3. 0.01 g = _____10_____ mg
4. 0.2 g = _____200_____ mg
5. 0.12 g = _____120_____ mg
6. 1 g = _____1000_____ mg
7. 0.6 g = _____600_____ mg
8. 0.5 g = _____500_____ mg

9. 0.3 g = _____300_____ mg
10. 0.2 g = _____200_____ mg
11. 0.1 g = _____100_____ mg
12. 0.06 g = _____60_____ mg
13. 0.03 g = _____30_____ mg
14. 0.015 g = _____15_____ mg
15. 0.01 g = _____10_____ mg

Apothecary System

Although the apothecary system was used in the past to write prescriptions, it has gradually been replaced by the metric system. Today, you rarely see medication orders in apothecary notation. Table 3-1 contains a brief overview of the apothecary system.

Apothecary Abbreviations

The apothecary system has specific abbreviations shown in Table 3-1. Roman numerals designate the amounts (Table 3-2).

Solid Apothecary Measure—The Grain

The only solid dosage measure in the apothecary system is the grain (abbreviated gr) followed by a Roman number (e.g., gr v). Arabic numbers also have been used (e.g., gr 5; 5 gr). Be careful not to confuse the apothecary *grain* (gr) with the metric *gram* (g, gm).

Solid Equivalents—Apothecary and Metric

Equivalents between the metric and apothecary systems are not exact (Table 3-3).
   Three equivalents require explanation:

gr x = 0.6 g = 600 mg or 650 mg

gr v = 0.3 g = 300 mg or 325 mg

gr i = 0.06 g = 60 mg or 65 mg

   Note that 15 grains = 1000 mg; 1 grain = 60 mg. If you multiply 15×60 the answer should be 1000 mg, but the answer is 900 mg. To remedy this discrepancy, some drug companies manufacture 1 grain to equal 65 mg. Both aspirin and acetaminophen are made this way (5 grains = 325 mg; 10 grains = 650 mg). If you're solving dosage problems where the order is written in one system and the stock comes in another system or conversion, use whichever equivalent is closer.

TABLE 3-1 Apothecary Abbreviations		
Apothecary Abbreviation	**Meaning**	**Explanation**
ʒ	Dram	This is a liquid measure. It is slightly less than a household teaspoon. (One dram equals 4 milliliters; ʒi = 4 mL.)
℥	Ounce	This is a liquid measure. It is slightly more than a household ounce. (One ounce equals 32 milliliters: ℥i = 32 mL.)
gr	Grain	Latin, *granum.* This solid measure was based on the weight of a grain of wheat in ancient times. There is no commonly used equivalent to the grain in the metric system.
gtt	Drop	Latin, *guttae.* This liquid measure was based on a drop of water. (One drop equals 1 minim.)
m (M, M_x)	Minim	Latin, *minim.* (One minim equals one drop: 1 m = 1 gtt.)
śś	One half	Latin, *semis*

TABLE 3-2   Roman Numerals and Arabic Numbers

Arabic	Roman
1	I or i
2	II or ii
3	III or iii
4	IV or iv
5	V or v
6	VI or vi
7	VII or vii
8	VIII or viii
9	IX or ix
10	X or x
15	XV or xv
20	XX or xx
40	XL or xl
50	L or l
60	LX or lx
100	C or c

TABLE 3-3   Metric and Apothecary Equivalents

Grain	Milligram	Gram*	Microgram
gr xv	1000 mg	1 g	
gr x	(650)† 600 mg	0.6 g	
gr vii śs	500 mg	0.5 g	
gr v	(325)† 300 mg	0.3 g	
gr iii	200 mg	0.2 g	
gr i śs or gr 1½	100 mg	0.1 g	
gr i	(65)† 60 mg	0.06 g	
gr śs or gr ½	30 mg	0.03 g	
gr ¼	15 mg	0.015 g	
gr ⅙	10 mg	0.01 g	
gr ¹⁄₁₀₀	0.6 mg		600 mcg
gr ¹⁄₁₅₀	0.4 mg		400 mcg
gr ¹⁄₂₀₀	0.3 mg		300 mcg

*g = gram.
†Alternative values.

SELF-TEST 8 Converting Grains to Milligrams

Fill in the blanks to convert gr to mg, and to convert mg or g to gr. For the correct answers in Arabic numbers, see the end of the chapter.

1. gr iss _____

2. gr v _____

3. gr ¹⁄₁₅₀ _____

4. gr 15 _____

5. gr 4 _____

6. gr ¼ _____

7. Aspirin gr x _____

8. Tylenol gr v _____

9. 3 g _____

10. 325 mg _____

11. 15 mg _____

12. 0.5 mg _____

13. 9 g _____

14. Tylenol 650 mg _____

15. Aspirin 325 mg _____

Household System

Household Measures

Household measures are occasionally used in preparing doses. These are the common ones and their abbreviations:

Teaspoon: tsp

Tablespoon: tbsp

Ounce: oz (or fl oz = fluid ounce)

Pint: pt

Quart: qt

Pound: lb

Household equivalents (approximate conversions):

1 tsp =	5 mL
1 tbsp =	15 mL
1 oz (or fl oz) =	30 mL
1 pt =	500 mL
1 quart =	1 L or 1000 mL
2.2 lb =	1 kg
1 inch =	2.5 cm (centimeters)

Metric Liquid Measures

These are the liquid measures in the metric system and their abbreviations:

Liter: L

Milliliter: mL (may be seen as ml)

Cubic centimeter: cc (The use of "cc" is discouraged however, because this abbreviation is not on The Joint Commission approved list.)

Liquid equivalents in the metric system are:

> 1 mL = 1 cc (acceptable in dosage; otherwise, the use of "cc" is discouraged
>   because this abbreviation is not on the Joint Commission's
>   approved list)
> 1 L = 1000 mL

Liquid Apothecary Measures

Although the apothecary system is rarely used, you may encounter these liquid apothecary measures and abbreviations:

Minim: M or Mx or m

Dram: ʒ or dr

Ounce: ℥ or oz

Drop: gtt

Liquid equivalents in the apothecary system and their abbreviations:

> 1 m (minim) = 1 gtt (drop)
> 1 dr (dram) = 4 mL
> 8 dr (drams) = 1 oz (fl oz)
> 1 minim = 1 drop

Conversions Among Liquid Measures

Figure 3-1 shows a medicine cup with metric, apothecary, and household equivalents. Figure 3-2 shows a 3-mL syringe. Note that 1 mL = approximately 16 minims.

> 5 mL = 1 tsp
> 15 mL = 1 tbsp = ½ fl oz = 4 drams
> 30 mL = 2 tbsp = 1 fl oz = 8 drams
> 500 mL = 1 pint
> 1000 mL (1 L) = 1 quart (2 pints)

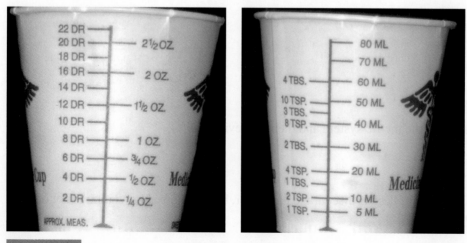

FIGURE 3-1

A medicine cup with apothecary, household, and metric equivalents.

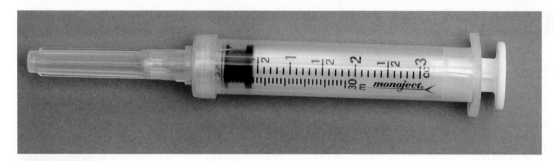

FIGURE 3-2

A 3-mL syringe with metric and apothecary measures. (© 2004 Lacey-Bordeaux Photography.)

Other Conversions

Temperature Conversions

Medication orders often use Centigrade temperature. To convert from Fahrenheit to Centigrade use this formula:

$$C = (F - 32) \times 5/9$$

To convert from Centigrade to Fahrenheit use this formula:

$$F = (C \times 9/5) + 32$$

Here is a table of approximate temperature equivalents:

Fahrenheit	Centigrade
212°	100°
105°	40.56°
104°	40°
103°	39.44°
102°	38.89°
101°	38.33°
100°	37.78°
99°	37.22°
98.6°	37°
97°	36.11°
96°	35.56°
32°	0°

Milliunit and Milliequivalent

A unit is a standard of measurement, and a milliunit is one-thousandth of a unit.

A drug used in obstetrics, Pitocin (oxytocin), is administered in milliunits per minute (see Chapter 9).

A milliequivalent is used to measure the amount of solute per liter. It is used when measuring different substances found in biological fluids, such as the amount of potassium in blood (normal value: 3.5 to 5.0 milliequivalents per liter). Some medications are administered in milliequivalents. Milliequivalents is abbreviated mEq or meq.

SELF-TEST 9   Liquid Equivalents and Mixed Conversions

Practice exercises in liquid equivalents and mixed conversions. For correct answers, see the end of the chapter. Some equivalencies may be approximate.

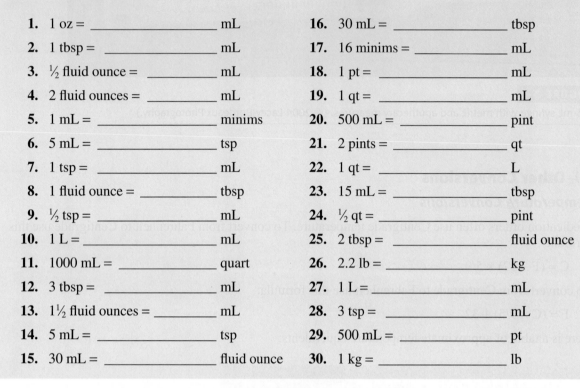

1. 1 oz = _____ mL
2. 1 tbsp = _____ mL
3. ½ fluid ounce = _____ mL
4. 2 fluid ounces = _____ mL
5. 1 mL = _____ minims
6. 5 mL = _____ tsp
7. 1 tsp = _____ mL
8. 1 fluid ounce = _____ tbsp
9. ½ tsp = _____ mL
10. 1 L = _____ mL
11. 1000 mL = _____ quart
12. 3 tbsp = _____ mL
13. 1½ fluid ounces = _____ mL
14. 5 mL = _____ tsp
15. 30 mL = _____ fluid ounce

16. 30 mL = _____ tbsp
17. 16 minims = _____ mL
18. 1 pt = _____ mL
19. 1 qt = _____ mL
20. 500 mL = _____ pint
21. 2 pints = _____ qt
22. 1 qt = _____ L
23. 15 mL = _____ tbsp
24. ½ qt = _____ pint
25. 2 tbsp = _____ fluid ounce
26. 2.2 lb = _____ kg
27. 1 L = _____ mL
28. 3 tsp = _____ mL
29. 500 mL = _____ pt
30. 1 kg = _____ lb

SELF-TEST 10   Temperature Conversions

Convert from Fahrenheit to Centigrade; Centigrade to Fahrenheit. Fot correct answers, see the end of the chapter.

1. 212° F = _____ C
2. 103° F = _____ C
3. 96° F = _____ C
4. 98.6° F = _____ C

5. 38.33° C = _____ F
6. 37.78° C = _____ F
7. 35.56° C = _____ F
8. 40.56° C = _____ F

Answers

Self-Test 1 Grams to Milligrams

1. 300	**4.** 1200	**7.** 80	**10.** 325
2. 1	**5.** 5000	**8.** 275	**11.** 2000
3. 20	**6.** 400	**9.** 40	**12.** 0.4

Self-Test 2 Milligrams to Grams

1. 0.004	**4.** 0.075	**7.** 0.05	**10.** 0.36
2. 0.12	**5.** 0.25	**8.** 0.6	**11.** 0.01
3. 0.04	**6.** 0.001	**9.** 0.005	**12.** 0.0001

Self-Test 3 Milligrams to Micrograms

1. 300	**4.** 80	**7.** 5000	**10.** 10000
2. 1	**5.** 1200	**8.** 700	**11.** 900
3. 20	**6.** 400	**9.** 40	**12.** 10

Self-Test 4 Micrograms to Milligrams

1. 0.8	**4.** 0.025	**7.** 0.05	**10.** 0.075
2. 0.004	**5.** 0.001	**8.** 0.75	**11.** 0.0001
3. 0.014	**6.** 0.2	**9.** 0.325	**12.** 0.15

Self-Test 5 Mixed Conversions

1. 0.0003	**4.** 100	**7.** 14	**9.** 200
2. 30	**5.** 0.1	**8.** 0.2	**10.** 650
3. 0.015	**6.** 0.05		

Self-Test 6 Common Equivalents

1. 1	**5.** 0.2	**9.** 0.015	**12.** 400
2. 0.6	**6.** 0.1	**10.** 0.01	**13.** 300
3. 0.5	**7.** 0.06	**11.** 600	**14.** 250
4. 0.3	**8.** 0.03		

Self-Test 7 Review of Grams to Milligrams

1. Multiply grams by 1000, move decimal point three places to the right, or use an arrow with the open part toward gram to show movement of decimal point three places.	**7.** 600
	8. 500
	9. 300
	10. 200
2. 1000	**11.** 100
3. 10	**12.** 60
4. 200	**13.** 30
5. 120	**14.** 15
6. 1000	**15.** 10

Self-Test 8 Converting Grains to mg

1. 100 mg	**5.** 240 mg	**9.** gr 45 or gr 50	**13.** gr 135
2. 300 mg	**6.** 15 mg	**10.** gr 5	**14.** gr 10
3. 0.4 mg	**7.** 650 mg	**11.** gr ¼	**15.** gr 5
4. 900 or 1000 mg	**8.** 325 mg	**12.** gr $\frac{1}{120}$	

Self-Test 9 Liquid Equivalents and Mixed Conversions

1. 30	**9.** 2.5	**17.** 1	**25.** 1
2. 15	**10.** 1000	**18.** 500	**26.** 1
3. 15	**11.** 1	**19.** 1000	**27.** 1000
4. 60	**12.** 45	**20.** 1	**28.** 15
5. 16	**13.** 45	**21.** 1	**29.** 1
6. 1	**14.** 1	**22.** 1	**30.** 2.2
7. 5	**15.** 1	**23.** 1	
8. 2	**16.** 2	**24.** 1	

Self-Test 10 Temperature Conversions

1. 100° C	**3.** 35.56° C	**5.** 100.99° F or 101° F	**7.** 96° F
2. 39.44° C	**4.** 37° C	**6.** 100° F	**8.** 105° F

Drug Labels and Packaging

Drug Labels

An understanding of drug labels and the ways in which drugs are packaged provides a background for dosage and administration.

Labels contain specific facts and appear on drugs intended to be administered as packaged: either in solid form or in liquid form. Occasionally the label does *not* include some details—such as route of administration, usual dose, and storage—because the container is too small. When you need more information than the label provides, consult a professional reference. Figure 4-1 shows a sample drug label.

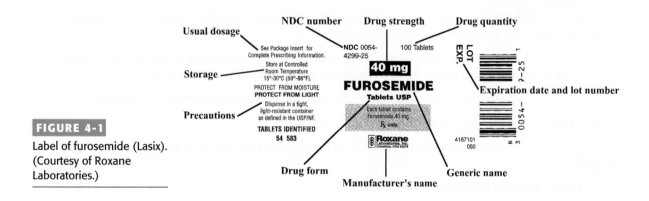

FIGURE 4-1

Label of furosemide (Lasix). (Courtesy of Roxane Laboratories.)

NDC NUMBER. The National Drug Code (NDC) is a number used by the pharmacist to identify the drug and the method of packaging.

- In Figure 4-1, the NDC is 0054-4299-25. The letters NSN (not shown) mean national supply number, a code for ordering the drug.

TOTAL AMOUNT OF DRUG IN THE CONTAINER. This information always appears on the label at either the top left, the top right, or at the bottom.

- Figure 4-1 indicates 100 tablets.

TRADE NAME. A drug's trade name (also called brand name or proprietary name) is usually followed by the federal registration symbol ® that follows the name. Several companies may manufacture the same drug, using different trade names. When a trade name appears on the label, it may be written either in all capital letters or with only the first letter capitalized.

• In Figure 4-1, Lasix is the trade name or brand name. It does not appear on this label.

GENERIC NAME. The generic name is the official accepted name of a drug, as listed in the United States Pharmacopeia (USP). A drug may have several trade names but only one official generic name. The generic name is not capitalized.

• The generic name given in Figure 4-1 is furosemide.

STRENGTH OF THE DRUG. For solid drugs, the label shows metric weights; for liquid drugs, the label states a solution of the drug in a solvent.

• In Figure 4-1, the strength is 40 mg.

FORM OF THE DRUG. The label specifies the type of preparation in the container.

• Figure 4-1 indicates that the drug is dispensed in tablets.

USUAL DOSAGE. The dosage information states how much drug is administered at a single time or during a 24-hour period. It also identifies who should receive the drug.

• Figure 4-1 tells the nurse where to find these details: "See Package Insert for Prescribing Information."

ROUTE OF ADMINISTRATION. The label specifies how the drug is to be given: orally, parenterally (through an injection of some type), or topically (applied to skin or mucous membranes). *If the label does not specify the route, the drug is in an oral form.*

• In Figure 4-1, the route is oral.

STORAGE. Certain conditions are necessary to protect the drug from losing its potency (effectiveness), so this information is crucial. Some drugs come in a dry form and must be dissolved, i.e., reconstituted. The drug may need one kind of storage when it's dry, and another kind after reconstitution.

• Figure 4-1 specifies storing the drug at controlled room temperature of 15 to 30°C (59–86°F).

PRECAUTIONS. The label may include specific instructions—related to safety, effectiveness, and/or administration—that the nurse must note and follow.

• Figure 4-1 shows these precautions: "Federal law prohibits dispensing without prescription. Protect from moisture. Protect from light. Dispense in a tight, light-resistant container."

MANUFACTURER'S NAME. If you have any question about the drug, direct them to this company.

• In Figure 4-1, the company is Roxane Laboratories, Inc.

EXPIRATION DATE. A drug expires on the last day of the indicated month. After that date, the drug cannot be used.

• Figure 4-1 does not show the expiration date.

LOT NUMBER. This number indicates the batch of drug from which this stock came.

• Figure 4-1 does not show the lot number.

ADDITIVES. The manufacturer may have added substances to the drug, for various reasons: to bind the drug, to make the drug dissolve more easily, to produce a specific pH, and so on. Information about such additives may appear on the label or in the literature accompanying the drug.

• Additives are not shown in Figure 4-1.

RECONSTITUTION.
• Some drugs that are typically dispensed in a dry (powder) form need to be reconstituted (dissolved).
• The drug label or drug insert provides specific directions about dissolving the powder.
• The manufacturer states the amount and type of liquid to use for dissolving the drug, as well as the resulting solution.

Example	Amoxicillin (Polymox) comes in powder form. Prepare suspension at time of dispensing. Add 88 mL water to the bottle. For ease in preparation, add the water in two portions. Shake well after each addition. This provides 150 mL suspension. Dosage is 125 mg amoxicillin per 5 mL solution.

SELF-TEST 1   Drug Labels

Read the label in Figure 4-2 and fill in the blanks. Answers are given at the end of the chapter.

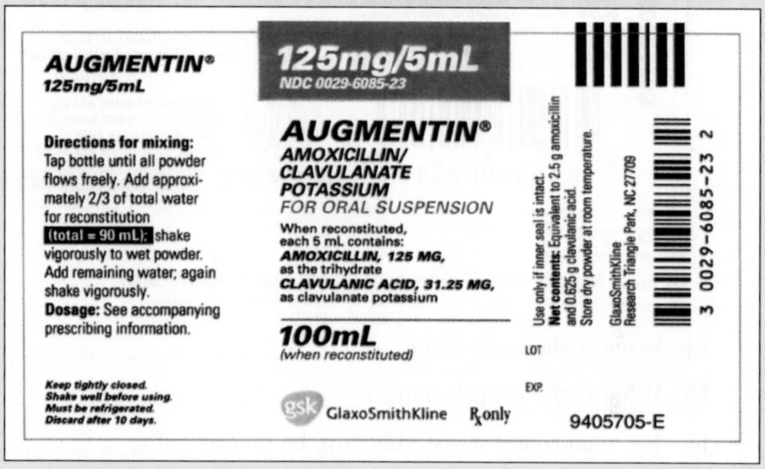

AUGMENTIN®
125mg/5mL

125mg/5mL
NDC 0029-6085-23

Directions for mixing:
Tap bottle until all powder flows freely. Add approximately 2/3 of total water for reconstitution (total = 90 mL); shake vigorously to wet powder. Add remaining water; again shake vigorously.
Dosage: See accompanying prescribing information.

AUGMENTIN®
AMOXICILLIN/
CLAVULANATE
POTASSIUM
FOR ORAL SUSPENSION
When reconstituted, each 5 mL contains:
AMOXICILLIN, 125 MG,
as the trihydrate
CLAVULANIC ACID, 31.25 MG,
as clavulanate potassium

100mL
(when reconstituted)

Use only if inner seal is intact.
Net contents: Equivalent to 2.5 g amoxicillin and 0.625 g clavulanic acid.
Store dry powder at room temperature.

GlaxoSmithKline
Research Triangle Park, NC 27709

3 0029-6085-23 2

LOT

EXP.

Keep tightly closed.
Shake well before using.
Must be refrigerated.
Discard after 10 days.

gsk GlaxoSmithKline   R℞only   9405705-E

FIGURE 4-2

Label of Augmentin for oral suspension. (Reproduced with permission of Glaxo-SmithKline.)

1. NDC number _____

2. Total amount of drug in the container _____

3. Trade name _____

4. Generic name _____

5. Strength of the drug _____

6. Form of the drug _____

7. Usual dosage _____

8. Route of administration _____

9. Storage _____

   _____

10. Directions for preparation _____

    _____

11. Precautions _____

    _____

12. Manufacturer _____

13. Expiration date _____

(continued)

SELF-TEST 1   Drug Labels (Continued)

Read the label in Figure 4-3 and fill in the blanks. Answers are given at the end of the chapter.

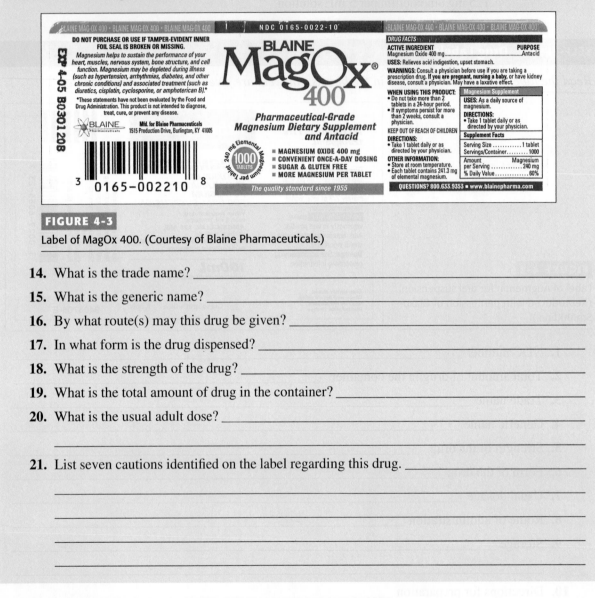

FIGURE 4-3

Label of MagOx 400. (Courtesy of Blaine Pharmaceuticals.)

14. What is the trade name? _____

15. What is the generic name? _____

16. By what route(s) may this drug be given? _____

17. In what form is the drug dispensed? _____

18. What is the strength of the drug? _____

19. What is the total amount of drug in the container? _____

20. What is the usual adult dose? _____

_____

21. List seven cautions identified on the label regarding this drug. _____

_____

_____

_____

_____

When a medication container holds a single drug, the written prescription indicates the dose in milligrams or grams, and calculation may be necessary.

Example

 a. Tylenol 0.6 g po q 4 h prn for temperature ↑ 101°

   Label: Tylenol 325 mg tablets

 b. Prednisone 20 mg po bid

   Label: Prednisone 10 mg tablets

 c. Digoxin 0.5 mg po daily

   Label: Digoxin 0.25 mg

 d. Cefozil 0.5 g po q 8°

   Label: 125 mg/5 mL

Some medication labels indicate more than one drug in the dose form. These combination drugs are ordered according to the number of tablets to give or the amount of liquid to pour.

Example

a. Order: Tylenol #3 tabs ii po q 4 h prn for pain

Label: acetaminophen 300 mg/codeine 30 mg tablet

b. Order: Robitussin DM 1 tsp po qid

Label: guaifenesin 100 mg/dextromethorphan 10 mg per 5 mL

c. Order: Talwin Compound 1 tab po q 6 h

Label: aspirin 325 mg/pentazocine 12.5 mg

d. Order: Phenergan VC Syrup 2 tsp po q 6 h while awake

Label: phenylephrine 5 mg/promethazine 6.25 mg per 5 mL

Drug Packaging

Drugs come in two types of packaging: *unit-dose* and *multidose.* Each type may contain a solid or liquid form of the drug for oral, parenteral, or topical use. Most institutions use a combination of unit-dose and multidose.

Unit-Dose Packaging

In an institutional setting, each dose is individually wrapped and labeled, and a 24-hour supply is prepared by the pharmacy and dispensed. A major value of unit-dose packaging is that two professionals—the pharmacist and the nurse—check the drug and the dose, thereby decreasing the possibility of error.

The medication may be stored in a medication cart, in a locked cabinet at the patient's bedside, or in a locked medication dispensing system, such as the Pyxis.

Unit-dose packaging does not relieve the nurse from responsibility to check the label three times and to calculate the amount of drug needed. Be aware that unit-dose drugs come in different strengths; and when trade names are ordered instead of generic names, there is always a chance of error. A dose may consist of one unit packet, two or more unit packets, or a fraction of one packet. Skilled-care nursing facilities often use a system that dispenses the unit-dose medication for one month (see Fig. 4-4).

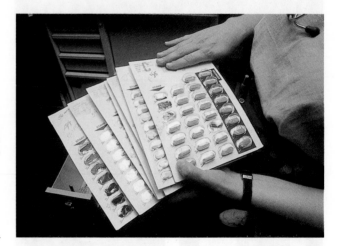

FIGURE 4-4

In long-term care settings, where medication prescriptions remain the same over weeks or months, "bingo" cards are a cost-effective method of dispensing medications. Each bubble contains one dose for the client. (Used with permission from Craven/Hirnle [2007] Fundamentals of Nursing. Philadelphia: Lippincott, Williams & Wilkins, p. 551.)

Example A nurse has a unit-dose 100-mg tablet. If an order calls for 50 mg, only half the tablet should be administered.

If a nurse has an order for 75 mg, and each unit packets contain 25-mg tablets, the nurse administers three tablets.

FOR THE ORAL ROUTE. For oral administration, unit-dose packaging comes in a number of forms:

1. Plastic bubble, foil, or paper wrappers containing tablets or capsules (Fig. 4-5A)

2. Plastic or glass containers that hold a single dose of a liquid or powder. The powder is reconstituted to a liquid form by following the directions given on the label (Fig. 4-5B).

3. A sealed medication cup containing a liquid. Once the nurse removes the cover the medication is ready to administer; the amount administered depends on the correct calculation of the dose (Fig. 4-5C).

FOR THE PARENTERAL ROUTE. These drugs—which may come in a solid or liquid form—are given by injection, via the route specified in the order (e.g., IM, Subcutaneous IVPB). Drugs packaged in the containers described below are sterile, and sterile technique is essential in their preparation and administration.

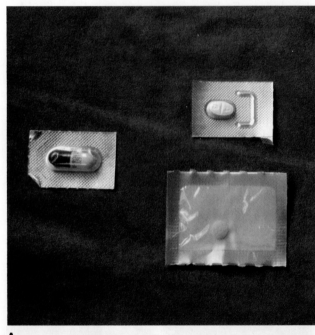

A

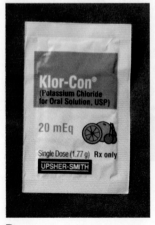

B

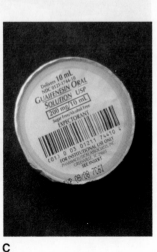

C

FIGURE 4-5

(**A**) Unit-dose tablets and capsules in foil wrappers. (**B**) Unit-dose powder in a sealed packet; it is placed in a container and diluted before giving. (**C**) Sealed cup containing a liquid medication. (Copyright © 2008 Lacey-Bordeaux Photography)

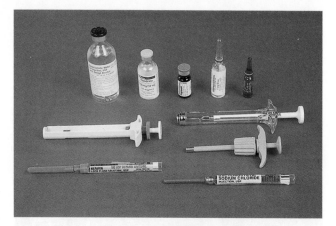

Parenteral route: (*top row*) vials and ampules; (*middle-bottom row*) prefilled cartridges and holders.

1. An *ampule* (ampoule) is a glass container that holds a single sterile dose of drug—either a liquid, a powder, or a crystal (Fig. 4-6). The container has a narrow neck that must be broken to reach the drug. Then the nurse uses a sterile syringe to withdraw the medication. Directions tell how to reconstitute the solid forms. Once the glass is broken, the drug cannot be kept sterile, so the nurse must be sure to discard any portion of the drug not immediately used.

2. A *vial* is a glass or plastic container with a sealed rubber top (Fig. 4-6). Medication in the container can be kept sterile. The container may have a sterile liquid or a sterile powder that the nurse must reconstitute with a sterile diluent and syringe. Since *single-dose vials* do not contain a preservative or a bacteriostatic agent, the nurse must discard any medication remaining after the dose is prepared.

3. Flexible *plastic bags* or *glass vials* may hold sterile medication for intravenous use (Fig. 4-7). The nurse administers the fluid via IV tubing connected to a needle or catheter placed in the patient's blood vessel.

4. *Prefilled syringes* contain sterile liquid medication that is ready to administer without further preparation. Although this type of unit-dose packaging is expensive, it can save lives in an emergency when speed is essential.

5. *Prefilled cartridges* are actually small vials with a needle attached. They fit into a metal or plastic holder and eject one unit-dose of a sterile drug in liquid form (Fig. 4-8).

FOR TOPICAL ADMINISTRATION. Drugs applied to the skin or mucous membranes can achieve a local effect. They can also achieve a systemic effect because they can be absorbed into the circulation.

1. *Transdermal patches* or *pads* are adhesive bandages placed on the skin (Fig. 4-9). They hold a drug form that is slowly absorbed into the circulation over a period ranging from hours to several days.

2. *Lozenges and pastilles* are disklike solids that slowly dissolve in the mouth (e.g., cough drops). Some drugs are prepared in a gum and are released by chewing (e.g., nicotine).

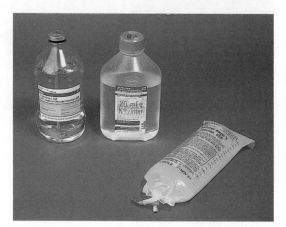

Plastic or glass containers hold medication for IV use.

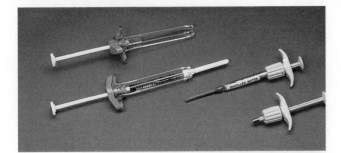

A

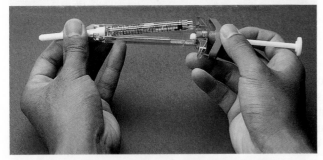

B

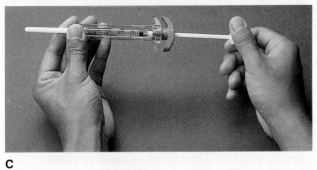

C

FIGURE 4-8

(**A**) Prefilled cartridges. (**B**) Inserting cartridge into injector device. (**C**) Cartridge is screwed into device, ready to administer drug.

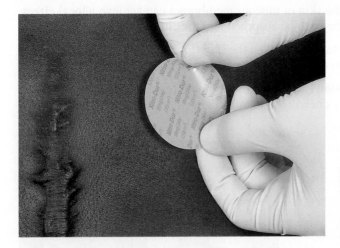

FIGURE 4-9

Transdermal patches or pads are placed on the skin. Drugs prepared in this manner include estrogen, fentanyl, testosterone, and nitroglycerin.

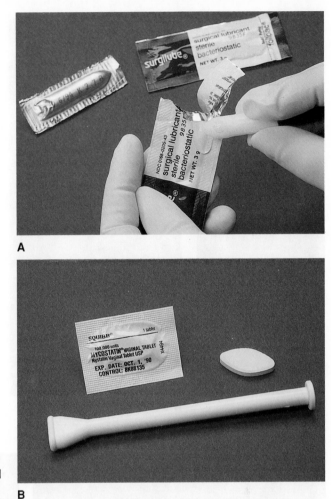

FIGURE 4-10

(**A**) Rectal suppository. (**B**) Vaginal suppository and applicator.

3. *Suppositories* in foil or plastic wrappers are molded forms that can be inserted into the rectum or vagina (Fig. 4-10). They hold medication in a substance (such as cocoa butter), that melts at body temperature and releases the drug. Suppositories may be used for unconscious patients or those unable to swallow.

4. *Plastic, disposable, squeezable containers* hold either prepared solutions for the vagina (douches) or enema solutions that are administered rectally (Fig. 4-11). To ease insertion, the containers for enemas have a lubricated nozzle. Squeezing the container forces the solution out.

Multidose Packaging

Within an institutional setting, such as a hospital, the nursing floor or unit may receive large stock containers of medications from which doses are poured. Although this type of packaging reduces the pharmacy's workload, it adds to preparation time and increases the possibility of error.

FOR THE ORAL ROUTE. Stock bottles contain a liquid or a solid form such as tablets, capsules, or powders. Large stock bottles hold medication that is dispensed over a period of days. When reconstituting the powders, the nurse must write the date and time of preparation on the container's label and must carefully note storage directions and expiration date. Caution: Powders, once dissolved, begin losing potency (Fig. 4-12A).

FOR THE PARENTERAL ROUTE. Multidose vials contain either a sterile liquid or a powder to be reconstituted using sterile technique. The nurse must write the date and time of preparation on the label and must note the expiration date and storage (Fig. 4-12B).

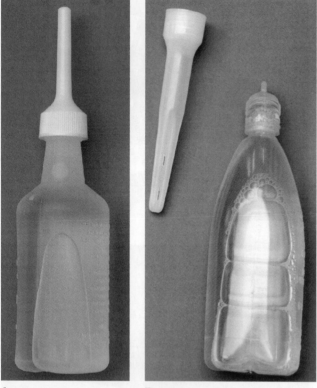

A   B

FIGURE 4-11

Unit-dose containers for rectal enema (**A**) and vaginal irrigation (**B**). (© 2004 Lacey-Bordeaux Photography.)

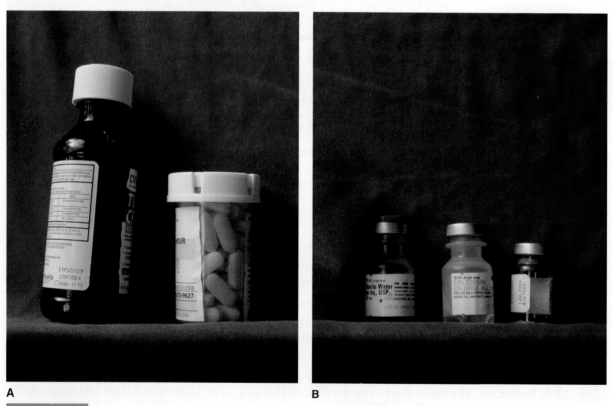

A   B

FIGURE 4-12

Multidose containers: (**A**) for the oral route; (**B**) for the parenteral route. (Copyright © 2008 Lacey-Bordeaux Photography)

FOR TOPICAL ADMINISTRATION. Since these containers are used over an extended period of time, it's important to avoid contaminating them. The nurse should label the container with the patient's name and reserve the container's use for only that patient. Here are some guidelines on using containers for topical medication:

1. Metal or plastic tubes often contain ointments or creams for application to the skin or mucous membranes. Squeezing the tubes releases the medication (Fig. 4-13A).

2. To avoid contamination of medicated creams, ointments, and pastes in jars, always use a sterile tongue blade or sterile glove to remove the medication.

3. When using dropper bottles for eye, ear, or nose medications, prevent cross-contamination by labeling each container with the patient's name and using the container only for that patient. The nurse must be careful to avoid touching mucous membranes with the dropper, because contamination of the dropper can cause pathogens to grow. Droppers come in two forms: monodrop containers, which are squeezed to release the medication, and containers with removable droppers. Separate, packaged droppers are also available to administer medications; these are sometimes calibrated (that is, marked in milliliters; Fig. 4-13B, C).

   Eye medications are labeled "ophthalmic" or "for the eye." Ear drugs are labeled "otic" or "auric" or "for the ear." Drugs for nasal administration are labeled "nose drops." Do not interchange these routes.

4. Lozenges and pastilles may be packaged in multidose as well as unit-dose containers.

5. Metered-dose inhalers (MDIs; Fig. 4-14) are aerosol devices with two parts: a canister under pressure and a mouthpiece. The canister contains multiple drug doses in either a liquid form or a microfine powder or crystal. The mouthpiece fits on the canister, and finger pressure on the mouthpiece opens a valve on the canister that discharges one dose. The physician's or healthcare provider's order states the number of inhalations or "puffs" to be taken. Medications for inhalation also may be packaged as liquids in vials or bottles, or as capsules containing powder for use with either a hand-held nebulizer (HHN) or an intermittent positive-pressure breathing apparatus (IPPB). Dry powder inhalers (DPI), such as Advair, contain a set number of doses and are administered in a similar way as metered-dose inhalers (Fig. 4-15).

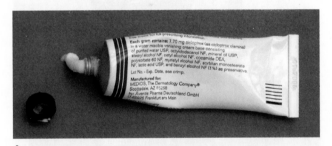

A

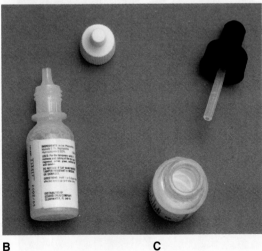

FIGURE 4-13

Topical multidose containers. (**A**) Tubes for creams or ointments. (**B**) Monodrop containers—the dropper is attached. (**C**) Removable dropper is sometimes calibrated for liquid measures. (© 2004 Lacey-Bordeaux Photography.)

B   C

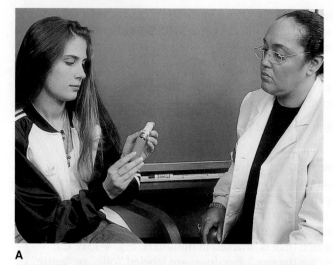

A

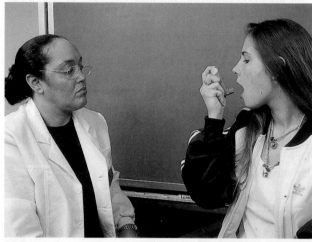

B

FIGURE 4-14

(**A**) Preparing the inhaler for use. (**B**) Administering medication.

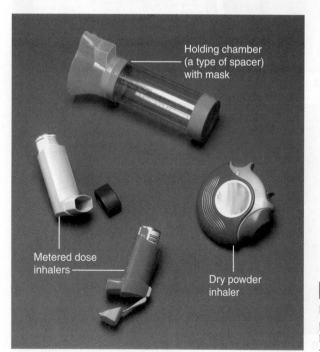

Holding chamber (a type of spacer) with mask

Metered dose inhalers

Dry powder inhaler

FIGURE 4-15

Examples of metered dose inhalers and spacers. (Used with permission from Taylor, C. [2008] Fundamentals of Nursing. Philadelphia: Lippincott Williams & Wilkins, p. 810.)

SELF-TEST 2 Drug Packaging

Match Column A with the letters in Column B to identify the meaning of terms used in drug packaging. Answers are given at the end of the chapter.

Column A

1. _____ unit-dose
2. _____ Ampule
3. _____ Parenteral
4. _____ Prefilled cartridge
5. _____ Reconstitution
6. _____ Topical
7. _____ Transdermal patch
8. _____ Vial
9. _____ Lozenge
10. _____ Cocoa butter

Column B

a. Dissolving a powder into solution

b. Glass or plastic container with a sealed rubber top

c. Route of administration to skin or mucous membranes

d. Individually wrapped and labeled drugs

e. Disklike solid that dissolves in the mouth

f. Suppository ingredient that melts at body temperature

g. General term for an injection route

h. Adhesive bandage applied to the skin that gradually releases a drug

i. Small vial, with a needle attached, that fits into a syringe holder

j. Glass container that must be broken to obtain the drug

Complete these statements related to drug packaging. Answers are given at the end of the chapter.

11. Date and time of reconstitution must be written _____

_____

_____

12. The best way to avoid cross-contamination of a multidose tube of ointment is to _____

_____

13. To remove medication from a jar of paste, the nurse should use _____

_____

14. Dropper bottles for eye medications will be labeled _____

_____

15. Doses of medication that require use of a metered-dose inhaler are ordered in _____

_____

16. Medications for the ear will be labeled _____

_____

17. The term *multidose* refers to _____

_____

(continued)

SELF-TEST 2   Drug Packaging (Continued)

18. The type of drug packaging that decreases the possibility of error is termed _____

_____

19. Drugs administered topically for a local effect may be absorbed and produce another effect that is called _____

_____

_____

20. The word *lozenge* describes _____

_____

_____

PROFICIENCY TEST 1 Labels and Packaging

Name: _____

Complete these questions. See Appendix A for answers.

1. Explain the difference between each of these pairs.
   a. 1. Unit-dose _____
      2. Multidose _____
   b. 1. Ampule_____
      2. Vial_____
   c. 1. Topical _____
      2. Parenteral _____
   d. 1. Trade name_____
      2. Generic name _____
   e. 1. Prefilled _____
      2. Reconstituted _____

2. Choose the correct answer.
   _____ a. A major advantage of the unit-dose system of drug administration is that
      1. the drug supply is always available
      2. no error is possible
      3. drugs are less expensive than stock bottles
      4. the pharmacist provides a second professional check
   _____ b. A major disadvantage of ampules over vials is that ampules
      1. are only glass
      2. when opened cannot be kept sterile
      3. contain only liquids
      4. cannot be used for injections
   _____ c. Which information is not found on the label for a drug to be given IVPB?
      1. Expiration date
      2. Indications (uses)
      3. Generic name
      4. Average dose
   _____ d. An order reads Valium 5 mg po now. A nurse correctly chooses diazepam. What name does diazepam represent?
      1. Generic
      2. Chemical
      3. Trade
      4. Proprietary
   _____ e. Which drug form is safest to administer to an unconscious patient?
      1. Suppository
      2. Syrup
      3. Capsule
      4. Aerosol

(continued)

PROFICIENCY TEST 1 **Labels and Packaging (Continued)**

3. Match the following:

1. _____ Avoid cross-contamination	**a.**	Topical application
2. _____ Removing medication from a jar	**b.**	Auric
3. _____ Eye medication	**c.**	Slow absorption over time
4. _____ Puffs ordered	**d.**	Reconstitution
5. _____ Date and time label	**e.**	Use a tongue blade
6. _____ Lozenge	**f.**	Cough drop
7. _____ Parenteral	**g.**	Individual nose droppers
8. _____ Local effect	**h.**	Ophthalmic
9. _____ Transdermal	**i.**	Inhalation
10. _____ Ear medication	**j.**	IM, Subcutaneous, IV

PROFICIENCY TEST 2   Interpreting a Label

*Name:*_____

Read the label and answer the questions. See Appendix A for answers.

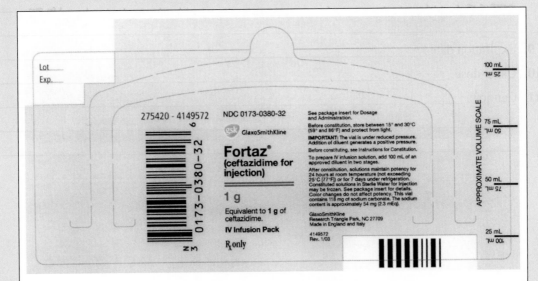

Table 5: Preparation of Fortaz Solutions			
Size	Amount of Diluent to Be Added (mL)	Approximate Available Volume (mL)	Approximate Ceftazidime Concentration (mg/mL)
Intramuscular			
500-mg vial	1.5	1.8	280
1-gram vial	3.0	3.6	280
Intravenous			
500-mg vial	5.0	5.3	100
1-gram vial	10.0	10.6	100
2-gram vial	10.0	11.5	170
Infusion pack			
1-gram vial	100*	100	10
2-gram vial	100*	100	20
Pharmacy bulk package			
6-gram vial	26	30	200

* Note: Addition should be in two stages (see Instructions for Constitution).

COMPATIBILITY AND STABILITY:
Intramuscular: Fortaz®, when constituted as directed with sterile water for injection, bacteriostatic water for injection, or 0.5% or 1% lidocaine hydrochloride injection, maintains satisfactory potency for 24 hours at room temperature or for 7 days under refrigeration. Solutions in sterile water for injection that are frozen immediately after constitution in the original container are stable for 3 months when stored at -20°C. Once thawed, solutions should not be refrozen. Thawed solutions may be stored for up to 8 hours at room temperature or for 4 days in a refrigerator.

Reproduced with permission of GlaxoSmithKline.

1. Trade name _____

2. Generic name _____

3. Route of administration _____

4. Total volume when reconstituted _____

5. Strength of reconstituted solution _____

6. Directions to reconstitute _____

_____

_____

_____

(continued)

PROFICIENCY TEST 2 **Interpreting a Label (Continued)**

7. Drug form as dispensed _____

8. Storage _____

_____

_____

9. Expiration date _____

10. Usual dose _____

11. Cautions _____

_____

_____

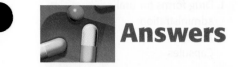 **Answers**

Self-Test 1 Drug Labels

1. 0029-6085-23
2. 100 mL when reconstituted
3. Augmentin
4. Amoxicillin/clavulanate potassium
5. 125 mg/5 mL
6. Dry powder
7. See accompanying literature
8. Oral
9. Store dry powder at room temperature. Must be refrigerated after reconstitution.
10. Tap bottle until all powder flows freely. Add approximately two thirds of total water for reconstitution (total = 90 mL); shake vigorously to wet powder. Add remaining water; again, shake vigorously.
11. See accompanying prescribing information. Keep tightly closed. Shake well before using. Must be refrigerated. Discard after 10 days. Use only if inner seal is intact.

12. GlaxoSmithKline
13. Not noted on this label; however, would be in the space marked "exp."
14. MagOx 400
15. Magnesium oxide
16. Oral
17. Tablet
18. 400 mg
19. 1000 tablets
20. Take one tablet daily or as directed by your physician.
21. Do not take more than two tablets in a 24-hour period. If symptoms persist for more than 2 weeks, consult a physician. Keep out of reach of children. Store at room temperature. Consult a physician if you're taking a prescription drug. If you are pregnant, nursing a baby, or have kidney disease, consult a physician. May have a laxative effect. Do not purchase or use if tamper-evident inner foil seal is broken or missing.

Self-Test 2 Drug Packaging

1. d
2. j
3. g
4. i
5. a
6. c
7. h
8. b
9. e
10. f
11. On the label of any powder that nurse dissolves. Powders begin to lose their potency as soon as they are placed in solution. By writing the date and time on the label, the nurse will be able to check for expiration time.

12. Label the tube with one patient's name and restrict its use to that one patient.
13. A sterile tongue blade or sterile gloves to prevent contamination of the jar contents.
14. "Ophthalmic" or "for the eye"
15. Number of inhalations or puffs
16. "Otic" or "auric"
17. Large stock containers that hold many doses of a drug
18. Unit-dose
19. A systemic effect; the drug reaches the circulation and is carried to other parts of the body.
20. A disklike solid that is slowly dissolved in the mouth (e.g., a cough drop)

CHAPTER

5

Drug Preparations and Equipment to Measure Doses

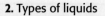

LEARNING OBJECTIVES

1. Drug forms for oral administration:
   Tablets
   Capsules
2. Types of liquids
3. Medicine cups
4. Parenteral preparations and syringes
5. Preparations for topical application
6. Rounding off dosage answers

Drugs are manufactured in different forms for oral, parenteral, and topical administration. This chapter focuses on the more common drug preparations used in the clinical area and on the equipment that nurses use to prepare accurate doses. (For more information on medication administration, see chapter 13.)

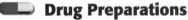 **Drug Preparations**

Oral Route

Oral drug forms are generally the easiest for the patient to take and the most convenient for the nurse to administer.

Tablets

- Tablets are made from powdered drugs that have been compressed or molded into solid shapes.

- Tablets may contain ingredients that bind the powder or aid in its gastrointestinal absorption (Fig. 5-1A).

- For a patient who has difficulty swallowing, you can crush plain tablets for oral administration. Several types of pill or tablet crushers are available.

Scored Tablets

- Scored tablets contain a line across the center, so you can easily break them into two halves.

- Do not break *unscored* tablets, because you can't be certain that the drug is evenly distributed (Fig. 5-1A).

- When in doubt about whether it's okay to break a tablet, check with the pharmacist.

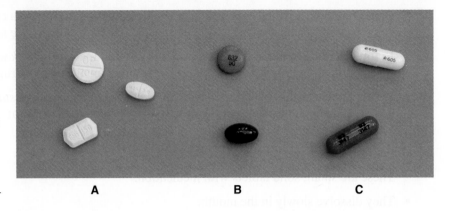

FIGURE 5-1
(**A**) Tablets that may be crushed or broken on the scored line.
(**B**) Tablets that may not be crushed. (**C**) Capsules. (© 2004 Lacey-Bordeaux Photography.)

A   B   C

Coated Tablets

- The coating makes these tablets smooth and easy to swallow.

- If necessary, you can crush some coated tablets.

- When in doubt about whether it's okay to break a coated tablet, check with the pharmacist.

Enteric-coated Tablets

- The enteric coating on these tablets protects the drug from being inactivated in the stomach. It also reduces the chance that the drug will irritate the gastric mucosa.

- Enteric-coated tablets dissolve in the more alkaline secretions of the intestine, rather than in the highly acidic stomach juices.

- Do not crush enteric-coated tablets (Fig. 5-1B).

Prolonged-release or Extended-release Tablets

- These tablets come in three types, with these abbreviations: XL, for extended length; CD, for controlled dose; SR, for sustained release.

- All three types disintegrate more slowly and have a longer duration of action than other tablets.

- With these tablets, a patient needs fewer doses: only one or two tablets each day.

- Do not crush prolonged-release tablets.

Sublingual Tablets

- Placed under the tongue, these tablets dissolve quickly.

- The patient absorbs the medication through the capillaries, so it reaches the patient's circulation without passing through the gastrointestinal tract.

Coded Tablets

- These tablets are easy to identify, because on their surface you can see either a number, a letter, or both (Fig. 5-1).

Capsules

- Capsules are gelatin containers that hold a drug in solid or liquid form.

- Avoid opening capsules. The drug is encased in the capsule for a good reason—possibly because contact with gastric juices will decrease the drug's potency or because the drug could irritate the stomach lining.

- Occasionally, if a patient has difficulty swallowing, you may open a capsule and combine its contents with a semisolid such as applesauce or custard. *But be sure to take this precaution:*

- Before deciding to mix a capsule's contents into food, *always check with the pharmacist* to find out whether the drug is available as a liquid or whether an alternative drug exists (Fig. 5-1C).

- Do not open capsules called *spansule, timespan, time release,* or *sustained release.* They are long-acting, and contain particles of the drug that are coated to dissolve at different times.

Lozenges

- These are small, solid tablets with medication.

- They dissolve slowly in the mouth.

- Many contain sugar or syrup and may be contraindicated (inappropriate) for patients with diabetes mellitus.

- They are often used for throat irritation.

Syrups

- Syrups are solutions of sugar in water, which disguise the medication's unpleasant taste.

- Because of the sugar they contain, syrups may be contraindicated for patients with diabetes mellitus.

Elixirs

- Elixirs are clear hydroalcoholic liquids that are sweetened.

- They may be contraindicated for patients with a history of alcoholism or diabetes mellitus.

Fluidextracts and Tinctures

- Fluidextracts and tinctures are alcoholic, liquid concentrations of a drug.

- Because these are very potent, they are ordered in small amounts.

- Tinctures are ordered in drops.

- Fluidextracts are the most concentrated of all liquids. The average dose of a fluidextract is 2 tsp or less.

Solutions

- Solutions are clear liquids that contain a drug dissolved in water.

Suspensions

- A suspension consists of solid particles of a drug, dispersed in a liquid.

- Because the particles settle to the bottom of the container upon standing, you must resuspend them to obtain an accurate dose.

- Therefore, before you pour any oral preparation, be sure to shake the bottle.

Magmas

- Magmas—for example, milk of magnesia—contain large, bulky particles.

Gels

- Gels—for example, magnesium hydroxide gel—contain small particles.

Emulsions

- Emulsions are creamy, white suspensions of fats or oils in an agent that reduces surface tension and thus makes the oil easier to swallow–for example, emulsified castor oil.

Powders

- Powders are dry, finely ground drugs, reconstituted according to directions.
- Oral antibiotics are frequently supplied as powders.
- In liquid form, powders become oral suspensions.
- Powders must be dissolved according to the manufacturer's instructions.
- When you reconstitute a powder, write these four facts on the label: the date, the time, your initials, and the solution you made.

Parenteral Route

The term *parenteral* does not actually indicate a specific route; rather, it's a general term meaning "by injection." The drug forms for parenteral administration include solutions, suspensions, and powders (as defined above). These are four common parenteral routes:

- ID (intradermal)
- Sub Q (subcutaneous)
- IM (intramuscular)
- IV (intravenous) and IVPB (intravenous piggyback)

Drug forms for parenteral use are sterile. To prepare and administer them, you need to use aseptic technique.

Topical Route

These are the commonly ordered preparations:

Aerosol Powders or Liquids

- Combined with a propellant, these are sprayed onto the skin.
- In nebulizers and inhalers, these are used in the mucous membranes of the respiratory tract.

Powders

- Powders, in dry form, may be applied to the skin.

Creams

- Creams are semisolid drug preparations.
- You can apply them externally to the skin or mucous membranes.
- Vaginal creams use a special applicator for insertion.

Ointments

- Ointments are semisolid preparations in a petroleum or lanolin base for topical use.
- Ointments used for the eye must be labeled "ophthalmic."

Pastes

- Pastes are thick ointments used to protect the skin.
- They absorb secretions and soften the skin.

Suppositories

- Suppositories are medication molded together with a firm base, such as cocoa butter, that melts at body temperature.
- They are shaped for insertion into the rectum, the vagina, and, less commonly, the urethra.

Transdermal Medications

- These medications consist of drug molecules, contained in a unique polymer patch that is applied to the skin just like an ordinary plastic bandage.
- Easy to apply, the patch is effective for hours or days at a time, because it is slowly released and absorbed through the skin.

Topical Drops (eye drops, nose drops, ear drops)

- These are water or saline drops.
- Medication is added for specific conditions.
- They are used in topical treatment of eyes, ears or nose.
- Specific techniques are used for administration.

The health provider's orders will indicate whether the topical medication should be applied to the skin, eye, ear, nose, vagina, or rectum.

SELF TEST 1   **Terms**

Match Column A with the letters in Column B to identify the meaning of the terms used for drug preparations. For correct answers, see the end of the chapter.

Column A	Column B
1. _____ Scored tablet	**a.** Coated drug particles dissolve at different times
2. _____ Enteric coated	**b.** The most concentrated of all liquids
3. _____ Spansule	**c.** Hydroalcoholic liquid ordered in drops
4. _____ Sublingual tablet	**d.** Large particles suspended in a liquid
5. _____ Capsule	**e.** A solid that can be broken in half
6. _____ Syrup	**f.** Route applied to skin or mucous membrane
7. _____ Elixir	**g.** Small particles suspended in a liquid
8. _____ Fluidextract	**h.** Medication that dissolves under the tongue
9. _____ Tincture	**i.** Gelatin containers for a solid or liquid drug
10. _____ Magma	**j.** Molded solid inserted into the rectum
11. _____ Gel	**k.** Drug dissolves in the more alkaline secretions of the intestine
12. _____ Topical	**l.** Sweetened hydroalcoholic liquid
13. _____ Suppository	**m.** Solution of sugar in water to improve the taste of a drug

Equipment to Measure Doses

Nurses do not use a scale to weigh oral solid doses such as the gram and the grain. Solids for oral administration come in tablets and capsules. Once you calculate the number to give, you pour the amount needed into a small container or cup and then discard the container after you've given the medication.

Liquids may be prepared as unit doses, ready for you to administer; or they may be stored in stock bottles, thus requiring calculation and measurement. Two practices will help you measure liquids accurately:

1. Pour liquids to a line. Never estimate a dose between two lines.

2. Pour liquids at eye level and on a flat surface (Fig. 5-2). The surface of the liquid has a natural curve called the meniscus. At eye level, the center of the curve should be on the measurement line, while the fluid at the sides of the container will appear to be above the line (Fig. 5-3).

To measure liquids, nurses typically use a medicine cup or a syringe.

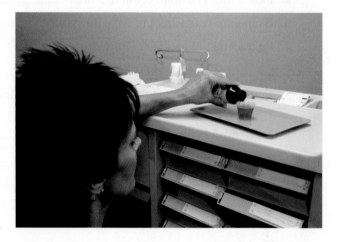

FIGURE 5-2

Liquids are poured at eye level. (Used with permission from Evans-Smith, P. [2005] *Taylor's clinical nursing skills.* Philadelphia: Lippincott, Williams & Wilkins, p. 117.)

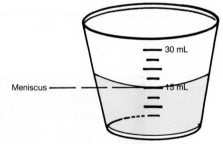

FIGURE 5-3

When viewing the liquid from eye level, the meniscus (lower curve of the fluid) should be on the line.

Medicine Cup

The medicine cup is a disposable container—made of plastic or paper—with markings that show equivalent measures for metric doses in milliliters, for apothecary doses in drams, and for household doses in tablespoons and teaspoons (Fig. 5-4).

The exercise below will help you apply your knowledge of liquid equivalents.

SELF TEST 2   Medicine Cup Measurements

Look at the medicine cup in Figure 5-4. Two sides are shown. Fill in answers related to this measuring device. Check your answers at the end of the chapter.

1. Find 30 mL. What other measures are equivalent to this?

    _____   _____   _____

2. Find 5 mL. Is a dram equal to 5 mL? _____

3. If an order reads dram ii, what line would you use to pour the dose? _____

4. Find 15 mL. What other equivalents equal this?

    _____   _____   _____

5. Consider the following answers to oral liquid dosage problems. What measurement line could you use?

    a. 10 mL Pour _____

    b. 4 tsp Pour _____

    c. ½ oz Pour _____

6. Suppose an answer to an oral liquid problem is 2 mL. Could you pour this dose into a medicine cup?

    Explain what you would do. _____

    _____

    _____

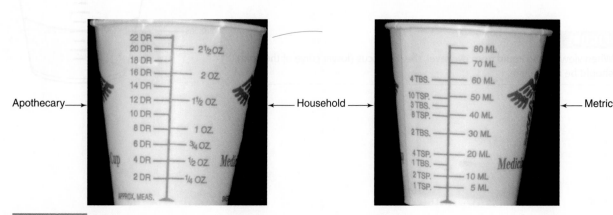

Apothecary →   ← Household →   ← Metric

22 DR
20 DR ── 2½ OZ
18 DR
16 DR ── 2 OZ
14 DR
12 DR ── 1½ OZ
10 DR
8 DR ── 1 OZ
6 DR ── ¾ OZ
4 DR ── ½ OZ
2 DR ── ¼ OZ
APPROX. MEAS.

── 80 ML
── 70 ML
4 TBS. ── 60 ML
10 TSP. ── 50 ML
3 TBS.
8 TSP. ── 40 ML
2 TBS. ── 30 ML
4 TSP. ── 20 ML
1 TBS.
2 TSP. ── 10 ML
1 TSP. ── 5 ML

FIGURE 5-4

A medicine cup for measurement of apothecary, household, or metric dose units.
(© 2004 Lacey-Bordeaux Photography.)

Syringes

Nurses use several different types of syringes to prepare routine parenteral doses. Each one serves a different purpose (Fig. 5-5).

Here are explanations for four types: the 3-mL syringe, the 1-mL syringe, and the insulin syringe—either the 100 units insulin syringe or low-dose 50 units insulin syringe.

SYRINGE. The syringe shown in Figure 5-6 is routinely used for injections. (Note: cc is the marking used on this syringe. Remember: cc = mL.) It has a 22-gauge needle, and the needle is 1½ inches long. The term *gauge* indicates the diameter (width) of the needle.

How to use a 3-mL syringe:

*   The markings on one side are in mL (cc) to the nearest tenth. Each line indicates 0.1 mL (cc).

*   The markings on the *opposite* side are in minims. Each line indicates 1 minim. (Note: Some syringes no longer show minims.)

*   When you're preparing a dose, hold the syringe with the needle up, and draw down the medication into the barrel. Suppose you're preparing a dose calculated to be 1.1 mL or 18 minims. Looking at Figure 5-6, count the lines to reach the correct dose.

SELF TEST 3 | **3-mL Syringe Amounts**

Use an arrow to indicate these amounts on the 3-mL syringe in Figure 5-6. Check your answers at the end of this chapter.

0.3 mL

25 m

1.2 mL

½ mL

2.7 mL

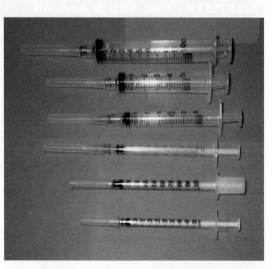

FIGURE 5-5

(*Top to bottom*) 12-mL syringe, 6-mL syringe, 3-mL syringe, 1-mL syringe (often called a *tuberculin syringe*), insulin 100 units syringe, and insulin 50 units syringe.

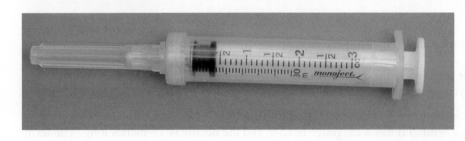

The 3-mL (cc) syringe shows markings for 0.7 mL (cc) and 0.8 mL (cc). What would you do if a dosage answer were 0.75 mL (cc)? Although you must not approximate doses between lines, you can handle the problem in two other ways.

1st way: Round off 0.75 mL (cc) to the nearest tenth. The answer would be 0.8 mL (cc), which can be drawn up to a line. (For details about rounding off numbers, see Chapter 1 and also later in this chapter.)

2nd way: Instead, use a *precision syringe,* which shows markings to the nearest hundredth.

PRECISION SYRINGE.   The 1-mL precision syringe has a 25-gauge needle that is ⅝-inches long. Of all the syringes nurses use, this one is the most accurate. It is sometimes called a tuberculin syringe. This syringe is marked in hundredths of a milliliter and in half minims (Fig. 5-7).

How to use a 1-mL precision syringe:

- The markings on one side are in minims. There is a short line between each half minim, and a long line indicating a whole minim.

- The markings on the *other* side are in milliliters. There are nine lines before 0.10. Each line is 0.01 mL.

- To prepare an injection, hold the syringe with the needle up, then draw down the medication into the barrel. Suppose you're preparing a dose calculated to be 0.25 mL. Looking at Figure 5-7, count the lines to reach the dose.

SELF TEST 4   **1-mL Syringe Amounts**

Use arrows to mark the following doses on the 1-mL precision syringe in Figure 5-7. Check your answers at the end of this chapter.

0.3 mL

0.45 mL

0.61 mL

0.95 mL

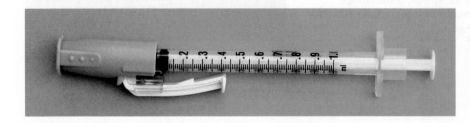

Rounding Off Numbers in Liquid Dosage Answers

When you're solving liquid injection problems, the answers are either in milliliters or (rarely) in minims. Sometimes the answer is not an even number—and if so, you must decide the degree of accuracy you can obtain. The degree of accuracy depends on the syringe you choose for giving the dose.

RULE	ROUNDING OFF NUMBERS

1. **When the last number is 5 or more, add 1 to the previous number.**
2. **When the number is 4 or less, drop the number.**

Example	
0.864 becomes 0.86	4.562 becomes 4.56
1.55 becomes 1.6	2.38 becomes 2.4
0.33 becomes 0.3	0.25 becomes 0.3

If you're using the 3-mL (cc) syringe, carry out decimals two places and then round off to the nearest tenth for milliliters. For answers in minims, carry out to the nearest tenth and then round off to the nearest whole number.

If you're using the 1-mL precision syringe, carry out decimals three places and then round off to the nearest hundredth for milliliters. For answers in minims, carry out to the nearest hundredth and then round off to the nearest tenth.

Note: Pediatric dosing may not use rounding, because these young patients need the exact dose. Always check with institutional policy and use correct pediatric equipment.

SELF TEST 5   3-mL Syringe—Rounding Answers

The following are possible answers to dosage problems that require use of a 3-mL syringe. Put a check (✓) next to the answer if it is acceptable. If it is not acceptable, change the answer to a correct form. Check your answers at the end of this chapter.

a. 0.1 mL _____	**e.** 0.2 mL _____	**i.** 0.4 mL _____
b. 1½ mL _____	**f.** 8½ minims _____	**j.** 0.65 mL _____
c. 0.83 mL _____	**g.** 1.7 mL _____	**k.** 3 minims _____
d. 0.98 minims _____	**h.** ½ mL _____	**l.** 5.5 minims _____

SELF TEST 6   1-mL Syringe—Rounding Answers

The following are possible answers to dosage problems that require the use of a 1-mL precision syringe. Put a check (✓) next to the answer if it is acceptable. If not acceptable, change the answer to a correct form. Check your answers at the end of this chapter.

a. 0.65 mL _____	**d.** 12.8 m _____	**g.** 0.758 mL _____
b. 12.5 minims _____	**e.** 0.346 mL _____	**h.** 5 minims _____
c. 0.04 mL _____	**f.** 0.290 mL _____	

INSULIN SYRINGE. The 1-mL syringe (100 units) is marked in *units* rather than in milliliters or minims. Use it only to prepare insulin. The physician or healthcare provider orders the type of insulin, the strength of insulin, and the number of units (Fig. 5-8).

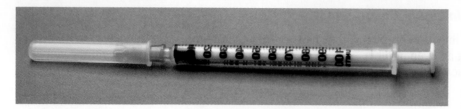

FIGURE 5-8

A 1-mL insulin syringe (© 2004 Lacey-Bordeaux Photography.)

Example

Order: 20 units NPH insulin every day subcutaneous.

Look at Figure 5-8. Between every 10 units, you'll see four short lines. These markings indicate that each line equals 2 units on this syringe. *Always check the markings on a syringe to be certain you understand what each line equals.*

Example

Order: 20 units NPH (unit-100) insulin every day subcutaneous.

To prepare this injection, hold the syringe with the needle up, then draw 20 units of insulin into the barrel.

SELF TEST 7 1-mL Insulin Syringe

Use arrows on the insulin syringe in Figure 5-8 to indicate the following amounts. Check your answers at the end of this chapter.

22 units

34 units

50 units

For odd-numbered insulin doses, do not use the syringe in Figure 5-8. Instead use a low-does insulin syringe. Make sure the doses are exact, not approximate.

LOW-DOSE INSULIN SYRINGE. The low-dose 50 units insulin syringe has a 28-gauge needle that is ½-inch long (Fig. 5-9). Notice that between every 5 units, the syringe shows four short lines. These markings indicate that each line equals 1 unit. The syringe is marked for 50 units, so you can use this syringe to draw up any dose of insulin up to 50 units.

SELF TEST 8 0.5-mL Insulin Syringe

Use arrows on the insulin syringe in Figure 5-9 to indicate the following amounts. Answers are given at the end of this chapter.

33 units

12 units

40 units

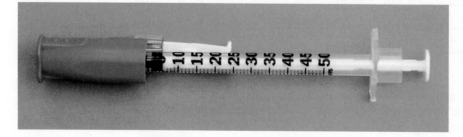

FIGURE 5-9

A ½-mL (low dose) insulin syringe for 50 units or less. (© 2004 Lacey-Bordeaux Photography.)

Needles for Intramuscular and Subcutaneous Injections

Each of the four syringes described above has a different injection needle.

Syringe	Gauge	Length, in.
3 mL	22	1½–3
1 mL	25	⅝–⅞
1 mL insulin	25–26	½–⅝
½ mL low-dose insulin	25–28	½–⅝

The term *gauge* (g) indicates the needle's diameter or width. The higher the gauge number, the finer or smaller the needle's diameter. In the gauges directly above, the low-dose insulin syringe needle has the smallest diameter (28 gauge), which makes it the finest needle in this group. A 16-gauge needle, used to transfuse blood cells, would be very wide and would have a wide opening.

The length of the needle you use depends on the route of injection. For deep intramuscular injections, you use a long needle. For subcutaneous injections, you use a short needle.

Choosing which type of needle to use for an adult or a child depends on three factors: the route of administration, the size and condition of the patient, and the amount of adipose tissue present at the site (Fig. 5-10).

Most hospitals use needleless systems to draw up parenteral medications and for intravenous therapy (Fig. 5-11). This helps to prevent accidental needle-sticks.

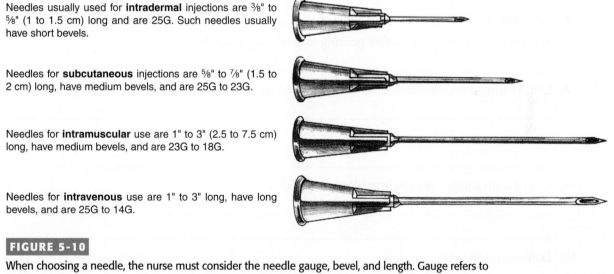

Needles usually used for **intradermal** injections are ⅜" to ⅝" (1 to 1.5 cm) long and are 25G. Such needles usually have short bevels.

Needles for **subcutaneous** injections are ⅝" to ⅞" (1.5 to 2 cm) long, have medium bevels, and are 25G to 23G.

Needles for **intramuscular** use are 1" to 3" (2.5 to 7.5 cm) long, have medium bevels, and are 23G to 18G.

Needles for **intravenous** use are 1" to 3" long, have long bevels, and are 25G to 14G.

FIGURE 5-10

When choosing a needle, the nurse must consider the needle gauge, bevel, and length. Gauge refers to the inside diameter of the needle; the smaller the gauge, the larger the diameter. Bevel refers to the angle at which the needle tip is opened, and length is the distance from the tip to the hub of the needle.

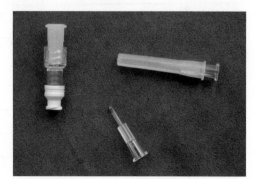

FIGURE 5-11

Needleless system. (Copyright © 2008 Lacey-Bordeaux Photography)

PROFICIENCY TEST 1 | **Drug Preparations and Equipment**

Name: _____

Complete these statements. See Appendix A for answers.

1. Elixirs may be contraindicated for patients with a history of _____

   or _____

2. The average dose of a fluidextract is _____

3. In giving medications parenterally, four common routes are _____ ,

   _____ , _____ , and _____

4. When a powder is reconstituted, what four facts must the nurse write on the label?

   a. _____

   b. _____

   c. _____

   d. _____

5. What route(s) require(s) aseptic technique in preparing and administering drugs?

   _____

6. An example of a drug listed as a magma is _____

7. What must you always do before pouring an oral suspension?

   _____

8. List six drug preparations that can be administered topically.

   _____   _____

   _____   _____

   _____   _____

9. List two advantages in using transdermal medications.

   _____

   _____

10. Define an ointment. _____

    _____

11. List two practices that help you pour oral liquids accurately.

    a. _____

    b. _____

12. Define the following:

    a. Meniscus _____

    _____

    b. Needle gauge _____

    _____

(continued)

PROFICIENCY TEST 1 | **Drug Preparations and Equipment (Continued)**

13. What factors determine the needle length chosen for an injection?

_____

_____

_____

14. List two rules for rounding off numbers.

   a. _____

_____

   b. _____

_____

15. What determines how dosage answers are rounded off?

_____

_____

_____

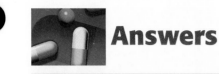

Answers

Self-Test 1 Terms

1. e   **5.** i   **8.** b   **11.** g

2. k   **6.** m   **9.** c   **12.** f

3. a   **7.** l   **10.** d   **13.** j

4. h

Self-Test 2 Medicine Cup Measurements

1. Other equivalents are 2 tbsp, 1 oz, 8 drams.

2. No, a dram is slightly less than 5 mL.

3. Use the 2-dram line.

4. Fifteen milliliters is equal to 1 tbsp, ½ oz, and 4 drams.

5. a. Pour 2 tsp.

   b. 4 tsp × 5 mL = 20 mL; use the 20-mL line

   c. ½ oz. Use the line for ½ oz.

6. No, there is no line for 2 mL. Use a syringe to obtain the 2 mL and then pour the amount into a medicine cup.

Self-Test 3 3-mL Syringe Amounts

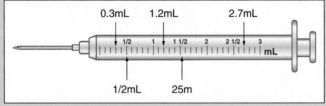

Self-Test 4 1-mL Syringe Amounts

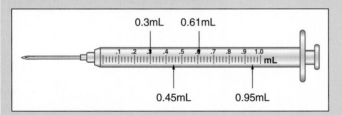

Self-Test 5 3-mL Syringe—Rounding Answers

a. 0.1 mL   ✓

b. 1½ mL   ✓

c. 0.83 mL   0.8 mL

d. 0.98 m   1 minim

e. 0.2 mL   ✓

f. 8½ m   9 m

g. 1.7 mL   ✓

h. ½ mL   ✓

i. 0.4 mL   ✓

j. 0.65 mL   0.7 mL

k. 3 minims   ✓

l. 5.5 minims   6 minims

Self-Test 6 1-mL Syringe—Rounding Answers

a. 0.65 mL   ✓

b. 12.5 m   ✓

c. 0.04 mL   ✓

d. 12.8 m   ✓

e. 0.346 mL   0.35 mL

f. 0.290 mL   0.29 mL

g. 0.758 mL   0.76 mL

h. 5 minims   ✓

Self-Test 7 1-mL Insulin Syringe

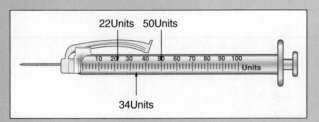

Self-Test 8 0.5-mL Insulin Syringe

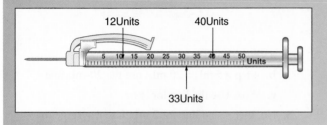

Calculation of Oral Medications— Solids and Liquids

LEARNING OBJECTIVES

1. Using proportion expressed as two ratios

2. Using proportion expressed as two fractions

3. Using the formula method

4. Converting order and supply to the same weight measure

5. Clearing decimal points before solving a problem

6. Using equivalents when conversions are needed

7. Interpreting special types of oral solid and liquid orders that do not require calculation

Drugs for oral administration are prepared by pharmaceutical companies as solids (tablets, capsules) and liquids. When the dose ordered by the physician or healthcare provider differs from the supply, the nurse calculates the amount to give the patient. The calculations can be solved in several ways. This chapter shows how to do the math in three ways: by two ratios, two fractions, and the formula method. Chapter 11 shows another way: dimensional analysis.

In dosage calculations, you start with three pieces of information:

1. The doctor's or healthcare provider's order

2. The quantity or strength of drug on hand

3. The solid or liquid form of the supply drug (i.e., the form the drug arrives in)

The unknown is the amount of drug to administer, usually designated as X or x. These letters represent the above information:

    D = desired dose (order)

    H = on hand or have

    S = supply

    X or x = unknown or answer (amount of drug to give)

Proportions Expressed as Two Fractions

Using fractions, set up proportions so that like units are across from each other (the units and the numerator match and the units and denominators match). The first fraction is the known equivalent.

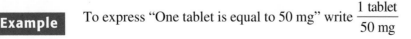

Example   To express "One tablet is equal to 50 mg" write $\dfrac{1 \text{ tablet}}{50 \text{ mg}}$

The second fraction is the unknown, the desired (ordered) dose. Example: x tablets is equal to 100 mg, written as $\dfrac{\text{x tablets}}{100 \text{ mg}}$

The completed proportion looks like

$$\frac{S}{H} = \frac{x}{D} \qquad \frac{\text{Supply}}{\text{Have}} = \frac{x}{\text{Desire}}$$

For the previous example, it would look like this: $\dfrac{1 \text{ tablet}}{50 \text{ mg}} = \dfrac{\text{x tablets}}{100 \text{ mg}}$

Next, solve for x. (For a review of how to solve proportions, refer to Chapter 1.)
In our current example, solving for x follows this process:

1. $\dfrac{1 \text{ tablet}}{50 \text{ mg}} = \dfrac{\text{x tablets}}{100 \text{ mg}}$

   $\dfrac{1 \text{ tablet}}{50 \text{ mg}} \times \dfrac{\text{x tablets}}{100 \text{ mg}}$

   $100 \times 1 = 50\text{x}$

2. $\dfrac{100 \times 1}{50} = \dfrac{50\text{x}}{50}$

3. $\dfrac{100}{50} = \dfrac{\cancel{50}\,\text{x}}{\cancel{50}}$

   $\dfrac{100}{50} = \text{x}$

Answer: 2 tablets = x

Proportions Expressed as Two Ratios

You can set up a ratio by using colons. Double colons separate the two ratios. The first ratio is the known equivalent; the second ratio is the desired (ordered) dose, the unknown. The ratio must always follow the same sequence.

The ratio will look like this:

   S : H : : x : D   Supply : Have : : x : Desire

For the previous example, your ratio would look like this:

   1 tablet : 50 mg : : x : 100 mg

Next, solve for x (For a review of how to solve ratios, refer to Chapter 1.)

1. 1 tablet : 50 mg : : x : 100 mg

2. $1 \times 100 = 50x$

3. $\dfrac{100}{50} = \dfrac{50x}{50}$

4. $\dfrac{100}{50} = x$

Answer: 2 tablets = x

Formula Method

The formula method is simpler than either of the above methods. Here's how the formula method is set up:

$$\frac{D}{H} \times S = x \qquad \frac{Desire}{Have} \times Supply = x$$

Using a formula eliminates the need for cross-multiplying, a potential source of error in calculation. When you use this method with oral solids, the supply is typically either 1 tablet or 1 capsule.

For the purposes of this book, we'll use these three methods—the formula method, the proportion method expressed as two fractions, and the proportion method expressed as two ratios. You just need to see which method makes the most sense to you, then learn it thoroughly and use it. If you want to look ahead to the method of dimensional analysis, see Chapter 11. Answers for the proficiency tests in each chapter will include our three methods plus dimensional analysis.

Oral Solids

Application of the Rule for Oral Solids

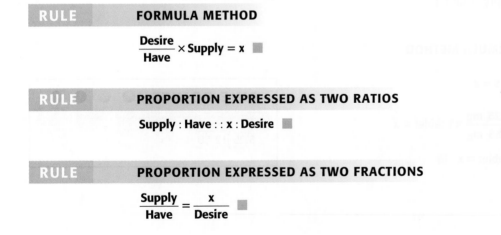

RULE   **FORMULA METHOD**

$$\frac{Desire}{Have} \times Supply = x \ \blacksquare$$

RULE   **PROPORTION EXPRESSED AS TWO RATIOS**

Supply : **Have** : : **x** : **Desire** ■

RULE   **PROPORTION EXPRESSED AS TWO FRACTIONS**

$$\frac{Supply}{Have} = \frac{x}{Desire} \ \blacksquare$$

Example   Order: Coreg (carvedilol) 6.25 mg po bid

Supply: Read the label

Store below 30°C (86°F).
Dispense in a tight, light-resistant container.
Protect from moisture.
Each Tiltab® tablet contains carvedilol, 12.5 mg.
Dosage: See accompanying prescribing information.
Important: Use safety closures when dispensing this product unless otherwise directed by physician or requested by purchaser.

GlaxoSmithKline
Research Triangle Park, NC 27709

12.5mg
NDC 0007-4141-20

COREG®
CARVEDILOL TABLETS

100 TILTAB® Tablets

gsk GlaxoSmithKline   R only

Used with permission of GlaxoSmithKline.

Desire: The order. In this example, desired is 6.25 mg.

Have: The strength of the drug supplied in the container. In the example, the label says that each tablet contains 12.5 mg.

Supply: The unit form in which the drug comes. Coreg comes in tablet form. Because tablets and capsules are single entities, the supply for oral solid drugs is always one.

Amount: How much supply to give. For oral solids the answer will be the number of tablets or capsules to administer.

When you're solving any problem, first check that the order and the supply are in the same weight measure. If they are not, you must convert one or the other amount to its equivalent. In this example, no equivalent is needed; both the order and the supply are in milligrams.

Example   Desire: Coreg (carvedilol) 6.25 mg po

Have: 12.5 mg

Supply: 1 tablet

RULE   **FORMULA METHOD**

$$\frac{D}{H} \times S = x$$

$$\frac{1}{2}\frac{6.25\ mg}{12.5\ mg} \times 1\ tablet = x$$

½ **tablet = x** ▪

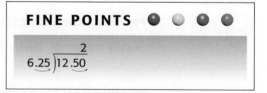

FINE POINTS ● ○ ● ●

$$6.25\overline{)12.50}\quad \overset{2}{}$$

RULE **PROPORTION EXPRESSED AS TWO RATIOS**

$$S : H :: x : D$$

1 tablet : 12.5 mg :: x : 6.25 mg

$$6.25 \times 1 = 12.5x$$

$$\frac{6.25}{12.5} = x$$

$$\frac{1}{2} \text{ tablet} = x \quad \blacksquare$$

RULE **PROPORTION EXPRESSED AS TWO FRACTIONS**

$$\frac{S}{H} = \frac{x}{Desire}$$

$$\frac{1 \text{ tablet}}{12.5 \text{ mg}} \times \frac{x}{6.25 \text{ mg}}$$

$$6.25 \times 1 = 12.5 \, x$$

$$\frac{6.25}{12.5} = x$$

$$\frac{1}{2} \text{ tablet} = x \quad \blacksquare$$

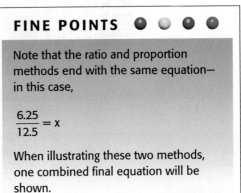

FINE POINTS ● ○ ● ●

Note that the ratio and proportion methods end with the same equation—in this case,

$$\frac{6.25}{12.5} = x$$

When illustrating these two methods, one combined final equation will be shown.

Clearing Decimals When Using the Formula Method

When the numerator and denominator in $\frac{D}{H}$ are decimals, add zeros to make the number of decimal places the same. Then drop the decimal points. This short arithmetic operation replaces long division:

$$\frac{\overset{\text{added}}{\overset{\downarrow}{0.5\underset{\smile}{0}\text{mg}}}}{0.2\underset{\smile}{5}\text{mg}} \quad \frac{\text{numerator}}{\text{denominator or divisor}}$$

In division, you must clear the denominator (divisor) of decimal points before you can carry out the arithmetic. Then you move the decimal point in the numerator the same number of places. (For further help in dividing decimals, refer to Chapter 1.)

Example Order: Lanoxin (digoxin) 0.125 mg po every day

Supply: Read the label

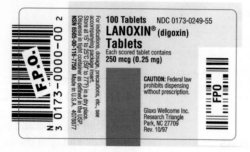

Used with permission of GlaxoSmithKline.

No equivalent is needed. It is stated on the label: 0.25 mg.

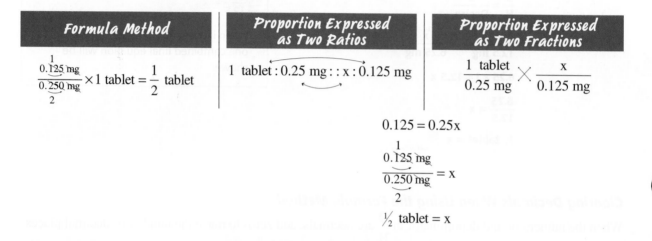

Formula Method	*Proportion Expressed as Two Ratios*	*Proportion Expressed as Two Fractions*
$\dfrac{\overset{1}{\cancel{0.125}\text{ mg}}}{\underset{2}{\cancel{0.250}\text{ mg}}} \times 1 \text{ tablet} = \dfrac{1}{2} \text{ tablet}$	$1 \text{ tablet} : 0.25 \text{ mg} :: x : 0.125 \text{ mg}$	$\dfrac{1 \text{ tablet}}{0.25 \text{ mg}} \times \dfrac{x}{0.125 \text{ mg}}$

$$0.125 = 0.25x$$

$$\frac{\overset{1}{\cancel{0.125}\text{ mg}}}{\underset{2}{\cancel{0.250}\text{ mg}}} = x$$

$$\tfrac{1}{2} \text{ tablet} = x$$

Example Order: Amoxil (amoxicillin) 1 g po q6h

Supply: 1 capsule equals 500 mg

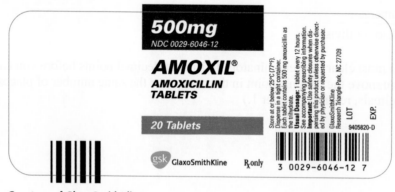

Courtesy of GlaxoSmithKline.

Equivalent: 1 g = 1000 mg

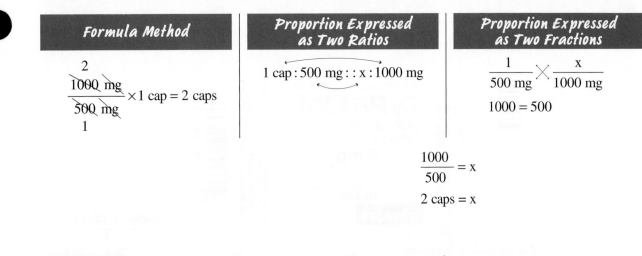

Formula Method	*Proportion Expressed as Two Ratios*	*Proportion Expressed as Two Fractions*

$$\frac{\overset{2}{\cancel{1000}\ \cancel{mg}}}{\underset{1}{\cancel{500}\ \cancel{mg}}} \times 1\ cap = 2\ caps$$

$$1\ cap : 500\ mg : : x : 1000\ mg$$

$$\frac{1}{500\ mg} \times \frac{x}{1000\ mg}$$

$$1000 = 500$$

$$\frac{1000}{500} = x$$

$$2\ caps = x$$

Example

Order: Synthroid (levothyroxine) 75 mcg po every day

Supply: Read the label

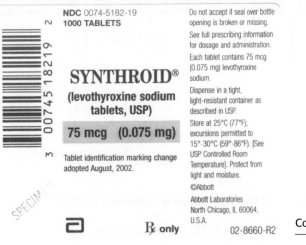

NDC 0074-5182-19
1000 TABLETS

SYNTHROID®
(levothyroxine sodium tablets, USP)

75 mcg   (0.075 mg)

Tablet identification marking change adopted August, 2002.

Do not accept if seal over bottle opening is broken or missing.

See full prescribing information for dosage and administration.

Each tablet contains 75 mcg (0.075 mg) levothyroxine sodium.

Dispense in a tight, light-resistant container as described in USP.

Store at 25°C (77°F); excursions permitted to 15°-30°C (59°-86°F). [See USP Controlled Room Temperature]. Protect from light and moisture.

©Abbott

Abbott Laboratories
North Chicago, IL 60064, U.S.A.

℞ only   02-8660-R2

Courtesy of Abbott Laboratories.

Note that the label gives the equivalent measure:

75 mcg = 0.075 mg

Because the order and the supply are in the same weight measure, no calculation is necessary. Give 1 tablet.

Example Order: Zyprexa (olanzapine) 7.5 mg po every day

Supply: Read the label

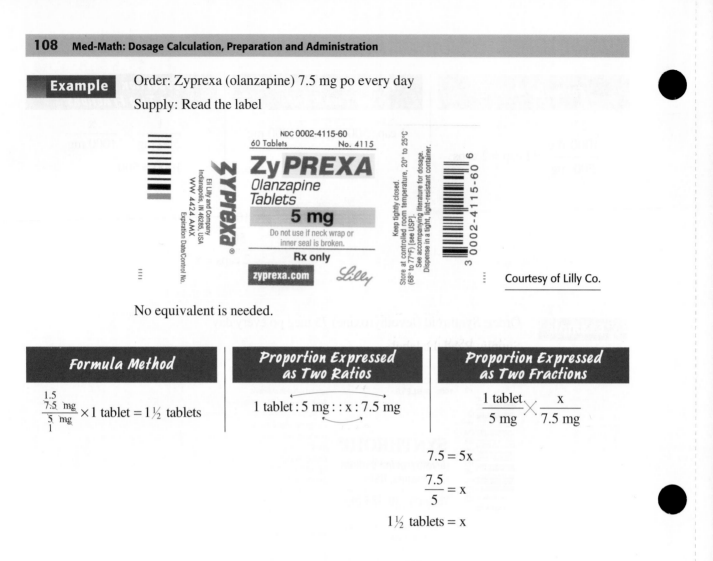

Courtesy of Lilly Co.

No equivalent is needed.

Formula Method	**Proportion Expressed as Two Ratios**	**Proportion Expressed as Two Fractions**
$\dfrac{\overset{1.5}{\cancel{7.5}} \text{ mg}}{\underset{1}{\cancel{5}} \text{ mg}} \times 1 \text{ tablet} = 1\frac{1}{2} \text{ tablets}$	$1 \text{ tablet} : 5 \text{ mg} :: x : 7.5 \text{ mg}$	$\dfrac{1 \text{ tablet}}{5 \text{ mg}} \times \dfrac{x}{7.5 \text{ mg}}$

$$7.5 = 5x$$

$$\frac{7.5}{5} = x$$

$$1\frac{1}{2} \text{ tablets} = x$$

Because the supply is scored you can administer 1½ tablets.

Example Order: Lamictal (lamotrigine) 200 mg po every day

Supply: Read the label

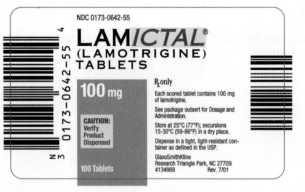

Courtesy of GlaxoSmithKline.

No equivalent is needed.

Formula Method	Proportion Expressed as Two Ratios	Proportion Expressed as Two Fractions
$\overset{2}{\underset{1}{\frac{200 \text{ mg}}{100 \text{ mg}}}} \times 1 \text{ tablet} = 2 \text{ tablets}$	1 tablet : 100 mg : : x : 200 mg	$\dfrac{S}{H} = \dfrac{x}{D}$ $\dfrac{1 \text{ tablet}}{100 \text{ mg}} \times \dfrac{x}{200 \text{ mg}}$

$$200 = 100x$$

$$\frac{200}{100} = x$$

$$2 \text{ tablets} = x$$

Example Order: Lasix (furosemide) 60 mg po every day

Supply: Read the label

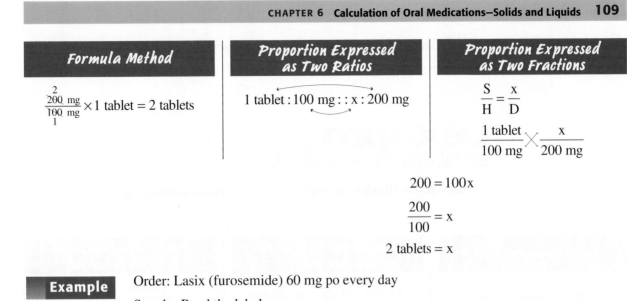

Courtesy of Boehringer Ingelheim Roxane.

No equivalent is needed.

Formula Method	Proportion Expressed as Two Ratios	Proportion Expressed as Two Fractions
$\overset{1.5}{\underset{1}{\frac{60 \text{ mg}}{40 \text{ mg}}}} \times 1 \text{ tablet} = 1\frac{1}{2} \text{ tablets}$	1 tablet : 40 mg : : x : 60 mg	$\dfrac{1 \text{ tablet}}{40 \text{ mg}} \times \dfrac{x}{60 \text{ mg}}$

$$60 = 40x$$

$$\frac{60}{40} = x$$

$$1\frac{1}{2} \text{ tablets} = x$$

The tablets are score so give 1½ tablets.

Example Order: Lexapro (escitalopram oxalate) 20 mg po every day

Supply: Read the label

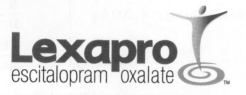

Equivalent to **10 mg** escitalopram

Courtesy of Pzifer Co.

Formula Method	Proportion Expressed as Two Ratios	Proportion Expressed as Two Fractions
$\dfrac{\overset{2}{20}\ mg}{\underset{1}{10}\ mg} \times 1\ tablet = 2\ tablets$	1 tablet : 10 mg : : x : 20 mg	$\dfrac{1\ tablet}{10\ mg} \times \dfrac{x}{20\ mg}$

$$20 = 10x$$

$$\frac{20}{10} = x$$

2 tablets

Example Order: Zyvox (linezolid) 0.6 gm PO q 12 hour

Supply: Read the label

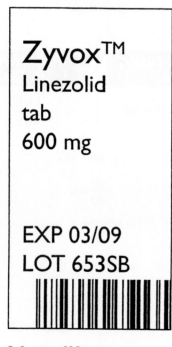

Zyvox™
Linezolid
tab
600 mg

EXP 03/09
LOT 653SB

0.6 gm = 600 mg

Formula Method	**Proportion Expressed as Two Ratios**	**Proportion Expressed as Two Fractions**
$\frac{600 \text{ mg}}{600 \text{ mg}} \times 1 \text{ tablet} = 1 \text{ tablet}$	1 tablet : 600 mg :: x : 600 mg	$\frac{1 \text{ tablet}}{600 \text{ mg}} \times \frac{x}{600 \text{ mg}}$

$$600 = 600x$$

$$\frac{600}{600} = x$$

$$1 \text{ tablet} = x$$

Example   Order: Lopressor (metoprolol) 25 mg PO bid
Supply: Read the label

METOPROLOL tablet
50 mg
AM010590

BES Laboratories INC

Formula Method	**Proportion Expressed as Two Ratios**	**Proportion Expressed as Two Fractions**
$\frac{50 \text{ mg}}{25 \text{ mg}} \times 1 \text{ tablet} = \frac{1}{2} \text{ tablet}$	1 tablet : 50 mg :: x : 25 mg	$\frac{1 \text{ tablet}}{50 \text{ mg}} \times \frac{x}{25 \text{ mg}}$

$$25 = 50x$$

$$\frac{25}{50} = x$$

$$\frac{1}{2} \text{ tablet} = x$$

SELF TEST 1 Oral Solids

Solve these practice problems. Answers are given at the end of the chapter. Remember the three methods:

Formula Method	Proportion Expressed as Two Ratios	Proportion Expressed as Two Fractions
$\dfrac{D}{H} \times S = x$	$S : H : : x : D$	$\dfrac{S}{H} \times \dfrac{x}{D}$

1. Order: Decadron (phenytoin) 1.5 mg po bid *2 tablets*
   Supply: tablets labeled 0.75 mg

2. Order: Lanoxin (digoxin) 0.25 mg po every day
   Supply: scored tablets labeled 0.5 mg *0.5 mg*

3. Order: Omnipen (ampicillin) 0.5 g po q6h = *500mg = 2 capsules*
   Supply: capsules labeled 250 mg

4. Order: Deltasone (prednisone) 10 mg po tid *4 tablets*
   Supply: tablets labeled 2.5 mg

5. Order: aspirin 650 mg po stat
   Supply: tablets labeled 325 mg *2 tablets*

6. Order: Procardia (nifedipine) 20 mg po bid *2 tablets*
   Supply: capsules labeled 10 mg

7. Order: Prolixin (fluphenazine) 10 mg po daily
   Supply: tablets labeled 2.5 mg

8. Order: penicillin G potassium 200,000 units po q8h
   Supply: scored tablets labeled 400,000 units

9. Order: Lanoxin (digoxin) 0.5 mg po every day
   Supply: scored tablets labeled 0.25 mg

10. Order: Capoten (captopril) 18.75 mg po tid
    Supply: scored tablets labeled 12.5 mg

11. Order: Seroquel (quetiapine) 300 mg po bid
    Supply: tablets labeled 200 mg

12. Order: Catapres (clonidine) 0.3 mg po hs
    Supply: tablets labeled 0.1 mg

13. Order: Capoten (captopril) 6.25 mg po bid
    Supply: scored tablets labeled 25 mg

14. Order: Catapres (clonidine) 400 mcg po every day
    Supply: tablets labeled 0.2 mg

15. Order: Coumadin (warfarin) 7.5 mg po every day
    Supply: scored tablets labeled 5 mg

16. Order: Micronase (glyburide) 0.625 mg every day
    Supply: scored tablets labeled 1.25 mg

(continued)

SELF TEST 1   **Oral Solids (Continued)**

17. Order: Naprosyn (naproxen) 0.5 g po every day
    Supply: scored tablets labeled 250 mg

18. Order: Hydrodiuril (hydrochlorothiazide) 37.5 mg po every day
    Supply: scored tablets labeled 25 mg

19. Order: Keflex (cephalexin) 1 g po q6h
    Supply: capsules labeled 500 mg

20. Order: Lioresal (baclofen) 25 mg po tid
    Supply: scored tablets labeled 10 mg

Special Types of Oral Solid Orders

Drugs that contain a number of active ingredients are ordered by the number to be administered and do not require calculation. Similarly, over-the-counter (OTC) medications are often ordered by how many are to be administered.

 Example

EXAMPLE 1
Vitamin B complex caplets 1 po every day

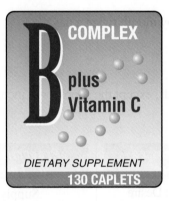

Interpret as: Give 1 caplet by mouth every day.

EXAMPLE 2

Aggrenox (aspirin/dipyridamole)
25 mg/200 mg capsules 1 capsule po bid

FINE POINTS ● ○ ● ●

Notice the label states how much of each drug makes up the drug. This is useful information, especially in medication administration and potential drug allergies.

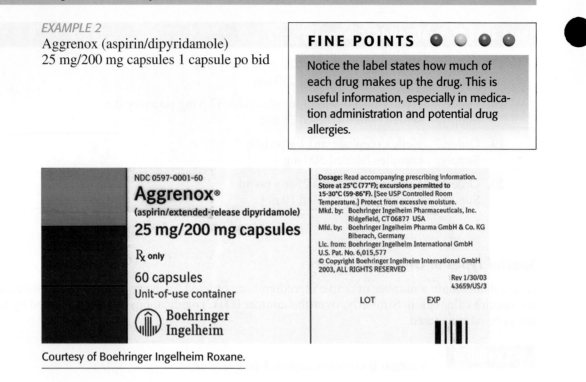

Courtesy of Boehringer Ingelheim Roxane.

Interpret as: Give 1 Aggrenox capsule by mouth twice a day.

Oral Liquids

For liquids, the three methods are set up just as for oral solids, except the supply will include a liquid measurement, usually milliliters (mL).

Formula Method	*Proportion Expressed as Two Ratios*	*Proportion Expressed as Two Fractions*
$\dfrac{\text{Desire}}{\text{Have}} \times \text{Supply} = \text{Amount (x)}$	Supply : Have : : x : Desire	$\dfrac{\text{Supply}}{\text{Have}} = \dfrac{\text{x}}{\text{Desire}}$

Example

Order: Zithromax (azithromycin)
oral susp 400 mg po every day × 4 days

Supply: Read the label

FINE POINTS ● ○ ● ●

Oral liquids may be measured using a medication cup, calibrated dropper, or needleless syringe.

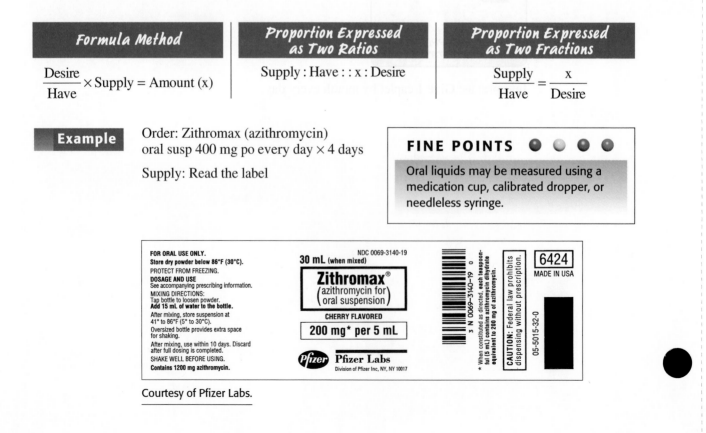

Courtesy of Pfizer Labs.

Formula Method	Proportion Expressed as Two Ratios	Proportion Expressed as Two Fractions

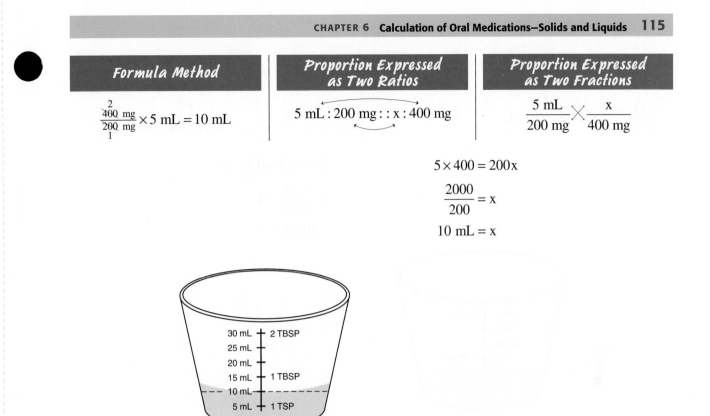

$$\frac{\overset{2}{\cancel{400}}\ mg}{\underset{1}{\cancel{200}}\ mg} \times 5\ mL = 10\ mL$$

$$5\ mL : 200\ mg : : x : 400\ mg$$

$$\frac{5\ mL}{200\ mg} \times \frac{x}{400\ mg}$$

$$5 \times 400 = 200x$$

$$\frac{2000}{200} = x$$

$$10\ mL = x$$

Administer 10 mL of Zithromax po every day for 4 days.

Before solving each problem, check to be certain that the order and your supply are in the same measure. If they are not, you must convert one or the other to its equivalent. Convert whichever one is easier for you to solve.

Example   Order: Lanoxin (digoxin) elixir 500 mcg × 1 dose

Supply: Read the label

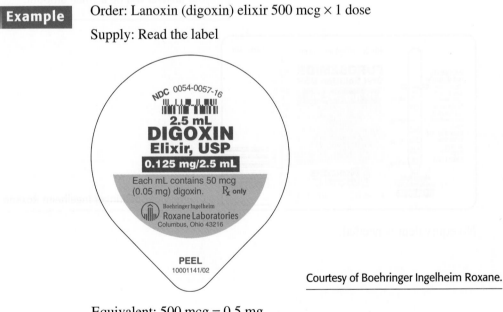

NDC 0054-0057-16

2.5 mL
DIGOXIN
Elixir, USP
0.125 mg/2.5 mL

Each mL contains 50 mcg
(0.05 mg) digoxin. R_x only

Boehringer Ingelheim
Roxane Laboratories
Columbus, Ohio 43216

PEEL
10001141/02

Courtesy of Boehringer Ingelheim Roxane.

Equivalent: 500 mcg = 0.5 mg

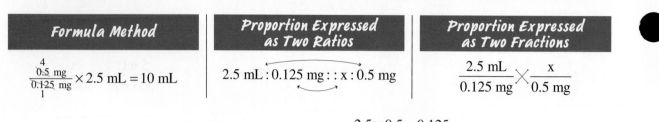

Formula Method	Proportion Expressed as Two Ratios	Proportion Expressed as Two Fractions

$$\frac{\overset{4}{\cancel{0.5}\text{ mg}}}{\underset{1}{\cancel{0.125}\text{ mg}}} \times 2.5\text{ mL} = 10\text{ mL}$$

$$2.5\text{ mL} : 0.125\text{ mg} :: x : 0.5\text{ mg}$$

$$\frac{2.5\text{ mL}}{0.125\text{ mg}} \times \frac{x}{0.5\text{ mg}}$$

$$2.5 \times 0.5 = 0.125\ x$$

$$\frac{1.25}{0.125} = x$$

$$10\text{ mL} = x$$

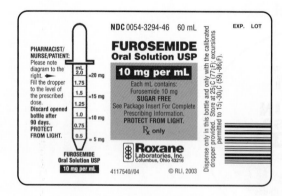

Administer 10 mL of digoxin × 1 dose.

Example Order: Lasix (furosemide) 34 mg po every day

Supply: Read the label

FINE POINTS ● ○ ● ●

Because the drug comes with a calibrated dropper, you are alerted that your answer will be a small amount.

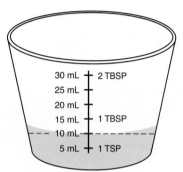

Courtesy of Boehringer Ingelheim Roxane.

No equivalent is needed.

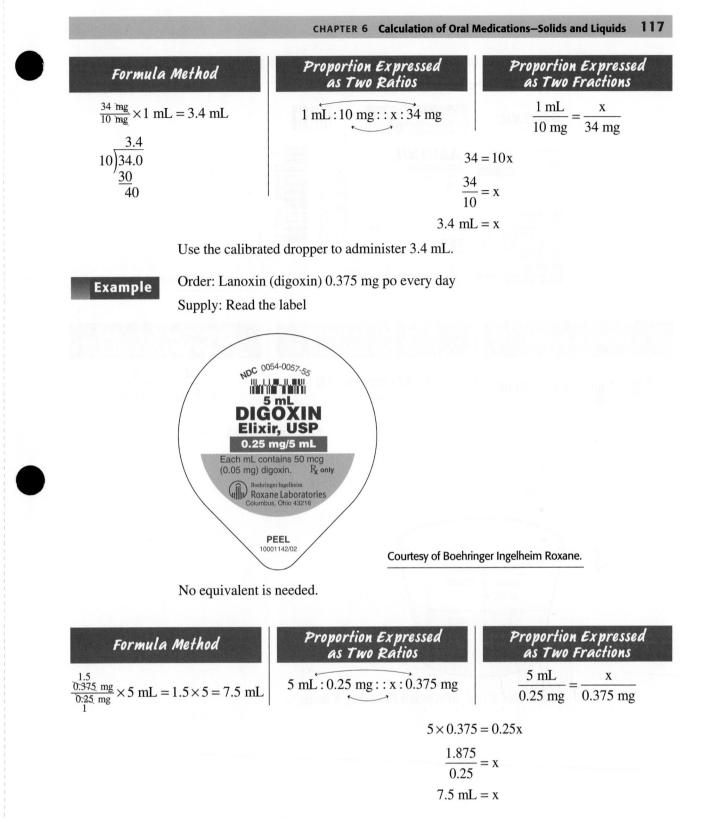

Formula Method	Proportion Expressed as Two Ratios	Proportion Expressed as Two Fractions
$\frac{34 \text{ mg}}{10 \text{ mg}} \times 1 \text{ mL} = 3.4 \text{ mL}$	$1 \text{ mL} : 10 \text{ mg} :: x : 34 \text{ mg}$	$\frac{1 \text{ mL}}{10 \text{ mg}} = \frac{x}{34 \text{ mg}}$

$$10\overline{)34.0}$$
$$\begin{array}{r} 3.4 \\ \hline 30 \\ \hline 40 \end{array}$$

$$34 = 10x$$

$$\frac{34}{10} = x$$

$$3.4 \text{ mL} = x$$

Use the calibrated dropper to administer 3.4 mL.

Example

Order: Lanoxin (digoxin) 0.375 mg po every day

Supply: Read the label

NDC 0054-0057-55

5 mL
DIGOXIN
Elixir, USP
0.25 mg/5 mL

Each mL contains 50 mcg
(0.05 mg) digoxin.   R$_x$ only

Boehringer Ingelheim
Roxane Laboratories
Columbus, Ohio 43216

PEEL
10001142/02

Courtesy of Boehringer Ingelheim Roxane.

No equivalent is needed.

Formula Method	Proportion Expressed as Two Ratios	Proportion Expressed as Two Fractions
$\frac{\overset{1.5}{\cancel{0.375} \text{ mg}}}{\underset{1}{\cancel{0.25} \text{ mg}}} \times 5 \text{ mL} = 1.5 \times 5 = 7.5 \text{ mL}$	$5 \text{ mL} : 0.25 \text{ mg} :: x : 0.375 \text{ mg}$	$\frac{5 \text{ mL}}{0.25 \text{ mg}} = \frac{x}{0.375 \text{ mg}}$

$$5 \times 0.375 = 0.25x$$

$$\frac{1.875}{0.25} = x$$

$$7.5 \text{ mL} = x$$

Use a needleless syringe to draw up 7.5 mL.

Example   Order: Amoxil (amoxicillin) oral suspension 500 mg po q8h

Supply: Read the label

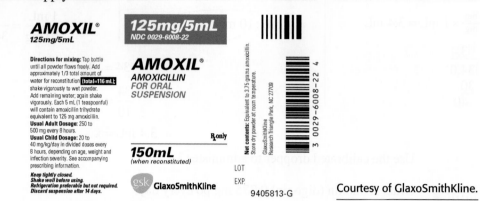

Courtesy of GlaxoSmithKline.

Formula Method	Proportion Expressed as Two Ratios	Proportion Expressed as Two Fractions

$$\frac{\overset{4}{\cancel{500}} \text{ mg}}{\underset{1}{\cancel{125}} \text{ mg}} \times 5 \text{ mL} = 4 \times 5 = 20 \text{ mL}$$

$$5 \text{ mL} : 125 \text{ mg} :: x : 500 \text{ mg}$$

$$\frac{5 \text{ mL}}{125 \text{ mg}} \times \frac{x}{500 \text{ mg}}$$

$$5 \times 500 = 125x$$

$$\frac{2500}{125} = x$$

$$20 \text{ mL} = x$$

Administer 20 mL of Amoxil PO every 8 hours

SELF TEST 2   Oral Liquids

Solve these oral liquid problems. Answers are given at the end of the chapter.

1. Order: EES (erythromycin) susp 0.75 g po qid
   Supply: liquid labeled 250 mg/mL

2. Order: ampicillin susp 500 mg po q8h
   Supply: liquid labeled 250 mg/5 mL

3. Order: Keflex (cephalexin) in oral suspension 0.35 g po q6h
   Supply: liquid labeled 125 mg/5 mL

4. Order: Sandimmune (cyclosporine) 150 mg po stat and every day
   Supply: liquid labeled 100 mg/mL in a bottle with a calibrated dropper

5. Order: Stelazine (trifluoperazine) 5 mg po bid
   Supply: liquid labeled 10 mg/mL

6. Order: Lanoxin (digoxin) 0.02 mg po every day
   Supply: pediatric elixir 0.05 mg/mL in a bottle with a dropper marked in tenths of a milliliter

7. Order: potassium chloride 30 mEq po every day
   Supply: liquid labeled 20 mEq/15 mL

8. Order: Lanoxin (digoxin) elixir 0.25 mg via nasogastric tube every day
   Supply: liquid labeled 0.25 mg/mL

9. Order: Risperdal (risperidone) 3 mg po bid
   Supply: liquid labeled 1 mg/mL

10. Order: Phenergan (promethazine) HCl syrup 12.5 mg po tid
    Supply: liquid labeled 6.25 mg/5 mL

11. Order: Vistaril (hydroxyzine) 50 mg po qid
    Supply: syrup labeled 10 mg per 5 mL

12. Order: Lasix (furosemide) 40 mg po q12h
    Supply: liquid labeled 10 mg/mL

13. Order: potassium chloride 10 mEq po bid
    Supply: liquid labeled 20 mEq/30 mL

14. Order: Compazine (prochlorperazine) 10 mg po tid
    Supply: syrup labeled 5 mg/5 mL

15. Order: phenobarbital 100 mg po hs
    Supply: elixir labeled 20 mg/5 mL

16. Order: Tylenol (acetaminophen) gr 10 po q4h prn
    Supply: elixir labeled 160 mg/5 mL

17. Order: Benadryl (diphenhydramine) 25 mg po q4h
    Supply: liquid labeled 12.5 mg/5 mL

18. Order: Thorazine (chlorpromazine) 50 mg po tid
    Supply: syrup labeled 10 mg/5 mL

19. Order: Colace (docusate) 100 mg po every day
    Supply: syrup labeled 50 mg/15 mL

20. Order: codeine 0.06 g po q4–6h prn
    Supply: liquid labeled 15 mg/5 mL

Special Types of Oral Liquid Orders

Some liquids, including OTC preparations and multivitamins, are ordered in the amount to be poured and administered. No calculation is required.

Example

EXAMPLE 1

Order: Robitussin (dextromethorphan) syrup 2 tsp q4h prn po

Supply: liquid labeled Robitussin syrup

No calculation is needed. Pour 2 tsp and take every 4 hours by mouth as necessary.

EXAMPLE 2

Order: milk of magnesia 30 mL tonight po

Supply: liquid labeled milk of magnesia

No calculation is required. Pour 30 mL milk of magnesia and give tonight by mouth.

Oral Solid and Liquid Problems Without Written Calculations

As you develop proficiency in solving problems, you will be able to calculate many answers "in your head" without written work.

SELF TEST 3 **Mental Drill Oral Solids**

Solve the problems "in your head" and write the amount to be given. Answers appear at the end of the chapter.

Order	Supply (scored tablets)	Answer
1. 20 mg	10 mg	_____
2. 0.125 mg	0.25 mg	_____
3. 0.25 mg	0.125 mg	_____
4. 200,000 units	100,000 units	_____
5. 0.5 mg	0.25 mg	_____
6. 0.2 g	400 mg	_____
7. 1 g	1000 mg	_____
8. 0.1 g	100 mg	_____
9. 0.01 g	20 mg	_____
10. 650 mg	325 mg	_____
11. 500 mg	250 mg	_____
12. gr i	60 mg	_____
13. 50 mg	0.1 g	_____
14. 4 mg	2 mg	_____

SELF TEST 4   Mental Drill Oral Liquids

Solve the problems "in your head" and write the amount to be given. Answers appear at the end of the chapter.

Order	Supply	Answer
1. 20 mg	10 mg/5 mL	_____
2. 10 mg	2 mg/5 mL	_____
3. 0.5 g	250 mg/5 mL	_____
4. 0.1 g	200 mg/10 mL	_____
5. 250 mg	0.1 g/6 mL	_____
6. 100 mg	50 mg/10 mL	_____
7. 12 mg	4 mg/5 mL	_____
8. 15 mg	30 mg/10 mL	_____
9. 15 mg	10 mg/4 mL	_____
10. 0.25 mg	0.5 mg/5 mL	_____

Putting it Together

Ms. CM is an 86 year old female who is being admitted with rapid atrial fibrillation that started about 11:00 P.M yesterday. No shortness of breath. Admitted for evaluation.

Past Medical History: hypertension, intermittent atrial fibrillation 3-4 years, chronic aortic insufficiency with dilated left ventricle; previous hospitalization several weeks ago with atrial fibrillation with a rapid ventricular rate. Other medical problems include moderate varicose veins, early dementia and chronic tobacco use.

No known drug allergies

Current Vital Signs: Blood pressure is 172/58, pulse 120-140/minute, respirations 20/minute, oxygen saturation 96% on 2 L n/c, afebrile

Medication Orders

Coumadin (warfarin) *anticoagulant* 7.5 mg PO daily

Prinivil (lisinopril) *antihypertensive* 20 mg PO q 12

Lanoxin (digoxin) *antiarrhythmic, increases cardiac contractility*

   Loading dose: 0.75 mg PO x1; 0.25 mg PO in 6 hours and 12 hours then

      0.125 mg PO daily PO, hold if HR<60

K Dur (potassium chloride) *potassium supplement* 30 mEq PO qd

Xanax (alprazolam) *antianxiety* 0.25-0.5 mg q 6 hr prn anxiety

(continued)

Putting it Together

Pepcid (famotidine) *histamine 2 blocker, decreases gastric acid* 20 mg PO

Tylenol (acetaminophen) *antiinflammatory* gr X q 4 hour prn mild pain

Tums (calcium carbonate) *mineral supplement, antacid* 1 gm PO daily

Calculations

1. Calculate how many tablets of Coumadin to administer. Available supply is 5 mg scored tablets.

2. Calculate how many tablets of Prinivil to administer. Available supply is 10 mg.

3. Calculate the loading dose of 0.75 mg of digoxin. Available supply is 500 mcg scored tablets and 250 mcg scored tablets. What are two options of administration?

4. Calculate the loading dose of 0.25 mg of digoxin. Available supply is 500 mcg scored tablets and 250 mcg scored tablets. What are two options of administration?

5. Calculate the maintenance dose of 0.125 mg of digoxin. Available supply is 500 mcg scored tablets and 250 mcg scored tablets. What are two options of administration?

6. K-dur 10 mEq is equal to 750 mg of potassium. How many mg of potassium would be in 15 mEq?

7. Calculate how many tablets of Xanax to administer with the range ordered. Available supply is 125 mcg tablets.

8. Calculate how many tsp of Pepcid to administer. Available supply is 40 mg in 5 mL.

9. Calculate how many tablets of Tylenol to administer. Available supply is 325 mg tablets.

10. Calculate how many tablets of Tums to administer. Available supply is 200 mg tablets.

Critical Thinking Questions

1. What medications would have a higher potential for error in calculation and why?

2. What medications have parameters for administration? Should any of these medications be held given the above scenario?

3. What are some alternatives to giving several tablets of a specific medication, i.e. 4 tablets to equal the ordered dose?

4. Are there any orders written incorrectly and why? What should you do to correct these?

5. This patient has difficulty with taking medications. What are some alternatives to administration?

Answers in Appendix B.

PROFICIENCY TEST 1   Calculation of Oral Doses

Name: _____

For liquid answers, draw a line on the medicine cup indicating the amount you would pour.
Answers are given in Appendix A.

1. Order: KCl elixir 20 mEq po bid
    Supply: liquid labeled 30 mEq/15 mL
    Answer   _____

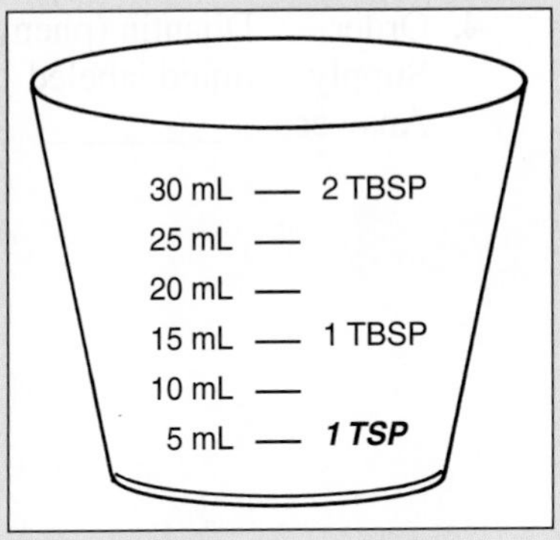

30 mL	2 TBSP
25 mL	
20 mL	
15 mL	1 TBSP
10 mL	
5 mL	*1 TSP*

2. Order: Dilantin (phenytoin) susp 150 mg po tid
    Supply: liquid labeled 75 mg/7.5 mL
    Answer   _____

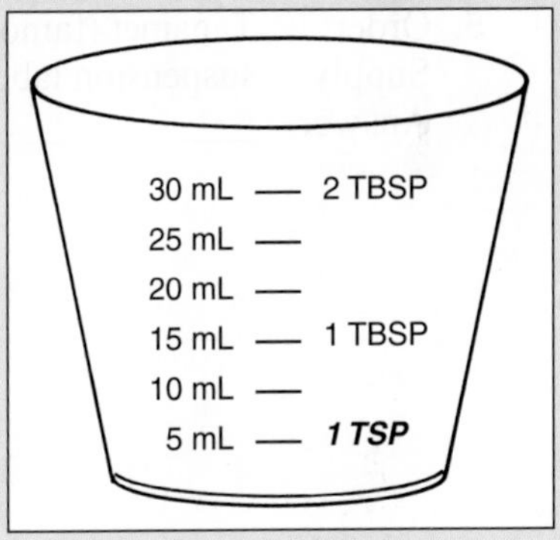

30 mL	2 TBSP
25 mL	
20 mL	
15 mL	1 TBSP
10 mL	
5 mL	*1 TSP*

3. Order: Lanoxin (digoxin) elixir 0.125 mg po every day
    Supply: liquid labeled 0.25 mg/10 mL
    Answer   _____

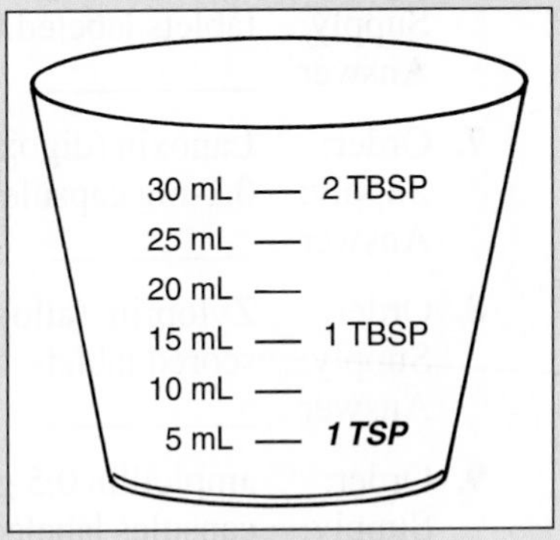

30 mL	2 TBSP
25 mL	
20 mL	
15 mL	1 TBSP
10 mL	
5 mL	*1 TSP*

(continued)

Name: _____

For liquid answers, draw a line on the medicine cup indicating the amount you would pour. Answers are given in Appendix A.

4. Order: Dilantin (phenytoin) oral susp 375 mg po tid
Supply: liquid labeled 125 mg/5 mL
Answer _____

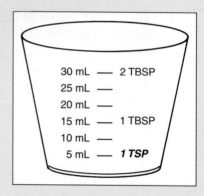

30 mL — 2 TBSP
25 mL —
20 mL —
15 mL — 1 TBSP
10 mL —
5 mL — *1 TSP*

5. Order: Tagamet (famotidine) 40 mg
Supply: suspension labeled 20 mg/2.5 mL
Answer _____

30 mL — 2 TBSP
25 mL —
20 mL —
15 mL — 1 TBSP
10 mL —
5 mL — *1 TSP*

6. Order: Lanoxin (digoxin) 0.5 mg po every day
Supply: tablets labeled 0.25 mg
Answer _____

7. Order: Lanoxin (digoxin) 100 mcg every day po
Supply: 0.1-mg capsules
Answer _____

8. Order: Zyloprim (allopurinol) 250 mg po every day
Supply: scored tablets 100 mg
Answer _____

9. Order: ampicillin 0.5 g po q6h
Supply: capsules labeled 250 mg
Answer _____

10. Order: Synthroid (levothyroxine) 0.3 mg po every day
Supply: tablets labeled 300 mcg scored
Answer _____

PROFICIENCY TEST 2   Calculation of Oral Doses (Test 2)

Name: _____

For liquid answers, draw a line on the medicine cup indicating the amount you would pour.
Answers are given in Appendix A.

1. Order: Advil (ibuprofen) 0.8 g po tid
   Supply: tablets labeled 400 mg
   Answer   _____

2. Order: Niazid (isoniazid) 0.3 g po every day
   Supply: tablets labeled 300 mg
   Answer   _____

3. Order: Tenormin (atenolol) 75 mg po bid
   Supply: 50 mg tablets
   Answer   _____

4. Order: Tylenol (acetaminophen) 0.65 g po q4h
   Supply: tablets labeled 325 mg
   Answer   _____

5. Order: Altace (ramipril) 10 mg po daily
   Supply: tablets labeled 2.5 mg
   Answer   _____

6. Order: Mycostatin (nystatin) oral susp 750,000 units
             po tid
   Supply: liquid labeled 100,000 units/mL
   Answer   _____

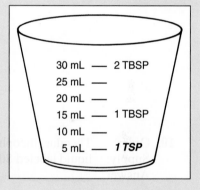

7. Order: oxacillin sodium 0.75 g po q6h
   Supply: liquid labeled 250 mg/5 mL
   Answer   _____

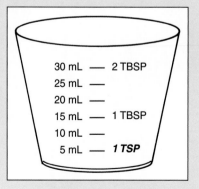

(continued)

PROFICIENCY TEST 2 **Calculation of Oral Doses (Test 2) (Continued)**

Name: _____

For liquid answers, draw a line on the medicine cup indicating the amount you would pour.
Answers are given in Appendix A.

8. Order: penicillin V potassium 500 mg po q6h
   Supply: liquid labeled 250 mg/5 mL
   Answer _____

| 30 mL — 2 TBSP |
| 25 mL — |
| 20 mL — |
| 15 mL — 1 TBSP |
| 10 mL — |
| 5 mL — *1 TSP* |

9. Order: Mylanta II 30 mL q4h prn
   Supply: liquid labeled Mylanta II
   Answer _____

| 30 mL — 2 TBSP |
| 25 mL — |
| 20 mL — |
| 15 mL — 1 TBSP |
| 10 mL — |
| 5 mL — *1 TSP* |

10. Order: Theodur (theophylline) 160 mg po q6h
   Supply: liquid labeled 80 mg/15 mL
   Answer _____

| 30 mL — 2 TBSP |
| 25 mL — |
| 20 mL — |
| 15 mL — 1 TBSP |
| 10 mL — |
| 5 mL — *1 TSP* |

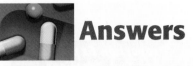 **Answers**

Self-Test 1 Oral Solids

Formula Method	Proportion Expressed as Two Ratios	Proportion Expressed as Two Fractions
$\dfrac{D}{H} \times S = x$	$S : H : : x : D$	$\dfrac{S}{H} = \dfrac{x}{D}$

1. No equivalent is needed.

Formula Method	Proportion Expressed as Two Ratios	Proportion Expressed as Two Fractions
$\dfrac{\overset{2}{1.50} \text{ mg}}{\underset{1}{0.75} \text{ mg}} \times 1 \text{ tablet} = 2 \text{ tablets}$	$1 \text{ tablet} : 0.75 \text{ mg} : : x : 1.5 \text{ mg}$	$\dfrac{1 \text{ tablet}}{0.75 \text{ mg}} \diagdown \dfrac{x}{1.5 \text{ mg}}$

$$1.5 = 0.75x$$

$$\frac{1.5}{0.75} = x$$

$$2 \text{ tablets} = x$$

2. No equivalent is needed.

Formula Method	Proportion Expressed as Two Ratios	Proportion Expressed as Two Fractions
$\dfrac{\overset{1}{0.25} \text{ mg}}{\underset{2}{0.50} \text{ mg}} \times 1 \text{ tablet} = \dfrac{1}{2} \text{ tablet}$	$1 \text{ tablet} : 0.5 \text{ mg} : : x : 0.25 \text{ mg}$	$\dfrac{1 \text{ tablet}}{0.5 \text{ mg}} \diagdown \dfrac{x}{0.25 \text{ mg}}$

$$0.25 = 0.5x$$

$$\frac{0.25}{0.5} = x$$

$$0.5 \text{ tablet} = x$$

or ½ tablet

3. Equivalent 0.5 g = 500 mg

Formula Method	Proportion Expressed as Two Ratios	Proportion Expressed as Two Fractions
$\dfrac{\overset{2}{500} \text{ mg}}{\underset{1}{250} \text{ mg}} \times 1 \text{ capsule} = 2 \text{ capsules}$	$1 \text{ capsule} : 250 \text{ mg} : : x : 500 \text{ mg}$	$\dfrac{1 \text{ capsule}}{250 \text{ mg}} \diagdown \dfrac{x}{500 \text{ mg}}$

$$\frac{500}{250} = x$$

$$2 \text{ capsules} = x$$

4. No equivalent is needed.

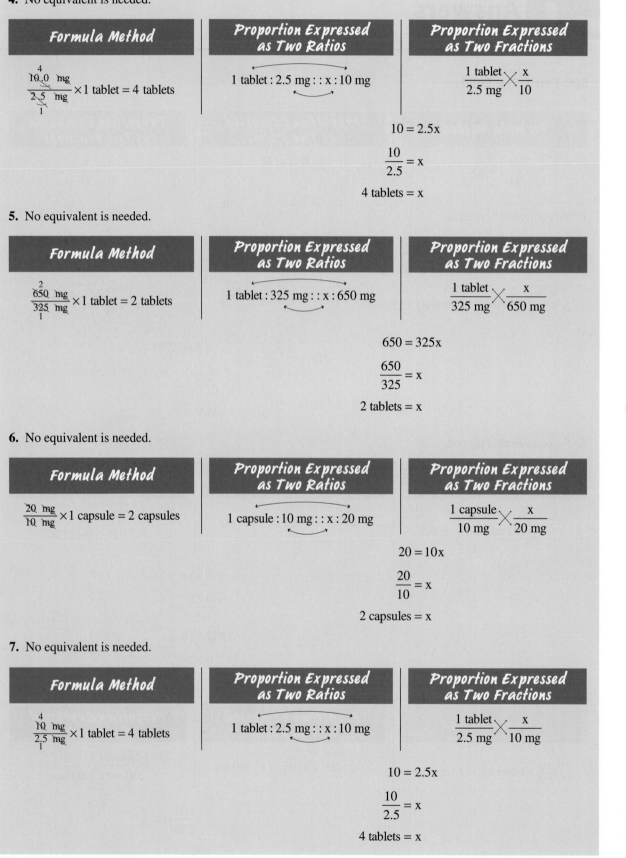

Formula Method	Proportion Expressed as Two Ratios	Proportion Expressed as Two Fractions
$\dfrac{\overset{4}{\cancel{10.0}}\ \text{mg}}{\underset{1}{\cancel{2.5}}\ \text{mg}} \times 1\ \text{tablet} = 4\ \text{tablets}$	1 tablet : 2.5 mg : : x : 10 mg	$\dfrac{1\ \text{tablet}}{2.5\ \text{mg}} \times \dfrac{x}{10}$

$$10 = 2.5x$$

$$\frac{10}{2.5} = x$$

$$4\ \text{tablets} = x$$

5. No equivalent is needed.

Formula Method	Proportion Expressed as Two Ratios	Proportion Expressed as Two Fractions
$\dfrac{\overset{2}{\cancel{650}}\ \text{mg}}{\underset{1}{\cancel{325}}\ \text{mg}} \times 1\ \text{tablet} = 2\ \text{tablets}$	1 tablet : 325 mg : : x : 650 mg	$\dfrac{1\ \text{tablet}}{325\ \text{mg}} \times \dfrac{x}{650\ \text{mg}}$

$$650 = 325x$$

$$\frac{650}{325} = x$$

$$2\ \text{tablets} = x$$

6. No equivalent is needed.

Formula Method	Proportion Expressed as Two Ratios	Proportion Expressed as Two Fractions
$\dfrac{\cancel{20}\ \text{mg}}{\cancel{10}\ \text{mg}} \times 1\ \text{capsule} = 2\ \text{capsules}$	1 capsule : 10 mg : : x : 20 mg	$\dfrac{1\ \text{capsule}}{10\ \text{mg}} \times \dfrac{x}{20\ \text{mg}}$

$$20 = 10x$$

$$\frac{20}{10} = x$$

$$2\ \text{capsules} = x$$

7. No equivalent is needed.

Formula Method	Proportion Expressed as Two Ratios	Proportion Expressed as Two Fractions
$\dfrac{\overset{4}{\cancel{10}}\ \text{mg}}{\underset{1}{\cancel{2.5}}\ \text{mg}} \times 1\ \text{tablet} = 4\ \text{tablets}$	1 tablet : 2.5 mg : : x : 10 mg	$\dfrac{1\ \text{tablet}}{2.5\ \text{mg}} \times \dfrac{x}{10\ \text{mg}}$

$$10 = 2.5x$$

$$\frac{10}{2.5} = x$$

$$4\ \text{tablets} = x$$

8. No equivalent is needed.

Formula Method	Proportion Expressed as Two Ratios	Proportion Expressed as Two Fractions
$\dfrac{\overset{1}{\cancel{200,000 \text{ units}}}}{\underset{2}{\cancel{400,000 \text{ units}}}} \times 1 \text{ tablet} = \dfrac{1}{2} \text{ tablet}$	1 tablet : 400,000 units : : x : 200,000	$\dfrac{1 \text{ tablet}}{400,000 \text{ units}} \bigtimes \dfrac{x}{200,000 \text{ units}}$

$$200,000 = 400,000x$$

$$\frac{200,000}{400,000} = x$$

0.5 tablet = x

or ½ tablet

9. No equivalent is needed.

Formula Method	Proportion Expressed as Two Ratios	Proportion Expressed as Two Fractions
$\dfrac{\overset{2}{\cancel{0.50 \text{ mg}}}}{\underset{1}{\cancel{0.25 \text{ mg}}}} \times 1 \text{ tablet} = 2 \text{ tablets}$	1 tablet : 0.25 mg : : x : 0.5 mg	$\dfrac{1 \text{ tablet}}{0.25 \text{ mg}} \bigtimes \dfrac{x}{0.5 \text{ mg}}$

$$0.5 = 0.25x$$

$$\frac{0.50}{0.25} = x$$

2 tablets = x

10. No equivalent is needed.

Formula Method	Proportion Expressed as Two Ratios	Proportion Expressed as Two Fractions
$\dfrac{\overset{1.5}{\cancel{18.75 \text{ mg}}}}{\underset{1}{\cancel{12.5 \text{ mg}}}} \times 1 \text{ tablet} = 1.5 \text{ tablets}$ or 1½ tablets	1 tablet : 12.5 mg : : x : 18.75 mg	$\dfrac{1 \text{ tablet}}{12.5 \text{ mg}} \bigtimes \dfrac{x}{18.75 \text{ mg}}$

$$18.75 = 12.5x$$

$$\frac{18.75}{12.5} = x$$

1.5 tablets = x

or 1½ tablets

11. No equivalent is needed.

Formula Method	Proportion Expressed as Two Ratios	Proportion Expressed as Two Fractions
$\dfrac{\cancel{300 \text{ mg}}}{\cancel{200 \text{ mg}}} \times 1 \text{ tablet} = 1\tfrac{1}{2} \text{ tablets}$	1 tablet : 200 mg : : x : 300 mg	$\dfrac{1 \text{ tablet}}{200 \text{ mg}} \bigtimes \dfrac{x}{300 \text{ mg}}$

$$300 = 200x$$

$$\frac{300}{200} = x$$

1½ tablets = x

12. No equivalent is needed.

Formula Method	Proportion Expressed as Two Ratios	Proportion Expressed as Two Fractions
$\dfrac{0.3 \text{ mg}}{0.1 \text{ mg}} \times 1 \text{ tablet} = x$ $3 \text{ tablets} = x$	1 tablet : 0.1 mg : : x : 0.3 mg	$\dfrac{1 \text{ tablet}}{0.1 \text{ mg}} \times \dfrac{x}{0.3 \text{ mg}}$

$$0.3 = 0.1x$$

$$\frac{0.3}{0.1} = x$$

$$3 \text{ tablets} = x$$

13. No equivalent is needed.

Formula Method	Proportion Expressed as Two Ratios	Proportion Expressed as Two Fractions
$\dfrac{\overset{0.25}{\cancel{6.25}} \text{ mg}}{\underset{1}{\cancel{25}} \text{ mg}} \times 1 \text{ tablet} = 0.25 \text{ tablet}$ (tablets can be quartered)	1 tablet : 25 mg : : x : 6.25 mg	$\dfrac{1 \text{ tablet}}{25 \text{ mg}} \times \dfrac{x}{6.25 \text{ mg}}$

$$6.25 \text{ mg} = 25x$$

$$\frac{6.25}{25} = x$$

$$0.25 \text{ or } \frac{1}{4} \text{ tablet}$$

14. Equivalent: 0.2 mg = 200 mcg

Formula Method	Proportion Expressed as Two Ratios	Proportion Expressed as Two Fractions
$\dfrac{\overset{2}{\cancel{400}} \text{ mcg}}{\underset{1}{\cancel{200}} \text{ mcg}} \times 1 \text{ tablet} = 2 \text{ tablets}$	1 tablet : 200 mcg : : x : 400 mcg	$\dfrac{1 \text{ tablet}}{200 \text{ mcg}} \times \dfrac{x}{400 \text{ mcg}}$

$$400 = 200x$$

$$\frac{400}{200} = x$$

$$2 \text{ tablets} = x$$

15. No equivalent is needed.

Formula Method	Proportion Expressed as Two Ratios	Proportion Expressed as Two Fractions
$\dfrac{\overset{1.5}{\cancel{7.5}} \text{ mg}}{\underset{1}{\cancel{5}} \text{ mg}} \times 1 \text{ tablet} = 1.5 \text{ tablets}$ or 1½ tablets	1 tablet : 5 mg : : x : 7.5 mg	$\dfrac{1 \text{ tablet}}{5 \text{ mg}} \times \dfrac{x}{7.5 \text{ mg}}$

$$7.5 \text{ mg} = 5x$$

$$\frac{7.5}{5} = x$$

$$1.5 \text{ or } 1\frac{1}{2} \text{ tablets}$$

16. No equivalent is needed.

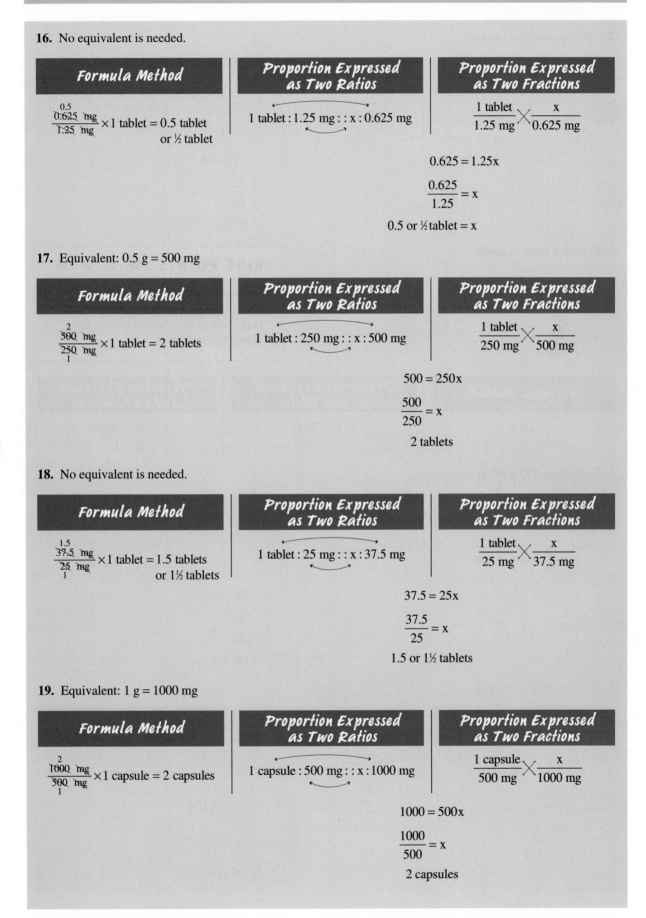

Formula Method	Proportion Expressed as Two Ratios	Proportion Expressed as Two Fractions
$\dfrac{\overset{0.5}{\cancel{0.625}\ \cancel{mg}}}{\cancel{1.25}\ \cancel{mg}} \times 1\ \text{tablet} = 0.5\ \text{tablet}$ or ½ tablet	1 tablet : 1.25 mg : : x : 0.625 mg	$\dfrac{1\ \text{tablet}}{1.25\ \text{mg}} \times \dfrac{x}{0.625\ \text{mg}}$

$$0.625 = 1.25x$$

$$\frac{0.625}{1.25} = x$$

0.5 or ½ tablet = x

17. Equivalent: 0.5 g = 500 mg

Formula Method	Proportion Expressed as Two Ratios	Proportion Expressed as Two Fractions
$\dfrac{\overset{2}{\cancel{500}\ \cancel{mg}}}{\underset{1}{\cancel{250}\ \cancel{mg}}} \times 1\ \text{tablet} = 2\ \text{tablets}$	1 tablet : 250 mg : : x : 500 mg	$\dfrac{1\ \text{tablet}}{250\ \text{mg}} \times \dfrac{x}{500\ \text{mg}}$

$$500 = 250x$$

$$\frac{500}{250} = x$$

2 tablets

18. No equivalent is needed.

Formula Method	Proportion Expressed as Two Ratios	Proportion Expressed as Two Fractions
$\dfrac{\overset{1.5}{\cancel{37.5}\ \cancel{mg}}}{\underset{1}{\cancel{25}\ \cancel{mg}}} \times 1\ \text{tablet} = 1.5\ \text{tablets}$ or 1½ tablets	1 tablet : 25 mg : : x : 37.5 mg	$\dfrac{1\ \text{tablet}}{25\ \text{mg}} \times \dfrac{x}{37.5\ \text{mg}}$

$$37.5 = 25x$$

$$\frac{37.5}{25} = x$$

1.5 or 1½ tablets

19. Equivalent: 1 g = 1000 mg

Formula Method	Proportion Expressed as Two Ratios	Proportion Expressed as Two Fractions
$\dfrac{\overset{2}{\cancel{1000}\ \cancel{mg}}}{\underset{1}{\cancel{500}\ \cancel{mg}}} \times 1\ \text{capsule} = 2\ \text{capsules}$	1 capsule : 500 mg : : x : 1000 mg	$\dfrac{1\ \text{capsule}}{500\ \text{mg}} \times \dfrac{x}{1000\ \text{mg}}$

$$1000 = 500x$$

$$\frac{1000}{500} = x$$

2 capsules

20. No equivalent is needed.

Formula Method	Proportion Expressed as Two Ratios	Proportion Expressed as Two Fractions
$\dfrac{\overset{2.5}{\cancel{25}}\ \cancel{mg}}{\underset{1}{\cancel{10}}\ \cancel{mg}} \times 1\ \text{tablet} = 2.5\ \text{tablets}$ or 2½ tablets	1 tablet : 10 mg : : x : 25 mg	$\dfrac{1\ \text{tablet}}{10\ \text{mg}} \times \dfrac{x}{25\ \text{mg}}$

$$25 = 10x$$

$$\frac{25}{10} = x$$

2.5 or 2½ tablets

Self-Test 2 Oral Liquids

FINE POINTS ● ○ ● ●

Calculations may be done in different ways. Answers should be the same regardless of the method chosen to solve the problem.

Formula Method	Proportion Expressed as Two Ratios	Proportion Expressed as Two Fractions
$\dfrac{D}{H} \times S = X$	S : H : : x : D	$\dfrac{S}{H} = \dfrac{x}{D}$

1. Equivalent 0.75 g = 750 mg

Formula Method	Proportion Expressed as Two Ratios	Proportion Expressed as Two Fractions
$\dfrac{\overset{3}{\cancel{750}}\ \cancel{mg}}{\underset{1}{\cancel{250}}\ \cancel{mg}} \times 1\ \text{mL} = 3\ \text{mL}$	1 mL : 250 mg : : x : 750 mg	$\dfrac{1\ \text{mL}}{250\ \text{mg}} \times \dfrac{x}{750\ \text{mg}}$

$$750 = 250x$$

$$\frac{750}{250} = x$$

3 mL = x

2. No equivalent is needed.

Formula Method	Proportion Expressed as Two Ratios	Proportion Expressed as Two Fractions
$\dfrac{\overset{2}{\cancel{500}}\ \cancel{mg}}{\underset{1}{\cancel{250}}\ \cancel{mg}} \times 5\ \text{mL} = 10\ \text{mL}$	5 mL : 250 mg : : x : 500 mg	$\dfrac{5\ \text{mL}}{250\ \text{mg}} \times \dfrac{x}{500\ \text{mg}}$

$$2500 = 250x$$

$$\frac{2500}{250} = x$$

10 mL = x

3. Equivalent 0.35 g = 350 mg

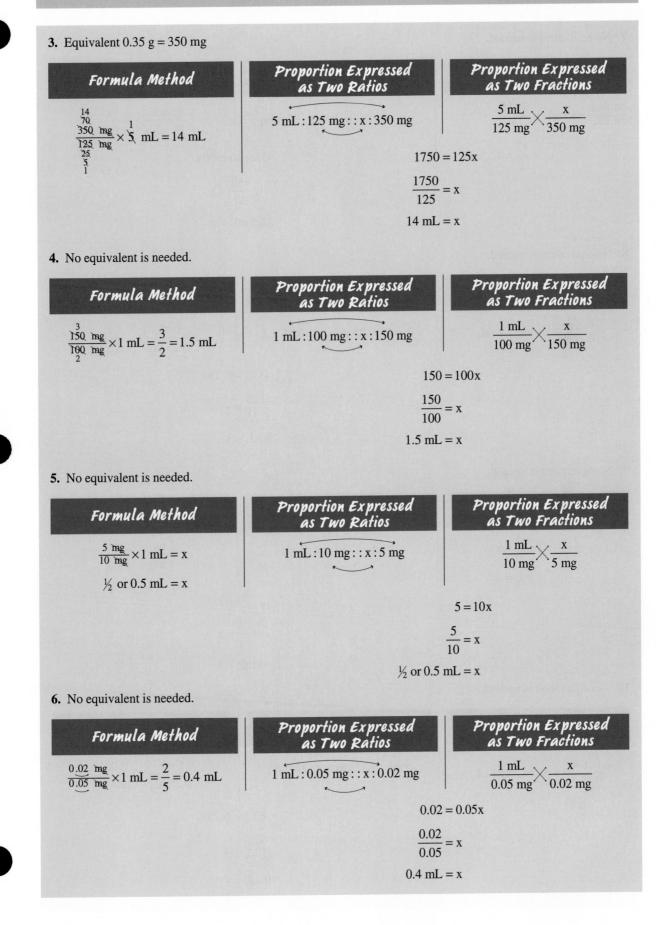

Formula Method	Proportion Expressed as Two Ratios	Proportion Expressed as Two Fractions
$\dfrac{\overset{14}{\overset{70}{\overset{350}{\cancel{125}}}} \text{ mg}}{\underset{1}{\underset{5}{\underset{25}{\cancel{125}}}} \text{ mg}} \times \overset{1}{\cancel{5}} \text{ mL} = 14 \text{ mL}$	5 mL : 125 mg : : x : 350 mg	$\dfrac{5 \text{ mL}}{125 \text{ mg}} \times \dfrac{\text{x}}{350 \text{ mg}}$

$$1750 = 125x$$
$$\frac{1750}{125} = x$$
$$14 \text{ mL} = x$$

4. No equivalent is needed.

Formula Method	Proportion Expressed as Two Ratios	Proportion Expressed as Two Fractions
$\dfrac{\overset{3}{\cancel{150}} \text{ mg}}{\underset{2}{\cancel{100}} \text{ mg}} \times 1 \text{ mL} = \dfrac{3}{2} = 1.5 \text{ mL}$	1 mL : 100 mg : : x : 150 mg	$\dfrac{1 \text{ mL}}{100 \text{ mg}} \times \dfrac{\text{x}}{150 \text{ mg}}$

$$150 = 100x$$
$$\frac{150}{100} = x$$
$$1.5 \text{ mL} = x$$

5. No equivalent is needed.

Formula Method	Proportion Expressed as Two Ratios	Proportion Expressed as Two Fractions
$\dfrac{5 \text{ mg}}{10 \text{ mg}} \times 1 \text{ mL} = x$ ½ or 0.5 mL = x	1 mL : 10 mg : : x : 5 mg	$\dfrac{1 \text{ mL}}{10 \text{ mg}} \times \dfrac{\text{x}}{5 \text{ mg}}$

$$5 = 10x$$
$$\frac{5}{10} = x$$
$$½ \text{ or } 0.5 \text{ mL} = x$$

6. No equivalent is needed.

Formula Method	Proportion Expressed as Two Ratios	Proportion Expressed as Two Fractions
$\dfrac{0.02 \text{ mg}}{0.05 \text{ mg}} \times 1 \text{ mL} = \dfrac{2}{5} = 0.4 \text{ mL}$	1 mL : 0.05 mg : : x : 0.02 mg	$\dfrac{1 \text{ mL}}{0.05 \text{ mg}} \times \dfrac{\text{x}}{0.02 \text{ mg}}$

$$0.02 = 0.05x$$
$$\frac{0.02}{0.05} = x$$
$$0.4 \text{ mL} = x$$

7. No equivalent is needed.

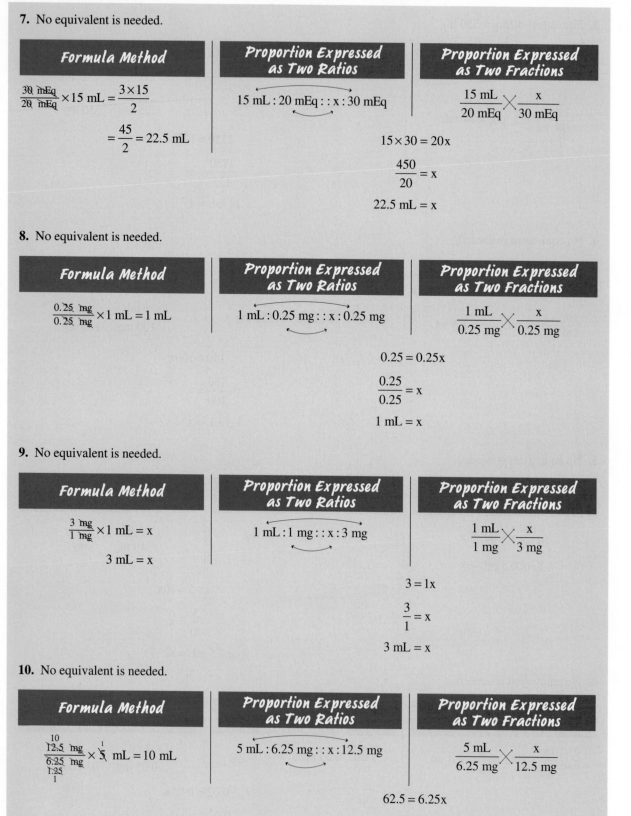

Formula Method	Proportion Expressed as Two Ratios	Proportion Expressed as Two Fractions
$\dfrac{30 \text{ mEq}}{20 \text{ mEq}} \times 15 \text{ mL} = \dfrac{3 \times 15}{2}$ $= \dfrac{45}{2} = 22.5 \text{ mL}$	15 mL : 20 mEq : : x : 30 mEq	$\dfrac{15 \text{ mL}}{20 \text{ mEq}} \times \dfrac{\text{x}}{30 \text{ mEq}}$

$$15 \times 30 = 20\text{x}$$
$$\frac{450}{20} = \text{x}$$
$$22.5 \text{ mL} = \text{x}$$

8. No equivalent is needed.

Formula Method	Proportion Expressed as Two Ratios	Proportion Expressed as Two Fractions
$\dfrac{0.25 \text{ mg}}{0.25 \text{ mg}} \times 1 \text{ mL} = 1 \text{ mL}$	1 mL : 0.25 mg : : x : 0.25 mg	$\dfrac{1 \text{ mL}}{0.25 \text{ mg}} \times \dfrac{\text{x}}{0.25 \text{ mg}}$

$$0.25 = 0.25\text{x}$$
$$\frac{0.25}{0.25} = \text{x}$$
$$1 \text{ mL} = \text{x}$$

9. No equivalent is needed.

Formula Method	Proportion Expressed as Two Ratios	Proportion Expressed as Two Fractions
$\dfrac{3 \text{ mg}}{1 \text{ mg}} \times 1 \text{ mL} = \text{x}$ $3 \text{ mL} = \text{x}$	1 mL : 1 mg : : x : 3 mg	$\dfrac{1 \text{ mL}}{1 \text{ mg}} \times \dfrac{\text{x}}{3 \text{ mg}}$

$$3 = 1\text{x}$$
$$\frac{3}{1} = \text{x}$$
$$3 \text{ mL} = \text{x}$$

10. No equivalent is needed.

Formula Method	Proportion Expressed as Two Ratios	Proportion Expressed as Two Fractions
$\dfrac{\overset{10}{\cancel{12.5} \text{ mg}}}{\underset{1}{\underset{1.25}{\cancel{6.25} \text{ mg}}}} \times \overset{1}{\cancel{5}} \text{ mL} = 10 \text{ mL}$	5 mL : 6.25 mg : : x : 12.5 mg	$\dfrac{5 \text{ mL}}{6.25 \text{ mg}} \times \dfrac{\text{x}}{12.5 \text{ mg}}$

$$62.5 = 6.25\text{x}$$
$$\frac{62.5}{6.25} = \text{x}$$
$$10 \text{ mL} = \text{x}$$

FINE POINTS ● ○ ● ●

Alternate arithmetic

$12.5 \times 5 = 62.5$

$$6.25 \overline{\smash{)}62.50} \quad \begin{array}{r} 10. \\ \end{array}$$
$$\underline{62\ 5}$$
$$0$$

11. No equivalent is needed.

Formula Method	Proportion Expressed as Two Ratios	Proportion Expressed as Two Fractions
$\dfrac{\overset{5}{\cancel{50}} \text{ mg}}{\underset{1}{\cancel{10}} \text{ mg}} \times 5 \text{ mL} = 25 \text{ mL}$	5 mL : 10 mg : : x : 50 mg	$\dfrac{5 \text{ mL}}{10 \text{ mg}} \times \dfrac{\text{x}}{50 \text{ mg}}$

$$5 \times 50 = 10x$$

$$\frac{250}{10} = x$$

$$25 \text{ mL} = x$$

12. No equivalent is needed.

Formula Method	Proportion Expressed as Two Ratios	Proportion Expressed as Two Fractions
$\dfrac{\overset{4}{\cancel{40}} \text{ mg}}{\underset{1}{\cancel{10}} \text{ mg}} \times 1 \text{ mL} = 4 \text{ mL}$	1 mL : 10 mg : : x : 40 mg	$\dfrac{1 \text{ mL}}{10 \text{ mg}} \times \dfrac{\text{x}}{40 \text{ mg}}$

$$40 = 10x$$

$$\frac{40}{10} = x$$

$$4 \text{ mL} = x$$

13. No equivalent is needed.

Formula Method	Proportion Expressed as Two Ratios	Proportion Expressed as Two Fractions
$\dfrac{\overset{1}{\cancel{10}} \text{ mEq}}{\underset{2}{\cancel{20}} \text{ mEq}} \times 30 \text{ mL} = \dfrac{30}{2} = 15 \text{ mL}$	30 mL : 20 mEq : : x : 10 mEq	$\dfrac{30 \text{ mL}}{20 \text{ mEq}} \times \dfrac{\text{x}}{10 \text{ mEq}}$

$$30 \times 10 = 20x$$

$$\frac{300}{20} = x$$

$$15 \text{ mL} = x$$

14. No equivalent is needed.

Formula Method	Proportion Expressed as Two Ratios	Proportion Expressed as Two Fractions
$\dfrac{\overset{2}{\cancel{10}\text{ mg}}}{\underset{1}{\cancel{5}\text{ mg}}} \times 5 \text{ mL} = 10 \text{ mL}$	$5 \text{ mL} : 5 \text{ mg} :: x : 10 \text{ mg}$	$\dfrac{5 \text{ mL}}{5 \text{ mg}} \times \dfrac{x}{10 \text{ mg}}$

$$10 \times 5 = 5x$$

$$\frac{50}{5} = x$$

$$10 \text{ mL} = x$$

15. No equivalent is needed.

Formula Method	Proportion Expressed as Two Ratios	Proportion Expressed as Two Fractions
$\dfrac{\overset{5}{\cancel{100}\text{ mg}}}{\underset{1}{\cancel{20}\text{ mg}}} \times 5 \text{ mL} = 25 \text{ mL}$	$5 \text{ mL} : 20 \text{ mg} :: x : 100 \text{ mg}$	$\dfrac{5 \text{ mL}}{20 \text{ mg}} \times \dfrac{x}{100 \text{ mg}}$

$$5 \times 100 = 20x$$

$$\frac{500}{20} = x$$

$$25 \text{ mL} = x$$

16. Equivalent: gr 10 = 650 mg

Formula Method	Proportion Expressed as Two Ratios	Proportion Expressed as Two Fractions
$\dfrac{650 \text{ mg}}{160 \text{ mg}} \times 5 \text{ mL} = \dfrac{3250}{160} = 20.31$ or 20 mL	$5 \text{ mL} : 160 \text{ mg} :: x : 650 \text{ mg}$	$\dfrac{5 \text{ mL}}{160 \text{ mg}} \times \dfrac{x}{650 \text{ mg}}$

$$650 \times 5 = 160x$$

$$\frac{3250}{160} = x$$

$$20.31 \text{ or } 20 \text{ mL}$$

17. No equivalent is needed.

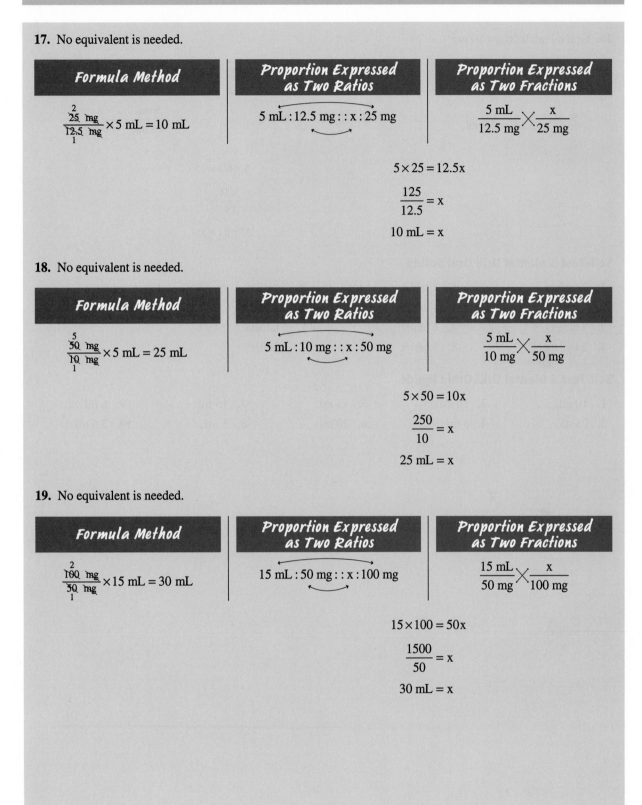

Formula Method	Proportion Expressed as Two Ratios	Proportion Expressed as Two Fractions
$\dfrac{\overset{2}{\cancel{25}}\ \cancel{mg}}{\underset{1}{\cancel{12.5}}\ \cancel{mg}} \times 5\ mL = 10\ mL$	$5\ mL : 12.5\ mg :: x : 25\ mg$	$\dfrac{5\ mL}{12.5\ mg} \times \dfrac{x}{25\ mg}$

$$5 \times 25 = 12.5x$$

$$\frac{125}{12.5} = x$$

$$10\ mL = x$$

18. No equivalent is needed.

Formula Method	Proportion Expressed as Two Ratios	Proportion Expressed as Two Fractions
$\dfrac{\overset{5}{\cancel{50}}\ \cancel{mg}}{\underset{1}{\cancel{10}}\ \cancel{mg}} \times 5\ mL = 25\ mL$	$5\ mL : 10\ mg :: x : 50\ mg$	$\dfrac{5\ mL}{10\ mg} \times \dfrac{x}{50\ mg}$

$$5 \times 50 = 10x$$

$$\frac{250}{10} = x$$

$$25\ mL = x$$

19. No equivalent is needed.

Formula Method	Proportion Expressed as Two Ratios	Proportion Expressed as Two Fractions
$\dfrac{\overset{2}{\cancel{100}}\ \cancel{mg}}{\underset{1}{\cancel{50}}\ \cancel{mg}} \times 15\ mL = 30\ mL$	$15\ mL : 50\ mg :: x : 100\ mg$	$\dfrac{15\ mL}{50\ mg} \times \dfrac{x}{100\ mg}$

$$15 \times 100 = 50x$$

$$\frac{1500}{50} = x$$

$$30\ mL = x$$

20. Equivalent: 0.06 g = 60 mg

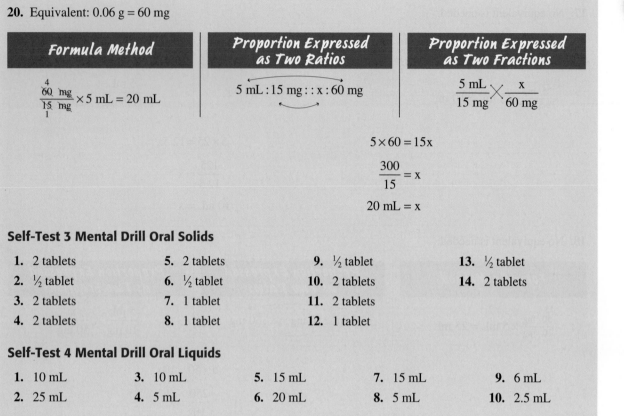

Formula Method	Proportion Expressed as Two Ratios	Proportion Expressed as Two Fractions

$$\frac{\overset{4}{\cancel{60}} \text{ mg}}{\underset{1}{\cancel{15}} \text{ mg}} \times 5 \text{ mL} = 20 \text{ mL}$$

$$5 \text{ mL} : 15 \text{ mg} :: x : 60 \text{ mg}$$

$$\frac{5 \text{ mL}}{15 \text{ mg}} \times \frac{x}{60 \text{ mg}}$$

$$5 \times 60 = 15x$$

$$\frac{300}{15} = x$$

$$20 \text{ mL} = x$$

Self-Test 3 Mental Drill Oral Solids

1. 2 tablets

2. ½ tablet

3. 2 tablets

4. 2 tablets

5. 2 tablets

6. ½ tablet

7. 1 tablet

8. 1 tablet

9. ½ tablet

10. 2 tablets

11. 2 tablets

12. 1 tablet

13. ½ tablet

14. 2 tablets

Self-Test 4 Mental Drill Oral Liquids

1. 10 mL

2. 25 mL

3. 10 mL

4. 5 mL

5. 15 mL

6. 20 mL

7. 15 mL

8. 5 mL

9. 6 mL

10. 2.5 mL

LEARNING OBJECTIVES

1. Solving injection-from-liquid problems

2. Syringes and marking

3. Insulin injections

4. Mixing insulins

5. Sliding-scale insulin calculations

6. Principles for reconstituting drugs from powder form

   Reading and understanding drug manufacturer's label and package insert directions

   Storing reconstituted drugs safely

   Labeling reconstituted drugs

Liquid drugs for injection are prepared by pharmaceutical companies as sterile solutions, powders, or suspensions. Aseptic techniques are used to prepare and administer them. As with oral medications, the nurse may have to calculate the correct dosage. The nurse must also follow correct administration techniques and special considerations (i.e., correct dilution, injection site, size of needle, speed of IV injection, etc.).

RULE **CALCULATING LIQUID INJECTIONS**

To solve liquid injection problems, use the same rule as for oral solids and liquids. ■

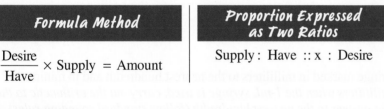

Formula Method	Proportion Expressed as Two Ratios	Proportion Expressed as Two Fractions
$\dfrac{\text{Desire}}{\text{Have}} \times \text{Supply} = \text{Amount}$	Supply : Have :: x : Desire	$\dfrac{\text{Supply}}{\text{Have}} = \dfrac{\text{x}}{\text{Desire}}$

Example Order: Stelazine (trifluoperazine) 1.5 mg IM q6h prn

Supply: Read the label

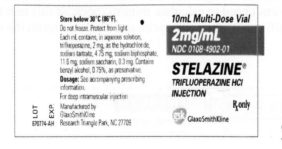

Store below 30°C (86°F).
Do not freeze. Protect from light.
Each mL contains, in aqueous solution, trifluoperazine, 2 mg, as the hydrochloride, sodium tartrate, 4.75 mg; sodium biphosphate, 11.6 mg; sodium saccharin, 0.3 mg. Contains benzyl alcohol, 0.75%, as preservative.
Dosage: See accompanying prescribing information.
For deep intramuscular injection
LOT
EXP.
670774-AH
Manufactured by
GlaxoSmithKline
Research Triangle Park, NC 27709

10mL Multi-Dose Vial
2mg/mL
NDC 0108-4902-01
STELAZINE®
TRIFLUOPERAZINE HCl
INJECTION
R only
GlaxoSmithKline

Courtesy of GlaxoSmithKline.

Desire: the amount ordered, here, 1.5 mg

Have: strength of the drug supplied, here, 2 mg

Supply: the unit form of the drug, here, 1 mL (For liquid calculations the supply is usually 1 mL)

Amount or *Answer:* how much liquid to give by injection in mL. "x" is used in all 3 methods.

Formula Method	Proportion Expressed as Two Ratios	Proportion Expressed as Two Fractions
$\dfrac{1.5 \text{ mg}}{2 \text{ mg}} \times 1 \text{ mL} = x$ $0.75 \text{ mL} = x$	$1 \text{ mL} : 2 \text{ mg} :: x : 1.5 \text{ mg}$	$\dfrac{1 \text{ mL}}{2 \text{ mg}} \times \dfrac{x}{1.5 \text{ mg}}$ $2x = 1.5$ $x = \dfrac{1.5}{2}$ $x = 0.75 \text{ mL}$

Calculating Injection Problems

3-mL Syringe

When you're calculating injection answers, the degree of accuracy depends on the syringe you use. Figure 7-1 shows a 3-mL syringe marked in milliliters to the nearest tenth and in minims to the nearest whole number. *To calculate milliliter answers for this 3-mL syringe, carry out the arithmetic to the hundredth place and then round off the answer to the nearest tenth (follow standard rounding rules).*

1.25 mL becomes 1.3 mL

1-mL Precision Syringe

Figure 7-2 shows a 1-mL precision syringe marked in milliliters to the nearest hundredth and in minims to the nearest half-minim. *To calculate milliliters when the 1-mL syringe is used, carry out the arithmetic to the thousandth place and then round off the answer to the nearest hundredth (follow standard rounding rules).*

0.978 mL becomes 0.98 mL

Each of the following examples provides a syringe. Calculate milliliters to the degree of accuracy required by the syringe markings. (You don't need to calculate minims, because this unit is rarely used; however, minim markings—M or m—still appear on many syringes.) Draw a line on the syringe to indicate your answer for milliliters.

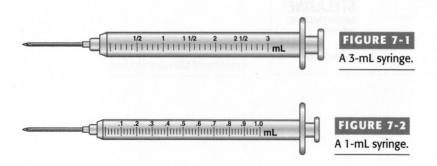

FIGURE 7-1
A 3-mL syringe.

FIGURE 7-2
A 1-mL syringe.

Example   Order: Demerol (meperidine HCl) 75 mg IM q4h prn

Supply: Read the label.

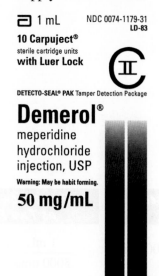

NDC 0074-1179-31
LD-83

1 mL

10 Carpuject®
sterile cartridge units
with Luer Lock

DETECTO-SEAL® PAK Tamper Detection Package

Demerol®
meperidine
hydrochloride
injection, USP

Warning: May be habit forming.

50 mg/mL

Courtesy of Abbott Laboratories.

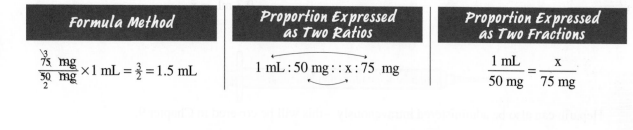

Formula Method	Proportion Expressed as Two Ratios	Proportion Expressed as Two Fractions
$\dfrac{\overset{3}{\cancel{75}}\ \text{mg}}{\underset{2}{\cancel{50}}\ \text{mg}} \times 1\ \text{mL} = \dfrac{3}{2} = 1.5\ \text{mL}$	$1\ \text{mL} : 50\ \text{mg} :: x : 75\ \text{mg}$	$\dfrac{1\ \text{mL}}{50\ \text{mg}} = \dfrac{x}{75\ \text{mg}}$

$$\frac{75}{50} = x$$

$$1.5\ \text{mL} = x$$
$$\text{or } 1\tfrac{1}{2}\ \text{mL}$$

Give 1.5 mL IM.

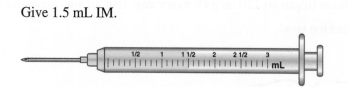

Example

Order: heparin sodium 1500 units subcutaneous bid

Supply: Read the label.

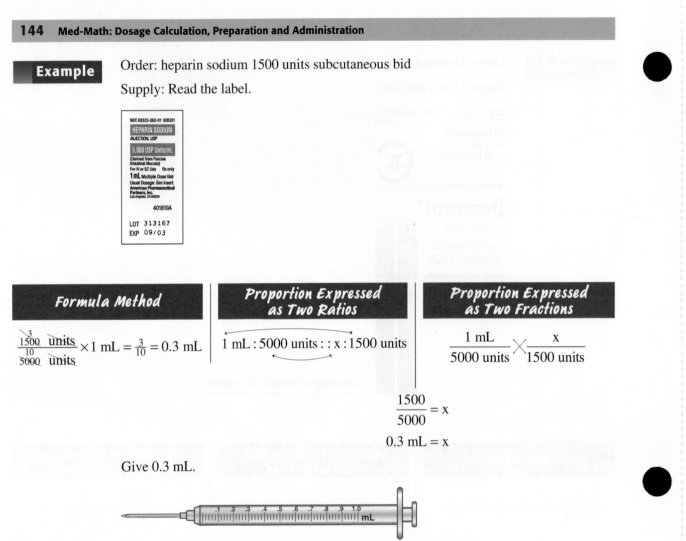

NDC 63323-262-01 926201

HEPARIN SODIUM
INJECTION, USP

5,000 USP Units/mL
(Derived from Porcine
Intestinal Mucosa)
For IV or SC Use   Rx only
1 mL Multiple Dose Vial
Usual Dosage: See insert.
**American Pharmaceutical
Partners, Inc.**
Los Angeles, CA 90024

401810A

LOT 313167
EXP 09/03

Formula Method	Proportion Expressed as Two Ratios	Proportion Expressed as Two Fractions
$\dfrac{\overset{3}{\cancel{1500}}\ \text{units}}{\underset{10}{\cancel{5000}}\ \text{units}} \times 1\ \text{mL} = \dfrac{3}{10} = 0.3\ \text{mL}$	1 mL : 5000 units : : x : 1500 units	$\dfrac{1\ \text{mL}}{5000\ \text{units}} \times \dfrac{\text{x}}{1500\ \text{units}}$

$$\frac{1500}{5000} = x$$

$$0.3\ \text{mL} = x$$

Give 0.3 mL.

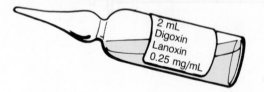

Heparin can also be administered intravenously—this will be covered in Chapter 9.

IV Medications

IV push (IVP) medications must be diluted and administered either according to directions in a nursing drug book or according to hospital policy. First, calculate the correct dose.

Example

Order: Lanoxin (digoxin) 120 mcg IV every day. Use a 1 mL precision syringe.

Supply: Read the label.

2 mL
Digoxin
Lanoxin
0.25 mg/mL

Conversion: 0.25 mg = 250 mcg

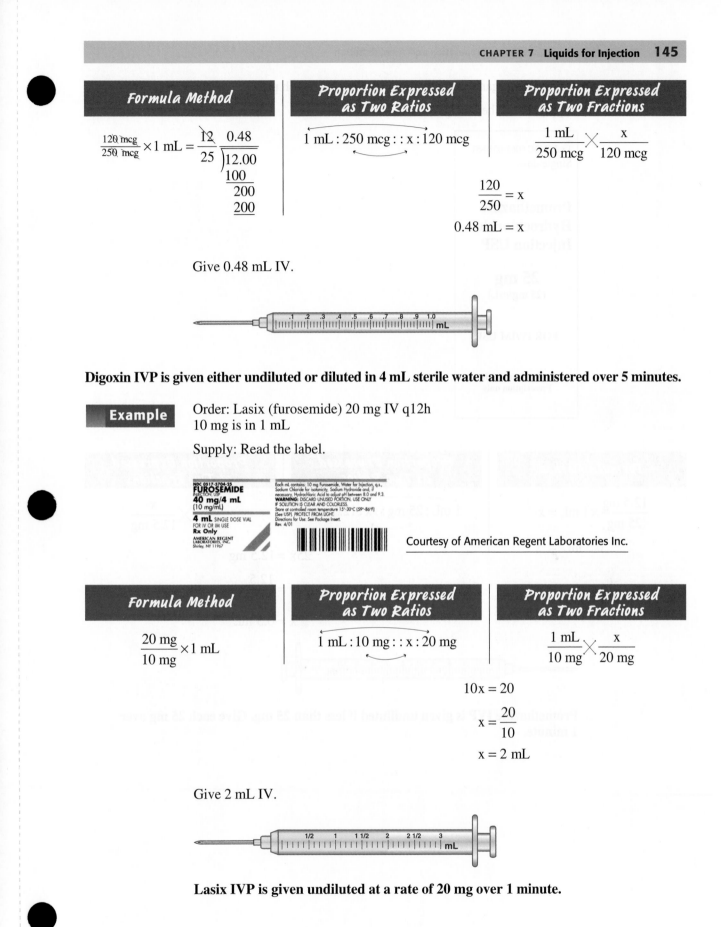

Formula Method	Proportion Expressed as Two Ratios	Proportion Expressed as Two Fractions
$\dfrac{120 \text{ mcg}}{250 \text{ mcg}} \times 1 \text{ mL} = \dfrac{12}{25} \overline{)\begin{array}{l}0.48 \\ 12.00 \\ \underline{100} \\ 200 \\ \underline{200} \end{array}}$	$1 \text{ mL} : 250 \text{ mcg} :: x : 120 \text{ mcg}$	$\dfrac{1 \text{ mL}}{250 \text{ mcg}} \times \dfrac{x}{120 \text{ mcg}}$

$$\frac{120}{250} = x$$

$$0.48 \text{ mL} = x$$

Give 0.48 mL IV.

Digoxin IVP is given either undiluted or diluted in 4 mL sterile water and administered over 5 minutes.

Example Order: Lasix (furosemide) 20 mg IV q12h
10 mg is in 1 mL

Supply: Read the label.

NDC 0517-5704-25
FUROSEMIDE
INJECTION, USP
40 mg/4 mL
(10 mg/mL)
4 mL SINGLE DOSE VIAL
FOR IV OR IM USE
Rx Only
AMERICAN REGENT
LABORATORIES, INC.
Shirley, NY 11967

Each mL contains: 10 mg Furosemide, Water for Injection, q.s.,
Sodium Chloride for isotonicity, Sodium Hydroxide and, if
necessary, Hydrochloric Acid to adjust pH between 8.0 and 9.3.
WARNING: DISCARD UNUSED PORTION. USE ONLY
IF SOLUTION IS CLEAR AND COLORLESS.
Store at controlled room temperature 15°-30°C (59°-86°F)
[See USP]. PROTECT FROM LIGHT.
Directions for Use: See Package Insert.
Rev. 4/01

Courtesy of American Regent Laboratories Inc.

Formula Method	Proportion Expressed as Two Ratios	Proportion Expressed as Two Fractions
$\dfrac{20 \text{ mg}}{10 \text{ mg}} \times 1 \text{ mL}$	$1 \text{ mL} : 10 \text{ mg} :: x : 20 \text{ mg}$	$\dfrac{1 \text{ mL}}{10 \text{ mg}} \times \dfrac{x}{20 \text{ mg}}$

$$10x = 20$$

$$x = \frac{20}{10}$$

$$x = 2 \text{ mL}$$

Give 2 mL IV.

Lasix IVP is given undiluted at a rate of 20 mg over 1 minute.

Example   Order: Phenergan (promethazine) 12.5 mg IV q4–6h prn

Supply: Read the label.

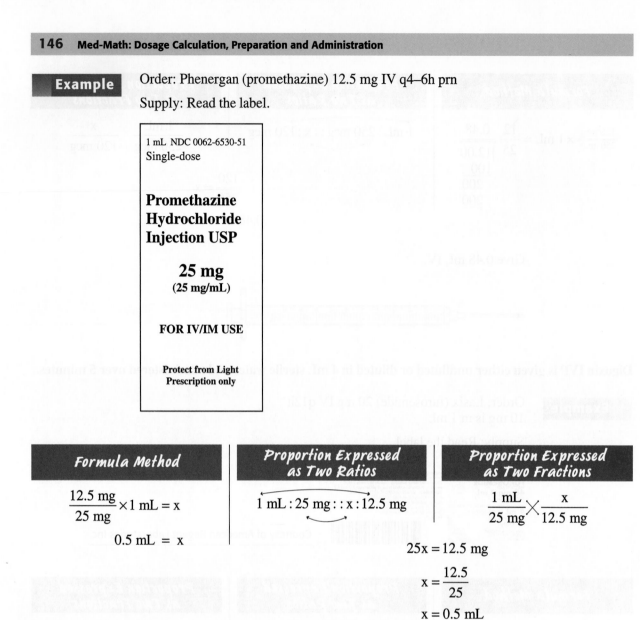

1 mL NDC 0062-6530-51
Single-dose

**Promethazine
Hydrochloride
Injection USP**

25 mg
(25 mg/mL)

FOR IV/IM USE

**Protect from Light
Prescription only**

Formula Method	Proportion Expressed as Two Ratios	Proportion Expressed as Two Fractions
$\dfrac{12.5 \text{ mg}}{25 \text{ mg}} \times 1 \text{ mL} = x$	1 mL : 25 mg : : x : 12.5 mg	$\dfrac{1 \text{ mL}}{25 \text{ mg}} \times \dfrac{x}{12.5 \text{ mg}}$
0.5 mL = x		

$$25x = 12.5 \text{ mg}$$

$$x = \frac{12.5}{25}$$

$$x = 0.5 \text{ mL}$$

Promethazine IVP is given undiluted if less than 25 mg. Give each 25 mg over 1 minute.

SELF-TEST 1   **Calculation of Liquids for Injection**

Practice calculations of injections from a liquid. Report your answer in milliliters; mark the syringe in milliliters. Answers appear at the end of the chapter.

1. Order: Clindamycin (cleocin) 0.3 g IM q6h
   Supply: liquid in a vial labeled 300 mg/2 mL

2. Order: morphine 12 mg IV stat
   Supply: vial of liquid labeled 15 mg/mL

3. Order: vitamin B$_{12}$ 1 mg IM every day
   Supply: vial of liquid labeled 1000 mcg/mL

4. Order: gentamicin 9 mg IM q8h
   Supply: pediatric ampule labeled 20 mg/2 mL

5. Order: Lanoxin (digoxin) 0.5 mg IV q6h × 3 doses
   Supply: vial labeled 0.25 mg/mL

6. Order: gentamicin 50 mg IM q8h
   Supply: vial labeled 40 mg/mL

(continued)

7. Order: phenobarbital 100 mg IM stat
Supply: ampule labeled 130 mg/mL

8. Order: Lanoxin (digoxin) 0.25 mg IV stat
Supply: ampule labeled 0.5 mg/2 mL

9. Order: heparin 6000 units subcutaneous q4h
Supply: vial labeled 10,000 units/mL

10. Order: Terbutaline (brethine) 0.25 mg subcutaneous for preterm contractions
Supply: ampule labeled 1 mg/1 mL

11. Order: Normadyne (labetolol) 20 mg IV stat
Supply: vial labeled 5 mg/mL

12. Order: Haldol (haloperidol) 2.5 mg IM q 4-8 hr
Supply: vial labeled 5 mg/Ml

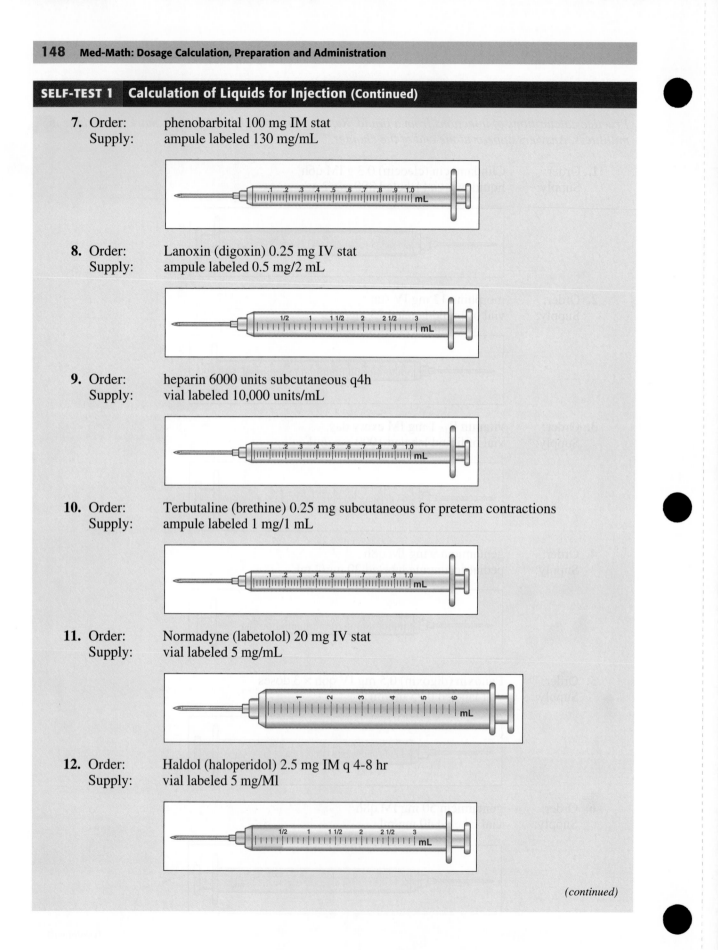

(continued)

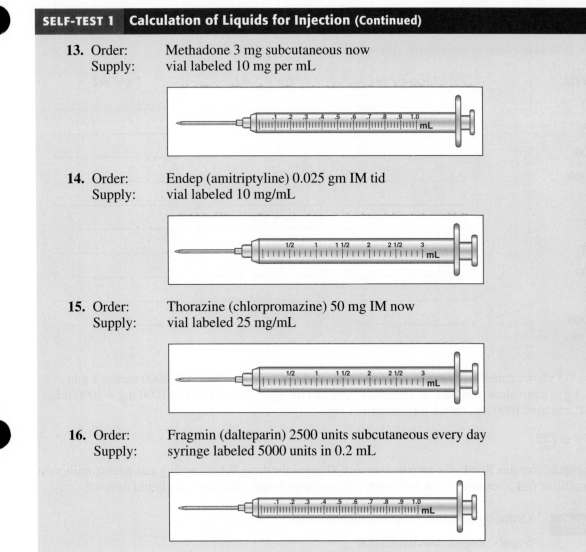

SELF-TEST 1 | **Calculation of Liquids for Injection (Continued)**

13. Order: Methadone 3 mg subcutaneous now
Supply: vial labeled 10 mg per mL

14. Order: Endep (amitriptyline) 0.025 gm IM tid
Supply: vial labeled 10 mg/mL

15. Order: Thorazine (chlorpromazine) 50 mg IM now
Supply: vial labeled 25 mg/mL

16. Order: Fragmin (dalteparin) 2500 units subcutaneous every day
Supply: syringe labeled 5000 units in 0.2 mL

Special Types of Problems in Injections From a Liquid

When Supply Is a Ratio

Labels may state the strength of a drug as a ratio.

Example | Adrenalin 1:1000

Ratios are always interpreted in the metric system as grams per milliliters. In the example given, 1:1000 means 1 g in 1000 mL. Ratios may be stated in three ways:

1 g per 1000 mL

1 g = 1000 mL

1 g/1000 mL

SELF-TEST 2 | **Ratios**

Write the following ratios in three ways. Answers appear at the end of the chapter.

RATIO	? g per ? mL	? g = ? mL	? g/? mL
1:20			
2:15			
1:500			
2:2000			
1:4			
2:25			
4:50			
1:100			
3:75			
5:1000			

Figure 7-3 shows epinephrine that is labeled 30 mL and is a 1:1000 solution. 1:1000 means 1 g in 1000 mL. 1 g is equivalent to 1000 mg. Therefore, you can interpret the solution as 1000 mg = 1000 mL. If 1000 mL contains 1000 mg, then 1 mL contains 1 mg.

$$\frac{1000 \text{ mg}}{1000 \text{ mL}} = \frac{1 \text{ mg}}{1 \text{ mL}}$$

Since the ampule contains 30 mL, the ampule contains 30 mg of the drug. When reading and writing milligram (mg) and milliliter (mL), remember that milligram is the solid measure; milliliter is the liquid measure.

Example

Order: epinephrine 1 mg subcutaneous stat

Supply: ampule labeled 1:1000

Equivalent: 1:1000 means

    1 g in 1000 mL

    1 g = 1000 mg

Therefore, 1000 mL contains 1000 mg.

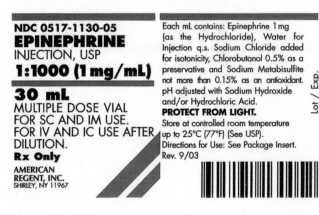

NDC 0517-1130-05
EPINEPHRINE
INJECTION, USP
1:1000 (1 mg/mL)
30 mL
MULTIPLE DOSE VIAL
FOR SC AND IM USE.
FOR IV AND IC USE AFTER DILUTION.
Rx Only
AMERICAN
REGENT, INC.
SHIRLEY, NY 11967

Each mL contains: Epinephrine 1 mg (as the Hydrochloride), Water for Injection q.s. Sodium Chloride added for isotonicity, Chlorobutanol 0.5% as a preservative and Sodium Metabisulfite not more than 0.15% as an antioxidant. pH adjusted with Sodium Hydroxide and/or Hydrochloric Acid.
PROTECT FROM LIGHT.
Store at controlled room temperature up to 25°C (77°F) (See USP). Directions for Use: See Package Insert. Rev. 9/03

Lot / Exp.

FIGURE 7-3

Epinephrine 1:1000. (Courtesy of American Regent Laboratories, Inc.)

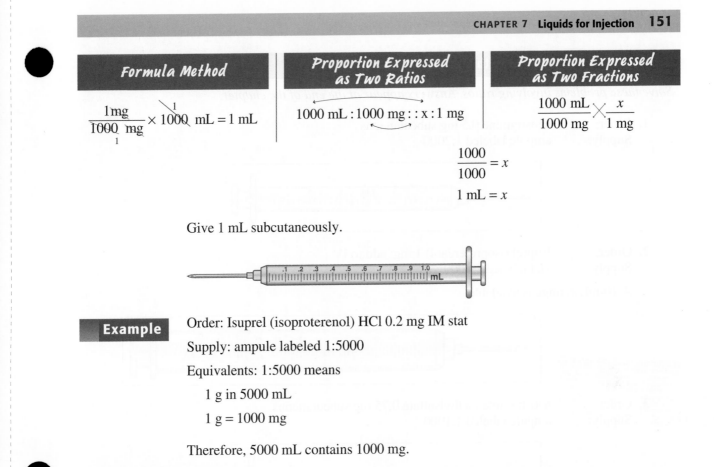

Formula Method	Proportion Expressed as Two Ratios	Proportion Expressed as Two Fractions
$\dfrac{1\,mg}{1000\,mg} \times 1000\,mL = 1\,mL$	$1000\,mL : 1000\,mg :: x : 1\,mg$	$\dfrac{1000\,mL}{1000\,mg} \times \dfrac{x}{1\,mg}$

$$\frac{1000}{1000} = x$$

$$1\,mL = x$$

Give 1 mL subcutaneously.

Example

Order: Isuprel (isoproterenol) HCl 0.2 mg IM stat

Supply: ampule labeled 1:5000

Equivalents: 1:5000 means

    1 g in 5000 mL

    1 g = 1000 mg

Therefore, 5000 mL contains 1000 mg.

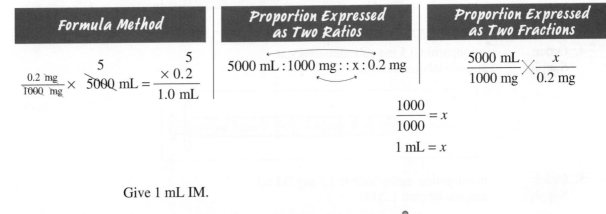

Formula Method	Proportion Expressed as Two Ratios	Proportion Expressed as Two Fractions
$\dfrac{0.2\,mg}{1000\,mg} \times 5000\,mL = \dfrac{\times 0.2}{1.0\,mL}$	$5000\,mL : 1000\,mg :: x : 0.2\,mg$	$\dfrac{5000\,mL}{1000\,mg} \times \dfrac{x}{0.2\,mg}$

$$\frac{1000}{1000} = x$$

$$1\,mL = x$$

Give 1 mL IM.

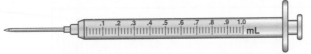

SELF-TEST 3   Using Ratios with Liquids for Injection

Solve these problems involving ratios. Answers appear at the end of the chapter.

1. Order: neostigmine 0.5 mg subcutaneous
    Supply: ampule labeled 1:2000

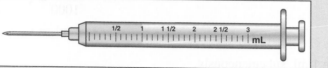

2. Order: Isuprel (isoproterenol) 1 mg: add to IV
    Supply: vial labeled 1:5000

A 10-mL syringe is available.

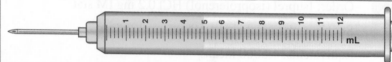

3. Order: neostigmine methylsulfate 0.75 mg subcutaneous
    Supply: ampule labeled 1:1000

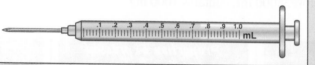

4. Order: epinephrine 0.5 mg subcutaneous stat
    Supply: ampule labeled 1:1000

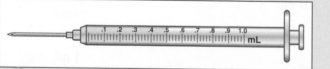

5. Order: neostigmine methylsulfate 1.5 mg IM tid
    Supply: ampule labeled 1:2000

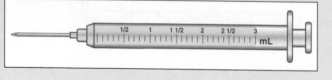

When Supply Is a Percent

Labels may state the strength of a drug as a percent. Percent means parts per hundred. *Percentages are always interpreted in the metric system as grams per 100 mL.*

Example   Lidocaine 2% = 2 g in 100 mL

Percents may be stated in three ways:

> 2 g per 100 mL
>
> 2 g = 100 mL
>
> 2 g/100 mL

SELF-TEST 4   Percentages

Write the following percentage in three ways. Answers appear at the end of the chapter.

PERCENTAGE	? g per 100 mL	? g = 100 mL	? g/100 mL
0.9%	_____	_____	_____
10%	_____	_____	_____
0.45%	_____	_____	_____
50%	_____	_____	_____
0.33%	_____	_____	_____
5%	_____	_____	_____
30%	_____	_____	_____
1.5%	_____	_____	_____
1%	_____	_____	_____
20%	_____	_____	_____

To solve percent problems, state the percent as the number of grams per mL.

Example   Order: lidocaine 30 mg for injection before suturing wound

Supply: Read the label.

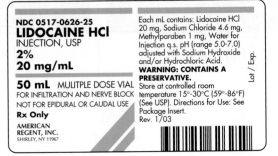

NDC 0517-0626-25
LIDOCAINE HCl
INJECTION, USP
2%
20 mg/mL

50 mL   MULITPLE DOSE VIAL
FOR INFILTRATION AND NERVE BLOCK
NOT FOR EPIDURAL OR CAUDAL USE
Rx Only
AMERICAN
REGENT, INC.
SHIRLEY, NY 11967

Each mL contains: Lidocaine HCl
20 mg, Sodium Chloride 4.6 mg,
Methylparaben 1 mg, Water for
Injection q.s. pH (range 5.0-7.0)
adjusted with Sodium Hydroxide
and/or Hydrochloric Acid.
**WARNING: CONTAINS A
PRESERVATIVE.**
Store at controlled room
temperature 15°-30°C (59°-86°F)
(See USP). Directions for Use: See
Package Insert.
Rev. 1/03

Lot / Exp.

Courtesy of American Regent Laboratories Inc.

Equivalents: 2% means

2 g in 100 mL

1 g = 1000 mg

2 g = 2000 mg

Supply is 2000 mg in 100 mL.

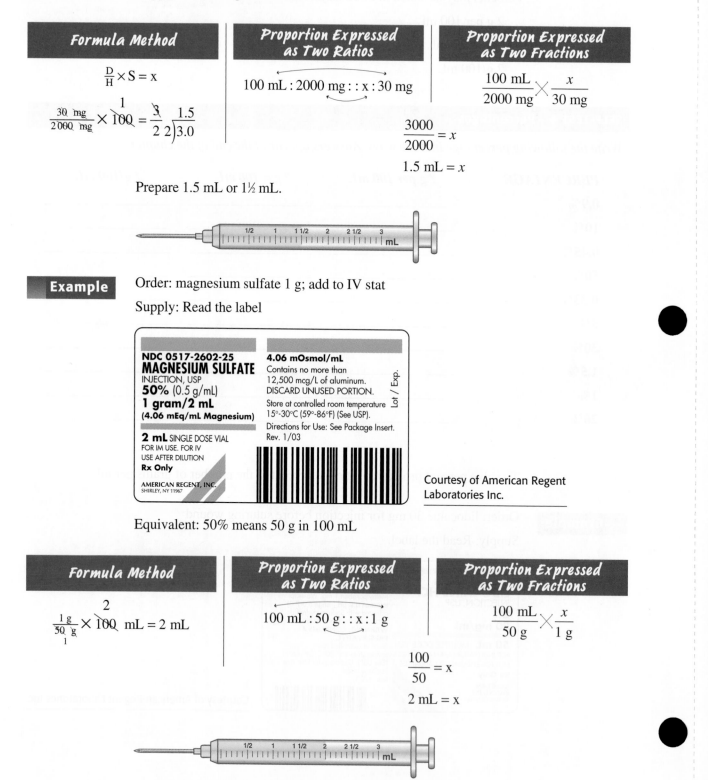

Formula Method	Proportion Expressed as Two Ratios	Proportion Expressed as Two Fractions
$\dfrac{D}{H} \times S = x$	100 mL : 2000 mg : : x : 30 mg	$\dfrac{100\ mL}{2000\ mg} \times \dfrac{x}{30\ mg}$
$\dfrac{30\ mg}{2000\ mg} \times 100 = \dfrac{3}{2}\ 2\overline{)3.0}$		$\dfrac{3000}{2000} = x$
		$1.5\ mL = x$

Prepare 1.5 mL or 1½ mL.

Example   Order: magnesium sulfate 1 g; add to IV stat

Supply: Read the label

NDC 0517-2602-25
MAGNESIUM SULFATE
INJECTION, USP
50% (0.5 g/mL)
1 gram/2 mL
(4.06 mEq/mL Magnesium)

2 mL SINGLE DOSE VIAL
FOR IM USE. FOR IV
USE AFTER DILUTION
Rx Only

AMERICAN REGENT, INC.
SHIRLEY, NY 11967

4.06 mOsmol/mL
Contains no more than
12,500 mcg/L of aluminum.
DISCARD UNUSED PORTION.
Store at controlled room temperature
15°-30°C (59°-86°F) (See USP).
Directions for Use: See Package Insert.
Rev. 1/03

Lot / Exp.

Courtesy of American Regent
Laboratories Inc.

Equivalent: 50% means 50 g in 100 mL

Formula Method	Proportion Expressed as Two Ratios	Proportion Expressed as Two Fractions
$\dfrac{1\ g}{50\ g} \times 100\ mL = 2\ mL$	100 mL : 50 g : : x : 1 g	$\dfrac{100\ mL}{50\ g} \times \dfrac{x}{1\ g}$
		$\dfrac{100}{50} = x$
		$2\ mL = x$

SELF-TEST 5   Using Percentages with Liquids for Injection

Solve these problems involving percentages. Answers appear at the end of the chapter. Answers are in milliliters (mL).

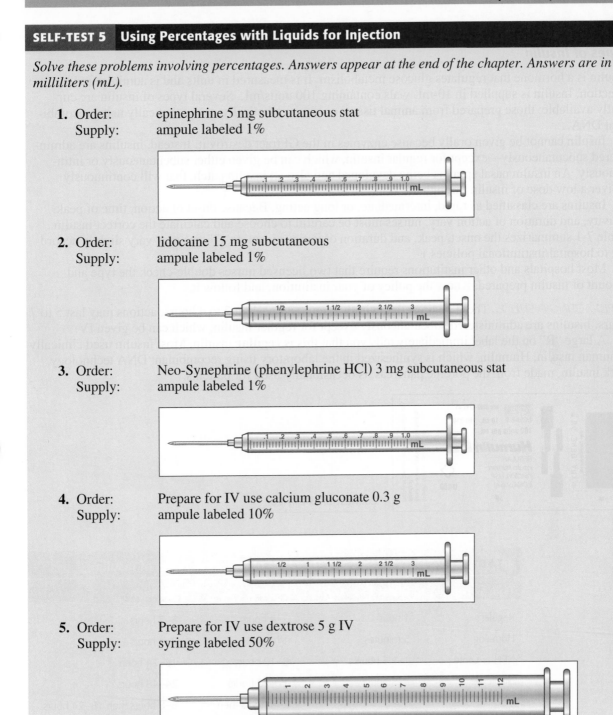

1. Order: epinephrine 5 mg subcutaneous stat
Supply: ampule labeled 1%

2. Order: lidocaine 15 mg subcutaneous
Supply: ampule labeled 1%

3. Order: Neo-Synephrine (phenylephrine HCl) 3 mg subcutaneous stat
Supply: ampule labeled 1%

4. Order: Prepare for IV use calcium gluconate 0.3 g
Supply: ampule labeled 10%

5. Order: Prepare for IV use dextrose 5 g IV
Supply: syringe labeled 50%

Insulin Injections

Types of Insulin

Insulin is a hormone that regulates glucose metabolism. It is measured in units and is administered by injection. Insulin is supplied in 10-mL vials containing 100 units/mL. Several types of insulin are currently available: those prepared from animal tissue, or semisynthetically, or synthetically using recombinant DNA.

Insulin cannot be given orally because enzymes in the GI tract destroy it. Instead, insulins are administered subcutaneously—except for regular insulin, which can be given either subcutaneously or intravenously. An insulin nasal spray is being developed and also an insulin patch, that will continuously deliver a low dose of insulin through the skin.

Insulins are classified as rapid, intermediate, or long acting. Because onset of action, time of peak activity, and duration of action vary, nurses must be careful to choose and calculate the correct insulin. Table 7-1 summarizes the onset, peak, and duration of various insulins. (Times may vary slightly according to hospital/institutional policies.)

Most hospitals and other institutions require that two licensed nurses double-check the type and amount of insulin prepared. Know the policy of your institution, and follow it.

RAPID-ACTING INSULINS. These begin acting within 1 hour and peak in 2 to 4 hours; actions may last 5 to 7 hours. Insulins are administered subcutaneously except for regular insulin, which can be given IV.

A large "R" on the label immediately tells you that this is **regular** insulin. Most insulin used clinically is human insulin, Humulin, which is synthesized in the laboratory using recombinant DNA technology. Pork insulin, made from the porcine pancreas, is occasionally used for patients.

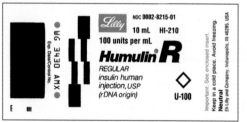

Courtesy of Eli Lilly Co.

TABLE 7-1	Onset, Peak, and Duration of Different Types of Insulin		
Type	**Onset**	**Peak**	**Duration**
Regular	1 hour	2–4 hours	5–7 hours
Humalog	5 minutes	1 hour	2–4 hours
NPH or Lente	1–2.5 hours	6–12 hours	18–24 hours
Ultralente	4–8 hours	12–20 hours	24–48 hours
Mixed insulins	30–60 minutes then 1–2 hours	2–4 hours then 6–12 hours	6–8 hours then 18–24 hours
Lantus	1 hour	None	24 hours

HUMALOG—A UNIQUE, RAPID-ACTING INSULIN. Humalog (lispro) is the newest human insulin product made by recombinant DNA technology. Like regular insulin, it lowers blood sugar, but much more rapidly. Humalog starts acting 5 minutes after injection, peaks in 1 hour, and lasts 2 to 4 hours.

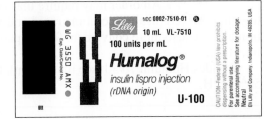

Courtesy of Eli Lilly Co.

LANTUS INSULIN. *Lantus insulin* is a newer agent that is given subcutaneously and must not be mixed with other insulins. Onset is 1 hour, it has no peak, and it lasts for 24 hours. This long duration makes it similar to normal insulin secretion.

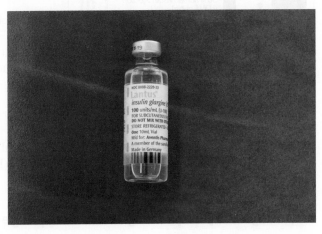

INTERMEDIATE-ACTING INSULINS. These begin action in 1 to 3 hours, peak around 6 to 12 hours, and may last 24 hours. On the label, the letters "N" or "L" or the term **isophane** indicate that regular insulin has been modified, through the addition of zinc and protamine (a basic protein), to delay absorption and prolong the time of action. These intermediate insulins can be prepared from either pork or Humulin R. The label may also show the letters NPH, which denote intermediate action: N means the solution is neutral pH; P indicates the protamine content; H stands for Hagedorn, the laboratory that first prepared this type of insulin.

Courtesy of Eli Lilly Co.

LONG-ACTING INSULINS. Like the intermediate-acting insulins these have been modified with the addition of zinc and protamine. They take 4 to 8 hours to act, peak in 12 to 20 hours, and can continue acting as long as 36 hours. Humulin U or Ultralente is an example of a long-acting insulin.

MIXED INSULINS. An order may require that you mix two insulins in one syringe and administer them together. Mixed insulins combine rapid and intermediate insulin. They save nursing time in preparation and are also more convenient for the patient, who must learn to draw up and self-administer an injection.

Besides Humulin 70/30 (see illustration), there is also a 50/50 insulin that is 50% regular insulin and 50% NPH.

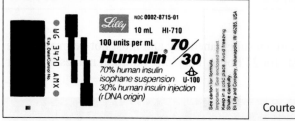

Courtesy of Eli Lilly Co.

Regular insulin should appear clear and colorless; it is the only insulin that may be given IV. Other insulins appear cloudy. Gently rotate (don't shake) cloudy insulin vials between your hands to resuspend the particles.

Types of Insulin Syringes

To administer insulin doses subcutaneously, use an insulin syringe. Two standard syringes measure U 100 insulin. The first measures doses up to 100 units (Fig. 7-4) and the second, called a *low-dose insulin syringe,* measures doses of 50 units or less (Fig. 7-5).

Preparing an Injection Using an Insulin Syringe

The physician or healthcare provider's order for insulin is written as units; the stock comes in 100 units/mL. Both syringes are calibrated (lined) for 100 units/mL.

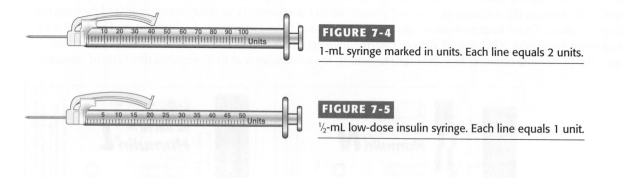

FIGURE 7-4
1-mL syringe marked in units. Each line equals 2 units.

FIGURE 7-5
½-mL low-dose insulin syringe. Each line equals 1 unit.

Example

Order: 60 units NPH subcutaneous every day

Supply: Read the label

Ask yourself three questions:

1. What is the order? NPH 60 units

2. What is the supply? NPH U 100/mL

3. Is a U 100 insulin syringe available? Yes.

Using aseptic technique, draw up the amount required into the syringe.

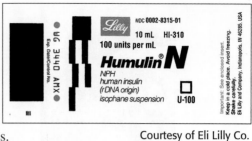

Courtesy of Eli Lilly Co.

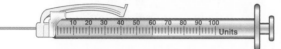

Example

Order: 35 units regular insulin subcutaneous stat

Supply: Read the label

Ask yourself three questions:

1. What is the order? regular insulin 35 units

2. What is the supply? U 100/mL regular insulin

3. What syringe should be used? low-dose insulin syringe

Using aseptic technique, draw up the amount required into the syringe.

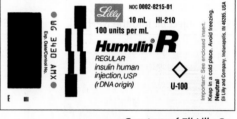

Courtesy of Eli Lilly Co.

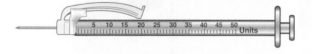

Mixing Two Insulins in One Syringe

Sometimes the physician or healthcare provider will order regular insulin to be mixed with another insulin and injected together at the same site. Remember two points:

1. Always draw up the regular insulin into the syringe first.

2. The total number of units in the syringe equals the two insulin orders added together.

Regular insulin is often ordered with NPH insulin. Since regular insulin is clear and NPH insulin is cloudy, the mnemonic "clear to cloudy" may help you to remember which insulin to draw up first.

To prepare two insulins with one syringe:

1. Inject into the NPH vial the amount of air equal to the amount of NPH insulin.

2. Inject into the regular vial the amount of air equal to the amount of regular insulin.

3. Withdraw the correct amount of regular insulin ("clear").

4. Withdraw the correct amount of NPH insulin ("cloudy").

5. The total number of units will be the regular insulin amount plus the NPH insulin amount.

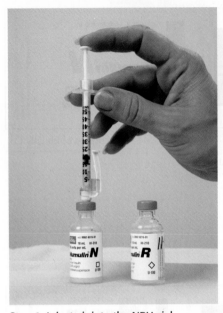

Step 1. Inject air into the NPH vial.

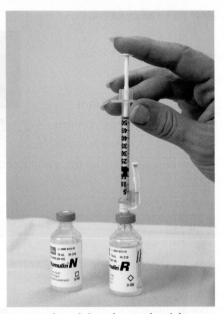

Step 2. Inject air into the regular vial.

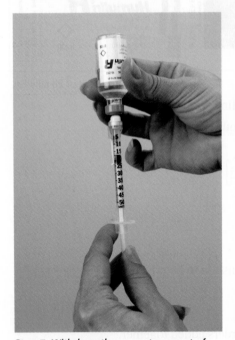

Step 3. Withdraw the correct amount of regular insulin.

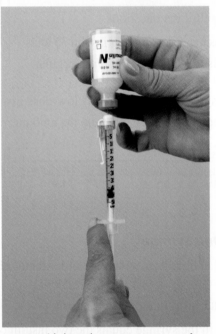

Step 4. Withdraw the correct amount of NPH insulin.

(Used with permission from Evans-Smith, P. [2005] *Taylor's clinical nursing skills.* Philadelphia: Lippincott Williams & Wilkins, p. 128–129.)

Example   Order: regular Humulin insulin 15 units ⎫
                    NPH Humulin insulin 10 units ⎭ every day subcutaneously

Supply: regular Humulin insulin 100 units/mL
           NPH Humulin insulin 100 units/mL

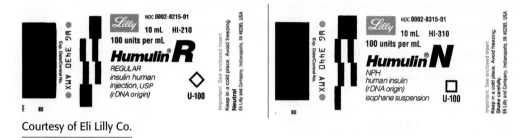

Courtesy of Eli Lilly Co.

1. What are the orders? regular (Humulin) insulin 15 units; NPH insulin 10 units (Humulin)

2. What is the supply? regular (Humulin) insulin unit-100/mL; NPH (Humulin) insulin unit-100/mL

3. Is there an insulin syringe? Yes

4. What will be the total units in the syringe? 25 units

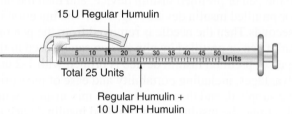

Sliding-Scale Regular Insulin Dosages

Sliding-scale insulin orders refer to a method of insulin administration that is based on the blood glucose result. The blood glucose result often comes from a finger-stick and uses some type of Accucheck monitor. The order will read something like this:

Accuchecks q 4 hours.

For BG 251-300 call physician.

For BG 201-250 give 5 units of regular insulin subcutaneous.

For BG 151-200 give 3 units of regular insulin subcutaneous.

For BG 101-150 give 2 units of regular insulin subcutaneous.

For BG 81-100 give 0 units of regular insulin subcutaneous.

For BG < 80 give 1 amp of D50 and call physician.

In this example, the nurse administers the blood glucose testing and, according to the results, gives the ordered amount of insulin.

Another type of formula is the calculation, somewhat like this:

Accuchecks q 4 hours.

For BG > 150, give number of units of regular insulin based on: BG-100/40

In this formula, the denominator can change depending on the order and how controlled the patient's blood sugar needs to be. A lower number in the denominator, i.e. BG-100/30, increases the amount of insulin the patient receives. This formula also applies when you are giving continuous IV infusion of regular insulin. (See Chapter 9.)

For either type of formula, most hospitals still require that another licensed person double-check both the calculation and the amount of insulin drawn into the syringe.

Order: S/S insulin (sliding-scale). BG-100/40 = number of units of regular insulin.

Blood glucose result: 340

Calculation: 340-100/40 =

140/40 =

3.5 units

Administer 4 units (dose rounds up in this example)

Since the insulin syringes do not have decimal markings, round the dose to a whole number. Always follow hospital/institutional policy on rounding insulin doses.

Insulin Pens and Prefilled Insulin Devices

Insulin pens and prefilled insulin devices contain insulin in a cartridge. The dosage is calculated in the same manner; a needle is attached to the pen or prefilled insulin device, and then the number of units is set with a small dial on the insulin pen or prefilled insulin device (Fig. 7-6). The injection is given subcutaneously, and held in place for 6-10 seconds. Then the needle is removed from the pen or prefilled insulin device and discarded safely. The insulin pen or prefilled insulin device can be used until the insulin cartridge is empty. Usually the insulin pen or prefilled insulin device is primed with 1-2 units before giving the actual dose. There are several advantages, including portability and ease of measuring an accurate dose. However, not all insulins can be supplied, and there is no way to mix insulins with an insulin pen or prefilled insulin device. In a hospital setting, the insulin pen or prefilled insulin device is supplied for only one patient and usually doses must be verified by two licensed nurses.

An insulin pump can administer insulin continuously by the subcutaneous route. A pump is placed near the abdominal area of the patient. The pump is preset at a certain rate to deliver the insulin via tubing through a needle inserted in the subcutaneous tissue. Settings can be adjusted to the patient's insulin needs. The site is usually changed every 2-3 days or as needed (Fig. 7-7).

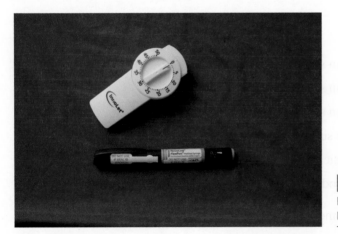

FIGURE 7-6

Insulin pen. (Copyright © 2008 Lacey-Bordeaux Photography)

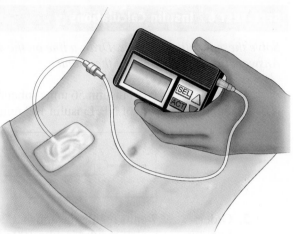

FIGURE 7-7

Insulin pump. (With permission from Taylor, C. [2008] Fundamentals of Nursing. Philadelphia: Lippincott, Williams, and Wilkins, p. 797).

Injections From Powders

Some medications are prepared in a dry form, powder, or crystal. As liquids they are unstable and lose potency over time. The drug must be reconstituted according to the manufacturer's directions, which will give the type and amount of diluent to use.

In some hospitals and other healthcare settings, the pharmacy is responsible for reconstituting medications. Sometimes, however, this task becomes the nurses' responsibility; that's why this book includes these kinds of dosage calculations. Many drugs are reconstituted using a special reconstitution device within an IV bag. (See Chapter 8 for more information.)

To solve injection-from-powder problems, you use the same rule as for oral medications and for injection from a liquid. This is because once the powder is dissolved, the powdered drug takes liquid form.

Application of the Rule for Injections From Powders

RULE

Formula Method	Proportion Expressed as Two Ratios	Proportion Expressed as Two Fractions
$\dfrac{\text{Desire}}{\text{Have}} \times \text{Supply} = \text{Amount}$	$\text{Supply} : \text{Desire} :: \text{x} : \text{Have}$	$\dfrac{\text{x}}{\text{Desire}} = \dfrac{\text{Supply}}{\text{Have}}$

(Powder examples follow Self-Test 6.)

SELF-TEST 6 | **Insulin Calculations**

Solve these insulin problems. Draw a line on the syringe to indicate the dose you would prepare. Answers appear at the end of the chapter.

1. Order: NPH insulin 56 units subcutaneous every day
   Supply: vial of NPH insulin 100 units/mL

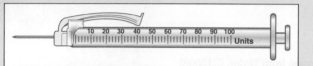

2. Order: 7 units regular insulin and 20 units NPH insulin subcutaneous every day 7 AM
   Supply: vial of regular insulin 100 units/mL and NPH 100 units/mL

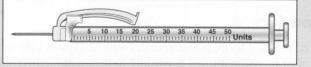

3. Order: regular Humulin insulin 4 units subcutaneous stat
   Supply: vial regular insulin 100 units/mL

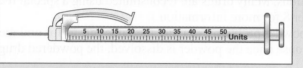

4. Order: Semilente insulin 28 units subcutaneous
   Supply: Semilente insulin prompt insulin zinc suspension 100 units/mL

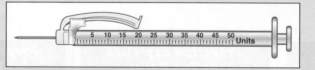

5. Order: 20 units of NPH subcutaneous every day
   Supply: vial of NPH 100 units/mL

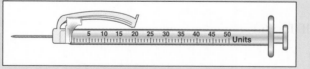

6. Order: regular insulin 16 units with NPH insulin 64 units subcutaneous every day
   Supply: vial of regular insulin 100 units/mL and vial of NPH 100 units/mL

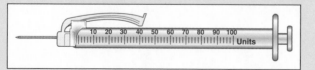

(continued)

SELF-TEST 6 | **Insulin Calculations (Continued)**

Use the following sliding scale to calculate the insulin dosages. Draw a line on the syringe to indicate the dose you would prepare.

Accuchecks q 4 hours.

For BG 251-300 call physician.

For BG 201-250 give 5 units of regular insulin subcutaneous.

For BG 151-200 give 3 units of regular insulin subcutaneous.

For BG 101-150 give 2 units of regular insulin subcutaneous.

For BG 81-100 give 0 units of regular insulin subcutaneous.

For BG < 80 give 1 amp of D50 and call physician.

7. Accucheck 110

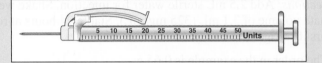

8. Accucheck 175

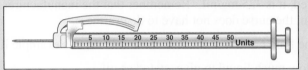

9. Accucheck 251

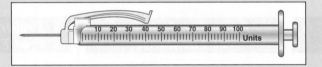

10. Accucheck 75

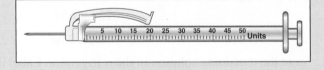

equivalent to
1gram cefonicid
NDC 0007-4353-01

EXP.

MONOCID®
STERILE CEFONICID
SODIUM
(LYOPHILIZED)

LOT

For IV or IM use

NSN 6505-01-189-4698
Before reconstitution protect from light and refrigerate
(2° to 8°C). **Usual Adult Dose:** 1 gram every 24 hours
as a single dose. See accompanying prescribing information.
For IV Infusion: See prescribing information.
For IM or IV Direct (Bolus) Injection: Add 2.5 mL Sterile
Water for Injection. Shake Well. Provides an approximate
volume of 3.1 mL(325 mg/mL). Properly reconstituted solutions of *Monocid* are stable 24 hours at room temperature
or 72 hours if refrigerated (5°C). **Caution:** Federal law
prohibits dispensing without prescription.
Glaxo SmithKline Pharmaceuticals
Philadelphia, PA 19101
694021-J

FIGURE 7-8

Label of Monocid (cefonicid
sodium). (Courtesy of Glaxo-
SmithKline Pharmaceuticals)

Example

Order: Monocid (cefonicid sodium) 0.65 g IM every day (Fig. 7-8).

Label directions: Add 2.5 mL sterile water for injection. Shake well. Provides an approximate volume of 3.1 mL (325 mg/mL). Stable 24 hours at room temperature or 72 hours if refrigerated (5°C).

Desire: The order in the example is 0.65 g.

Have: The strength of the drug supplied. The example is 1 g as a dry powder; when reconstituted, it is 325 mg/mL. Remember that the manufacturer gives the strength of the solution; the nurse does not have to determine it.

Supply: The fluid portion of the solution made. In this example it is 1 mL = 325 mg.

Answer: How much liquid to give, stated as mL.

Equivalent: 0.65 g = 650 mg

Formula Method	Proportion Expressed as Two Ratios	Proportion Expressed as Two Fractions
$\frac{D}{H} \times S = x \frac{\overset{2}{650} \text{ mg}}{\underset{1}{325} \text{ mg}} \times 1 \text{ mL} = 2 \text{ mL}$	1 mL : 325 mg : : x mL : 650 mg	$\frac{x \text{ mL}}{650 \text{ mg}} \times \frac{1 \text{ mL}}{325 \text{ mg}}$

$$325x = 650$$

$$x = 2 \text{ mL}$$

Give 2 mL. Store the remaining solution in the refrigerator. Label the vial with the date, the time, the solution made (325 mg/mL), the expiration date, and the initials of the nurse who dissolved the powder.

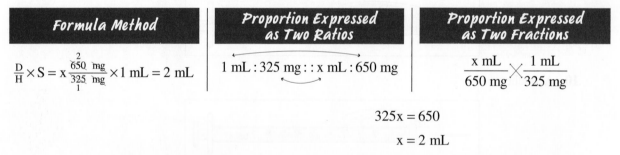

325 mg/mL
10/15/07 1600
SB
Expires 10/18/07

Distinctive Features of Injections From Powders

Aseptic technique is used to prepare and administer the medication, which is given parenterally (usually IM, IV, or IVPB). The dry drug is supplied in vials of powder or crystals and may come in different strengths. Because powders deteriorate in solution, choose the strength closest to the amount ordered.

The powder is usually diluted with one of the following:

Sterile water for injection

Bacteriostatic water for injection with a preservative added

Normal saline for injection (0.9% sodium chloride)

Directions will state which fluids may be used. Read this information carefully because some fluids may be incompatible (i.e., unsuitable) as diluents. When the powder goes into solution, *displacement* occurs. This means that as the powder dissolves, it increases the volume added to the vial. There is no uniformity in the way powders go into solution.

Refer to the label in Figure 7-8 again. The manufacturer tells the nurse to add 2.5 mL sterile water to provide an approximate volume of 3.1 mL. In this example, 0.6 mL is the displacement volume. *Injections-from-powder problems are solved by using the solution made, not the displacement volume.* The manufacturer will give the solution.

| **Example** | The package insert information concerning the dilution of Cefobid (cefoperazone) injection is reproduced in Figure 7-9. Examine the directions with the intention of solving the following problem, then read the explanation: |

Order: Cefobid (cefoperazone) 0.5 g IM q12h

Supply: 1-g vial of powder

Search the directions for three pieces of information to dissolve your supply, which is 1 gram:

1. Type of fluid needed to dissolve the powder

2. Amount of fluid to add

3. Solution made

Explanation

1. Figure 7-9 gives *Solutions for Initial Reconstitution:* sterile water for injection, bacteriostatic water for injection, and 0.9% sodium chloride injection. Choose one.

2. The heading *Preparation for Intramuscular Injection* states that when a concentration of 250 mg or more is to be administered, a 2% lidocaine solution should be used together with sterile water for injection in a two-step dilution.

3. Two tables are given. The upper table has the two-step dilution; the lower one does not. Because the order requires two steps, use the directions in the top table.

4. Two strengths of powder are listed in the upper table. Look at the extreme left. They are for a 1-g vial and a 2-g vial. Our supply is a 1-g vial. Follow directions for 1 g.

5. The next heading is *Final Cefoperazone Concentration.* Two possibilities are given for the dilution: 333 mg/mL and 250 mg/mL. Because the order calls for 0.5 g, choose 250 mg/mL. 0.5 grams = 500 mg so you will need 2 mL of solution.

6. To make the solution of 250 mg/mL, add the following: 2.8 mL sterile water and 1.0 mL 2% lidocaine.

7. The last column on the right, headed *Withdrawable Volume,* lists 4 mL. Ignore this column; it does not affect the answer: When you add 2.8 mL and 1.0 mL, you expect to have 3.8 mL. The package insert states you will end up with 4 mL. The manufacturer is giving the displacement.

RECONSTITUTION

The following solutions may be used for the initial reconstitution of CEFOBID sterile powder:

Table 1. Solutions for Initial Reconstitution

5% Dextrose Injection (USP)	0.9% Sodium Chloride Injection (USP)
5% Dextrose and 0.9% Sodium Chloride Injection (USP)	Normosol® M and Dextrose Injection
5% Dextrose and 0.2% Sodium Chloride Injection (USP)	Normosol® R
10% Dextrose Injection (USP)	Sterile Water for Injection*
Bacteriostatic Water for Injection [Benzyl Alcohol or Parabens] (USP)*†	

* Not to be used as a vehicle for intravenous infusion.
† Preparation containing Benzyl Alcohol should not be used in neonates.

Preparation for Intramuscular Injection

Any suitable solution listed above may be used to prepare CEFOBID sterile powder for intramuscular injection. When concentrations of 250 mg/ml or more are to be administered, a lidocaine solution should be used. These solutions should be prepared using a combination of Sterile Water for Injection and 2% Lidocaine Hydrochloride Injection (USP) that approximates a 0.5% Lidocaine Hydrochloride Solution. A two-step dilution process as follows is recommended: First, add the required amount of Sterile Water for Injection and agitate until CEFOBID powder is completely dissolved. Second, add the required amount of 2% lidocaine and mix.

	Final Cefoperazone Concentration	Step 1 Volume of Sterile Water	Step 2 Volume of 2% Lidocaine	Withdrawable Volume*†
1 g vial	333 mg/ml	2.0 ml	0.6 ml	3 ml
	250 mg/ml	2.8 ml	1.0 ml	4 ml
2 g vial	333 mg/ml	3.8 ml	1.2 ml	6 ml
	250 mg/ml	5.4 ml	1.8 ml	8 ml

When a diluent other than Lidocaine HCl Injection (USP) is used reconstitute as follows:

	Cefoperazone Concentration	Volume of Diluent to be Added	Withdrawable Volume*
1 g vial	333 mg/ml	2.6 ml	3 ml
	250 mg/ml	3.8 ml	4 ml
2 g vial	333 mg/ml	5.0 ml	6 ml
	250 mg/ml	7.2 ml	8 ml

* There is sufficient excess present to allow for withdrawal of the stated volume.
† Final lidocaine concentration will approximate that obtained if a 0.5% Lidocaine Hydrochloride Solution is used as diluent.

STORAGE AND STABILITY

CEFOBID sterile powder is to be stored at or below 25°C (77°F) and protected from light prior to reconstitution. After reconstitution, protection from light is not necessary.

The following parenteral diluents and approximate concentrations of CEFOBID provide stable solutions under the following conditions for the indicated time periods. (After the indicated time periods, unused portions of solutions should be discarded.)

Controlled Room Temperature (15Υ–25ΥC/59Υ–77ΥF)

24 Hours — Approximate

Bacteriostatic Water for Injection [Benzyl Alcohol or Parabens] (USP)	300 mg/ml
5% Dextrose Injection (USP)	2 mg to 50 mg/ml
5% Dextrose and Lactated Ringer's Injection	2 mg to 50 mg/ml
5% Dextrose and 0.9% Sodium Chloride Injection (USP)	2 mg to 50 mg/ml
5% Dextrose and 0.2% Sodium Chloride Injection (USP)	2 mg to 50 mg/ml
10% Dextrose Injection (USP)	2 mg to 50 mg/ml
Lactated Ringer's Injection (USP)	2 mg/ml
0.5% Lidocaine Hydrochloride Injection (USP)	300 mg/ml
0.9% Sodium Chloride Injection (USP)	2 mg to 300 mg/ml
Normosol® M and 5% Dextrose Injection	2 mg to 50 mg/ml
Normosol® R	2 mg to 50 mg/ml
Sterile Water for Injection	300 mg/ml

Reconstituted CEFOBID solutions may be stored in glass or plastic syringes, or in glass or flexible plastic parenteral solution containers.

Refrigerator Temperature (2Υ–8ΥC/36Υ–46ΥF)

5 Days — Approximate Concentrations

Bacteriostatic Water for Injection [Benzyl Alcohol or Parabens] (USP)	300 mg/ml
5% Dextrose Injection (USP)	2 mg to 50 mg/ml
5% Dextrose and 0.9% Sodium Chloride Injection (USP)	2 mg to 50 mg/ml
5% Dextrose and 0.2% Sodium Chloride Injection (USP)	2 mg to 50 mg/ml
Lactated Ringer's Injection (USP)	2 mg/ml
0.5% Lidocaine Hydrochloride Injection (USP)	300 mg/ml
0.9% Sodium Chloride Injection (USP)	2 mg to 300 mg/ml
Normosol® M and 5% Dextrose Injection	2 mg to 50 mg/ml
Normosol® R	2 mg to 50 mg/ml
Sterile Water for Injection	300 mg/ml

Reconstituted CEFOBID solutions may be stored in glass or plastic syringes, or in glass or flexible plastic parenteral solution containers.

FIGURE 7-9

Reconstitution directions for Cefobid (cefoperazone sodium). (Courtesy of Pfizer Laboratories.)

8. You now have all the information needed to prepare the dose ordered. Your solution is 250 mg/mL. Equivalent: 0.5 g = 500 mg.

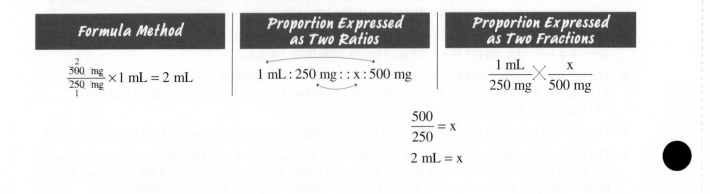

Formula Method	*Proportion Expressed as Two Ratios*	*Proportion Expressed as Two Fractions*
$\dfrac{\overset{2}{500}\ \text{mg}}{\underset{1}{250}\ \text{mg}} \times 1\ \text{mL} = 2\ \text{mL}$	$1\ \text{mL} : 250\ \text{mg} :: x : 500\ \text{mg}$	$\dfrac{1\ \text{mL}}{250\ \text{mg}} \times \dfrac{x}{500\ \text{mg}}$

$$\frac{500}{250} = x$$

$$2\ \text{mL} = x$$

Give 2 mL IM.

9. Write on the label the solution you made, the date, time, expiration date, and your initials.

10. Note the storage directions and stability expiration.

Where to Find Information About Reconstitution of Powders

Information about reconstitution of powders may be found from

- The label on the vial of powder
- The package insert that comes with the vial of powder
- Nursing drug handbooks
- Other references such as the *Physician's Desk Reference (PDR)*

STEPS FOR RECONSTITUTING POWDERS WITH DIRECTIONS

1. Read the order.
2. Identify the supply.
3. Dilute the fluid.
4. Identify the solution and new supply.
5. Apply the rule and arithmetic.
6. Obtain the amount to give.
7. Write on the label the solution made, date, time, expiration date, and your initials.
8. Store according to directions.

Example

Order: Ancef (cefazolin sodium) 0.3 g IM (Fig. 7-10)

Supply: 500 mg powder

Diluting fluid: 2.0 mL sterile water for injection

Solution and new supply: 225 mg/mL

RECONSTITUTION
Preparation of Parenteral Solution
Parenteral drug products should be SHAKEN WELL when reconstituted, and inspected visually for particulate matter prior to administration. If particulate matter is evident in reconstituted fluids, the drug solutions should be discarded. When reconstituted or diluted according to the instructions below, Ancef (sterile cefazolin sodium, SK&F) is stable for 24 hours at room temperature or for 96 hours if stored under refrigeration. Reconstituted solutions may range in color from pale yellow to yellow without a change in potency.
Single-Dose Vials
For I.M. injection, I.V. direct (bolus) injection, or I.V. infusion, reconstitute with Sterile Water for Injection according to the following table. SHAKE WELL.

Vial Size	Amount of Diluent	Approximate Concentration	Approximate Available Volume
250 mg.	2.0 ml.	125 mg./ml.	2.0 ml.
500 mg.	2.0 ml.	225 mg./ml.	2.2 ml.
1 gram	2.5 ml.	330 mg./ml.	3.0 ml.

FIGURE 7-10

Reconstitution directions for Ancef (cefazolin sodium). (Courtesy of GlaxoSmithKline.)

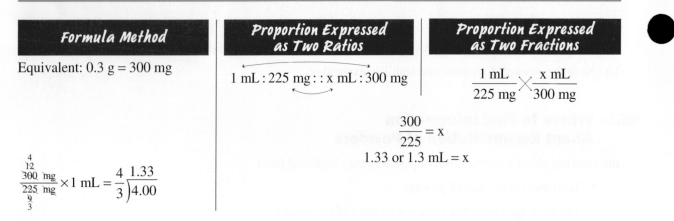

Formula Method	Proportion Expressed as Two Ratios	Proportion Expressed as Two Fractions
Equivalent: 0.3 g = 300 mg	1 mL : 225 mg : : x mL : 300 mg	$\dfrac{1 \text{ mL}}{225 \text{ mg}} \times \dfrac{x \text{ mL}}{300 \text{ mg}}$

$$\frac{300}{225} = x$$

1.33 or 1.3 mL = x

$$\frac{\overset{4}{\overset{12}{\cancel{300}}} \text{ mg}}{\underset{3}{\underset{9}{\cancel{225}}} \text{ mg}} \times 1 \text{ mL} = \frac{4}{3} \overset{1.33}{\overline{)4.00}}$$

Give 1.3 mL IM.

Write on label: 225 mg/mL, date, time, expiration date, initials.

Storage: Refrigerate; stable for 96 hours.

Example   Order: penicillin G potassium 1 million units IM q6h (Fig. 7-11)

Fig. 11

Supply powder: 5 million-unit vial

Diluting fluid and number of milliliters: Use sterile water for injection. Write out the directions for the 5 million-unit vial (supply).

23 mL will provide 200,000 units/mL.

18 mL will provide 250,000 units/mL.

8 mL will provide 500,000 units/mL.

3 mL will provide 1 million units/mL.

Choose 3 mL to dilute the powder.

Solution and new supply: 1 million units/mL.

PENICILLIN G POTASSIUM for injection
Preparation of Solutions
Use sterile water for injection
      RECONSTITUTION
1,000,000 u vial

Diluent	Desired Concentration
9.6 ml	100,000 u/ml
4.6 ml	200,000 u/ml
3.6 ml	250,000 u/ml

5,000,000 u vial

Diluent	Desired Concentration
23 ml	200,000 u/ml
18 ml	250,000 u/ml
8 ml	500,000 u/ml
3 ml	1,000,000 u/ml

Storage
Prepared solutions may be kept in the refrigerator one week.

FIGURE 7-11

Preparation of solution for the 1,000,000-unit and the 5,000,000-unit vials of penicillin G potassium.

Formula Method	**Proportion Expressed as Two Ratios**	**Proportion Expressed as Two Fractions**
$\dfrac{1 \text{ million units}}{1 \text{ million units}} \times 1 \text{ mL} = 1 \text{ mL}$	1 mL : 1 million : : x mL : 1 million units units	$\dfrac{1 \text{ mL}}{1 \text{ million units}} \times \dfrac{\text{x}}{1 \text{ million units}}$

$$\frac{1 \text{ million}}{1 \text{ million}} = x$$

$$1 \text{ mL} = x$$

Give 1 mL IM.

Write on label: 1 million units/mL, date, time, expiration date, initials

Storage: Refrigerate; stable for 1 week

Note: This solution (1 million units/mL) may be so concentrated that it is painful when injected. To make a less painful solution, you can dilute the powder with 8 mL to make 500,000 units/mL and give 2 mL to the patient.

Here are a few tips before you begin Self-Test 7.

- When reading the directions for reconstitution, look first at the solutions you can make. Think the problem through mentally and choose one dilution, so that you will have a focus as you read.

- If your answer is more than 3 mL for an IM injection, consider using two syringes and injecting in two different sites.

- Experience in administering injections will guide you in choosing the solution's concentration. Stronger concentrations, although smaller in volume, may be more painful; a more dilute solution may be more suitable despite its larger volume.

- Each powder problem is unique. Carefully read the directions.

- Choose one diluting fluid for injection: generally sterile water or 0.9% sodium chloride. You do not need to list all of the fluids in your answer.

- For the following practice problems and self-tests, assume that the doses ordered and the order are correct. Chapter 12 discusses the nurse's responsibilities in drug knowledge. Dosages for infants and children are discussed in Chapter 10.

SELF-TEST 7 Injections from Powders

Solve the following problems in injections from powders and write your answers using the steps. Answers appear at the end of the chapter.

1. Order: Ceptaz (ceftazidime) 1 g IM q6h (Fig. 7-12)
Supply: 1 g powder

a. Diluting fluid and number of milliliters:
b. Solution and new supply:
c. Rule and arithmetic:
d. Answer:
e. Write on label:
f. Storage:

CEFTAZIDIME INJECTION

Reconstitution
Single dose vials: Reconstitute with sterile water. Shake well.

Vial Size	Diluent	Approx. Avail. Volume	Approx. Avg. Concentration
IM or IV bolus injection			
1 gram	3.0 mL	3.6 mL	280 mg/mL
IV infusion			
1 gram	10 mL	10.6 mL	95 mg/mL
2 gram	10 mL	11.2 mL	180 mg/mL

Stable for 18 hours at room temperature or seven days if refrigerated.

FIGURE 7-12
Label and reconstitution directions for Ceptaz (ceftazidime).

2. Order: Omnipen (ampicillin sodium) 250 mg IM q6h (Fig. 7-13)
Supply: 500-mg vial of powder

a. Diluting fluid and number of milliliters:
b. Solution and new supply:
c. Rule and arithmetic:
d. Answer:
e. Write on label:
f. Storage:

AMPICILLIN
Reconstitution
Dissolve contents of a vial with the amount of Sterile Water or Bacteriostatic Water.

Amount Ordered	Recommended Amount of Diluent	Withdraw Volume	Concentration in mg/ml
500 mg	1.8 ml	2.0 ml	250 mg
1.0 Gram	3.4 ml	4.0 ml	250 mg
2.0 gram	6.8 ml	8.0 ml	250 mg

Storage
Use within one hour of reconstitution.

FIGURE 7-13
Reconstitution directions for Omnipen (ampicillin sodium) for IM or IV injection.

(continued)

3. Order: Ancef (cefazolin sodium) 225 mg IM q6h (Fig. 7-14)
Supply: On the shelf there are three vial sizes of powder: 250 mg, 500 mg, 1 g

    a. Supply chosen:
    b. Diluting fluid and number of milliliters:
    c. Solution and new supply:
    d. Rule and arithmetic:
    e. Answer:
    f. Write on label:
    g. Storage:

RECONSTITUTION
Preparation of Parenteral Solution
Parenteral drug products should be SHAKEN WELL when reconstituted, and inspected visually for particulate matter prior to administration. If particulate matter is evident in reconstituted fluids, the drug solutions should be discarded. When reconstituted or diluted according to the instructions below, Ancef (sterile cefazolin sodium, SK&F) is stable for 24 hours at room temperature or for 96 hours if stored under refrigeration. Reconstituted solutions may range in color from pale yellow to yellow without a change in potency.
Single-Dose Vials
For I.M. injection, I.V. direct (bolus) injection, or I.V. infusion, reconstitute with Sterile Water for Injection according to the following table. SHAKE WELL.

Vial Size	Amount of Diluent	Approximate Concentration	Approximate Available Volume
250 mg.	2.0 ml.	125 mg./ml.	2.0 ml.
500 mg.	2.0 ml.	225 mg./ml.	2.2 ml.
1 gram	2.5 ml.	330 mg./ml.	3.0 ml.

FIGURE 7-14

Reconstitution directions for Ancef (cefazolin sodium). (Courtesy of GlaxoSmithKline.)

4. Order: Fortaz (ceftazidime) 500 mg IM q6h (Fig. 7-15)
Supply: 1 g powder

    a. Diluting fluid and number of milliliters:
    b. Solution and new supply:
    c. Rule and arithmetic:
    d. Answer:
    e. Write on label:
    f. Storage:

5. Order: Mefoxin (cefoxitin sodium) 200 mg IM q4h
Supply: vial of powder labeled 1 g

Refer to Figure 7-16.

    a. Diluting fluid and number of milliliters:
    b. Solution made and new supply:
    c. Rule and arithmetic:
    d. Answer:
    e. Write on label:
    f. Storage:

(continued)

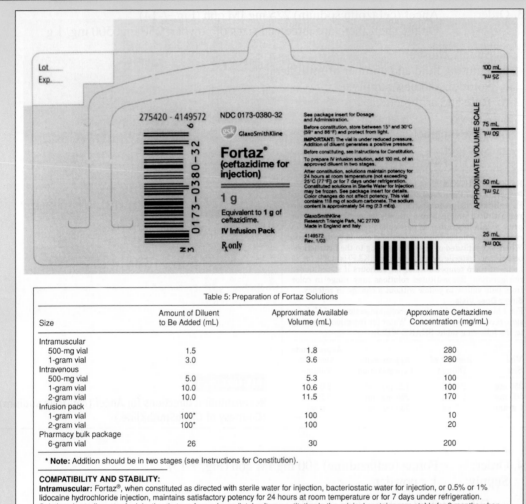

Table 5: Preparation of Fortaz Solutions

Size	Amount of Diluent to Be Added (mL)	Approximate Available Volume (mL)	Approximate Ceftazidime Concentration (mg/mL)
Intramuscular			
500-mg vial	1.5	1.8	280
1-gram vial	3.0	3.6	280
Intravenous			
500-mg vial	5.0	5.3	100
1-gram vial	10.0	10.6	100
2-gram vial	10.0	11.5	170
Infusion pack			
1-gram vial	100*	100	10
2-gram vial	100*	100	20
Pharmacy bulk package			
6-gram vial	26	30	200

* **Note:** Addition should be in two stages (see Instructions for Constitution).

COMPATIBILITY AND STABILITY:
Intramuscular: Fortaz®, when constituted as directed with sterile water for injection, bacteriostatic water for injection, or 0.5% or 1% lidocaine hydrochloride injection, maintains satisfactory potency for 24 hours at room temperature or for 7 days under refrigeration. Solutions in sterile water for injection that are frozen immediately after constitution in the original container are stable for 3 months when stored at -20°C. Once thawed, solutions should not be refrozen. thawed solutions may be stored for up to 8 hours at room temperature or for 4 days in a refrigerator.

FIGURE 7-15

Preparation of Fortaz (ceftazidime) solutions. (Reproduced with permission of GlaxoSmithKline.)

For the next set of problems, you must choose the direction you need to give the ordered dose. Directions for these problems are located throughout Chapter 7. For each problem provide the answer for

a. Diluting fluid and number of milliliters
b. Solution made and new supply
c. Answer
d. Label

6. Order: Ceptaz (ceftazidime sodium) 90 mg IM q12h
Supply: vial of powder labeled Ceptaz 1 g (refer to Fig. 7-12)

SELF-TEST 7 **Injections from Powders (Continued)**

Table 3 — Preparation of Solution

Strength	Amount of Diluent to be Added (mL) + +	Approximate Withdrawable Volume (mL)	Approximate Average Concentration (mg/mL)
1 gram Vial	2 (Intramuscular)	2.5	400
2 gram Vial	4 (Intramuscular)	5	400
1 gram Vial	10 (IV)	10.5	95
2 gram Vial	10 or 20 (IV)	11.1 or 21.0	180 or 95
1 gram Infusion Bottle	50 or 100 (IV)	50 or 100	20 or 10
2 gram Infusion Bottle	50 or 100 (IV)	50 or 100	40 or 20
10 gram Bulk	43 or 93 (IV)	49 or 98.5	200 or 100

+ +Shake to dissolve and let stand until clear.

Intramuscular
MEFOXIN, as constituted with Sterile Water for Injection, Bacteriostatic Water for Injection, or 0.5 percent or 1 percent lidocaine hydrochloride solution (without epinephrine), maintains satisfactory potency for 24 hours at room temperature, for one week under refrigeration (below 5°C), and for at least 30 weeks in the frozen state.

FIGURE 7-16

Directions to reconstitute Mefoxin (cefoxitin sodium). (Courtesy of Merck Co. Inc.)

7. Order: Ancef (cefazolin sodium) 0.45 g IM q12h
   Supply: vial of powder labeled cefazolin sodium 500 mg (refer to Fig. 7-14)

8. Order: ampicillin sodium 400 mg IM q6h (refer to Fig. 7-13)
   Supply: 500 mg

9. Order: Fortaz (ceftazidime) 0.5 g IM q6h (refer to Fig. 7-15)
   Supply: 1 g

10. Order: Mefoxin (cefoxitin sodium) 0.5 g IM q12h
   Supply: vial of powder labeled Mefoxin 1 g (refer to Fig. 7-16)

CRITICAL THINKING: TEST YOUR CLINICAL SAVVY

You are a nursing student about to graduate from one of the most prestigious nursing schools in America. On your last day of clinical, you are to give insulin to the last patient in your nursing school career. The patient has been insulin dependent for 15 years. The ordered dose is 30 units of NPH insulin and 20 units of regular insulin. Unfortunately, the hospital has run out of insulin syringes. Your instructor is going to check your insulin before you administer it.

1. How many milliliters would you need for the total dose of insulin?
2. Could you use a 1-mL syringe to draw up insulin? If so, how would this be done and what would be the precautions?
3. What would be the danger in using a 1-mL syringe?
4. Could you use a 3-mL syringe? A 5-mL syringe?
5. What would be the danger in using a 3-mL or 5-mL syringe?
6. What amount of insulin would be safe to draw up in a 1-mL syringe?

CRITICAL THINKING: TEST YOUR CLINICAL SAVVY

You are working in a medical-surgical unit of a large city hospital. A patient is to receive 500,000 units of penicillin G potassium, IV, q 12 hours. Normally a vial containing 1 million units is considered stock drug (reconstituted: 250,000 units = 1 mL). Because of a nationwide shortage, a vial with 5 million units of penicillin G potassium is supplied (reconstituted 1,000,000 units = 1 mL).

1. What should you do to ensure no mistakes are made for the initial dosing and for subsequent dosing of penicillin?
2. What is the danger in administering too much of any drug?
3. What is the danger in administering too much penicillin and/or potassium?

Putting it Together

Mr. B. is a 54 year old male with known asthma, recently hospitalized for hematuria and discharged three days ago. Since then he has had dyspnea with wheezing and a dry cough. He has been using nebulized bronchodilators without any relief. Has sinus congestion, no headache, some subjective fevers. No history of pulmonary embolism or DVT. Admitted now for treatment and evaluation of dyspnea.

Past Medical History: renal cell carcinoma, hypertension, asthma, type 2 diabetes, hypercholesterolemia. Previous surgeries: hemorrhoidectomy, hiatal hernia repair, nephrectomy. Obstructive sleep apnea. Social history: life long smoker, no alcohol. Lives with his son.

Allergies: Keflex causing rash. Augmentin causing rash. Phenergan causing leg spasm.

Current Vital Signs: Pulse is 96, BP 170/100, RR of 18, sat 96% afebrile.

Medication Orders

Lasix (furosemide) *diuretic* 40 mg IV q 12 h

Epogen (epoetin) *erythropoietin* 8000 units subcutaneous Tuesday/Thursday/Saturday

Heparin *anticoagulant* 2500 units subcutaneous q 8h

Theodur (theophylline) *bronchodilator* 300 mg PO q 12 hr

Flovent (fluticasone) *corticosteroid* 1 puff bid

Norvasc (amlodipine) *antihypertensive* 10 mg PO daily

Mevacor (lovastatin) *antihyperlipidemic* 50 mg PO daily

Solu-Medrol (methylprednisolone) *corticosteroid, glucocorticoid* 100 mg IVP daily

Phenergan (promethazine) *antiemetic* 12.5 mg IV q 6 h prn nausea.

Vancocin (vancomycin) *antiinfective* 1 GM IV q 12 hr

Vasotec (enalapril) *antihypertensive* 0.625 mg IV q 6h over 5 minutes prn SBP >160

Accuchecks ac and hs. For BG >150 Sliding scale: BG-50/20 = units regular insulin subcutaneous

Putting it Together

Calculations

1. Calculate how many mL of Lasix to administer. Available supply is 10 mg/mL.

2. Calculate how many mL of Heparin to administer. Available supply is 5000 units/mL.

3. Calculate how many mL of Epogen to administer. Available supply is 20000 units/mL.

4. Calculate how much (if any) insulin to give for blood glucose of 200.

5. Calculate how many mL of Solu-Medrol to administer. Available supply is 125 mg in 2 mL.

6. Calculate how many mL to administer of Phenergan. Available supply is 25 mg/mL.

7. What prn medication should be given (if any) for the patient's blood pressure? Calculate how many mL if available supply is 1.25 mg/mL.

8. Calculate the amount of VAncomycin to add to an IV piggy back for infusion. Available supply is 500 mg/mL after reconstitution.

Critical Thinking Questions

1. What are precautions that need to be taken with IV push drugs?

2. What are precautions that need to be taken with insulin calculations and administration?

3. What are common mistakes that could happen with insulin dosages?

4. What are common mistakes that could happen with heparin dosages?

5. Why would this patient be on insulin coverage if the patient is type 2 ("non-insulin dependent") diabetic?

6. What medications should be held and why?

Answers in Appendix B.

Name: _____

Solve these injection problems. Draw a line on the syringe indicating the amount you would prepare in milliliters. See Appendix A for answers.

1. Order: sodium amytal 0.1 g IM at 7 AM
   Supply: ampule of liquid labeled 200 mg/3 mL

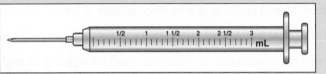

2. Order: morphine sulfate 5 mg IV stat
   Supply: vial of liquid labeled 15 mg/mL

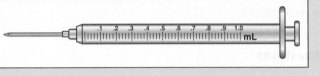

3. Order: Benadryl (diphenhydramine) 25 mg IM q4h prn
   Supply: ampule of liquid labeled 50 mg (2-mL size)

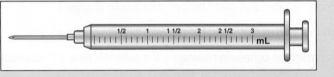

4. Order: NPH insulin 15 units and Humulin insulin 5 units subcutaneous every day 7 AM
   Supply: vials of NPH insulin 100 units/mL and Humulin insulin 100 units/mL

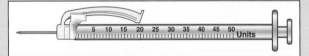

5. Order: add 20 mEq potassium chloride to IV stat
   Supply: vial of liquid labeled 40 mEq (3 g) per 20 mL

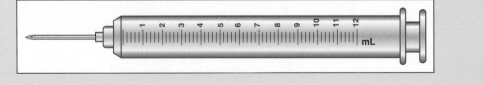

(continued)

6. Order: scopolamine 0.6 mg subcutaneous stat
   Supply: vial labeled 0.4 mg/mL

7. Order: atropine sulfate 0.8 mg IV at 7 AM
   Supply: vial labeled 0.4 mg/mL

8. Order: add 0.5 g dextrose 25% to IV stat
   Supply: vial of liquid labeled infant 25% dextrose injection 250 mg/mL

9. Order: Vitamin C (ascorbic acid) 200 mg IM bid
   Supply: ampule labeled 500 mg/2 mL

10. Order: epinephrine 7.5 mg subcutaneous stat
   Supply: ampule labeled 1:100

11. Order: Valium (diazepam) 10 mg IV now
   Supply: vial labeled 5 mg/mL

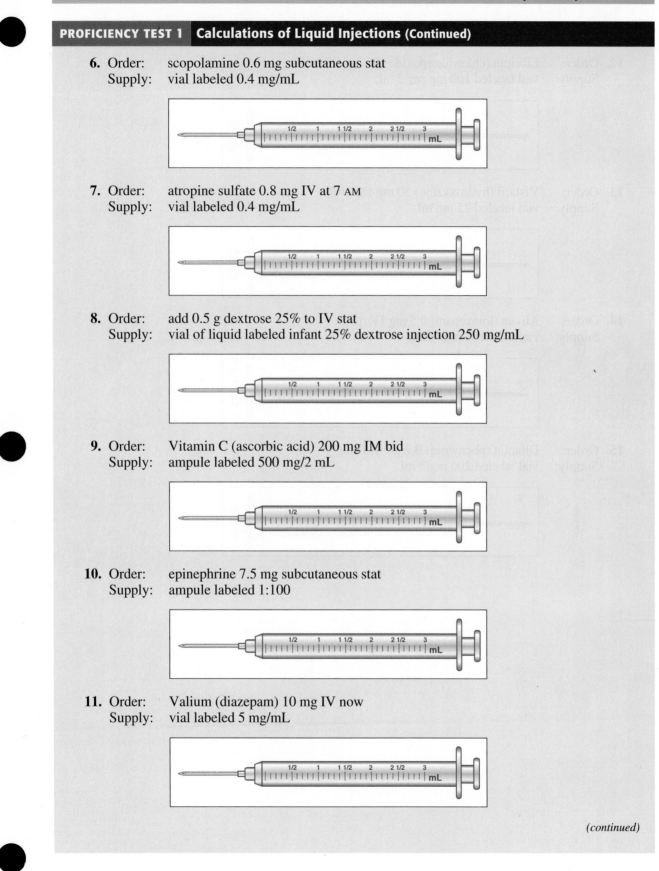

(continued)

12. Order: Librium (chlordiazepoxide) 25 mg IM bid
     Supply: vial labeled 100 mg per 2 mL

13. Order: Vistaril (hydroxyzine) 50 mg IM bid
     Supply: vial labeled 25 mg/mL

14. Order: Ativan (lorazepam) 0.5 mg IV q 4hr
     Supply: vial labeled 2 mg/mL

15. Order: Dilantin (phenytoin) 0.2 gm IM stat
     Supply: vial labeled 200 mg/2 mL

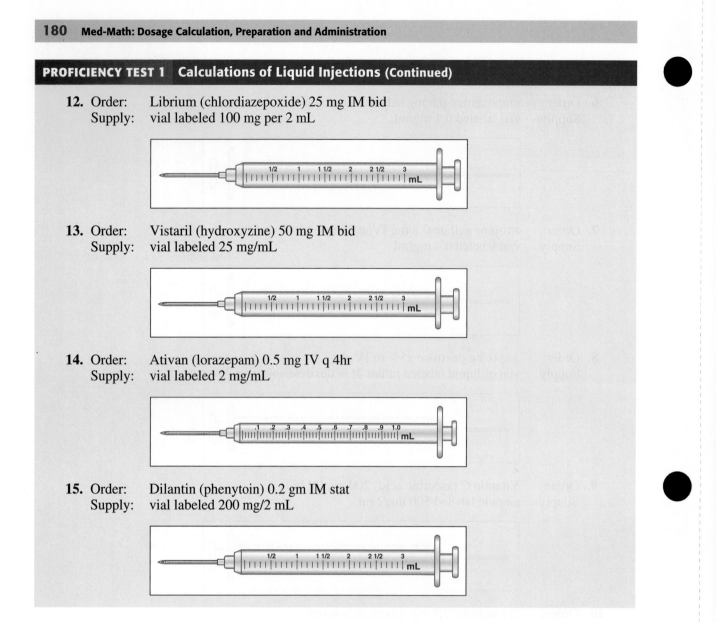

PROFICIENCY TEST 2 | **Calculations of Liquid Injections**

Name: _____

Solve these problems for injections from a liquid. Draw a line on the syringe indicating the amount you would prepare in milliliters. See Appendix A for answers.

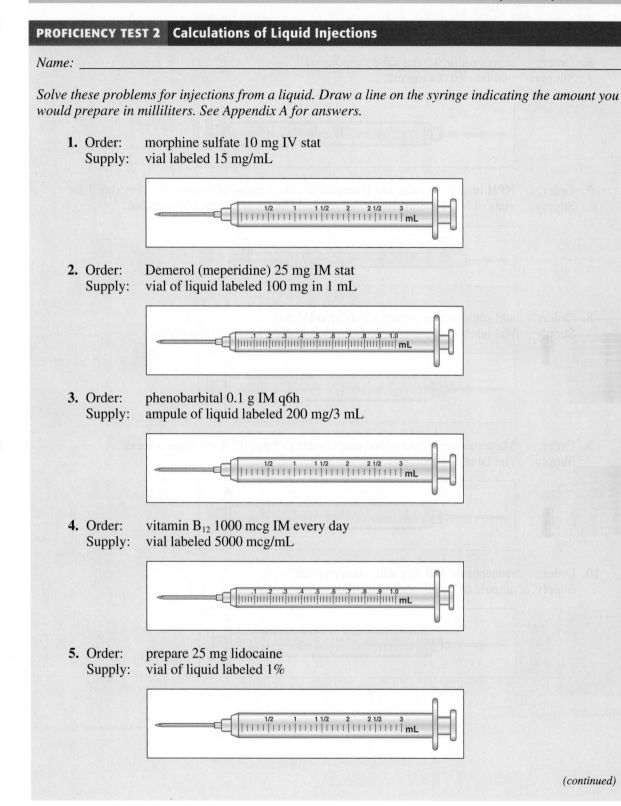

1. Order: morphine sulfate 10 mg IV stat
   Supply: vial labeled 15 mg/mL

2. Order: Demerol (meperidine) 25 mg IM stat
   Supply: vial of liquid labeled 100 mg in 1 mL

3. Order: phenobarbital 0.1 g IM q6h
   Supply: ampule of liquid labeled 200 mg/3 mL

4. Order: vitamin B$_{12}$ 1000 mcg IM every day
   Supply: vial labeled 5000 mcg/mL

5. Order: prepare 25 mg lidocaine
   Supply: vial of liquid labeled 1%

(continued)

PROFICIENCY TEST 2 **Calculations of Liquid Injections (Continued)**

6. Order: scopolamine 0.5 mg subcutaneous stat
 Supply: vial labeled 0.4 mg/mL

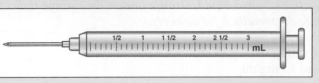

7. Order: NPH insulin 10 units and Humulin insulin 3 units subcutaneous every day 7 AM
 Supply: vials of NPH insulin 100 units/mL and Humulin insulin 100 units/mL

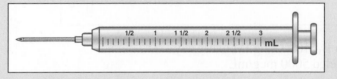

8. Order: add sodium bicarbonate 1.2 mEq to IV stat
 Supply: vial labeled infant 4.2% sodium bicarbonate 5 mEq (0.5 mEq/mL)

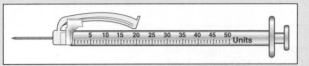

9. Order: Masteron (dromostanolone proprionate) 75 mg IM three times a week
 Supply: vial labeled 50 mg/mL

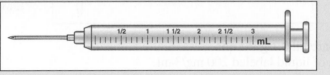

10. Order: epinephrine 500 mcg subcutaneous stat
 Supply: ampule of liquid labeled 1:1000

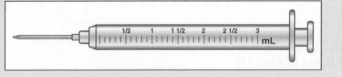

PROFICIENCY TEST 3 **Calculations of Liquid Injections**

Name: _____

Aim for 90% or better on this test. Assume you have only a 3-mL syringe. See Appendix A for answers.

1. Order: Lanoxin (digoxin) 0.25 mg IM every day   *x = 1mL*
   Supply: ampule labeled 0.5 mg/2 mL

2. Order: Benadryl (diphenhydramine hydrochloride) 40 mg IM stat
   Supply: ampule labeled 50 mg (2-mL size)   *x = 1.6mL*

3. Order: morphine sulfate 8 mg IV q4h prn   *x = 0.53mL*
   Supply: vial labeled 15 mg/mL

4. Order: Demerol (meperidine) 25 mg IM q4h prn   *x = 0.25 mL*
   Supply: vial labeled 100 mg/mL

5. Order: Vitamin C (ascorbic acid) 200 mg IM every day   *x = 0.8mL*
   Supply: ampule labeled 500 mg/2 mL

6. Order: vitamin B_{12} 1500 mcg every day IM
   Supply: vial labeled 5000 mcg/mL

7. Order: atropine sulfate 0.6 mg IV at 7:30 AM
   Supply: vial labeled 0.4 mg/mL

8. Order: sodium amytal 0.1 g IM stat
   Supply: ampule 200 mg/3 mL

9. Order: Dilaudid (hydromorphone HCl) 1.5 mg IM q4h prn
   Supply: vial labeled 2 mg/mL

10. Order: penicillin G procaine 600,000 units IM q12h
    Supply: vial labeled 500,000 USP units/mL

11. Order: add nitroglycerin 200 mcg to IV stat
    Supply: vial labeled 0.8 mg/mL

12. Order: neostigmine methylsulfate 500 mcg subcutaneous
    Supply: ampule labeled 1:4000

13. Order: Levo-Dromoran (levorphanol tartrate) 3 mg subcutaneous
    Supply: vial labeled 2 mg/mL

14. Order: epinephrine 0.4 mg subcutaneous stat
    Supply: ampule labeled 1:1000 (2-mL size)

15. Order: magnesium sulfate 500 mg IM
    Supply: ampule labeled 50% (2-mL size)

(continued)

PROFICIENCY TEST 3 **Calculations of Liquid Injections (Continued)**

16. Order: Numorphan (oxymorphone HCl) 0.75 mg subcutaneous
 Supply: vial labeled 1.5 mg/mL

17. Order: add lidocaine 100 mg to IV stat
 Supply: ampule labeled 20%

18. Order: Lanoxin (digoxin) 0.125 mg IV 10 AM
 Supply: ampule labeled 0.25 mg/2 mL

19. Order: Nubain (nalbuphine HCl) 12 mg IM
 Supply: vial 10 mg/mL

20. Order: add 10 mEq KCl to IV
 Supply: vial 40 mEq/20 mL

PROFICIENCY TEST 4 | **Mental Drill in Liquids-for-Injection Problems**

Name: _____

As you develop proficiency in solving problems, you will be able to calculate many answers without written work. This drill combines your knowledge of equivalents and dosages. Solve these problems mentally and write only the amount to give. See Appendix A for answers.

Order	*Supply*	*Give*
1. 0.5 g IM	250 mg/mL	_____
2. 10 mEq IV	40 mEq/20 mL	_____
3. 0.5 mg IM	0.25 mg/mL	_____
4. 100 mg IM	0.2 g/2 mL	_____
5. 50 mg IM	100 mg = 1 mL	_____
6. 0.25 mg IM	0.5 mg/2 mL	_____
7. 0.3 mg subcutaneous	0.4 mg/mL	_____
8. 1 mg subcutaneous	1:1000 solution	_____
9. 1 g IV	5% solution	_____
10. 0.1 g IM	200 mg/5 mL	_____
11. 400,000 units IM	500,000 units/mL	_____
12. 0.5 mg IM	0.5 mg/2 mL	_____
13. 1 g IV	50% solution	_____
14. 75 mg IM	100 mg/2 mL	_____
15. 15 mg IM	1:100 solution	_____
16. 35 mg IM	100 mg/mL	_____
17. 0.6 mg subcutaneous	0.4 mg per mL	_____
18. 0.15 g IM	0.2 g/2 mL	_____

Name: _____

Solve the problems. See Appendix A for answers.

1. Order:　Fortaz (ceftazidime) 250 mg IM q8h
   Supply:　vial of powder labeled 1-g powder (refer to Fig. 7-15)

   a. Diluting fluid and number of milliliters:
   b. Solution and new supply:
   c. Rule and arithmetic:
   d. Amount to give:
   e. Write on label:
   f. Storage:

2. Order:　Ticar (ticarcillin disodium) 1 g IM
   Supply:　vial of powder labeled Ticar 1 g (Fig. 7-17)

   a. Diluting fluid and number of milliliters:
   b. Solution and new stock:
   c. Rule and arithmetic:
   d. Amount to give:
   e. Write on label:
   f. Storage:

DIRECTIONS FOR USE
　—1 Gm, 3 Gm and 6 Gm Standard Vials—
INTRAMUSCULAR USE: (Concentration of approximately 385 mg/ml).
For initial reconstitution use Sterile Water for Injection, USP, Sodium Chloride Injection, USP or 1% Lidocaine Hydrochloride solution* (without epinephrine).
Each gram of Ticarcillin should be reconstituted with 2 ml of Sterile Water for Injection, U.S.P., Sodium Chloride Injection, U.S.P. or 1% Lidocaine Hydrochloride solution* (without epinephrine) and **used promptly.** Each 2.6 ml of the resulting solution will then contain 1 Gm of Ticarcillin.
*[For full product information, refer to manufacturer's package insert for Lidocaine Hydrochloride.]
As with all intramuscular preparations, TICAR (Ticarcillin Disodium) should be injected well within the body of a relatively large muscle, using usual techniques and precautions.

FIGURE 7-17

Directions for use of ticarcillin disodium (Ticar). (Courtesy of GlaxoSmithKline.)

3. Order:　ampicillin sodium 300 mg IM q8h
   Supply:　vial of 500 mg powder (Fig. 7-18)

   a. Diluting fluid and number of milliliters:
   b. Solution and new supply:
   c. Rule and arithmetic:
   d. Amount to give:
   e. Write on label:
   f. Storage:

4. Order:　Mefoxin (cefoxitin) 300 mg IM q4h
   　　　　　Supply: vial of powder 1 g (Fig. 7-19)

   a. Diluting fluid and number of milliliters:
   b. Solution and new supply:
   c. Rule and arithmetic:

(continued)

PROFICIENCY TEST 5 | **Injections from Powders (Continued)**

Intramuscular Use: 125 mg vial: Add 1 ml Sterile Water for Injection, USP, or Bacteriostatic Water for Injection, USP (TUBEX® Sterile Cartridge-Needle Unit) to give a final concentration of 125 mg per ml. For fractional doses, withdraw the ampicillin sodium solution as follows:

Dose	Withdraw
25 mg	0.2 ml
50 mg	0.4 ml
75 mg	0.6 ml
100 mg	0.8 ml
125 mg	1 ml

250 mg vial: Add 0.9 ml Sterile Water for Injection, USP, or Bacteriostatic Water for Injection, USP (TUBEX) to give a final concentration of 250 mg/ml. For fractional doses, withdraw the ampicillin sodium solution as follows:

Dose	Withdraw
125 mg	0.5 ml
150 mg	0.6 ml
175 mg	0.7 ml
200 mg	0.8 ml
225 mg	0.9 ml
250 mg	1 ml

For dilution of 500-mg, 1-gram, and 2-gram vials, dissolve contents of a vial with the amount of Sterile water for Injection, USP, or Bacteriostatic Water for Injection, USP, listed in the table below:

Label Claim	Recommended Amount of Diluent	Withdrawable Volume	Concentration in mg/ml
500 mg	1.8 ml	2.0 ml	250 mg
1.0 gram	3.4 ml	4.0 ml	250 mg
2.0 gram	6.8 ml	8.0 ml	250 mg

While the 1-gram and 2-gram vials are primarily for intravenous use, they may be administered intramuscularly when the 250-mg or 500-mg vials are unavailable. In such instances, dissolve in 3.4 or 6.8 ml Sterile Water for Injection, USP, or Bacteriostatic Water for Injection, USP, to give a final concentration of 250 mg/ml

The above solutions must be used within one hour after reconstitution.

FIGURE 7-18

Reconstitution directions for ampicillin sodium for IM or IV injection.

	— Preparation of Solution		
Strength	Amount of Diluent to be Added (mL) + +	Approximate Withdrawable Volume (mL)	Approximate Average Concentration (mg/mL)
1 gram Vial	2 (Intramuscular)	2.5	400
2 gram Vial	4 (Intramuscular)	5	400
1 gram Vial	10 (IV)	10.5	95
2 gram Vial	10 or 20 (IV)	11.1 or 21.0	180 or 95
1 gram Infusion Bottle	50 or 100 (IV)	50 or 100	20 or 10
2 gram Infusion Bottle	50 or 100 (IV)	50 or 100	40 or 20
10 gram Bulk	43 or 93 (IV)	49 or 98.5	200 or 100

+ + Shake to dissolve and let stand until clear.

Intramuscular
MEFOXIN, as constituted with Sterile Water for Injection, Bacteriostatic Water for Injection, or 0.5 percent or 1 percent lidocaine hydrochloride solution (without epinephrine), maintains satisfactory potency for 24 hours at room temperature, for one week under refrigeration (below 5°C), and for at least 30 weeks in the frozen state.

FIGURE 7-19

Directions to reconstitute Mefoxin (cefoxitin sodium). (Courtesy of Merck Co. Inc.)

    d. Amount to give:
    e. Write on label:
    f. Storage:

5. Order: Ancef (cefazolin sodium) 0.33 g IM q8h
          Supply: vial of powder labeled 1 g (see Fig. 7-10)

    a. Diluting fluid and number of milliliters:
    b. Solution and new supply:
    c. Rule and arithmetic:
    d. Amount to give:
    e. Write on label:
    f. Storage:

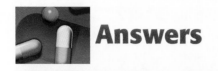

Answers

Self-Test 1 Calculation of Liquids for Injection

1. Equivalent: 0.3 g = 300 mg

Formula Method	Proportion Expressed as Two Ratios	Proportion Expressed as Two Fractions
$\dfrac{\overset{1}{\cancel{300}}\ \text{mg}}{\underset{1}{\cancel{300}}\ \text{mg}} \times 2\ \text{mL} = 2\ \text{mL}$	2 mL : 300 mg : : x : 300 mg	$\dfrac{2\ \text{mL}}{300\ \text{mg}} \times \dfrac{x}{300\ \text{mg}}$

$$\frac{600}{300} = x$$

$$2\ \text{mL} = x$$

Give 2 mL IM.

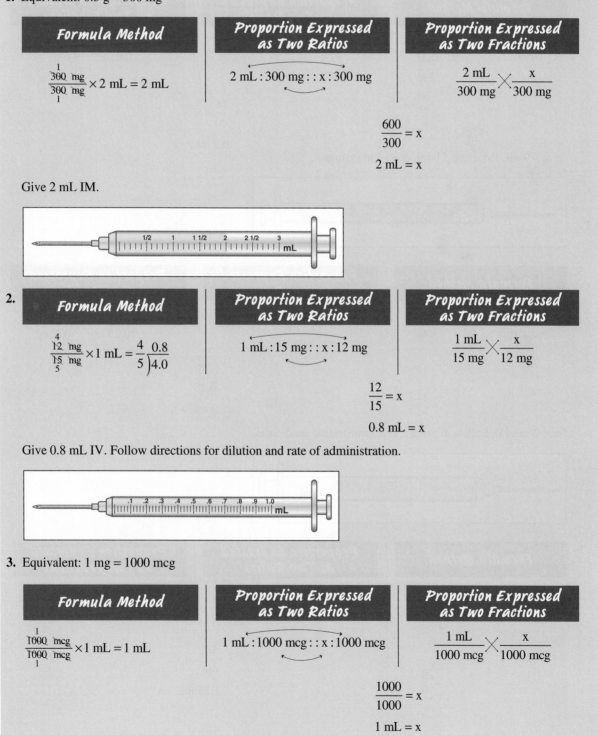

2.

Formula Method	Proportion Expressed as Two Ratios	Proportion Expressed as Two Fractions
$\dfrac{\overset{4}{\cancel{12}}\ \text{mg}}{\underset{5}{\cancel{15}}\ \text{mg}} \times 1\ \text{mL} = \dfrac{4}{5}\ \overset{0.8}{\overline{)4.0}}$	1 mL : 15 mg : : x : 12 mg	$\dfrac{1\ \text{mL}}{15\ \text{mg}} \times \dfrac{x}{12\ \text{mg}}$

$$\frac{12}{15} = x$$

$$0.8\ \text{mL} = x$$

Give 0.8 mL IV. Follow directions for dilution and rate of administration.

3. Equivalent: 1 mg = 1000 mcg

Formula Method	Proportion Expressed as Two Ratios	Proportion Expressed as Two Fractions
$\dfrac{\overset{1}{\cancel{1000}}\ \text{mcg}}{\underset{1}{\cancel{1000}}\ \text{mcg}} \times 1\ \text{mL} = 1\ \text{mL}$	1 mL : 1000 mcg : : x : 1000 mcg	$\dfrac{1\ \text{mL}}{1000\ \text{mcg}} \times \dfrac{x}{1000\ \text{mcg}}$

$$\frac{1000}{1000} = x$$

$$1\ \text{mL} = x$$

Give 1 mL IM.

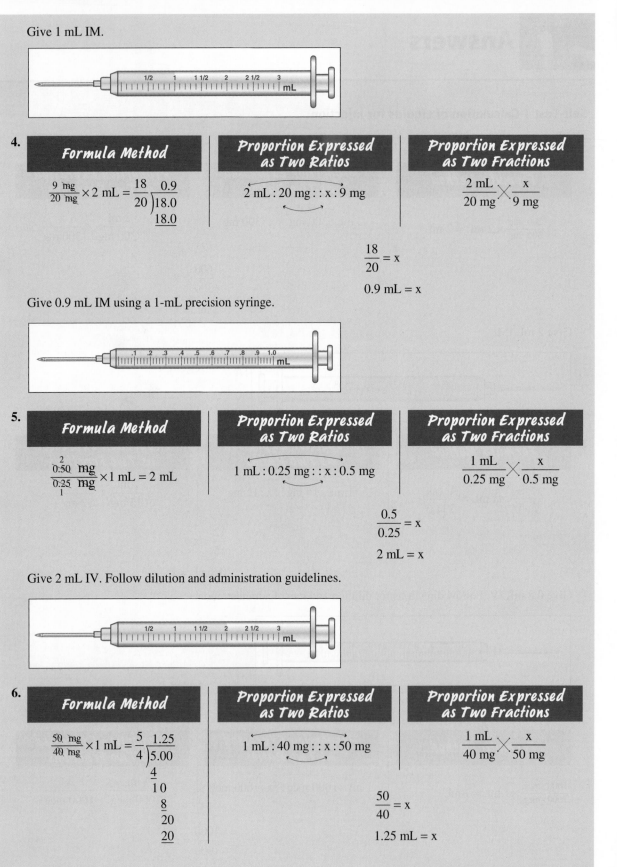

4.

Formula Method	Proportion Expressed as Two Ratios	Proportion Expressed as Two Fractions
$\dfrac{9 \text{ mg}}{20 \text{ mg}} \times 2 \text{ mL} = \dfrac{18}{20} \overline{)\dfrac{0.9}{18.0}}$ $\underline{18.0}$	2 mL : 20 mg : : x : 9 mg	$\dfrac{2 \text{ mL}}{20 \text{ mg}} \times \dfrac{\text{x}}{9 \text{ mg}}$

$$\frac{18}{20} = x$$

$$0.9 \text{ mL} = x$$

Give 0.9 mL IM using a 1-mL precision syringe.

5.

Formula Method	Proportion Expressed as Two Ratios	Proportion Expressed as Two Fractions
$\dfrac{\overset{2}{0.50} \text{ mg}}{\underset{1}{0.25} \text{ mg}} \times 1 \text{ mL} = 2 \text{ mL}$	1 mL : 0.25 mg : : x : 0.5 mg	$\dfrac{1 \text{ mL}}{0.25 \text{ mg}} \times \dfrac{\text{x}}{0.5 \text{ mg}}$

$$\frac{0.5}{0.25} = x$$

$$2 \text{ mL} = x$$

Give 2 mL IV. Follow dilution and administration guidelines.

6.

Formula Method	Proportion Expressed as Two Ratios	Proportion Expressed as Two Fractions
$\dfrac{50 \text{ mg}}{40 \text{ mg}} \times 1 \text{ mL} = \dfrac{5}{4} \overline{)\dfrac{1.25}{5.00}}$ $\underline{4}$ $\quad 1\ 0$ $\quad \underline{8}$ $\quad\ 20$ $\quad\ \underline{20}$	1 mL : 40 mg : : x : 50 mg	$\dfrac{1 \text{ mL}}{40 \text{ mg}} \times \dfrac{\text{x}}{50 \text{ mg}}$

$$\frac{50}{40} = x$$

$$1.25 \text{ mL} = x$$

Give 1.3 mL IM.

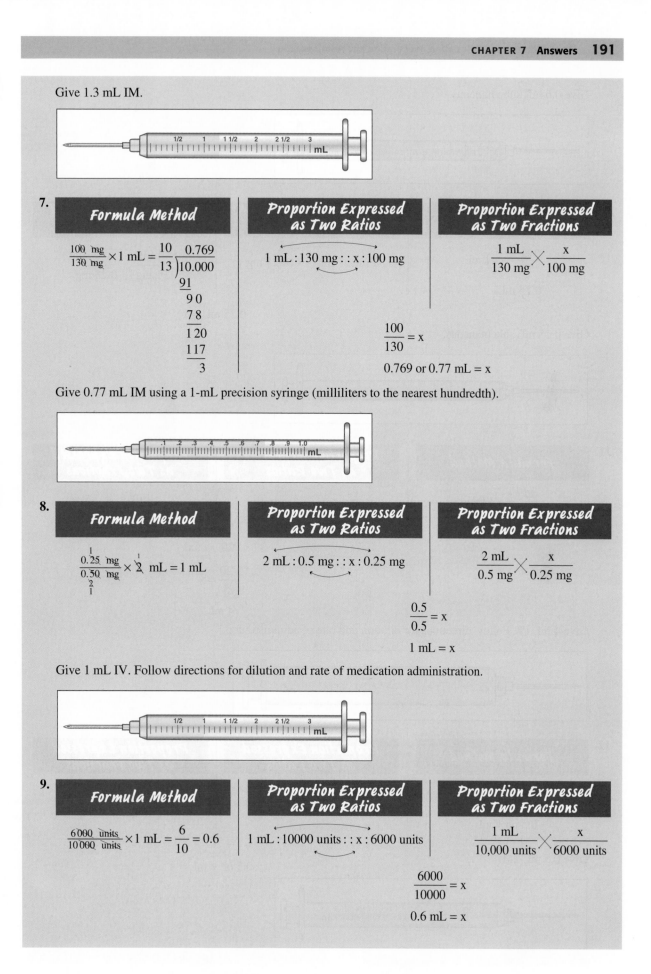

7.

Formula Method	Proportion Expressed as Two Ratios	Proportion Expressed as Two Fractions
$\dfrac{100 \text{ mg}}{130 \text{ mg}} \times 1 \text{ mL} = \dfrac{10}{13}$ $\begin{array}{r} 0.769 \\ 13\overline{)10.000} \\ \underline{91} \\ 9\,0 \\ \underline{7\,8} \\ 1\,20 \\ \underline{1\,17} \\ 3 \end{array}$	1 mL : 130 mg :: x : 100 mg	$\dfrac{1 \text{ mL}}{130 \text{ mg}} \times \dfrac{\text{x}}{100 \text{ mg}}$

$$\frac{100}{130} = x$$

0.769 or 0.77 mL = x

Give 0.77 mL IM using a 1-mL precision syringe (milliliters to the nearest hundredth).

8.

Formula Method	Proportion Expressed as Two Ratios	Proportion Expressed as Two Fractions
$\dfrac{\overset{1}{0.25} \text{ mg}}{\underset{\underset{1}{2}}{0.50} \text{ mg}} \times \overset{1}{2} \text{ mL} = 1 \text{ mL}$	2 mL : 0.5 mg :: x : 0.25 mg	$\dfrac{2 \text{ mL}}{0.5 \text{ mg}} \times \dfrac{\text{x}}{0.25 \text{ mg}}$

$$\frac{0.5}{0.5} = x$$

1 mL = x

Give 1 mL IV. Follow directions for dilution and rate of medication administration.

9.

Formula Method	Proportion Expressed as Two Ratios	Proportion Expressed as Two Fractions
$\dfrac{6000 \text{ units}}{10\,000 \text{ units}} \times 1 \text{ mL} = \dfrac{6}{10} = 0.6$	1 mL : 10000 units :: x : 6000 units	$\dfrac{1 \text{ mL}}{10,000 \text{ units}} \times \dfrac{\text{x}}{6000 \text{ units}}$

$$\frac{6000}{10000} = x$$

0.6 mL = x

Give 0.6 mL subcutaneous.

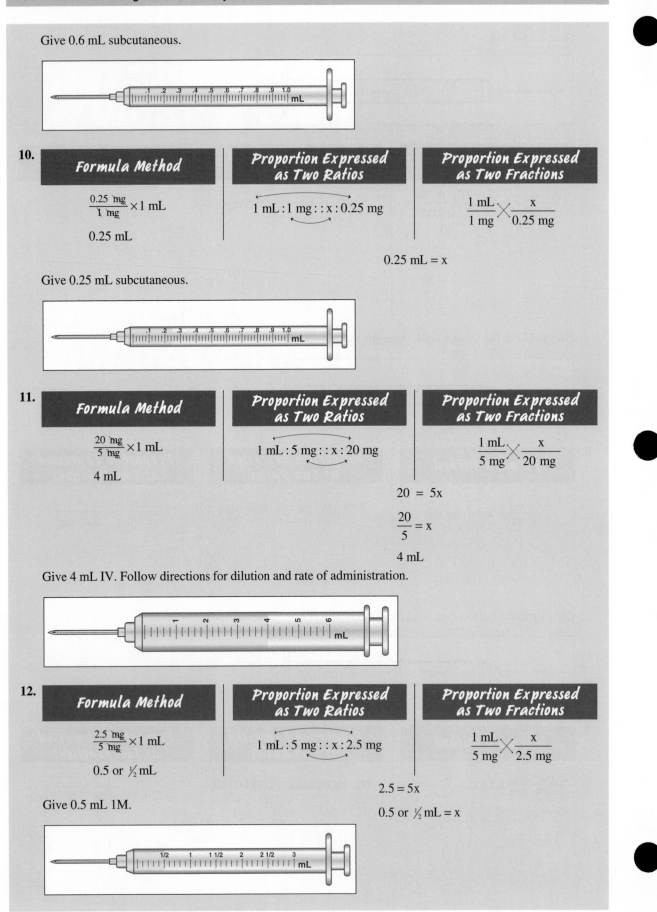

10.

Formula Method	Proportion Expressed as Two Ratios	Proportion Expressed as Two Fractions

$$\frac{0.25 \text{ mg}}{1 \text{ mg}} \times 1 \text{ mL}$$

0.25 mL

1 mL : 1 mg : : x : 0.25 mg

$$\frac{1 \text{ mL}}{1 \text{ mg}} \times \frac{x}{0.25 \text{ mg}}$$

0.25 mL = x

Give 0.25 mL subcutaneous.

11.

Formula Method	Proportion Expressed as Two Ratios	Proportion Expressed as Two Fractions

$$\frac{20 \text{ mg}}{5 \text{ mg}} \times 1 \text{ mL}$$

4 mL

1 mL : 5 mg : : x : 20 mg

$$\frac{1 \text{ mL}}{5 \text{ mg}} \times \frac{x}{20 \text{ mg}}$$

$$20 = 5x$$

$$\frac{20}{5} = x$$

4 mL

Give 4 mL IV. Follow directions for dilution and rate of administration.

12.

Formula Method	Proportion Expressed as Two Ratios	Proportion Expressed as Two Fractions

$$\frac{2.5 \text{ mg}}{5 \text{ mg}} \times 1 \text{ mL}$$

0.5 or ½ mL

1 mL : 5 mg : : x : 2.5 mg

$$\frac{1 \text{ mL}}{5 \text{ mg}} \times \frac{x}{2.5 \text{ mg}}$$

$$2.5 = 5x$$

0.5 or ½ mL = x

Give 0.5 mL 1M.

13.

Formula Method	Proportion Expressed as Two Ratios	Proportion Expressed as Two Fractions
$\dfrac{3 \text{ mg}}{10 \text{ mg}} \times 1 \text{ mL} = x$	1 mL : 10 mg :: x : 3 mg	$\dfrac{1 \text{ mL}}{10 \text{ mg}} \times \dfrac{x}{3 \text{ mg}}$
0.3 mL		

$$3 = 10\,x$$
$$\frac{3}{10} = x$$
$$0.3 = x$$

Give 0.3 mL subcutaneously.

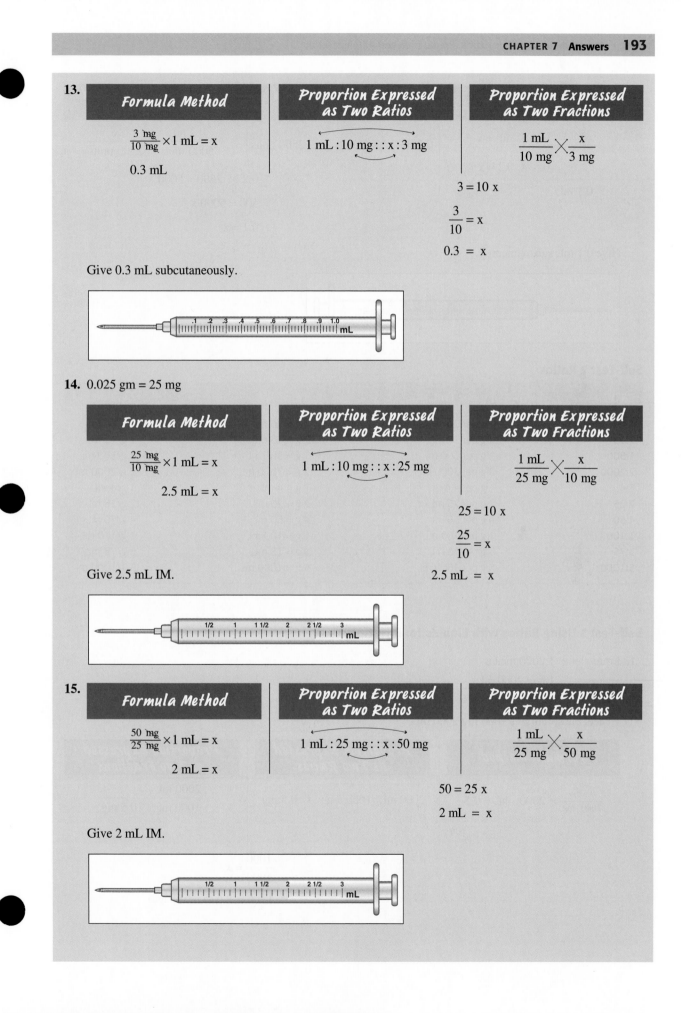

14. 0.025 gm = 25 mg

Formula Method	Proportion Expressed as Two Ratios	Proportion Expressed as Two Fractions
$\dfrac{25 \text{ mg}}{10 \text{ mg}} \times 1 \text{ mL} = x$	1 mL : 10 mg :: x : 25 mg	$\dfrac{1 \text{ mL}}{25 \text{ mg}} \times \dfrac{x}{10 \text{ mg}}$
2.5 mL = x		

$$25 = 10\,x$$
$$\frac{25}{10} = x$$

Give 2.5 mL IM. $2.5 \text{ mL} = x$

15.

Formula Method	Proportion Expressed as Two Ratios	Proportion Expressed as Two Fractions
$\dfrac{50 \text{ mg}}{25 \text{ mg}} \times 1 \text{ mL} = x$	1 mL : 25 mg :: x : 50 mg	$\dfrac{1 \text{ mL}}{25 \text{ mg}} \times \dfrac{x}{50 \text{ mg}}$
2 mL = x		

$$50 = 25\,x$$
$$2 \text{ mL} = x$$

Give 2 mL IM.

16.

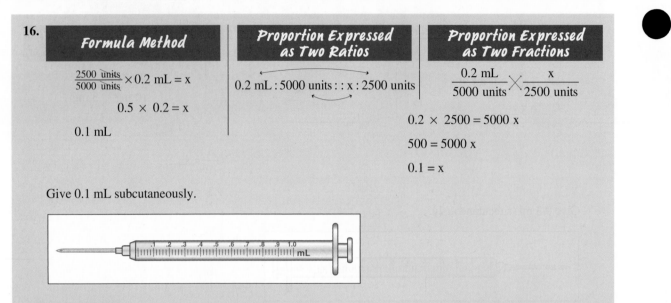

Formula Method	Proportion Expressed as Two Ratios	Proportion Expressed as Two Fractions
$\dfrac{2500 \text{ units}}{5000 \text{ units}} \times 0.2 \text{ mL} = x$	0.2 mL : 5000 units : : x : 2500 units	$\dfrac{0.2 \text{ mL}}{5000 \text{ units}} \times \dfrac{x}{2500 \text{ units}}$
$0.5 \times 0.2 = x$		$0.2 \times 2500 = 5000 \, x$
0.1 mL		$500 = 5000 \, x$
		$0.1 = x$

Give 0.1 mL subcutaneously.

Self-Test 2 Ratios

RATIO	? g per ? mL	? g = ? mL	? g/? mL
1:20	1 g per 20 mL	1 g = 20 mL	1 g/20 mL
2:15	2 g per 15 mL	2 g = 15 mL	2 g/15 mL
1:500	1 g per 500 mL	1 g = 500 mL	1 g/500 mL
2:2000	2 g per 2000 mL	2 g = 2000 mL	2 g/2000 mL
1:4	1 g per 4 mL	1 g = 4 mL	1 g/4 mL
2:25	2 g per 25 mL	2 g = 25 mL	2 g/25 mL
4:50	4 g per 50 mL	4 g = 50 mL	4 g/50 mL
1:100	1 g per 100 mL	1 g = 100 mL	1 g/100 mL
3:75	3 g per 75 mL	3 g = 75 mL	3 g/75 mL
5:1000	5 g per 1000 mL	5 g = 1000 mL	5 g/1000 mL

Self-Test 3 Using Ratios with Liquids for Injection

1. Equivalent: 1:2000 means

    1 g in 2000 mL

    1 g = 1000 mg

Hence, the solution is 1000 mg/2000 mL.

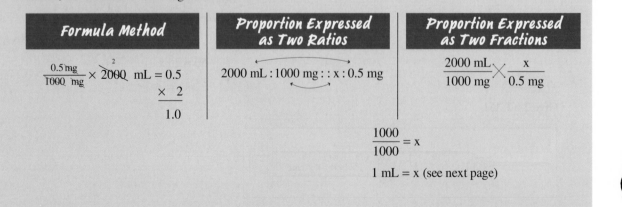

Formula Method	Proportion Expressed as Two Ratios	Proportion Expressed as Two Fractions
$\dfrac{0.5 \text{ mg}}{1000 \text{ mg}} \times \overset{2}{2000} \text{ mL} = 0.5$	2000 mL : 1000 mg : : x : 0.5 mg	$\dfrac{2000 \text{ mL}}{1000 \text{ mg}} \times \dfrac{x}{0.5 \text{ mg}}$
$\dfrac{\times \ 2}{1.0}$		
		$\dfrac{1000}{1000} = x$
		1 mL = x (see next page)

Give 1 mL subcutaneous.

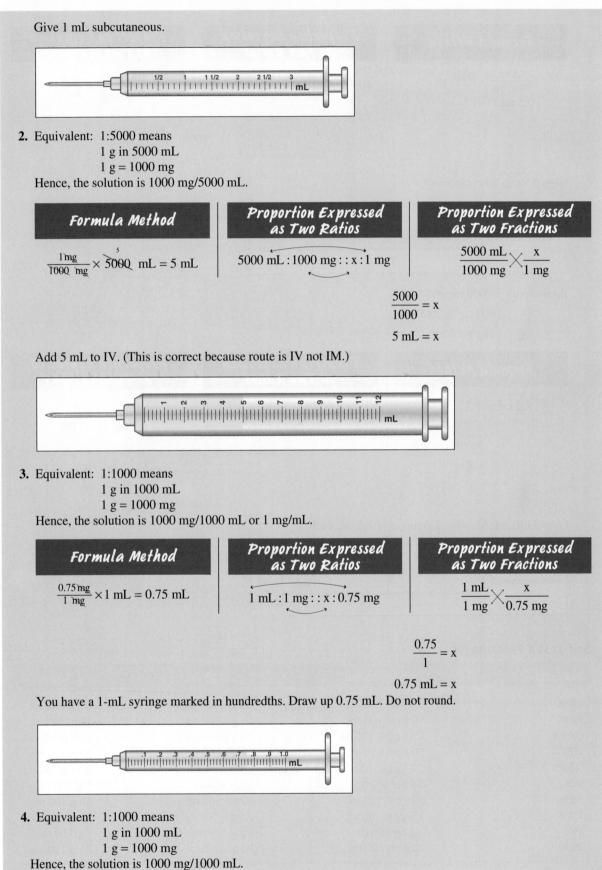

2. Equivalent: 1:5000 means
   1 g in 5000 mL
   1 g = 1000 mg
Hence, the solution is 1000 mg/5000 mL.

Formula Method	Proportion Expressed as Two Ratios	Proportion Expressed as Two Fractions
$\dfrac{1 \text{ mg}}{1000 \text{ mg}} \times \overset{5}{5000} \text{ mL} = 5 \text{ mL}$	5000 mL : 1000 mg :: x : 1 mg	$\dfrac{5000 \text{ mL}}{1000 \text{ mg}} \times \dfrac{x}{1 \text{ mg}}$

$$\frac{5000}{1000} = x$$

$$5 \text{ mL} = x$$

Add 5 mL to IV. (This is correct because route is IV not IM.)

3. Equivalent: 1:1000 means
   1 g in 1000 mL
   1 g = 1000 mg
Hence, the solution is 1000 mg/1000 mL or 1 mg/mL.

Formula Method	Proportion Expressed as Two Ratios	Proportion Expressed as Two Fractions
$\dfrac{0.75 \text{ mg}}{1 \text{ mg}} \times 1 \text{ mL} = 0.75 \text{ mL}$	1 mL : 1 mg :: x : 0.75 mg	$\dfrac{1 \text{ mL}}{1 \text{ mg}} \times \dfrac{x}{0.75 \text{ mg}}$

$$\frac{0.75}{1} = x$$

$$0.75 \text{ mL} = x$$

You have a 1-mL syringe marked in hundredths. Draw up 0.75 mL. Do not round.

4. Equivalent: 1:1000 means
   1 g in 1000 mL
   1 g = 1000 mg
Hence, the solution is 1000 mg/1000 mL.

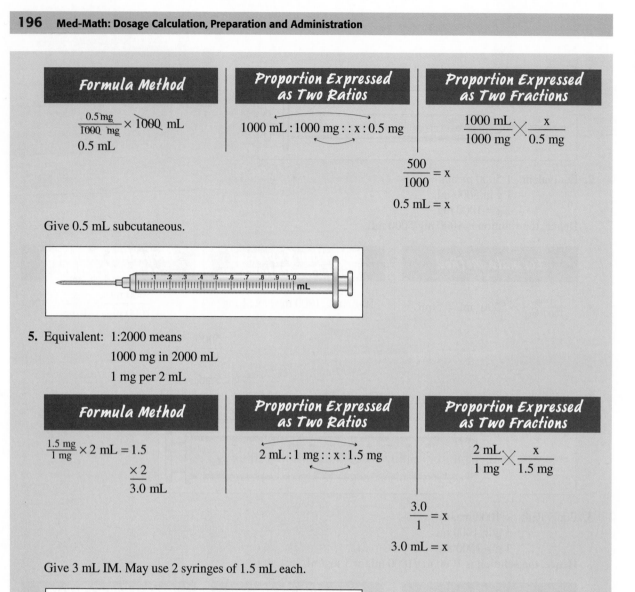

Formula Method	Proportion Expressed as Two Ratios	Proportion Expressed as Two Fractions
$\frac{0.5 \text{ mg}}{1000 \text{ mg}} \times 1000 \text{ mL}$ 0.5 mL	$1000 \text{ mL} : 1000 \text{ mg} :: x : 0.5 \text{ mg}$	$\frac{1000 \text{ mL}}{1000 \text{ mg}} \times \frac{x}{0.5 \text{ mg}}$ $\frac{500}{1000} = x$ $0.5 \text{ mL} = x$

Give 0.5 mL subcutaneous.

5. Equivalent: 1:2000 means
    1000 mg in 2000 mL
    1 mg per 2 mL

Formula Method	Proportion Expressed as Two Ratios	Proportion Expressed as Two Fractions
$\frac{1.5 \text{ mg}}{1 \text{ mg}} \times 2 \text{ mL} = 1.5$ $\frac{\times 2}{3.0 \text{ mL}}$	$2 \text{ mL} : 1 \text{ mg} :: x : 1.5 \text{ mg}$	$\frac{2 \text{ mL}}{1 \text{ mg}} \times \frac{x}{1.5 \text{ mg}}$ $\frac{3.0}{1} = x$ $3.0 \text{ mL} = x$

Give 3 mL IM. May use 2 syringes of 1.5 mL each.

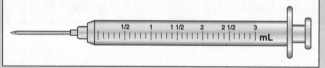

Self-Test 4 Percentages

PERCENTAGE	? g per 100 mL	? g = 100 mL	? g/100 mL
0.9%	0.9 g per 100 mL	0.9 g = 100 mL	0.9 g/100 mL
10%	10 g per 100 mL	10 g = 100 mL	10 g/100 mL
0.45%	0.45 g per 100 mL	0.45 g = 100 mL	0.45 g/100 mL
50%	50 g per 100 mL	50 g = 100 mL	50 g/100 mL
0.33%	0.33 g per 100 mL	0.33 g = 100 mL	0.33 g/100 mL
5%	5 g per 100 mL	5 g = 100 mL	5 g/100 mL
30%	30 g per 100 mL	30 g = 100 mL	30 g/100 mL
1.5%	1.5 g per 100 mL	1.5 g = 100 mL	1.5 g/100 mL
1%	1 g per 100 mL	1 g = 100 mL	1 g/100 mL
20%	20 g per 100 mL	20 g = 100 mL	20 g/100 mL

Self-Test 5 Using Percentages with Liquids for Injection

1. Equivalent: 1% 1 g in 100 mL

    1 g = 1000 mg

    Hence, the solution is 1000 mg/100 mL.

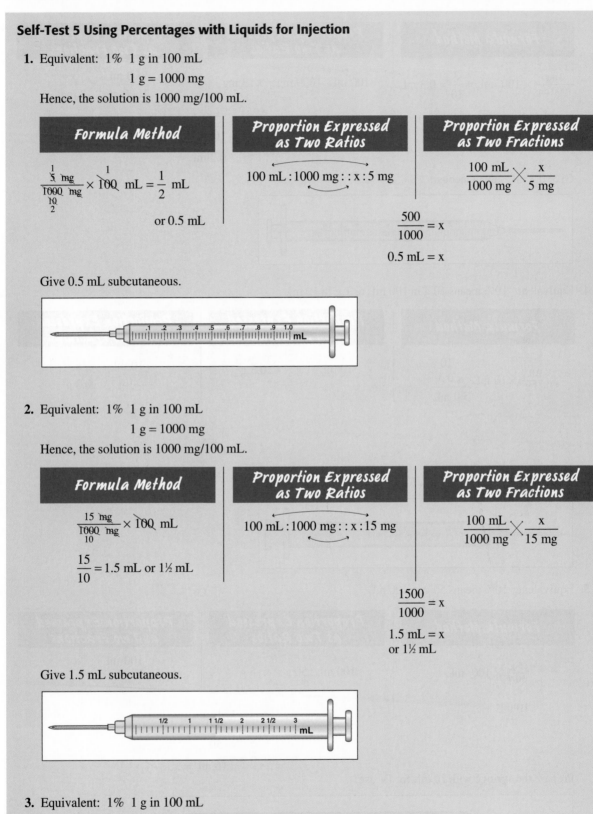

Formula Method	Proportion Expressed as Two Ratios	Proportion Expressed as Two Fractions
$\dfrac{\overset{1}{\cancel{5}}\text{ mg}}{\underset{\underset{2}{10}}{\cancel{1000}}\text{ mg}} \times \overset{1}{\cancel{100}}\text{ mL} = \dfrac{1}{2}\text{ mL}$ or 0.5 mL	100 mL : 1000 mg : : x : 5 mg	$\dfrac{100\text{ mL}}{1000\text{ mg}}\times\dfrac{\text{x}}{5\text{ mg}}$

$$\frac{500}{1000} = x$$

$$0.5\text{ mL} = x$$

Give 0.5 mL subcutaneous.

2. Equivalent: 1% 1 g in 100 mL

    1 g = 1000 mg

    Hence, the solution is 1000 mg/100 mL.

Formula Method	Proportion Expressed as Two Ratios	Proportion Expressed as Two Fractions
$\dfrac{15\text{ mg}}{\underset{10}{\cancel{1000}}\text{ mg}} \times \overset{}{\cancel{100}}\text{ mL}$ $\dfrac{15}{10} = 1.5\text{ mL or } 1\tfrac{1}{2}\text{ mL}$	100 mL : 1000 mg : : x : 15 mg	$\dfrac{100\text{ mL}}{1000\text{ mg}}\times\dfrac{\text{x}}{15\text{ mg}}$

$$\frac{1500}{1000} = x$$

$$1.5\text{ mL} = x$$
or $1\tfrac{1}{2}$ mL

Give 1.5 mL subcutaneous.

3. Equivalent: 1% 1 g in 100 mL

    1 g = 1000 mg

    Hence, the solution is 1000 mg/100 mL.

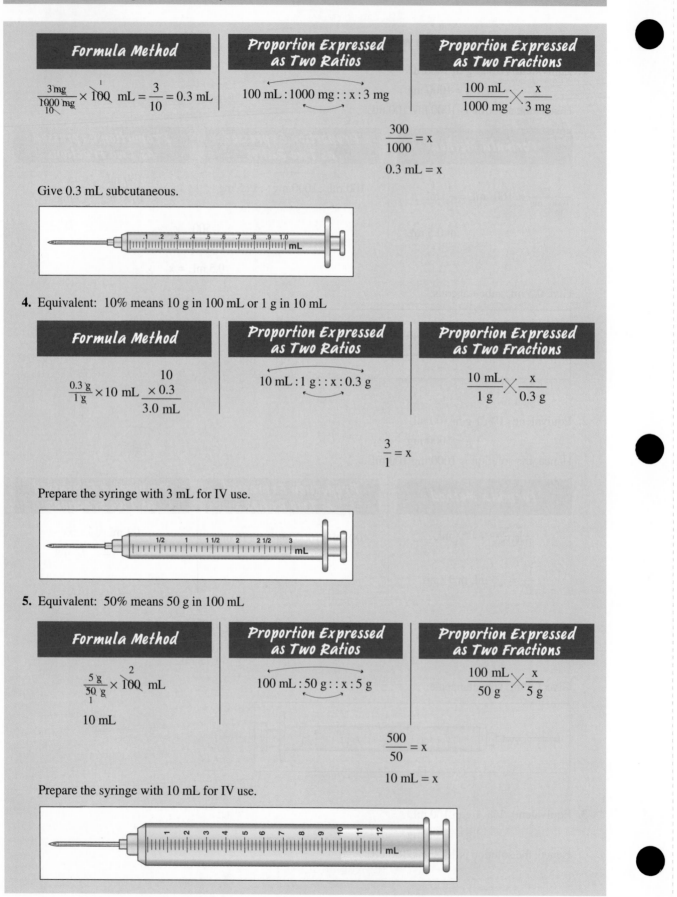

Formula Method	Proportion Expressed as Two Ratios	Proportion Expressed as Two Fractions
$\dfrac{3\,mg}{\underset{10}{1000\,mg}} \times \overset{1}{100}\ mL = \dfrac{3}{10} = 0.3\,mL$	$100\,mL : 1000\,mg :: x : 3\,mg$	$\dfrac{100\,mL}{1000\,mg} \times \dfrac{x}{3\,mg}$

$$\frac{300}{1000} = x$$

$$0.3\,mL = x$$

Give 0.3 mL subcutaneous.

4. Equivalent: 10% means 10 g in 100 mL or 1 g in 10 mL

Formula Method	Proportion Expressed as Two Ratios	Proportion Expressed as Two Fractions
$\dfrac{0.3\,g}{1\,g} \times 10\,mL \quad \dfrac{\overset{10}{\times 0.3}}{3.0\,mL}$	$10\,mL : 1\,g :: x : 0.3\,g$	$\dfrac{10\,mL}{1\,g} \times \dfrac{x}{0.3\,g}$

$$\frac{3}{1} = x$$

Prepare the syringe with 3 mL for IV use.

5. Equivalent: 50% means 50 g in 100 mL

Formula Method	Proportion Expressed as Two Ratios	Proportion Expressed as Two Fractions
$\dfrac{5\,g}{\underset{1}{50\,g}} \times \overset{2}{100}\ mL$ $10\,mL$	$100\,mL : 50\,g :: x : 5\,g$	$\dfrac{100\,mL}{50\,g} \times \dfrac{x}{5\,g}$

$$\frac{500}{50} = x$$

$$10\,mL = x$$

Prepare the syringe with 10 mL for IV use.

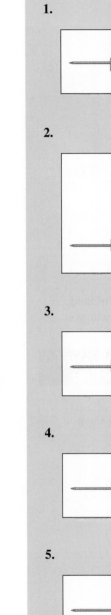

Self-Test 6 Insulin Calculations

1.

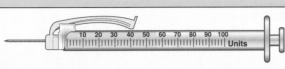

2.

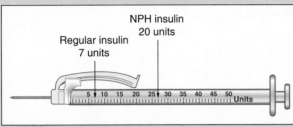

3.

4.

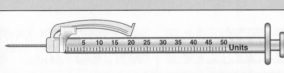

5.

6.

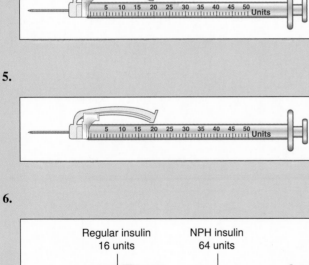

7.

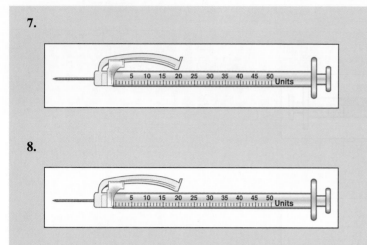

8.

9. Call physician.

10. Give 1 amp D50 and call physician.

Self-Test 7 Injections from Powders

1. You want 1 g. The supply is 1 g. When you dilute the powder, you will give the whole amount of fluid, *whatever the amount is.* The manufacturer states it will be 1g in 3.6 mL. If you solve the arithmetic you have

Formula Method	Proportion Expressed as Two Ratios	Proportion Expressed as Two Fractions
$\dfrac{1000 \text{ mg}}{280 \text{ mg}} \times 1 \text{ mL} = \dfrac{100}{28}$ $\begin{array}{r} 3.57 \\ 28\overline{)100.00} \\ \underline{84} \\ 160 \\ \underline{140} \\ 200 \\ \underline{196} \end{array}$ $= 3.6 \text{ mL} = x$	$1 \text{ mL} : 280 \text{ mg} :: x \text{ mL} : 1000 \text{ mg}$ $\dfrac{1000}{280} = x$ $3.6 \text{ mL} = x$	$\dfrac{1 \text{ mL}}{280 \text{ mg}} \times \dfrac{x}{1000 \text{ mg}}$

   a. 3 mL sterile water for injection

   b. 1 g in 3.6 mL; 280 mg/mL

   c. Not necessary

   d. Give 3.6 mL in two syringes.

   e. Discard the vial; it is empty.

   f. Discard the vial in appropriate receptacle.

2. a. 1.8 mL sterile water for injection

   b. 250 mg/mL

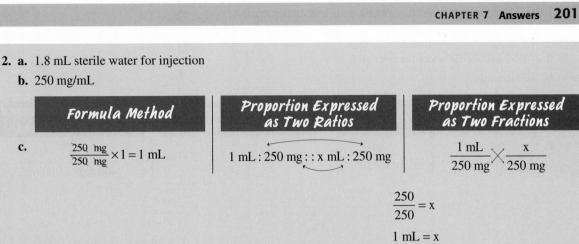

Formula Method	Proportion Expressed as Two Ratios	Proportion Expressed as Two Fractions
c. $\dfrac{250\ \text{mg}}{250\ \text{mg}} \times 1 = 1\ \text{mL}$	1 mL : 250 mg : : x mL : 250 mg	$\dfrac{1\ \text{mL}}{250\ \text{mg}} \times \dfrac{x}{250\ \text{mg}}$

$$\frac{250}{250} = x$$

$$1\ \text{mL} = x$$

   d. Give 1 mL IM.

   e. "The above solutions must be used within 1 hour after reconstitution." You must discard the remaining fluid.

   f. None

3. a. Choose 500 mg powder. (Can you see why?)

   b. Add 2 mL sterile water for injection.

   c. 225 mg/mL

   d. Not necessary: You want 225 mg; you made 225 mg/mL.

   e. Give 1 mL IM.

   f. 225 mg/mL, date, time, expiration date: 96 hours after reconstitution, initials

   g. Refrigerate; stable for 96 hours

4. a. 3.0 mL sterile water for injection

   b. 280 mg/mL

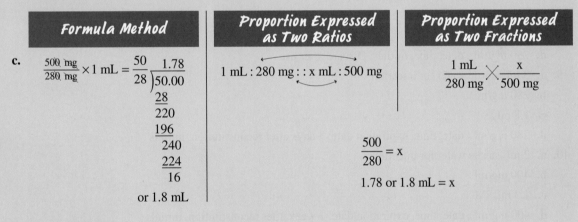

Formula Method	Proportion Expressed as Two Ratios	Proportion Expressed as Two Fractions
c. $\dfrac{500\ \text{mg}}{280\ \text{mg}} \times 1\ \text{mL} = \dfrac{50}{28}$ $28\overline{)50.00}$ $\underline{28}$ 220 $\underline{196}$ 240 $\underline{224}$ 16 or 1.8 mL	1 mL : 280 mg : : x mL : 500 mg	$\dfrac{1\ \text{mL}}{280\ \text{mg}} \times \dfrac{x}{500\ \text{mg}}$

$$\frac{500}{280} = x$$

1.78 or 1.8 mL = x

   d. Give 1.8 mL IM.

   e. 280 mg/mL, date, time, expiration date: 7 days after reconstitution, initials

   f. Refrigerate; stable for 7 days

5. **a.** Add 2 mL sterile water for injection.

   b. 400 mg/mL

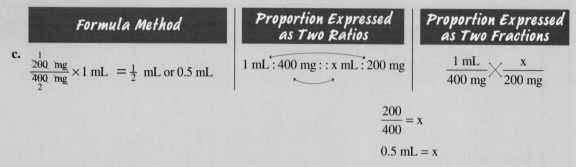

Formula Method	Proportion Expressed as Two Ratios	Proportion Expressed as Two Fractions

c. $\dfrac{\overset{1}{\cancel{200}}\ \cancel{mg}}{\underset{2}{\cancel{400}}\ \cancel{mg}} \times 1\ mL = \dfrac{1}{2}\ mL$ or 0.5 mL | $1\ mL : 400\ mg :: x\ mL : 200\ mg$ | $\dfrac{1\ mL}{400\ mg} \times \dfrac{x}{200\ mg}$

$$\dfrac{200}{400} = x$$

$$0.5\ mL = x$$

   d. Give ½ mL (0.5 mL).

   e. 400 mg/mL, date, time, expiration date: 1 week after reconstitution, initials

   f. Refrigerate; stable for 1 week

6. **a.** 3.0 mL sterile water for injection

   b. 280 mg/mL

   c. Give 0.3 mL IM (3-mL syringe) or 0.32 mL (1-mL precision syringe).

   d. 280 mg/mL, date, time, expiration date: 1 week after reconstitution, initials

7. **a.** 2 mL sterile water for injection

   b. 225 mg/mL

   c. 2 mL IM

   d. 225 mg/mL, date, time, expiration date: 96 hours after reconstitution, initials

8. **a.** 1.8 mL sterile water for injection

   b. 250 mg/mL

   c. 1.6 mL

   d. 250 mg/mL, date, time, initials. Discard after use.

9. **a.** 3 mL sterile water for injection

   b. 280 mg/mL

   c. 1.8 mL

   d. 280 mg/mL, date, time, expiration date: 7 days after reconstitution, initials

10. **a.** 2 mL sterile water for injection

   b. 400 mg/mL

   c. 1.3 mL IM

   d. 400 mg/mL, date, time, expiration date: 1 week after reconstitution, initials

Calculation of Basic IV Drip Rates

LEARNING OBJECTIVES

1. IV fluids
2. IV drip factors
3. Infusion pumps
4. Labeling IVs
5. Calculating basic IV drip rates
   mL over a number of hours
   mL/hr
   gtt/min
6. Determining hours an IV will run
7. Choosing infusion set tubing
8. Adding medications to continuous IVs
9. Intermittent piggyback drip rates (IVPB)
10. Enteral Feeding

Administration of parenteral fluids and medications by the IV route is common medical practice and is a specialty within nursing and health care. Texts such as *Plumer's Principles and Practice of Intravenous Therapy* (Lippincott, 2006) present detailed and extensive information. This chapter presents basic knowledge—types of fluids, equipment, calculation of drip rates, and recording intake. Chapter 9 presents rules and calculations for special types of IV orders.

Types of Intravenous Fluids

Intravenous fluids are packaged in sterile plastic bags or glass bottles. The nurse selects the IV fluid ordered and prepares the solution. It is essential to choose the correct IV fluid to avoid serious fluid and electrolyte imbalance that may occur from infusing the wrong solution.

If you have any doubt about the correct IV solution, always double-check with another healthcare professional.

Common abbreviations for IV fluids are D, dextrose; W, water; and NS, normal (or isotonic) saline. An order often indicates a percent of these. For example, D5W means 5% dextrose in water; 0.9%NS means 0.9% saline in water.

Example	Written Order	Supply Label
	1000 mL D5W	1000 mL D5%W
	500 mL D5S	500 mL D5% 0.9%NS
	250 mL D5½NS	250 mL D5% 0.45%NS
	500 mL D5⅓NS	500 mL D5% 0.33%NS
	500 mL NS	500 mL 0.9%NS
	1000 mL ½NS	1000 mL 0.45%NS

Kinds of Intravenous Drip Factors

IV fluids are administered through infusion sets. These consist of plastic tubing attached at one end to the IV bag, and at the other end to a needle or catheter inserted into a blood vessel. The top of the infusion set contains a chamber. Sets with a small needle in the chamber are called microdrip, because their drops are small. To deliver 1 mL fluid to the patient, 60 drops must drip in the chamber (60 gtt = 1 mL). All microdrip sets deliver 60 gtt/mL.

Infusion sets without a small needle in the chamber are called macrodrip (Fig. 8-1). Drops per milliliter differ according to the manufacturer. For example, Baxter-Travenol macrodrip sets deliver 10 gtt/mL, so 10 drops must drip in the chamber (10 gtt = 1 mL); and Abbott sets deliver 15 gtts/mL, so 15 drops must drip in the chamber (15 gtt = 1 mL). The package label states the drops per milliliter (gtt/mL). Sometimes the drop factor is also stated on the top part of the chamber. To calculate IV drip rates, you must know this information.

The tubing for these sets includes a roller clamp that you can open or close to regulate the drip rate; use a watch or a clock with a second hand to count the number of drops per minute in the chamber (Fig. 8-2).

Infusion Pumps

Electric infusion pumps also deliver IV fluid. Some are easy to operate; others are more elaborate. You must enter two pieces of information: the total number of milliliters to be infused and the number of milliliters per hour. Pumps used in specialty units also allow you to input the name of the medication, the concentration of the medication, the amount of fluid, and the patient's weight. The infusion rate can be set in mL/hr and the pump automatically calculates the dose in mg, mcg, etc. The pump can also calculate the dosage based on weight. Figure 8-3 shows the face of an infusion pump, with

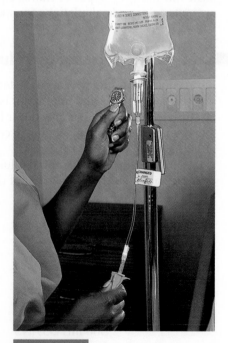

FIGURE 8-2

Timing the IV drip rate. (© B. Proud.) (With permission From Taylor, C., Lillis, C., & LeMone, P. [2004]. *Photo atlas of medication administration.* Philadelphia: Lippincott Williams & Wilkins, p. 46.)

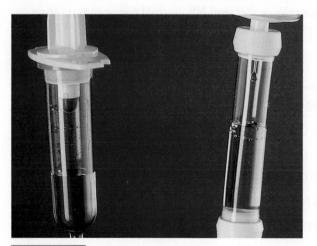

FIGURE 8-1

Drip chambers for macrodrip and microdrip IV tubing.

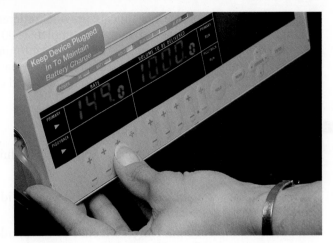

FIGURE 8-3

IV rate is programmed into the infusion pump in mL/hr.

IV tubing connected. If an order reads "500 mL D5W IV. Run 50 mL/hr," you press the buttons on the pump that read:

- Volume for Infusion
- 500 mL
- Rate for Infusion
- 50 mL
- On.

The pump automatically delivers 50 mL/hr and runs over a 10-hour period.

IV pumps can also run intravenous piggybacks (IVPB). If an order reads "Ampicillin 2 g IVPB in 100 mL NS over 1 hour," you press the buttons on the pump that read:

- Secondary Volume
- 100 mL
- Secondary Rate
- 100 mL
- On.

The pump interrupts the main IV to administer the IVPB over 1 hour, then resumes the primary flow.

Labeling IVs

Every IV must be identified so that any professional can check both the fluid that is infusing and the drip rate. A typical order includes the following information:

Patient name, room, bed number, date, and time

Order: 500 mL D5W½NS. Run 50 mL/hr.

Label			
Patient	James Latham	Room	1411B
Date, Time	6/26, 1000A	Rate	50 gtt/min
Order	500 mL D5½NS	Run	50 mL/hr
Time	10 A–8 P	Initials	CB

Note that the physician or healthcare provider ordered 50 mL/hr. Because the IV fluid amount is 500 mL, the infusion will take 10 hours to complete (500 divided by 50 = 10); the time is 10 AM to 8 PM (10 hours). With microdrip tubing, 50 mL/hr = 50 gtt/min, the nurse sets the rate. (Instructions for calculating IV drip rates appear in the next section.) Your goal is to deliver the amount of fluid ordered, in the time ordered, and with a drip rate that is continuous and even.

Calculating Basic IV Drip Rates

Routine IV orders specify the number of milliliters of fluid and the duration of administration:

Example	250 mL D5W IV at 250 mL/hr	Fluid amount: 250 mL	Time: 1 hour
	1000 mL Ringer's lactate IV 8 AM–8 PM	Fluid amount: 1000 mL	Time: 12 hours
	500 mL D5½NS with 20 mEq KCl IV to run 75 mL/hr on a pump	Fluid amount: 500 mL	Time: 75 mL/hour

The equipment that you use determines the drip factor and the calculations needed. An infusion pump is set in mL/hr, so your dosage calculations are in mL/hr as well. IV tubing sets infuse at gtt/min, and the infusion rate depends on the drip rate of the tubing used. Although many institutions use only infusion pumps today, occasionally you will need to calculate and infuse intravenous fluid using the drip rate calculation.

RULE	**SOLVING IV CALCULATIONS WITH MICRO- AND MACRODRIP TUBING**

The terms "drop factor," "drip factor," "gtt factor," and "tubing drip factor" are all used to explain how many gtts per mL the tubing delivers. In this text, we will use "tubing factor" or "TF" to mean all these terms. ■

Calculation:

$$\frac{\text{Number of milliliters to infuse} \times \text{TF}}{\text{Number of minutes to infuse}} = \text{drops per minute or gtts/min}$$

For example, the order is to infuse 120 mL of IV fluid over 60 minutes with a tubing factor of 10 gtts/mL. The calculation is:

$$\frac{120 \text{ mL} \times 10 \text{gtts/mL}}{60 \text{ minutes}} = 20 \text{ gtts/minute}$$

Explanation:

TF: the tubing drip factor—either microdrip (60 gtt = 1 mL) or macrodrip

Depending on the manufacturer, macrodrip could be 10 gtt = 1 mL, 15 gtt = 1 mL, or 20 gtt = 1 mL.

min: the number of minutes, specified in every IV order. If the order reads "hour" then you convert to minutes by multiplying by 60 (60 minutes = 1 hour).

gtt/min: the drip factor, calculated to deliver an even flow of fluid over a specified time. To regulate the drip rate, use a second hand on a watch or a clock. If the drip rate is calculated to be 20 gtt/min, open the clamp and regulate the drip until you reach that amount. Usually you break this amount down into seconds, rather than counting for a full minute. For this example, 20 gtt/min becomes approximately 3 gtt every 20 seconds (divide 20 by 60, since a minute contains 60 seconds).

The problems requiring calculation in this text will supply the drip factor. When you're working in the clinical area, you must read the package label to identify the gtt/mL.

Solving IV Calculations Using an Infusion Pump

Infusion pumps are always calculated in mL/hr. Here's how to calculate the example from above, infusing 120 mL of IV fluid over 60 minutes:

$$\frac{\text{Total number of milliliters ordered}}{\text{Number of hours to run}} = \text{mL/hr}$$

The calculation looks like this:

$$\frac{120 \text{ mL}}{1 \text{ hr}} = 120 \text{ mL/hr}$$

Note that 60 minutes was changed to 1 hour (60 minutes = 1 hour).

After calculating, connect the intravenous fluids to the infusion pump with the appropriate tubing, set the pump at 120 mL/hr, and start the infusion.

Explanation:

mL: The physician or healthcare provider will indicate the number of milliliters to be infused in the order.

# hr: The number of hours to run depends on the way the order is written. For example, if the order is written
  q8h = 8 hours at a time
  10 AM–4 PM = 6 hours
  60 minutes = 1 hour
  90 minutes = 1.5 hours (to get the number of hours, divide minutes by 60)

Alternate Way:

Here's a formula you can use to calculate what rate to set on the infusion pump:

$$\frac{\text{Number of milliliters to infuse} \times \text{TF}}{\text{Number of minutes to infuse}} = \text{drops per minute or gtts/min}$$

With infusion pumps, the tubing factor is always 60 gtts/mL. For the calculation "infuse 120 mL of intravenous fluid over 60 minutes using an infusion pump," the formula looks like this:

$$\frac{120 \text{ mL} \times 60 \text{ gtts/mL}}{60 \text{ minutes}}$$

Drip rates are rounded to the nearest whole number, unless using an infusion pump that can infuse in tenths or hundredths (i.e., 8.25 mL/hr). Usually these infusion pumps are used in a specialty setting such as critical care or pediatrics.

Applying the Rule

Example

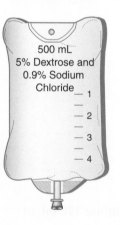

Order: 1000 mL Ringer's lactate IV 8 AM–8 PM

Available: an infusion pump

8 AM to 8 PM indicates the IV will run for 12 hours. The infusion pump regulates the rate in milliliters per hour.

$$\frac{\text{number mL}}{\text{number hr}} = \text{mL/hr}$$

$$\frac{1000 \text{ mL}}{12 \text{ hr}} = \frac{1000}{12}$$

$$12\overline{)1000.0} \quad 83.3$$
$$\underline{96}$$
$$40$$
$$\underline{36}$$
$$40$$
$$36$$

Label the IV.

Set the pump as follows:

Total number mL: 1000

mL/hr: 83

Example

Order: 500 mL D5NS IV 12 NOON–4 PM

Available: microdrip at 60 gtt/mL; macrodrip at 20 gtt/mL

The IV will run 4 hours or 240 minutes (4 × 60 minutes). Because no pump is available, the nurse must choose the drip factor. Solve for both drip factors and choose one.

Macrodrip

$$\frac{500 \text{ mL} \times \overset{1}{\cancel{20}}}{\underset{12}{\cancel{240}}} = 12\overline{)500.0} \quad 41.6$$
$$\underline{48}$$
$$20$$
$$\underline{12}$$
$$80$$

Macrodrip at 42 gtt/min

Microdrip

$$\frac{\overset{1}{500 \times \overset{\cancel{60}}{}}}{\underset{4}{240}} = 4\overline{\smash{)}\begin{array}{l}125 \\ 500 \\ \underline{4} \\ 10 \\ \underline{8} \\ 20\end{array}}$$

Microdrip at 125 gtt/min

Answers are macrodrip at 42 gtt/min and microdrip at 125 gtt/min. Choose one. (See the explanation for choosing the infusion set, after this discussion.)

Label the IV.

Set the drip rate.

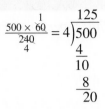

Example

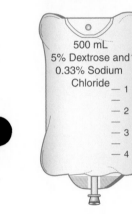

Order: 500 mL D5⅓NS IV KVO for 24°

Available: microdrip at 60 gtt/mL; macrodrip 10 gtt/mL

Because no pump is available, choose the IV set. The IV will run 24 hours or 1400 minutes (24 × 60 minutes). Work out the problem for micro- and macrodrip and make a nursing judgment about which tubing to use.

Macrodrip

$$\frac{500 \text{ mL} \times \overset{1}{\cancel{10}} \text{ gtts}}{\underset{140}{\cancel{1400}} \text{ minutes}} = 140\overline{\smash{)}\begin{array}{l}3.5 \\ 500.0 \\ \underline{420} \\ 800 \\ \underline{700}\end{array}}$$

Macrodrip at 4 gtt/min

Microdrip

$$\frac{500 \text{ mL} \times \cancel{60} \text{ gtt}}{\cancel{1400} \text{ minutes}} = \frac{3000}{140} \quad 140\overline{\smash{)}\begin{array}{l}21.4 \\ 3000.0 \\ \underline{280} \\ 200 \\ \underline{140} \\ 600\end{array}}$$

Microdrip at 21 gtt/min

A 4-gtt/min macrodrip is too slow. Choose microdrip. (See the explanation on p. 212 for choosing the infusion set.)

Label the IV.

Select a microdrip infusion set.

Set the drip rate at 21 gtt/min.

SELF-TEST 1 Calculation of Drip Factors

Calculate the drip factor for the following IV orders given in milliliters per hour or gtts per minute. Answers are given at the end of the chapter.

1. Order: 150 mL D5W 0.33NS IV q8h
   Available: infusion pump

2. Order: 250 mL D5W; run at 25 mL/hr
   Available: infusion pump

3. Order: 1000 mL D5NS; run 100 mL/hr
   Available: macrodrip (20 gtt/mL); microdrip (60 gtt/mL)

4. Order: 180 mL D5⅓NS 12 NOON–6 PM
   Available: macrodrip (10 gtt/mL); microdrip (60 gtt/mL)

5. Order: 1000 mL D5W 0.45NS IV 4 PM–12 MIDNIGHT
   Available: macrodrip (15 gtt/mL); microdrip (60 gtt/mL)

6. Order: 250 mL D5W IV q8h
   Available: infusion pump

7. Order: 500 mL NS IV over 2 h
   Available: infusion pump

8. Order: 1000 mL D5NS IV 4 AM–4 PM
   Available: macrodrip (15 gtt/mL); microdrip (60 gtt/mL)

9. Order: 1000 mL D5W 0.45 NS IV; run 150 mL/hr
   Available: macrodrip (10 gtt/mL); microdrip (60 gtt/mL)

10. Order: 150 mL 0.9 NS IV; over 1 h
    Available: macrodrip (20 gtt/mL); microdrip (60 gtt/mL)

Determining Hours an IV Will Run

Knowing how to calculate approximately how long an IV will last helps you in your work, because you can use that amount of time to prepare the next IV or note any new orders.

$$\frac{\text{number of milliliters ordered}}{\text{number of milliliters per hour}} = \text{number of hours to run}$$

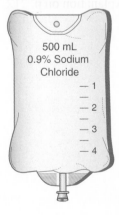

Example

500 mL
0.9% Sodium
Chloride
— 1
— 2
— 3
— 4

Order: 500 mL NS IV; infuse at 75 mL/hr

Rule: $\frac{\text{number mL}}{\text{number mL/hr}} = \text{hr}$

$$\frac{500 \text{ mL}}{75 \text{ mL/hr}} = 75\overline{\smash{)}500.00} \; \begin{array}{r} 6.67 \\ \end{array}$$

$$\begin{array}{r} \underline{450} \\ 50\ 0 \\ \underline{45\ 0} \\ 5\ 00 \end{array}$$

The IV will last approximately 6.7 hours.

Example

Order: 1000 mL D5½ NS IV 8 AM–8 PM

No math necessary; 8 AM–8 PM = 12 hours

The IV will last 12 hours.

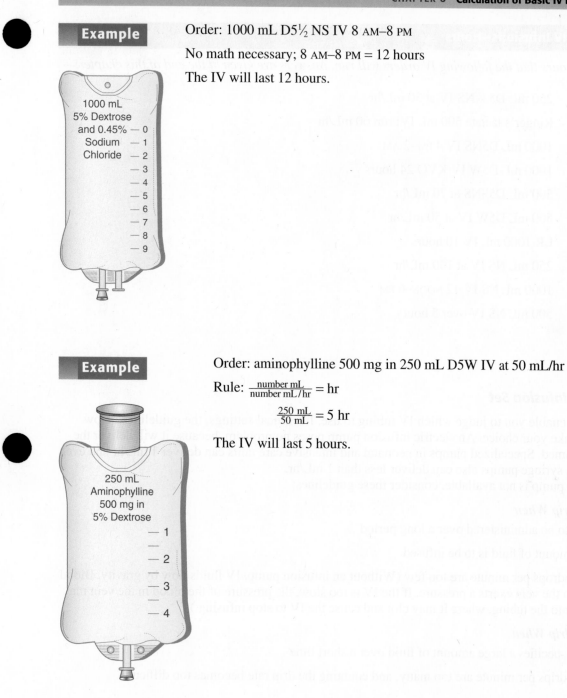

Example

Order: aminophylline 500 mg in 250 mL D5W IV at 50 mL/hr

Rule: $\frac{\text{number mL}}{\text{number mL/hr}} = \text{hr}$

$\frac{250 \text{ mL}}{50 \text{ mL}} = 5 \text{ hr}$

The IV will last 5 hours.

SELF-TEST 2   IV Infusions—Hours

Calculate the hours that the following IV orders will run. Answers are given at the end of this chapter.

1. Order: 250 mL D5 ½ NS IV at 30 mL/hr

2. Order: Ringer's lactate 500 mL IV; run 60 mL/hr

3. Order: 1000 mL D5NS IV 4 PM–2 AM

4. Order: 1000 mL D5W IV KVO 24 hours

5. Order: 500 mL D5½NS at 70 mL/hr

6. Order: 500 mL D5W IV at 50 mL/hr

7. Order: LR 1000 mL IV 10 hours

8. Order: 250 mL NS IV at 100 mL/hr

9. Order: 1000 mL NS IV 12 NOON–6 PM

10. Order: 500 mL NS IV over 5 hours

Choosing the Infusion Set

Experience will enable you to judge which IV tubing to use. In clinical settings, the guidelines below will help you make your choice. An electric infusion pump poses no problem, because it will deliver the amount programmed. Specialized pumps in neonatal and intensive care units can deliver 1 mL/hr and even less. Specialized syringe pumps also can deliver less than 1 mL/hr.

When an IV pump is not available, consider these guidelines:

Use Microdrip When

• the IV is to be administered over a long period

• a small amount of fluid is to be infused

• the macrodrops per minute are too few (Without an infusion pump, IV fluids flow by gravity. Blood flowing in the vein exerts a pressure. If the IV is too slow, the pressure of the blood in the vein may back up into the tubing, where it may clot and cause the IV to stop infusing.)

Use Macrodrip When

• the order specifies a large amount of fluid over a short time

• the microdrips per minute are too many, and counting the drip rate becomes too difficult

Need for Continuous Observation

Many factors may interfere with the drip rate. When you are not using an infusion pump, gravity will cause the IV to vary from its starting rate; you will need to check the IV frequently. You'll need to monitor other conditions as well. As the amount of fluid decreases in the IV bag, pressure changes occur—and they, too, may affect the rate. The patient's movements can kink the tube and shut off the flow; they can change the position of the needle or catheter in the vein. The needle can become lodged against the side of the blood vessel, thereby altering the flow, or it may be forced out of the vessel, allowing fluid to enter the tissues (infiltration). (Signs of possible infiltration are swelling, pain,

Medications for Intermittent Intravenous Administration

Some IV medications are administered not continuously but only intermittently, such as q4h, q6h, or q8h. This route is termed *intravenous piggyback* or IVPB (Fig. 8-5). The term admixture refers to the premixed IVPB.

Most of these drugs are prepared in powder form. The manufacturer specifies the type and amount of diluent needed to reconstitute the drug; later, the nurse connects the IVPB (containing the reconstituted drug) by IV tubing to the main IV line. Some IVPB medications come pre-mixed from the manufacturer. For other medications, the institutional pharmacy may reconstitute and prepare IVPB solutions in a sterile environment using a laminar flow hood. This procedure saves nursing time, because when the nurse is ready to administer the drugs, they have already been prepared, labeled, and screened for incompatibilities. Nevertheless, the nurse still bears considerable responsibility: You must check the diluent and volume. You must also check the dose and the expiration date of the reconstituted solution; note whether the IVPB should be refrigerated before use, or whether it can remain at room temperature until hung. Finally, you must calculate the drip rate and record this information on the IVPB label before hanging the bag.

The physician or healthcare provider may write a detailed order, such as "Vancomycin 0.5 g IVPB in 100 mL D5W over 1 hr." More often, however, the physician or healthcare provider writes only the drug, route, and time interval, relying on the nurse to research the manufacturer's directions for the amount and type of diluent and the time for the infusion to run (e.g., Order: cefazolin 1 g IVPB q6h).

Explanation

To solve IVPB problems, you use a calculation much like the one you used for the IV:

$$\frac{mL \times TF}{min} = gtt/min$$

mL: The label or the package insert will state the type and amount of diluent. Nurses' drug references and the *Physicians Drug Reference* also contain this information.

TF: The tubing for IVPB is called a secondary administration set and has a macrodrip factor. It is shorter than main line IV tubing. In the clinical setting, check the label for the tubing drip factor.

min: The manufacturer may or may not indicate the number of minutes needed for the IVPB medication to be infused. When the number is not given, follow this general rule for adults: allow 30 minutes for every 50 mL solution.

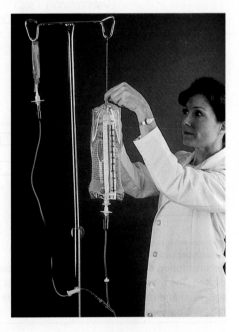

FIGURE 8-5

Photo of a primary IV line (*right*) and an IVPB (or secondary) line (*left*). Fluid flows continuously through the primary line into the patient's vein. At timed intervals, medication placed in an intravenous piggyback bag (IVPB) is attached by tubing to the primary IV for delivery to the patient. The primary fluid is lowered and the IVPB fluid flows. After the IVPB has infused, the primary fluid begins infusing again. An IV infusion pump may also be used, and medication in the IVPB is infused through the pump.

Example

Order: cefazolin 1 g IVPB q6h

Supply: **package insert** IVPB dilution of cefazolin sodium. Reconstitute with 50 to 100 mL of sodium chloride injection or other solution listed under administration. Other solutions listed include D5W, D10W, D5LR, and D5NS.

Use 50 mL D5W. It is the most common IVPB diluent and we have 50-mL bags. No time for infusion is given in the directions for IVPB. Use 30 minutes for 50 mL.

Here's the calculation

$$\frac{mL \times TF}{min} = gtt/min$$

mL = 50 mL D5W

TF = 10 gtt/mL (For a secondary asministration, no set time for administration is given. Follow the general adult rule of 30 minutes for every 50 mL.)

min = 30

$$\frac{50 \times 10}{30} = 16.6 = 17 \ gtt/min$$

Before hanging the IVPB, reconstitute the drug. You have a vial of powder labeled 1 g, and you need the whole amount. You have a 50-mL bag of D5W, and you need that whole amount as well. To mix the powder and the diluent, use a reconstitution device—a sterile implement containing two needles that connects the vial and the 50-mL bag. With this device, you can dilute the powder and place it in the IV bag without using a syringe (Fig. 8-6). Some manufacturers now enclose a reconstitution device with the IV bag. Once the powder is reconstituted, label the IV bag.

The order is q6h, and generally the administration times are 6 AM, 12 NOON, 6 PM, 12 MIDNIGHT. The time of infusion is 30 minutes, and for this label, will run from 12 NOON to 12:30 PM.

Rather than spending valuable time looking through package inserts for directions, check the concise information in drug references such as *Lippincott's Nursing Drug Guide.*

Medication Added		
Patient *Tom Smith*		**Room** *1503*
Date *cefazolin 1 g*		**Flow Rate** *17 gtt/min*
Base solution *50 mL D5W*		**Initials** *RT*
Time to Run *12 NOON–12:30 PM*		**Date** *6/14*

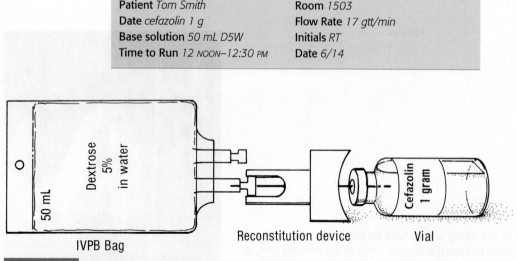

FIGURE 8-6

Reconstitution device. The IVPB bag is squeezed, forcing fluid into the vial of powder, which is then diluted. The three parts are turned to a vertical position—vial up, IVPB bag down. The IVPB bag is squeezed and released. This creates a negative pressure, allowing the diluted medication to flow into the IVPB bag.

Example

Order: Vancomycin 1 g IVPB 7 AM

Supply: 500 mg powder

Package insert directions: 250 mL (1 g)/D5W

Run over 2 hours (1 g). Refrigerate for 7 days.

$$\frac{mL \times TF}{min} = gtt/min$$

$$\frac{250 \times 10}{120} = \frac{250}{12} \quad 12\overline{)250.0} \frac{20.8}{} = 21 \ gtt/min$$

Use a reconstitution device to add 1 g vancomycin (two vials of 500 mg) to 250 mL D5W. Label the IV. Set the rate at 21 gtt/min. The IVPB will run 2 hours.

When you're using an infusion pump for IVPB, solve the problem by setting 60 gtt as the tubing factor. Most infusion pumps have a special setting for "secondary IV administration." Choose this setting, then program the rate in mL/hr. After the IVPB has infused, the pump then either switches back to the primary IV infusion or begins beeping, letting you know that the infusion is complete.

SELF-TEST 4 | **IVPB Drip Factors**

Solve these drip factors for IVPB problems. Answers are given at the end of this chapter.

1. Order: Zovirax (acyclovir) 500 mg IVPB q8h
   Supply: 500 mg powder
   Package directions: 100 mL/D5W. Infuse 1 hour/once a day
   Available: macrodrip tubing at 10 gtt/mL

2. Order: Ceptaz (ceftazidime) 1 g IVPB q12h
   Supply: 1 g powder
   Package directions: 50 mL (1 g)/D5W. Infuse in 15–30 minutes/store for 7 days
                      (REFRIGERATED)
   Available: macrodrip tubing at 10 gtt/mL

3. Order: Claforan (cefotaxime) 1 g IVPB q6h
   Supply: 1 g powder
   Package directions: 50 mL (1 g)/D5W. Infuse in 15–30 minutes/store for 5 days
                      (REFRIGERATED)
   Available: macrodrip tubing at 10 gtt/mL

4. Order: Omnipen (ampicillin) 500 mg IV q6h
   Supply: 2 g in 5 mL
   Package directions: 50 mL (500 mg)/D5W. Infuse in 15–30 minutes
   Available: microdrip tubing at 60 gtt/mL

5. Order: Nebcin (tobramycin) 50 mg IV q8h
   Supply: 80 mg in 2 mL
   Package directions: 100 mL (50 mg)/D5W. Infuse in 60 minutes
   Available: macrodrip tubing at 15 gtt/mL

6. Order: Timentin (ticarcillin) 500 mg IV q6h
   Supply: 1 g in 5 mL
   Package directions: 50 mL (500 mg)/D5W. Infuse in 30 minutes
   Available: macrodrip tubing at 15 gtt/mL

Ambulatory Infusion Device

An ambulatory infusion device such as the one pictured in Figure 8-7 is used when a patient is receiving long term antibiotic or other infusion therapy. The device is filled with the medication and a vacuum within the container infuses the medication over a specific time frame when the device is attached to the patient's IV. This is convenient for the patient, so that they may go home from the hospital on infusion therapy and continue in daily activities. The patient may have a peripheral IV site that has to be changed every 3–4 days, or may have a long term indwelling IV catheter, such as a PICC (peripherally inserted central catheter) line.

Enteral Nutrition

Enteral feeding is used when a patient cannot eat, or cannot eat enough. A tube is passed through the nasal or oral cavity to the stomach or duodenum (nasogastric, N/G tube, or oralgastric, O/G tube), or it is placed more permanently, as with a percutaneous endoscopic gastrostomy (PEG) tube, gastrostomy tube (G tube) or jejunostomy tube (J tube). Commercial tube feedings are used as well (Fig. 8-8); these formulas, though varied, usually carry a high caloric component. They may also include high fiber and high protein and may vary according to a patient's disease state.

Tube feedings are administered with a pump that regulates the amount of feeding. The feedings may be *intermittent*, delivering the formula at regular periods of time; *cyclic*, giving the formula over several hours of the day (over 12–16 hours); or *continuous*, infusing the formula constantly (Fig. 8–9).

Enteral feedings require careful monitoring to avoid complications and to ensure the patient's safety. Full-strength tube feeding is recommended, although diluted tube feedings are still used. The section below discusses common dilutions and the way to calculate the dose. For more information on enteral feedings, consult a basic nursing book such as *Fundamentals of Nursing*, by Taylor, Lillis, LeMone, and Lynn (Lippincott, 2008).

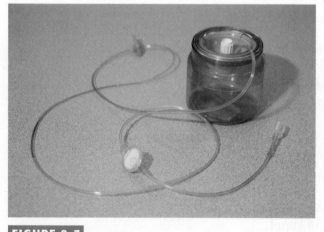

FIGURE 8-7
Ambulatory infusion device.

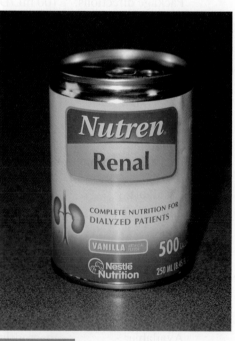

FIGURE 8-8
Comercially prepared tube feeding.

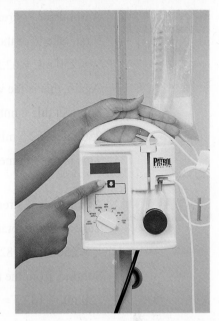

FIGURE 8-9

Feeding pump for infusion of tube feeding. (Used with permission from Craven, R. and Hirnle, C. [2007]. Fundamentals of Nursing [5th ed.]. Philadelphia: Lippincott, Williams & Williams, p. 995.)

Calculation of Tube Feedings

An order for tube feedings will read:

> Administer Isocal full strength at 60 mL/hr. Check for residual every 4 hours. Flush tube with 50 mL of water every 4 hours.

This order does not require calculation.

Add Isocal to a tube feeding bag, and set the tube feeding pump at 60 mL/hr.

Complete the other orders per protocol.

Follow hospital protocol for changing of tube feeding bag and tubing.

Example   Administer ½ strength Isocal at 60 mL/hr. The total volume will equal 250 mL.

For this problem, begin by taking ½ of the total volume to infuse:

½ × 250 mL = 125 mL

This number tells you how much formula to add to the tube feeding bag.

Next, subtract that number from the total volume.

250 mL − 125 mL = 125 mL

This new number tells you how much water to add to the tube feeding bag.

Now that you have diluted the formula to ½ strength, infuse it at 60 mL/hr.

Example   Administer ¼ strength Isocal at 60 mL/hr. Total volume to equal 250 mL.

First, take ¼ of the total volume:

¼ × 250 mL = 62.5 mL

Again, this is the volume of formula to add to the tube feeding bag.

Subtract this number from the total volume:

250 mL − 62.5 mL = 182.5 mL

This is the volume of water to dilute.

Example   Administer ¾ strength Isocal at 60 mL/hr. Total volume to equal 250 mL.

Take ¾ of the total volume:

¾ × 250 mL = 182.5 mL of Isocal

Subtract from the total:

250 mL − 182.5 = 62.5 mL of water to dilute.

SELF-TEST 5   Calculation of Tube Feedings

Solve these problems stating how much of the feeding and how much water to add. Answers are at the end of the chapter.

1. ¾ strength Isocal must be prepared. Total volume is 275 mL. How much Isocal is to be mixed with how much water?

2. 75 mL of 75% Magnacal must be prepared. How much Magnacal is to be mixed with how much water?

3. ½ strength Osmolite must be prepared. 100 mL is the total volume. How much Osmolite is to be mixed with how much water?

4. ¼ strength Ensure must be prepared. Total volume is 85 mL. How much Ensure is to be mixed with how much water?

5. 25% Renalcal must be prepared. 400 mL is the total volume. How much Renalcal is to be mixed with how much water?

6. 50% Suplena must be prepared. 400 mL is the total volume. How much Suplena is to be mixed with how much water?

Recording Intake

Keep an accurate account of parenteral intake as well as liquids taken orally and/or enterally (e.g., tube feedings). Each institution provides a flow sheet to record fluid input over a specified period of time. Usually when an IVPB is infusing, the primary IV stops infusing. After the IVPB is completed, the primary IV flow rate begins again. (Refer to Fig. 8-5.)

SELF-TEST 6   Fluid Intake

Answer the following questions regarding fluid intake. Answers are given at the end of this chapter.

1. A total of 900 mL of an IV solution is to infuse at 100 mL/hr. If it is 9 AM when the infusion starts, at what time will it be completed?

2. A patient is receiving an antibiotic IVPB in 75 mL q6h to run over 1 hour plus a maintenance IV of 125 mL/hr. What is the 24-hour intake parenterally?

3. An IV of 1000 mL D5NS is infusing at 10 microdrips per minute. What is the parenteral intake for 8 hours?

4. A doctor orders 500 mL aminophylline 0.5 g to infuse at 50 mL/hr. How many mg will the patient receive each hour?

5. A total of 20,000 units of heparin is added to 500 mL D5W, and the order is to infuse IV at 30 mL/hr. How many hours will the IV run?

6. A patient is receiving an antibiotic IVPB in 50 mL q8h to run over 1 hour plus a maintenance IV of 100 mL/hr. What is the 24-hour intake parenterally?

7. A total of 500 mL of an IV solution is to infuse at 50 mL/hr. If it is 6 AM when the infusion starts, at what time is it completed?

8. IV of D5W 1000 mL is infusing at 125 mL/hr. How many hours will the IV run?

9. A patient is receiving an antibiotic IVPB in 250 mL q6h. What is the 24-hour intake parenterally?

10. A physician orders 100 units regular insulin in 100 mL to infuse at 10 mL/hr. How many units will the patient receive each hour?

SELF-TEST 7   IV Drip Rates

Solve these problems related to intravenous and IVPB drip rates. Answers are given at the end of the chapter.

1. Order: 1500 mL D5W 8 AM–8 PM
    Available: macrodrip tubing (10 gtt/mL)   *21 gtts/min*
    What is the drip rate?

2. Order: 250 mL D5 ½ NS IV KVO (give over 12 hours)
    Available: microdrip tubing
    What is the drip rate?   *21 gtts/min*

3. Order: 150 mL D5 ⅓ NS IV; run 20 mL/hr
    Available: infusion pump

    a. What is the drip rate?   *20 mL/hr*
    b. How long will the IV last?   *7.5 hrs*

4. Order: 1000 mL D5NS with 15 mEq KCl IV; run 100 mL/hr
    Available: macrotubing (20 gtt/mL) and microdrip

    a. How many hours will this run?   *10 hrs*
    b. How many milliliters of KCl will you add to the IV if KCl comes in a vial labeled
        40 mEq/20 mL?
    c. What tubing will you use?
    d. What are the gtt/min?

5. Order: aminophylline 1 g in 500 mL D5W IV at 75 mL/hr
    Available: vial of aminophylline 1 g in 10 mL; infusion pump

    a. How many mL of aminophylline should be added to the IV?
    b. How will you set the drip rate?

6. Order: Amikin (amikacin) 0.4 g IVPB q8h
    Supply: 2-mL vial labeled 250 mg/mL
    Package directions: 100 mL/D5W 30 minutes
    Available: macrodrip tubing 10 gtt/mL

    a. How many mL of amikacin should be added to the IV?
    b. What are the gtt/min?

7. Order: 500 mL D5 ½ NS IV q8h
    Available: microdrip tubing
    What are the gtt/min?

8. Order: 1000 mL D5W IV q24h
    Available: macrodrip tubing (15 gtt/mL)
    What is the drip rate?

9. Order: Heparin 25,000 units in 250 mL NS at 20 mL/hr
    How long will the IV last?

10. Order: 500 mL NS over 4 h
    Available: macrodrip tubing (20 gtt/mL)
    What is the drip rate?

SELF-TEST 8   IV Problems

Solve these problems related to drip rates. Answers are given at the end of this chapter.

1. Order: aqueous penicillin G 1 milliunits in 100 mL D5W IVPB q6h over 40 minutes
      (macrodrip tubing at 10 gtt/mL) (milliunits = million units)

   Supply: vial labeled 5 million units of powder. Directions say to inject 18 mL sterile water
      for injection to yield 20 mL solution. Reconstituted solution is stable for 1 week.

   a. How would you prepare the penicillin?
   b. What solution will you make?
   c. What amount of penicillin solution should be placed into the bag of 100 mL D5W?
   d. What is the drip factor for the IVPB?

2. A total of 1000 mL of an IV solution is to infuse at 100 mL/hr. If the infusion starts at 8 AM,
   at what time will it be completed?

3. Order: gentamicin 60 mg IVPB in 50 mL D5W over 30 minutes using macrodrip
      (20 gtt/mL)

   Supply: vial of gentamicin 40 mg/mL; 50-mL bag of D5W; order is correct

   a. How many mL of gentamicin will you add to the 50-mL bag of D5W?
   b. What is the drip factor for the IVPB?

4. Calculate the drip factor for 1500 mL D5 ½ NS to run 12 hours by macrodrip (10 gtt/mL).

5. Intralipid, 500 mL q6h, is ordered for a patient together with a primary IV that is infusing at
   80 mL/hr. Calculate the 24-hour parenteral intake. (Total will be amount of lipids plus primary
   IV amount.)

6. Order: 1000 mL D5W with 20 mEq KCl and 500 mg vitamin C at 60 mL/hr. No infusion
      pump is available.

   a. Approximately how many hours will the IV run?
   b. Which tubing will you choose—macrodrip at 10 gtt/mL or microdrip at 60 gtt/mL?
   c. What are the drops per minute for the tubing that you choose?

Putting it Together

Mrs. Richardson is a 41 year female admitted with nausea, vomiting and diarrhea. In the emergency room, she had a fever, leukocytosis, and potassium of 5.5.

Past Medical History: end stage renal disease, diabetes mellitus, hypertension

Post left upper extremity graft placement.

No known drug allergies.

Current Vital Signs: BP 82/50, pulse is 111/minute, respirations 20/minute, oxygen saturation 86% on room air. Temp is 98.6, on admission was 101.7

Medication Orders

Gentamicin *anti-infective* 100 mg IV in 100 mL over 1 hour daily

Cubicin (daptomycin) *anti-infective* 500 mg in 100 mL NS every 24 hours over 30 min

Zosyn (piperacillin and tazobactam) *anti-infective* 3.375 gm in 50 mL IV in NS every 6 hours

Procardia (nifedipine) XL *anti-hypertensive* 90 mg PO q 24 hr

Prinivil (lisinopril) *anti-hypertensive* 20 mg PO every day

NS 1000 mL at 40 mL/hr IV

Fragmin (dalteparin) *anticoagulant* 2500 units subcutaneous qd

Reglan (metoclopramide) *anti-nausea*, *prokinetic agent* 20 mg IV prn q 6 h for nausea and vomiting. For doses over 10 mg must be IVPB

Calculations

1. Calculate the infusion rate for the Gentamicin with microdrip and macrodrip (20 gtts/mL) tubing.

2. Calculate the infusion rate for the Cubicin with microdrip and macrodrip (20 gtts/mL) tubing.

3. Calculate the infusion rate for Zosyn with microdrip and macrodrip (15 gtts/mL) tubing.

4. Calculate how many hours a 1000 mL of NS solution at 40 mL/hr will infuse. Use an infusion pump.

5. Calculate the total intake for 24 hours, including the primary IV and all antibiotics.

Critical Thinking Questions

1. What medications (PO or IV) should be held and why?

2. Why would a patient receive 3 antibiotics instead of only 1 antibiotic?

3. After 6 hours, the NS has only infused 150 mL. How much should have infused? What are some reasons that the IV solution has not infused more? Should the nurse increase the rate of the infusion in order to "catch up" on the total amout needed?

4. Is the Reglan to be infused as an IVPB? How much solution should it be mixed with and how long to infuse?

Answers in Appendix B.

Name: _____

There are 10 questions related to IV and IVPB and enteral feeding calculations. Answers are given in Appendix A.

1. Order: 1000 mL D5NS; run 150 mL/hr IV
   Supply: IV bag of 1000 mL D5NS

   a. Approximately how many hours will the IV run?
   b. Which tubing will you choose—macrodrip (10 gtt/mL) or microdrip (60 gtt/mL)?
   c. What will be the drip rate?

2. Order: 100 mL Ringer's solution 12 NOON–6 PM IV

   a. What size tubing will you use?
   b. What are the gtt/min?

3. Order: 150 mL NS IV over 3 hours
   Supply: bag of 250 mL normal saline for IV and macrotubing, 15 gtt/mL; microtubing, 60 gtt/mL

   a. What would you do to obtain 150 mL NS?
   b. What IV tubing would you use?
   c. What are the gtt/min?

4. Order: 500 mL D5W IV KVO. Solve for 24 hours. An infusion pump is available. What should be the setting on the infusion pump?

5. Order: Vibramycin (doxycycline) 100 mg IVPB every day
   Supply: 100 mg powder
   Package directions: 250 mL/D5W to infuse over 1 hour; macrodrip tubing 10 gtt/mL

   a. State the amount and type of IV fluid you will use and the time for infusion you will use.
   b. What are the gtt/min?

6. Order: aminophylline 500 mg in 250 mL D5W to run 8 hours IV
   Available: vial of aminophylline labeled 1 g in 10 mL; microdrip tubing

   a. How much aminophylline is needed?
   b. What is the drip rate?

7. A patient is receiving a primary IV at the rate of 125 mL/hr. The doctor orders cefoxitin 1 g in 75 mL D5W q6h to run over 1 hour
   Calculate the 24-hour parenteral intake.

8. Order: 1000 mL D5 ½ NS to run at 90 mL/hr; infusion pump available

   a. What will be the pump setting?
   b. Approximately how long will the IV run?

9. A doctor orders 500 mL aminophylline 0.5 g to infuse at 50 mL/hr. How many milligrams will the patient receive each hour?

10. Order: Bactrim (trimethoprim and sulfamethoxazole) 5 mL IVPB q6h
    Supply: vial of 5 mL; one 5-mL vial per 75 mL D5W run over 60 to 90 minutes.
    The main IV line is connected to an infusion pump. What will you do? Refer to Figure 8-4.

    a. State the type and amount of IV fluid you would use and the time for infusion.
    b. How would you program the infusion pump?

(continued)

11. ¾ strength Isocal must be prepared. 150 mL is the total volume. How much Isocal is to be mixed with how much water?

12. ½ strength Vivonex must be prepared. 500 mL is the total volume. How much Vivonex is to be mixed with how much water?

13. 25% strength Osmolite must be prepared. 400 mL is the total volume. How much Osmolite is to be mixed with how much water?

14. Full strength Isocal must be prepared. 500 mL is the total volume. How much Isocal is to be mixed with how much water?

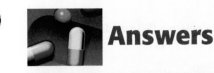

Answers

Self-Test 1 Calculation of Drip Factors

1. This is a continuous IV of 150 mL every 8 hours. There is a pump available.
   Minutes = 8 × 60 = 480.

$$\frac{150 \text{ mL} \times \overset{1}{\cancel{60}} \text{ gtt}}{\underset{8}{\cancel{480}} \text{ min}} = \frac{150 \text{ mL}}{8} \quad 8\overline{\smash{)}150.0} \;\; {\scriptstyle 18.7}$$

$$\begin{array}{r} 8 \\ \hline 70 \\ 64 \\ \hline 60 \end{array}$$

   Label the IV. Set the pump: total number
   mL = 150; mL/hr = 19.

2. This is a continuous IV. A pump is available. The order states mL/hr. There is no calculation needed. Label the IV. Set the pump as follows: total number mL = 250; mL/hr = 25.

3. mL/hr = The order gives 100 mL/hr; mL/hr = gtt/min microdrip, so you know the microdrip is 100 gtt/min. Work out the macrodrip factor and choose the tubing.

   Macrodrip

$$\frac{\text{mL/hr} \times \text{TF}}{\text{number min}} = \text{gtt/min}$$

$$\frac{100 \times \overset{1}{\underset{3}{\cancel{20}}}}{\underset{3}{\cancel{60}} \text{ min}} = \frac{100}{3} = 33.3$$

   Macrodrip at 33 gtt/min

   Microdrip at 100 gtt/min (mL/hr = gtt/min)

   Either drip rate could be used. Label the IV.

4. This is a small volume over several hours; use microdrip. Macrodrip would be too slow (5 gtt/min). Minutes = 6 hours × 60 = 360.

$$\frac{\text{mL/hr} \times \text{TF}}{\text{min}} = \text{gtt/min}$$

$$\frac{180 \text{ mL} \times \overset{1}{\cancel{60}} \text{ gtt}}{\underset{6}{\cancel{360}} \text{ min}} = \frac{180}{6} \quad 6\overline{\smash{)}180} \;\; {\scriptstyle 30}$$

$$\begin{array}{r} 18 \\ \hline 0 \end{array}$$

   Microdrip is 30 gtt/min because mL/hr = gtt/min.

5. This is a large volume over several hours. Solve using two steps and decide.

   Microdrip

$$\frac{\text{mL/hr} \times \text{TF}}{\text{min}} = \text{gtt/min}$$

$$\frac{1000 \text{ mL} \times \overset{1}{\cancel{60}} \text{ gtt}}{\underset{8}{\cancel{480}} \text{ min}} = \frac{1000}{8} \quad 8\overline{\smash{)}1000.0} \;\; {\scriptstyle 125.}$$

$$\begin{array}{r} 8 \\ \hline 20 \\ 16 \\ \hline 40 \end{array}$$

   microdrip will be 125 gtt/min because mL/hr = gtt/min.

   Macrodrip

$$\frac{125 \times \overset{1}{\cancel{15}}}{\underset{4}{\cancel{60}} \text{ min}} = \frac{125}{4} \quad 4\overline{\smash{)}125.0} \;\; {\scriptstyle 31.2}$$

$$\begin{array}{r} 12 \\ \hline 5 \\ 4 \\ \hline 10 \\ 8 \end{array}$$

   Macrodrip at 31 gtt/min

   Microdrip at 125 gtt/min

   Use macrodrip.

   Label the IV.

6. This is a continuous IV of 250 mL every 8 hours. There is a pump available. It will run 8 hours.
   Minutes = 8 × 60 = 480 minutes.

$$\frac{250 \times \overset{1}{\cancel{60}}}{\underset{8}{\cancel{480}} \text{ min}} = \frac{250 \text{ mL}}{8} \quad 8\overline{\smash{)}250.0} \;\; {\scriptstyle 31.2} \text{ mL/hr}$$

$$\begin{array}{r} 24 \\ \hline 10 \\ 8 \\ \hline 2.0 \end{array}$$

   Label the IV. Set the pump: total number
   mL = 250; mL/hr = 31.

7. This is a continuous IV of 500 mL over 2 hours. There is a pump available.

It will run 2 hours. Minutes = $2 \times 60 = 120$.

$$\frac{500 \text{ mL} \times \overset{1}{\cancel{60}}\text{gtt}}{\underset{2}{\cancel{120}} \text{ min}} = \frac{\cancel{500} \text{ mL}}{2} \quad \begin{array}{r} 250.0 \text{ mL/hr} \\ 2 \overline{)500.0} \\ \underline{4} \\ 10 \\ \underline{10} \\ 0 \end{array}$$

Label the IV. Set the pump: total number mL = 500; mL/hr = 250.

8. This is a large volume over several hours; macrodrip. Solve using two steps.

$$\frac{\text{mL/hr} \times \text{TF}}{\text{min}} = \text{gtt/min}$$

Macrodrip

$$\frac{1000 \times \overset{1}{\cancel{15}}}{\underset{48}{\cancel{720}} \text{ min}} = 48 \begin{array}{r} 20.8 \\ \overline{)1000.0} \\ \underline{96} \\ 400 \\ \underline{384} \\ 6 \end{array}$$

Microdrip

$$\frac{1000 \times \overset{1}{\cancel{60}}}{\underset{12}{\cancel{720}} \text{ min}} = 12 \begin{array}{r} 83 \\ \overline{)1000} \\ \underline{96} \\ 40 \\ \underline{36} \\ 4 \end{array}$$

Macrodrip at 21 gtt/min, microdrip at 83 gtt/min

Use macrodrip.

Label the IV.

9. This is a large volume at a fast rate. Use macrodrip. Solve using step 2 only.

$$\frac{\text{mL/hr} \times \text{TF}}{\text{min}} = \text{gtt/min}$$

$$\frac{150 \times \overset{1}{\cancel{10}}}{\underset{6}{\cancel{60}} \text{ min}} = \frac{150}{6} \begin{array}{r} 25.0 \text{ gtt/min} \\ \overline{)150.0} \\ \underline{12} \\ 30 \\ \underline{30} \\ 0 \end{array}$$

Macrodrip at 25 gtt/min, microdrip at 150 gtt/min

Use macrodrip.

Label the IV.

10. This is a large volume over a short time. Use macrodrip tubing. The rate is 150 mL/hr (150 mL over 1 hour). Use step 2 only.

$$\frac{\text{mL/hr} \times \text{TF}}{\text{min}} = \text{gtt/min}$$

$$\frac{150 \times \overset{1}{\cancel{20}}}{\underset{3}{\cancel{60}} \text{ min}} = \frac{150}{3} \begin{array}{r} 50 \text{ gtt/min} \\ \overline{)150.0} \\ \underline{15} \\ 0 \end{array}$$

Macrodrip at 50 gtt/min, microdrip at 150 gtt/min

Use macrodrip.

Label the IV.

Self-Test 2 IV Infusions—Hours

1. 8.3 hours approximately $\left(\frac{250}{30} = 8.3\right)$

2. 8.3 hours approximately $\left(\frac{500}{60} = 8.3\right)$

3. 10 hours (no math)

4. 24 hours (no math)

5. 7.1 hours approximately $\left(\frac{500}{70} = 7.1\right)$

6. 10 hours $\left(\frac{500}{50} = 10\right)$

7. 10 hours (no math)

8. 2.5 hours $\left(\frac{250}{100} = 2.5\right)$

9. 6 hours (no math)

10. 5 hours (no math)

Self-Test 3 IV Infusion Rates

1. You want vitamin C 500 mg and the supply is 500 mg in 2 mL. Use a syringe to add the 2 mL to 500 mL D5W. You have microdrip available. The IV is to run at 60 mL/hr. Remember mL/hr = gtt/min for microdrip. No math necessary. Set the microdrip at 60 gtt/min. Label the IV.

$$\frac{60\ mL \times \cancel{60}\ gtt}{\cancel{60}\ min} = 60\ mL/hr$$

2. You want 250 mg hydrocortisone sodium succinate, and it comes 250 mg with a 2-mL diluent. Use a syringe to reconstitute the hydrocortisone with 2 mL diluent and add it to the IV. 8 AM– 12 MIDNIGHT is 16 hours.

mL/hr = gtt/min for microdrip. No math for microdrip. Microdrip = 63 gtt/min. Label the IV. Minutes = 60 × 16 = 960.

$$\frac{1000\ mL \times \overset{1}{\cancel{60}}\ gtt}{\underset{16}{\cancel{960}}\ min} = 16\overline{)1000.0}$$

$$\begin{array}{r} 62.5 \\ 16\overline{)1000.0} \\ \underline{96} \\ 40 \\ \underline{32} \\ 80 \\ \underline{80} \end{array}$$

3. You want 250 mg aminophylline. Supply is 500 mg/10 mL.

Formula Method	Proportion Expressed as Two Ratios	Proportion Expressed as Two Fractions
$\dfrac{250\ mg}{500\ mg} \times 10\ mL = 5\ mL$	10mL : 500 mg : : x mL : 250 mg	$\dfrac{10\ mL}{500\ mg} \diagup \dfrac{x}{250\ mg}$

$$\frac{2500}{500} = x$$
$$5 = x$$

Add 5 mL aminophylline to 250 mL D5W. Order is 50 mL/hr. You have an infusion pump. No math. Set the pump as follows: total number mL = 250; mL/hr = 50.

4. You want KCl 10 mEq. Supply is 20 mEq/10 mL.

Formula Method	Proportion Expressed as Two Ratios	Proportion Expressed as Two Fractions
$\dfrac{10\ mEq}{20\ mEq} \times 10\ mL = 5\ mL$	10 mL : 10 mEq : : x mL : 20 mEq	$\dfrac{10\ mL}{20\ mEq} \diagup \dfrac{x}{10\ mEq}$

$$\frac{100}{20} = x$$
$$5\ mL = x$$

Add 5 mL KCl to 250 mL D5W½NS. 12 NOON–6 PM is 6 hours. 6 hours = 6 × 60 = 360 minutes.

$$\frac{250\ mL \times \overset{1}{\cancel{60}}\ gtt}{\underset{6}{\cancel{360}}\ min} = \frac{\cancel{250}}{6} \quad \begin{array}{r} 41.6 \\ 6\overline{)250.0} \\ \underline{24} \\ 10 \\ \underline{6} \\ 4\ 0 \\ \underline{3\ 6} \end{array} = 42\ mL/hr$$

mL/hr = gtt/min microdrip

Set the microdrip at 42 gtt/min.

Label the IV.

Self-Test 4 IVPB Drip Factors

1. Zovirax (acyclovir) comes in 500 mg powder. Use a reconstitution device to add the powder to 100 mL D5W; min = 60; TF = 10 gtt/mL for IVPB.

   Rule: $\frac{mL \times TF}{min} = gtt/min$

   $$\frac{100 \times 10}{60 \; min} = \frac{100}{6} \overline{)\frac{16.6}{100.0}} = 17 \; gtt/min$$

   Label the IVPB.

   Set the rate at 17 gtt/min.

2. Ceptaz (ceftazidime) comes in a 1-g powder

   Use a reconstitution device to add the powder to 50 mL D5W; min, 30; TF, 10 gtt/mL for IVPB

   Rule: $\frac{mL \times TF}{min} = gtt/min$

   $$\frac{50 \times 10}{30 \; min} = \frac{50}{3} = 16.6 = 17 \; gtt/min$$

   Label the IVPB.

   Set the rate at 17 gtt/min.

3. Claforan (cefotaxime) comes as a 1-g powder

   Use a reconstitution device to add the powder to 50 mL D5W; min, 30; TF, 10 gtt/mL for IVPB

   $\frac{mL \times TF}{min} = gtt/min$

   $$\frac{50 \times 10}{30 \; min} = 16.6 = 17 gtt/min$$

   Label the IVPB

   Set the rate at 17 gtt/min.

4. Omnipen (ampicillin) comes as a 2-g powder.

   Reconstitute in 4.5 mL diluent = total volume 5 mL (2 g = 5 mL, 2000 mg = 5 mL)

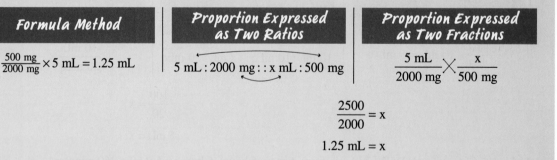

Formula Method	Proportion Expressed as Two Ratios	Proportion Expressed as Two Fractions
$\frac{500 \; mg}{2000 \; mg} \times 5 \; mL = 1.25 \; mL$	5 mL : 2000 mg : : x mL : 500 mg	$\frac{5 \; mL}{2000 \; mg} \times \frac{x}{500 \; mg}$

$$\frac{2500}{2000} = x$$

$$1.25 \; mL = x$$

   Add 1.25 mL to 50 mL D5W. Total min = 30; TF = 60 gtt/mL.

   $\frac{mL \times TF}{min} = gtt/min$

   $$\frac{50 \times \overset{2}{60}}{\underset{1}{30} \; min} = 100 \; gtt/min$$

   Label the IVPB.

   Set the rate at 100 gtt/min.

5. Nebcin (tobramycin) comes as 80-mg. Reconstitute in 2 mL diluent = 2 mL (80 mg = 2 mL)

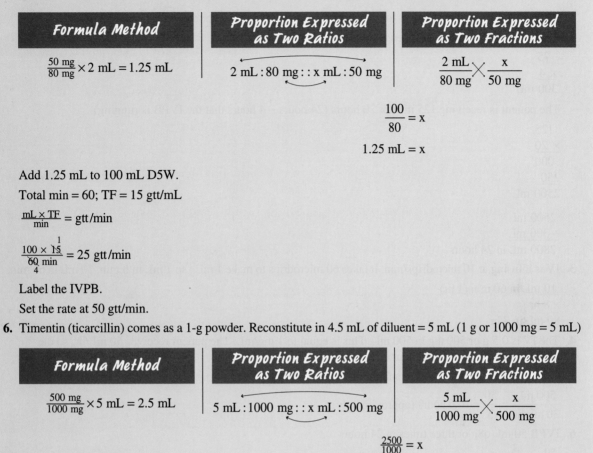

Formula Method	Proportion Expressed as Two Ratios	Proportion Expressed as Two Fractions
$\frac{50 \text{ mg}}{80 \text{ mg}} \times 2 \text{ mL} = 1.25 \text{ mL}$	2 mL : 80 mg : : x mL : 50 mg	$\frac{2 \text{ mL}}{80 \text{ mg}} \times \frac{x}{50 \text{ mg}}$

$$\frac{100}{80} = x$$

$$1.25 \text{ mL} = x$$

Add 1.25 mL to 100 mL D5W.

Total min = 60; TF = 15 gtt/mL

$$\frac{\text{mL} \times \text{TF}}{\text{min}} = \text{gtt/min}$$

$$\frac{100 \times \overset{1}{\cancel{15}}}{\underset{4}{\cancel{60}} \text{ min}} = 25 \text{ gtt/min}$$

Label the IVPB.

Set the rate at 50 gtt/min.

6. Timentin (ticarcillin) comes as a 1-g powder. Reconstitute in 4.5 mL of diluent = 5 mL (1 g or 1000 mg = 5 mL)

Formula Method	Proportion Expressed as Two Ratios	Proportion Expressed as Two Fractions
$\frac{500 \text{ mg}}{1000 \text{ mg}} \times 5 \text{ mL} = 2.5 \text{ mL}$	5 mL : 1000 mg : : x mL : 500 mg	$\frac{5 \text{ mL}}{1000 \text{ mg}} \times \frac{x}{500 \text{ mg}}$

$$\frac{2500}{1000} = x$$

$$2.5 \text{ mL} = x$$

Add 2.5 mL to 50 mL D5W.

Total min, 30; TF, 15 gtt/mL

$$\frac{\text{mL} \times \text{TF}}{\text{min}} = \text{gtt/min}$$

$$\frac{50 \times \overset{1}{\cancel{15}}}{\underset{2}{\cancel{30}} \text{ min}} = 25 \text{ gtt/min}$$

Self-Test 5 Calculation of Tube Feedings

1. 206.25 mL of Isocal. 68.75 mL water.

2. 56.25 mL Magnacal. 18.75 mL water.

3. 50 mL Osmolite. 50 mL water.

4. 21.25 mL Ensure. 63.75 mL water.

5. 100 mL Renalcal. 300 mL water.

6. 200 mL Suplena. 200 mL water.

Self-Test 6 Fluid Intake

1. 900 mL at 100 mL/hr = 9 hours to run. If the IV starts at 9 AM, + 9 hours = 6 PM.

2. IVPB is 75 mL q6h or four times in 24 hours

$$\begin{array}{r} 75 \\ \times\ 4 \\ \hline 300\ \text{mL} \end{array}$$

   The patient is receiving 125 mL for 20 hours (24 hours − 4 hours that the IVPB is running).

$$\begin{array}{r} 125 \\ \times\ 20 \\ \hline 000 \\ 250 \\ \hline 2500\ \text{mL} \end{array}$$

$$\begin{array}{r} 2500\ \text{mL} \\ +\ 300\ \text{mL} \\ \hline 2800\ \text{mL in 24 hours} \end{array}$$

3. IV is infusing at 10 microdrips/min. It takes 60 microdrips to make 1 mL., so 1 mL in 6 min, 10 mL in 60 min.

   10 mL in 60 min (1 hr)

$$\begin{array}{r} \times\ 8\ \text{hr} \\ \hline 80\ \text{mL in 8 hr} \end{array}$$

4. The IV is 0.5 g or 500 mg in 500 mL. This is equal to 1 mg/mL. The patient receives 50 mL/hr, so the patient receives 50 mg each hour.

5. The IV is infusing at 30 mL/hr and the solution is 500 mL.

$$\frac{500\ \text{mL}}{30\ \text{mL/hr}} = \frac{50}{3} = 16.6\ \text{hours (approximately)}$$

6. IVPB 50 mL q8h or three times in 24 hours

$$\begin{array}{r} 50 \\ \times\ 3 \\ \hline 150\ \text{mL} \end{array}$$

   The patient is receiving 100 mL for 21 hours (24 hours − 3 hours that the IVPB is running).

$$\begin{array}{r} 100 \\ \times\ 21 \\ \hline 100 \\ +\ 200 \\ \hline 2100\ \text{mL} \end{array}$$

$$\begin{array}{r} 2100\ \text{mL} \\ +\ 150\ \text{mL} \\ \hline 2250\ \text{mL in 24 hours} \end{array}$$

7. 500 mL at 50 mL/hr = 10 hours to run. If the IV starts at 6 AM + 10 hours = 4 PM.

8. The IV is infusing at 125 mL/hr and the solution is 1000 mL.

$$\frac{1000\ \text{mL}}{125\ \text{mL/hr}} = 8\ \text{hours}$$

9. IVPB is 250 mL q6h or four times in 24 hours

$$\begin{array}{r} 250 \\ \times\ 4 \\ \hline 1000\ \text{mL in 24 hours} \end{array}$$

10. The IV is 100 units in 100 mL or 1 unit/mL. The patient receives 10 mL/hr so the patient receives 10 units/hr.

Self-Test 7 IV Drip Rates

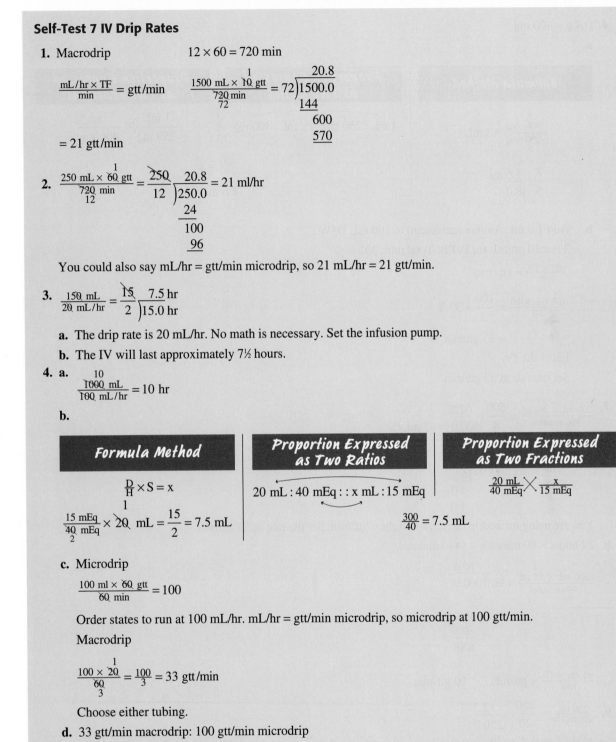

1. Macrodrip $12 \times 60 = 720$ min

$$\frac{mL/hr \times TF}{min} = gtt/min \qquad \frac{1500 \; mL \times \overset{1}{\cancel{10}} \; gtt}{\underset{72}{\cancel{720}} \; min} = 72 \overset{\displaystyle 20.8}{\overline{)1500.0}}$$

$$\begin{array}{r} 144 \\ \hline 600 \\ 570 \\ \hline \end{array}$$

$= 21$ gtt/min

2. $\dfrac{250 \; mL \times \overset{1}{\cancel{60}} \; gtt}{\underset{12}{\cancel{720}} \; min} = \dfrac{\cancel{250}}{12} \; 12\overset{\displaystyle 20.8}{\overline{)250.0}} = 21$ ml/hr

$$\begin{array}{r} 24 \\ \hline 100 \\ 96 \\ \hline \end{array}$$

You could also say mL/hr = gtt/min microdrip, so 21 mL/hr = 21 gtt/min.

3. $\dfrac{\cancel{150} \; mL}{\cancel{20} \; mL/hr} = \dfrac{\cancel{15}}{2} \; 2\overset{\displaystyle 7.5 \; hr}{\overline{)15.0 \; hr}}$

   a. The drip rate is 20 mL/hr. No math is necessary. Set the infusion pump.
   b. The IV will last approximately 7½ hours.

4. a. $\dfrac{\overset{10}{\cancel{1000}} \; mL}{\cancel{100} \; mL/hr} = 10$ hr

   b.

Formula Method	Proportion Expressed as Two Ratios	Proportion Expressed as Two Fractions
$\dfrac{D}{H} \times S = x$		$\dfrac{20 \; mL}{40 \; mEq} \diagup \dfrac{x}{15 \; mEq}$
$\dfrac{15 \; mEq}{\underset{2}{\cancel{40}} \; mEq} \times \overset{1}{\cancel{20}} \; mL = \dfrac{15}{2} = 7.5$ mL	$20 \; mL : 40 \; mEq :: x \; mL : 15 \; mEq$	$\dfrac{300}{40} = 7.5$ mL

   c. Microdrip

   $$\frac{100 \; ml \times \cancel{60} \; gtt}{\cancel{60} \; min} = 100$$

   Order states to run at 100 mL/hr. mL/hr = gtt/min microdrip, so microdrip at 100 gtt/min.

   Macrodrip

   $$\frac{100 \times \overset{1}{\cancel{20}}}{\underset{3}{\cancel{60}}} = \frac{100}{3} = 33 \; gtt/min$$

   Choose either tubing.
   d. 33 gtt/min macrodrip: 100 gtt/min microdrip

5. a. You desire 1 g. Aminophylline comes 1 g in 10 mL. Add 10 mL to the IV of 500 mL D5W and label.
   b. You have an infusion pump; there is no math.
      Set the pump:
      total mL = 500; mL/hr = 75

6. 0.4 g = 400 mg

a.

Formula Method	Proportion Expressed as Two Ratios	Proportion Expressed as Two Fractions
$$\dfrac{\overset{8}{\cancel{400}}\ \text{mg}}{\underset{5}{\cancel{250}}\ \text{mg}} \times 1\ \text{mL}$$	1 mL : 250 mg : : x mL : 400 mg	$$\dfrac{1\ \text{mL}}{250\ \text{mg}} \times \dfrac{\text{x}}{400\ \text{mg}}$$

$$\dfrac{\cancel{8}}{5}\overline{)8.0}\quad 1.6\ \text{mL}$$

$$\dfrac{400}{250} = \text{x}$$

1.6 mL

b. Add 1.6 mL Amikin (amikacin) to 100 mL D5W.

TF = 10 gtt/mL for IVPB. Total min, 30

$$\dfrac{\text{mL} \times \text{TF}}{\text{min}} = \text{gtt/min}$$

$$\dfrac{100\ \text{mL} \times 1\cancel{0}}{3\cancel{0}} = \dfrac{100}{3} = 33.3$$

$$= 33\ \text{gtt/min}$$

Label the IV.

Set the rate at 33 gtt/min.

7. $$\dfrac{500\ \text{mL} \times \overset{1}{\cancel{60}}\ \text{gtt}}{\underset{8}{\cancel{480}}\ \text{minutes}} = \dfrac{500}{8}\ \overline{)500.0}\quad \begin{array}{r}62.5\\\end{array} = 63\ \text{mL/hr}$$

$$\begin{array}{r} 48 \\ \overline{20} \\ 16 \\ \overline{4\,0} \\ 4\,0 \end{array}$$

You are using microdrip tubing, so mL/hr = gtt/min. Set the rate at 63 gtt/min.

8. 24 hours × 60 minutes = 1440 minutes.

$$\dfrac{1000\ \text{mL} \times \overset{1}{\cancel{15}}\ \text{gtt}}{\underset{96}{\cancel{1440}}\ \text{minutes}} = 96\ \overline{)1000.0}\quad \begin{array}{r}10.4\\\end{array}$$

$$\begin{array}{r} 96 \\ \overline{40} \\ 0 \\ \overline{400} \end{array}$$

$$\dfrac{\text{mL/hr} \times \text{TF}}{\text{min}} = \text{gtt/min}\qquad 10\ \text{gtt/min}$$

9. $$\dfrac{250\ \text{mL}}{20\ \text{mL/hr}} = \dfrac{250}{20}\ \overline{)250.0}\quad \begin{array}{r}12.5\\\end{array}$$

$$\begin{array}{r} 20 \\ \overline{50} \\ 40 \\ \overline{10\,0} \end{array}$$

The IV will last 12.5 hours.

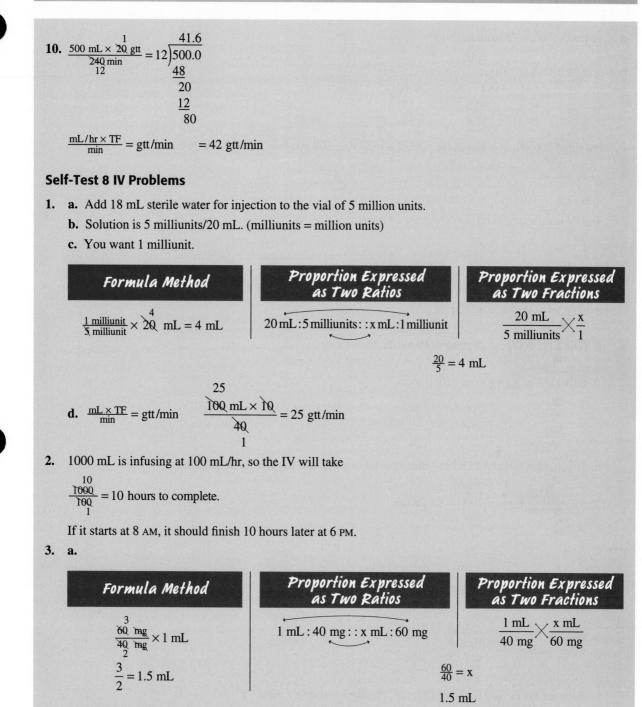

10. $\dfrac{500 \text{ mL} \times \overset{1}{\cancel{20}} \text{ gtt}}{\underset{12}{\cancel{240} \text{ min}}} = 12\overline{)\begin{array}{l}41.6 \\ 500.0 \\ \underline{48} \\ 20 \\ \underline{12} \\ 80\end{array}}$

$\dfrac{\text{mL/hr} \times \text{TF}}{\text{min}} = \text{gtt/min} \qquad = 42 \text{ gtt/min}$

Self-Test 8 IV Problems

1. **a.** Add 18 mL sterile water for injection to the vial of 5 million units.
    b. Solution is 5 milliunits/20 mL. (milliunits = million units)
    c. You want 1 milliunit.

Formula Method	Proportion Expressed as Two Ratios	Proportion Expressed as Two Fractions
$\dfrac{1 \text{ milliunit}}{5 \text{ milliunit}} \times \overset{4}{\cancel{20}} \text{ mL} = 4 \text{ mL}$	$20 \text{ mL} : 5 \text{ milliunits} :: x \text{ mL} : 1 \text{ milliunit}$	$\dfrac{20 \text{ mL}}{5 \text{ milliunits}} \times \dfrac{x}{1}$

$\dfrac{20}{5} = 4 \text{ mL}$

d. $\dfrac{\text{mL} \times \text{TF}}{\text{min}} = \text{gtt/min}$ $\dfrac{\overset{25}{\cancel{100}} \text{ mL} \times \overset{}{\cancel{10}}}{\underset{1}{\cancel{40}}} = 25 \text{ gtt/min}$

2. 1000 mL is infusing at 100 mL/hr, so the IV will take

$\dfrac{\overset{10}{\cancel{1000}}}{\underset{1}{\cancel{100}}} = 10 \text{ hours to complete.}$

If it starts at 8 AM, it should finish 10 hours later at 6 PM.

3. **a.**

Formula Method	Proportion Expressed as Two Ratios	Proportion Expressed as Two Fractions
$\dfrac{\overset{3}{\cancel{60}} \text{ mg}}{\underset{2}{\cancel{40}} \text{ mg}} \times 1 \text{ mL}$ $\dfrac{3}{2} = 1.5 \text{ mL}$	$1 \text{ mL} : 40 \text{ mg} :: x \text{ mL} : 60 \text{ mg}$	$\dfrac{1 \text{ mL}}{40 \text{ mg}} \times \dfrac{x \text{ mL}}{60 \text{ mg}}$ $\dfrac{60}{40} = x$ 1.5 mL

Add 1.5 mL gentamicin.

b. $\dfrac{\text{mL} \times \text{TF}}{\text{min}} = \text{gtt/min}$

$\dfrac{50 \text{ mL} \times \cancel{20}}{\cancel{30} \text{ min}} = \dfrac{\overset{}{\cancel{100}}}{3} \quad 3\overline{)\begin{array}{l}33.3 \\ 100.00\end{array}} = 33 \text{ gtt/min}$

4. $12 \text{ hours} \times 60 = 720 \text{ minutes}$

$$\frac{1500 \text{ mL} \times \overset{1}{\cancel{10}} \text{ gtt}}{\underset{72}{\cancel{720}} \text{ min}} = 72\overline{)1500.0}$$

$$\begin{array}{r} 20.8 \\ 72\overline{)1500.0} \\ \underline{194} \\ 60\ 0 \\ \underline{57\ 6} \end{array}$$

5. Intralipid 500 mL q6h means the patient is receiving 500 mL four times every 24 hours

$$\begin{array}{r} 500 \\ \times\ \ 4 \\ \hline 2000 \text{ mL} \end{array}$$

The IV is infusing 80 mL/hr. There are 24 hours in a day, so

$$\begin{array}{r} 24 \\ \times\ 80 \\ \hline 1920 \end{array}$$

$$\begin{array}{r} 2000 \text{ mL} \\ \text{Adding these we have } +1920 \text{ mL} \\ \hline 3920 \text{ mL} \end{array}$$

6. a. You have 1000 mL running at 60 mL/hr, therefore

$$\begin{array}{r} 16.6 \\ 60\overline{)1000.0} \\ \underline{60} \\ 400 \\ \underline{360} \\ 40\ 0 \end{array} = \text{approximtely } 16\tfrac{1}{2} \text{ hours}$$

b. If you want 60 mL/hr and use microdrip tubing, the drip factor will be 60 gtt/min:

$$\frac{1000 \text{ mL} \times \overset{1}{\cancel{60}} \text{ gtt}}{\underset{16}{\cancel{960}} \text{ minutes}} = 16\overline{)1000} = 63 \text{ gtt/min}$$

$$\begin{array}{r} 62.5 \\ 16\overline{)1000} \\ \underline{96} \\ 40 \\ \underline{32} \\ 80 \end{array}$$

If you use macrodrip tubing you have

$16 \text{ hours} \times 60 \text{ min} = 960 \text{ minutes.}$

$$\frac{1000 \text{ mL} \times \overset{1}{\cancel{10}} \text{ gtt}}{\underset{96}{\cancel{960}} \text{ minutes}} = 96\overline{)1000.0}$$

$$\begin{array}{r} 10.4 \\ 96\overline{)1000.0} \\ \underline{96} \\ 400 \end{array}$$

Because the IV will run over 16 hours, choose *microdrip tubing*.

c. The drip factor will be 60 gtt/min. *Note:* It is not incorrect to choose the macrodrip at 10 gtt/min. However, because the IV will run so many hours, a good flow might help to keep the IV running.

CHAPTER
9

Special Types of Intravenous Calculations

In Chapter 8 we studied calculations for microdrip and macrodrip factors, the use of the infusion pump, and IVPB orders. In this chapter we consider calculations for orders written in units, milliunits, milligrams, and micrograms; special types of calculations in relation to continuous heparin infusion and continuous insulin infusion; methods of calculating the safety of doses based on kilograms of body weight and body surface area (BSA); and the handling of orders for patient-controlled analgesia (PCA).

This chapter's dosage calculations are for medications mixed in IV fluids and delivered as continuous infusions. Administering these medications via infusion pumps ensures a correct rate and accuracy of dose (Fig. 9-1). Many infusion pumps can deliver rates less than 1 (e.g., 0.5 mL/hr, 0.25 mL/hr, etc.), and they also can be programmed with the amount of drug, amount of solution, patient's weight, and time unit (minutes or hours). Once the pump is set at an infusion rate, the pump calculates how much drug the patient is receiving. The nurse, however, still bears the responsibility for double-checking the calculation and entering the correct information on the infusion pump.

Because many of the medications that infuse via continuous infusions are very potent, small changes in the infusion rate can greatly affect the body's physiologic response. In particular, vasopressor drugs such as Dopamine, Epinephrine, Dobutamine, and Levoped can affect the patient's blood pressure and heart rate, even in small doses. In most hospital settings, the pharmacy prepares medications and IV solutions.

 Amount of Drug in a Solution

These calculations can be complicated. One helpful technique is reduction: Start with the entire amount of drug mixed in solution, and then reduce it to the amount of the drug in only 1 mL of solution.

Here's an example:

Heparin is mixed 25,000 units in 500 mL D5W.

How much heparin is in 1 mL of fluid?

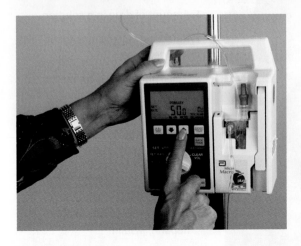

FIGURE 9-1

Infusion pump. (With permission from Evans-Smith, P. [2005]. *Taylor's clinical nursing skills.* Philadelphia: Lippincott Williams & Wilkins.)

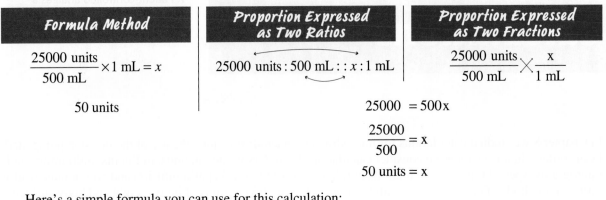

Formula Method	*Proportion Expressed as Two Ratios*	*Proportion Expressed as Two Fractions*
$\dfrac{25000 \text{ units}}{500 \text{ mL}} \times 1 \text{ mL} = x$	$25000 \text{ units} : 500 \text{ mL} :: x : 1 \text{ mL}$	$\dfrac{25000 \text{ units}}{500 \text{ mL}} \times \dfrac{x}{1 \text{ mL}}$
50 units		

$$25000 = 500x$$

$$\frac{25000}{500} = x$$

$$50 \text{ units} = x$$

Here's a simple formula you can use for this calculation:

$$\frac{\text{Amount of Drug}}{\text{Amount of Fluid (mL)}} = \text{amount of drug in 1 mL}$$

Medications Ordered in Units/hr or mg/hr

Sometimes patient medications are administered as continuous IVs. For these medications, solutions are standardized to decrease the possibility of error. Check the guidelines (institutional or drug references) to verify dose, dilution, and rate. If any doubts exist, consult with the prescribing physician or healthcare provider.

Units/hr–Rule and Calculation

The order will indicate the amount of drug to be added to the IV fluid and also the amount to administer.

Example   Order: heparin, infuse 800 units/hr

Available: heparin 40,000 units in 1000 mL D5W infusion pump

You know the solution and the amount to administer. Because you'll be using an infusion pump, the answer will be in mL/hr.

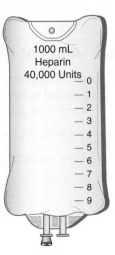

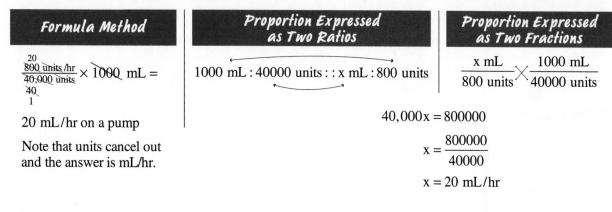

Formula Method	Proportion Expressed as Two Ratios	Proportion Expressed as Two Fractions
$\dfrac{\overset{20}{\cancel{800 \text{ units/hr}}}}{\underset{\underset{1}{40}}{\cancel{40,000 \text{ units}}}} \times 1000 \text{ mL} =$	$1000 \text{ mL} : 40000 \text{ units} :: x \text{ mL} : 800 \text{ units}$	$\dfrac{x \text{ mL}}{800 \text{ units}} \times \dfrac{1000 \text{ mL}}{40000 \text{ units}}$

20 mL/hr on a pump

Note that units cancel out
and the answer is mL/hr.

$$40,000x = 800000$$

$$x = \frac{800000}{40000}$$

$$x = 20 \text{ mL/hr}$$

How many hours will the IV run?

$\dfrac{\text{number mL}}{\text{number mL/hr}}$

$\dfrac{1000 \text{ mL}}{20 \text{ mL/hr}} = 50 \text{ hours}$

Note: Most hospitals require changing the IV fluids every 24 hours.

Example   Order: heparin sodium 1100 units/hr IV

Supply: infusion pump, standard solution (premixed by the
pharmacy) of 25,000 units in 250 mL D5W

With an infusion pump, the answer will be in mL/hr.

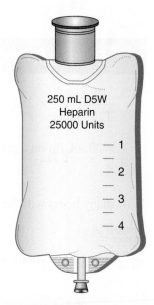

250 mL D5W
Heparin
25000 Units

— 1
— 2
— 3
— 4

Formula Method	Proportion Expressed as Two Ratios	Proportion Expressed as Two Fractions
$\dfrac{1100 \text{ units/hr} \times 250 \text{ mL}}{\underset{\underset{1}{\cancel{100}}}{\cancel{25,000 \text{ units}}}} =$	$250 \text{ mL} : 25000 \text{ units} :: x \text{ mL} : 1100 \text{ units}$	$\dfrac{x \text{ mL}}{1100 \text{ units}} \times \dfrac{250 \text{ mL}}{25000 \text{ units}}$

11 mL/hr on a pump

$$x \text{ mL} = \frac{275000}{25000}$$

$$x = 11 \text{ mL/hr}$$

How many hours will the IV run?

$\dfrac{\text{number mL}}{\text{number mL/hr}}$

$\dfrac{250 \text{ mL}}{11 \text{ mL/hr}} = 22.75 \text{ or } 23 \text{ hours}$

Example   Order: regular insulin 10 units/hr IV

Available: infusion pump, standard solution of 125 units regular insulin in 250 mL NS

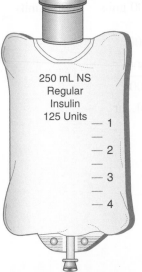

250 mL NS
Regular
Insulin
125 Units
— 1
— 2
— 3
— 4

Formula Method	*Proportion Expressed as Two Ratios*	*Proportion Expressed as Two Fractions*
$\dfrac{10 \text{ units}}{125 \text{ units}} \times \overset{2}{250} \text{ mL}$ $= 20 \text{ mL/hr on a pump}$	$250 \text{ mL} : 125 \text{ units} :: x \text{ mL} : 10 \text{ units}$	$\dfrac{x \text{ mL}}{10} \times \dfrac{2500}{125}$ $x \text{ mL} = \dfrac{2500}{125 \text{ units}}$ $x = 20 \text{ mL/hr}$

How many hours will the IV run?

$\dfrac{\text{number mL}}{\text{number mL/hr}}$

$\dfrac{250 \text{ mL}}{20 \text{ mL/hr}} = 12.5$ or approximately 13 hours

mg/hr; g/hr–Rule and Calculation

The order will indicate the amount of drug added to the IV fluid and the amount to administer.

Example   Order: calcium gluconate 2 g in 100 mL D5W; run 0.25 g/hr IV via infusion pump.

Because we know the solution and the amount of drug per hour, we can solve the problem and administer the drug in mL/hr per infusion pump. Round the final answer to the nearest whole number.

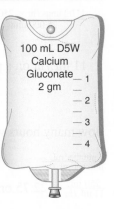

100 mL D5W
Calcium
Gluconate
2 gm
— 1
— 2
— 3
— 4

Formula Method	Proportion Expressed as Two Ratios	Proportion Expressed as Two Fractions
$\dfrac{0.25\,\text{g/hr}}{\underset{1}{\overset{}{2\,\text{g}}}} \times \overset{50}{\cancel{100}}\ \text{mL} = 12.5$ 13 mL/hr on a pump	$100\ \text{mL} : 2\ \text{g} :: x\ \text{mL} : 0.25\ \text{g}$ $x = \dfrac{25}{2}$ $x = 12.5$ or $13\ \text{mL/hr}$	$\dfrac{x\ \text{mL}}{0.25\ \text{g/hr}} \times \dfrac{100\ \text{mL}}{2\ \text{g}}$

How many hours will the IV run?

$\dfrac{\text{number mL}}{\text{number mL/hr}}$

$\dfrac{100\ \text{mL}}{13\ \text{mL/hr}} = 7.6$ or approximately 8 hours

Example   Order: aminophylline 250 mg in 250 mL D5W; run 65 mg/hr IV per infusion pump.

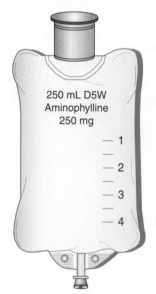

250 mL D5W
Aminophylline
250 mg

— 1
— 2
— 3
— 4

Formula Method	Proportion Expressed as Two Ratios	Proportion Expressed as Two Fractions
$\dfrac{65\ \text{mg/hr}}{\underset{1}{\overset{}{250\ \text{mg}}}} \times \overset{1}{\cancel{250}}\ \text{mL}$ $= 65\ \text{mL/hr}$ on a pump	$250\ \text{mL} : 250\ \text{mg} :: x\ \text{mL} : 65\ \text{mg}$ $x = \dfrac{65 \times \cancel{250}}{\cancel{250}}$ $x = 65\ \text{mL/hr}$	$\dfrac{x\ \text{mL}}{65\ \text{mg}} \times \dfrac{250\ \text{mL}}{250\ \text{mg}}$

How many hours will the IV run?

$\dfrac{\text{number mL}}{\text{number mL/hr}}$

$\dfrac{250\ \text{mL}}{65\ \text{mL/hr}} = 3.8$ or approximately 4 hours

Solve the following problems. Answers appear at the end of this chapter.

1. Order: heparin sodium 800 units/hr IV
   Supply: infusion pump, standard solution of 25,000 units in 250 mL D5W

   a. What is the rate?
   b. How many hours will the IV run?

2. Order: Zovirax (acyclovir) 500 mg in 100 mL D5W IV over 1 hr
   Supply: pump, Zovirax (acyclovir) 500 mg in 100 mL
   What is the rate?

3. Order: Amicar (aminocaproic acid) 24 g in 1000 mL D5W over 24 hr IV
   Supply: infusion pump, vials of Amicar (aminocaproic acid) labeled 5 g per 20 mL
   What is the rate?

4. Order: Cardizem (diltiazem) 125 mg in 100 mL D5W at 10 mg/hr IV
   Supply: infusion pump, vial of Cardizem (diltiazem) labeled 5 mg/mL
   What is the rate?

5. Order: Lasix (furosemide) 100 mg in 100 mL D5W; infuse 4 mg/hr
   Supply: infusion pump, vial of Lasix (furosemide) labeled 10 mg/mL
   What is the rate?

6. Order: regular insulin 15 units/hr IV
   Supply: standard solution of 125 units in 250 mL NS, infusion pump

   a. What is the drip rate?
   b. How many hours will this IV run?

7. Order: nitroglycerin 50 mg in 250 mL D5W over 24 hr via pump
   What is the drip rate?

8. Order: heparin 1200 units/hr IV
   Supply: infusion pump, standard solution of 25,000 units in 500 mL D5W

   a. What is the rate?
   b. How many hours will the IV run?

9. Order: regular insulin 23 units/hr IV
   Supply: infusion pump, standard solution of 250 units in 250 mL NS

   a. What is the rate?
   b. How many hours will the IV run?

10. Order: Streptase (streptokinase) 100,000 international units/hr for 24 hr IV
    Supply: infusion pump, standard solution of 750,000 international units in 250 mL NS
    What is the rate?

mg/min—Rule and Calculation

The order will indicate the amount of drug added to IV fluid and also the amount of drug to administer. These medications are administered through an IV infusion pump in mL/hr.

Example Order: Bretylol (bretylium) 1 mg/min IV

Supply: infusion pump, standard solution of 1 g in 500 mL D5W (1000 mg in 500 mL)

The order calls for 1 mg/min. You need milliliters per hour for the pump.

Convert the order to mg/hr, by multiplying the drug amount by 60 (60 minutes =1 hour). 1 mg/min × 60 = 60 mg/hr

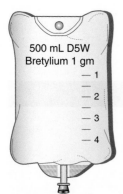

500 mL D5W
Bretylium 1 gm
— 1
— 2
— 3
— 4

Formula Method	Proportion Expressed as Two Ratios	Proportion Expressed as Two Fractions
$\dfrac{\overset{30}{\cancel{60}\ \text{mg/hr}}}{\underset{\underset{1}{2}}{\cancel{1000}\ \text{mg}}} \times \overset{}{\cancel{500}}\ \text{mL} = 30\ \text{mL/hr}$	500 mL : 1000 mg : : x mL : 60 mg	$\dfrac{\text{x mL}}{60\ \text{mg}} \diagdown \dfrac{500\ \text{mL}}{1000\ \text{mg}}$

$$x = \frac{30000}{1000}$$

$$x = 30\ \text{mL/hr}$$

Set pump at 30 mL/hr.

How many hours will the IV run?

$\dfrac{\text{number mL}}{\text{number mL/hr}}$

$\dfrac{500\text{mL}}{30\text{mL/hr}} = 16.6$ or approximately 17 hours

Example Order: lidocaine 2 mg/min IV

Supply: infusion pump, standard solution of 2 g in 500 mL D5W (2000 mg in 500 mL)

The order calls for 2 mg/min. We need mL/hr for the pump.

Multiply 2 mg/min × 60 = 120 mg/hr

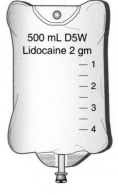

500 mL D5W
Lidocaine 2 gm
— 1
— 2
— 3
— 4

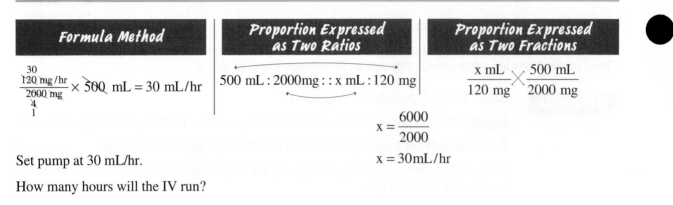

Formula Method	*Proportion Expressed as Two Ratios*	*Proportion Expressed as Two Fractions*

$$\frac{\overset{30}{\cancel{120 \text{ mg/hr}}}}{\underset{\underset{1}{4}}{\cancel{2000 \text{ mg}}}} \times \cancel{500} \text{ mL} = 30 \text{ mL/hr}$$

$$500 \text{ mL} : 2000 \text{mg} :: x \text{ mL} : 120 \text{ mg}$$

$$\frac{x \text{ mL}}{120 \text{ mg}} \times \frac{500 \text{ mL}}{2000 \text{ mg}}$$

$$x = \frac{6000}{2000}$$

$$x = 30 \text{mL/hr}$$

Set pump at 30 mL/hr.

How many hours will the IV run?

$$\frac{\text{number mL}}{\text{number mL/hr}}$$

$$\frac{500 \text{ mL}}{30 \text{mL/hr}} = 16.6 \text{ or approximately 17 hours}$$

SELF-TEST 2   **Infusion Rates for Drugs Ordered in mg/min**

Solve the following problems. Answers appear at the end of the chapter.

1. Order: lidocaine 1 mg/min IV
   Supply: 2 g in 250 mL D5W, infusion pump

   a. What is the drip rate?
   b. How many hours will the IV run?

2. Order: Pronestyl (procainamide) 3 mg/min IV
   Supply: Pronestyl (procainamide) 1 g in 250 D5W, infusion pump

   a. What is the drip rate?
   b. How many hours will the IV run?

3. Order: Bretylol (bretylium) 2 mg/min IV
   Supply: Bretylol (bretylium) 1 g in 500 mL D5W, infusion pump

   a. What is the drip rate?
   b. How many hours will the IV run?

4. Order: Cordarone (amiodarone) 1 mg/min for 6 hr
   Supply: Cordarone (amiodarone) 450 mg in 250 mL D5W, infusion pump
   What is the drip rate?

5. Order: Pronestyl (procainamide) 1 mg/min IV
   Supply: Pronestyl (procainamide) 2 g in 500 mL D5W, infusion pump

   a. What is the drip rate?
   b. How many hours will the IV run?

Medications Ordered in mcg/min, mcg/kg/min, or milliunits/min

Intensive care units administer powerful drugs in extremely small amounts called micrograms (1 mg = 1000 mcg). The orders for these drugs often use the patient's weight as a determinant, because these drugs are so potent.

> **Example** Order: renal dose dopamine 2 mcg/kg/min
>
> Order: titrate levophed to maintain arterial mean pressure above 65 mm Hg and below 95 mm Hg

This section shows how to calculate doses in micrograms and in milliunits, and how to use kilograms in determining doses.

mcg/min—Rule and Calculation

Drugs ordered in mcg/min are standardized solutions prepared by a pharmacist. They are administered using infusion pumps that deliver medication in mL/hr.

To calculate drugs ordered in mcg/min, first determine how much of the drug is in 1 mL of solution (see beginning of this chapter). If the drug is supplied in mg, convert it to mcg; then divide that amount by 60 to get mcg/min. The final number tells you how much of the drug is in 1 mL of fluid. You can then use one of the three methods to solve for the infusion rate, on the basis of the ordered dosage.

Solving mcg/min requires four steps:

1. Reduce the numbers in the standard solution to mg/mL.

2. Change mg to mcg.

3. Divide by 60 to get mcg/min.

4. Use either the formula, ratio, or proportion method to solve for mL/hr.

> **Example** Order: Intropin (dopamine) 400 mcg/min IV
>
> Supply: infusion pump, standard solution 400 mg in 250 mL D5W
>
> **Step 1.** Reduce the numbers in the standard solution.
>
> $$\frac{400 \text{ mg}}{250 \text{ mL}} = 1.6 \text{ mg in 1 mL}$$
>
> **Step 2.** Change mg to mcg.
>
> $$1.6 \text{ mg x } 1000 = 1600 \text{ mg/1 mL}$$
>
> **Step 3.** Divide by 60 to get mcg/min.
>
> $$\frac{1600 \text{ mcg}}{60 \text{ min}} = 26.67 \ \text{mcg/min}$$
>
> (round to hundredths)
>
> **Step 4.** Solve for mL/hr (Round to nearest whole number).

250 mL D5W
Dopamine
400 mg

— 1
— 2
— 3
— 4

Formula Method	**Proportion Expressed as Two Ratios**	**Proportion Expressed as Two Fractions**
$\frac{400 \text{ mcg/min}}{26.67 \text{ mcg/min}} \times 1 \text{ mL}$ $= 15 \text{ mL/hr}$	$1 \text{ mL} : 26.67 \text{ mcg/min} :: x \text{ mL} : 400 \text{ mcg/min}$	$\dfrac{1 \text{ mL}}{26.67 \text{ mcg/min}} \times \dfrac{x \text{ mL}}{400 \text{ mcg/min}}$

$$400 = 26.67x$$
$$\tfrac{400}{26.67} = 15 \text{ mL/hr}$$

To set the infusion pump, program the following

- Total number mL ordered

- mL/hr to run

Set the pump: total number mL = 250 (standard solution); mL/hr = 15

Example   Order: Aramine (metaraminol) 60 mcg/min IV

Supply: infusion pump, standard solution 50 mg in 250 mL D5W

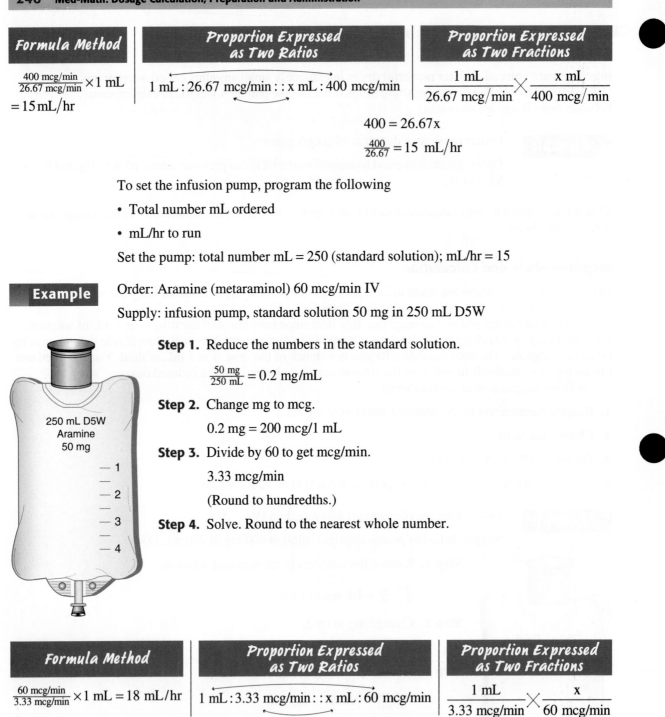

Step 1. Reduce the numbers in the standard solution.

$$\tfrac{50 \text{ mg}}{250 \text{ mL}} = 0.2 \text{ mg/mL}$$

Step 2. Change mg to mcg.

0.2 mg = 200 mcg/1 mL

Step 3. Divide by 60 to get mcg/min.

3.33 mcg/min

(Round to hundredths.)

Step 4. Solve. Round to the nearest whole number.

(bag label: 250 mL D5W / Aramine / 50 mg)

Formula Method	**Proportion Expressed as Two Ratios**	**Proportion Expressed as Two Fractions**
$\frac{60 \text{ mcg/min}}{3.33 \text{ mcg/min}} \times 1 \text{ mL} = 18 \text{ mL/hr}$	$1 \text{ mL} : 3.33 \text{ mcg/min} :: x \text{ mL} : 60 \text{ mcg/min}$	$\dfrac{1 \text{ mL}}{3.33 \text{ mcg/min}} \times \dfrac{x}{60 \text{ mcg/min}}$

$$60 = 3.33x$$
$$\frac{60}{3.33} = 18 \text{ mL/hr}$$

Set the pump: total number mL = 250 (standard solutions); mL/hr = 18

mcg/kg/min–Rule and Calculation

Example

Order: Intropin (dopamine) 2 mcg/kg/min

Supply: infusion pump, standard solution 200 mg in 250 mL D5W; client weighs 176 lb

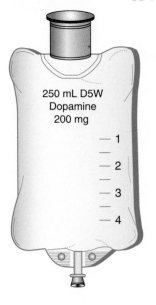

250 mL D5W
Dopamine
200 mg

— 1

— 2

— 3

— 4

Note that this order is somewhat different. You are to give 2 mcg/kg body weight. First you weigh the patient and then convert pounds to kilograms; if the weight is in kilograms, then multiply the number of kilograms by 2 mcg. Once you have determined this answer, follow the steps described earlier.

The patient weighs 176 lb.

$$\frac{176 \text{ lb}}{2.2} \qquad \frac{80}{\overline{)176.0}} = 80 \text{ kg}$$

$$\begin{array}{r} 80 \text{ kg} \\ \times\ 2 \text{ mcg} \\ \hline 160 \text{ mcg} \end{array}$$ The order now is 160 mcg/min.

1. Reduce the numbers in the standard solution.

   $$\frac{200 \text{ mg}}{250 \text{ mL}} = 0.8 \text{ mg/mL}$$

2. Change mg to mcg.

   $$0.8 = 800 \text{ mcg/mL}$$

3. Divide by 60 to get mcg/kg/min.

   $$\frac{800}{60} = 13.33$$

   (Round to hundredths.)

4. Solve. Round to the nearest whole number.

Formula Method	Proportion Expressed as Two Ratios	Proportion Expressed as Two Fractions
$\frac{160 \text{ mcg/min}}{13.33 \text{ mcg/min}} \times 1 \text{ mL} = 12 \text{mL/hr}$	1 mL : 13.33 mcg/min :: x mL : 160 mcg/min	$\frac{x \text{ mL}}{160 \text{ mg/min}} \times \frac{1 \text{ mL}}{13.33 \text{ mcg/min}}$

$$160 = 13.33x$$

$$\frac{160}{13.33} = 12 \text{ mL}$$

Set the pump: total number mL = 250 (standard solution); mL/hr = 12 mL/hr

Milliunits/min—Rule and Calculation

In obstetrics, a Pitocin (oxytocin) drip can initiate labor. The standard solution is 15 units in 250 mL. Because 1 unit = 1000 milliunits, you solve these problems in the same way as mcg/min.

Example

Order: Pitocin (oxytocin) drip 2 milliunits/min IV

Supply: infusion pump, standard solution 15 units in NS 250 mL

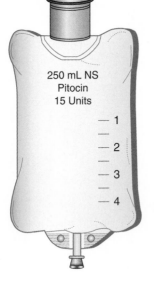

1. Reduce the numbers in the standard solution.

$$\frac{15 \text{ units}}{250 \text{ mL}} = 0.06 \text{ units/mL}$$

2. Change units of pitocin to milliunits.

1 unit = 1000 milliunits

0.06 x 1000 = 60 milliunits/mL

3. Divide by 60 to get milliunits/min.

$$\frac{60}{60} = 1 \text{ milliunit/min.}$$

4. Solve. Round to the nearest whole number.

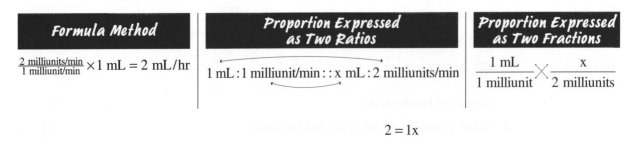

Formula Method	Proportion Expressed as Two Ratios	Proportion Expressed as Two Fractions
$\frac{2 \text{ milliunits/min}}{1 \text{ milliunit/min}} \times 1 \text{ mL} = 2 \text{ mL/hr}$	1 mL : 1 milliunit/min : : x mL : 2 milliunits/min	$\frac{1 \text{ mL}}{1 \text{ milliunit}} \times \frac{x}{2 \text{ milliunits}}$

$$2 = 1x$$
$$x = 2 \text{ mL/hr}$$

Set the pump: total number mL = 250 mL; mL/hr = 2 mL/hr

SELF-TEST 3 **Infusion Rates for Drugs Ordered in mcg/min, mcg/kg/min, milliunits/min**

Calculate the number of mL to infuse and the rate of infusion. Answers appear at the end of the chapter.

1. Order: Intropin (dopamine) double strength, 800 mcg/min IV
    Supply: standard solution 800 mg in 250 mL D5W, infusion pump

2. Order: Levophed (norepinephrine), 12 mcg/min IV
    Supply: standard solution of 4 mg in 250 mL D5W, infusion pump

3. Order: Dobutrex (dobutamine) 5 mcg/kg/min IV
    Supply: patient weight, 220 lb; standard solution of 1 g in 250 mL D5W, infusion pump

4. Order: Dobutrex (dobutamine) 7 mcg/kg/min IV
    Supply: patient weight, 70 kg; standard solution of 500 mg in 250 mL D5W, infusion pump

5. Order: nitroglycerin 10 mcg/min IV
    Supply: standard solution of 50 mg in 250 mL D5W, infusion pump

6. Order: Pitocin drip (oxytocin) 1 milliunit/min IV
    Supply: infusion pump, standard solution 15 units in 250 mL NS

7. Order: Isuprel (isoproterenol) titrated at 4 mcg/min IV
    Supply: infusion pump, solution 2 mg/in 250 mL D5W

8. Order: Brevibloc (esmolol) 50 mcg/kg/min IV
    Supply: infusion pump, 2.5 g in 250 mL D5W; weight, 58 kg

9. Order: Nipride (nitroprusside) 2 mcg/kg/min IV
    Supply: patient weight, 80 kg; nipride 50 mg in 250 mL D5W, infusion pump

10. Order: Inocor (amrinone) 200 mcg/min
    Supply: Inocor (amrinone) 0.1 g in 100 mL NS, infusion pump

Body Surface Nomogram

Antineoplastic drugs used in cancer chemotherapy have a narrow therapeutic range. Calculation of these drugs is based on BSA in square meters—a method considered more precise than mg/kg/body weight. Body surface area is the measured or calculated area of the body.

There are several mathematical formulas to calculate body surface area. One often used is:

$$\sqrt{\frac{weight\,(kg) \times height\,(cm)}{3600}} = BSA$$

Average BSA:

"Normal" BSA: 1.7 m².

Average BSA for men: 1.9 m²

Average BSA for women: 1.6 m²

You can estimate BSA by using a three-column chart called a nomogram (Fig. 9-2). Mark the patient's height in the first column, and the patient's weight in the third column. Then draw a line between these two marks. The point at which the line intersects the middle column indicates estimated body surface in meters squared. You'll use a different BSA chart for children, because of differences in growth (see Chapter 10).

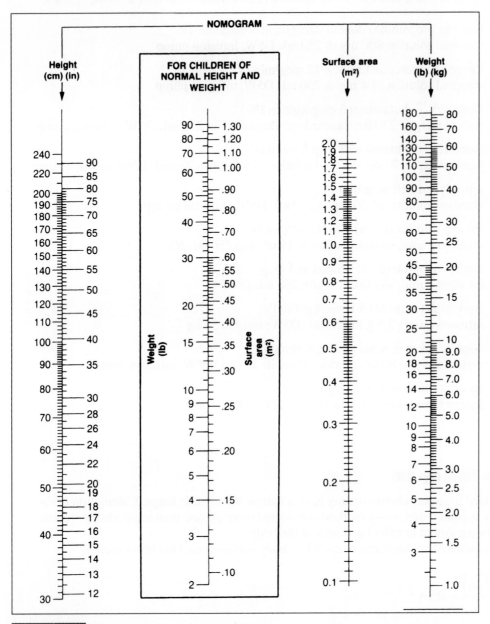

FIGURE 9-2

Body surface area (BSA) is critical when calculating dosages for pediatric patients or for drugs that are extremely potent and need to be given in precise amounts. The nomogram shown here lets you plot the patient's height and weight to determine the BSA. Here's how it works:

1. Locate the patient's height in the left column of the nomogram and the weight in the right column.

2. Use a ruler to draw a straight line connecting the two points. The point where the line intersects the surface area column indicates the patient's BSA in square meters.

3. For an average-sized child, use the simplified nomogram in the box. Just find the child's weight in pounds on the left side of the scale, and then read the corresponding BSA on the right side.

FIGURE 9-3

Portion of doctor's order form for chemotherapy. The doctor or health care provider writes the patient's height and weight and calculates the BSA as 2.1 m². The protocol dosage is the guide used to determine the patient's dose. For mitomycin, the protocol is 12 mg/m² × 2 m² = 24 mg. For 5FU, the protocol dose is 1000 mg/m² × 2 m² = 2000 mg.

DIAGNOSIS: Anal Cancer PROTOCOL NAME/NUMBER:

PATIENT'S HEIGHT: 6'2 cm WEIGHT: 186 Kg or BSA: 2.1 m²

VENOUS ACCESS: DEEP ☐ PERIPHERAL ☒

everyday

DRUG	PROTOCOL DOSAGE	PATIENTS DOSAGE	ROUTE AND DILUENT	FREQUENCY AND / OR DOSAGE	# OF DAYS
1. Mitomycin	12 mg/m²	24 mg	IVP × 1 m 9/08		
2. 5FU	1000 mg/m²	2000 mg	in 1000 mL of NS as a continuous infusion everyday × 4 days on 9/08, 9/09, 9/10, 9/11		
3.					

The oncologist, a physician who specializes in treating cancer, lists the patient's height, weight, and BSA; gives the protocol (drug requirement based on BSA in m²); and then gives the order.

Figure 9-3 shows a partial order sheet for chemotherapy. Both the pharmacist and the nurse validate the order before preparation.

To determine BSA in m², you can use a special calculator, obtained from companies manufacturing antineoplastics. Many websites also calculate BSA; see, for example, www.halls.md/body-surface-area/bsa.htm.

m²—Rule and Calculation

Oncology drugs are prepared by a pharmacist or specially trained technician who is gowned, gloved, and masked, and works under a laminar flow hood; these precautions protect the pharmacist or technician and also ensures sterility. When the medication reaches the unit, the nurse bears two responsibilities: checking the doses for accuracy before administration and using an infusion pump for IV orders.

Example

Hgt, 6′0″; wgt, 175 lb; BSA, 2.0 m²

Order: Platinol (cisplatin) 160 mg (80 mg/m²) IV in 1 L NS with 2 mg magnesium sulfate over 2 hr

1. Check the BSA using the nomogram in Figure 9-2. It is correct. Protocol calls for 80 mg/m²; 160 mg is correct.
2. The IV is prepared by the pharmacy. Determine the rate of infusion.
   1 L = 1000 mL

$$\frac{\text{number mL}}{\text{number hr}} = \text{mL/hr} \qquad \frac{\overset{500}{\cancel{1000}}}{\underset{1}{\cancel{2}}} = 500 \text{ mL/hr}$$

Set the pump: total number mL, 1000; mL/hr, 500

SELF-TEST 4 **Use of Nomogram**

Solve the following problems. Answers appear at the end of this chapter. Use the nomogram in Figure 9-2 to double-check the BSA.

1. Hgt, 6'0"; wt, 165 lb; BSA, 1.96 m^2
   Order: Doxil (doxorubicin) 39 mg (20 mg/m^2) in D5W 250 mL to infuse over ½ hr

   a. Is dose correct?
   b. How should the pump be set?

2. Hgt, 165 cm; wt, 70 kg; BSA, 1.77 m^2
   Order: Lomustine (CCNU) 230 mg po (130 mg/m^2) once q6 weeks

   a. Is dose correct?
   b. Lomustine (CCNU) comes in tabs of 100 mg and 10 mg. What is the dose?

3. Hgt, 6'2"; wt, 170 lb; BSA, 2.0 m^2
   Order: Cerubidine (daunorubicin) 80 mg (40 mg/m^2) in D5W over 1 hr IV
   Supply: IV bag labeled 80 mg in 80 mL D5W; infuse in rapidly flowing IV

   a. Is dose correct?
   b. How should the pump be set? (See IVPB administration in Chapter 8.)

4. Hgt, 65"; wt, 175 lb; BSA, 2.0 m^2
   Order: Vepesid (etoposide) 400 mg po every day × 3 (200 mg/m^2)
   Supply: capsules of 50 mg

   a. Is dose correct?
   b. How many capsules should be poured?

5. Hgt, 5'3"; wgt, 120 lb; BSA, 1.6 m^2
   Order: Taxol (paclitaxel) 216 mg (135 mg/m^2) in D5W ½ L glass bottle over 3 hr

   a. Is dose correct?
   b. How should the pump be set?

Patient-Controlled Analgesia (PCA)

PCA, an IV method of pain control, allows a patient to self-administer a preset dose of pain medication. The physician or healthcare provider prescribes the narcotic dose and concentration, the basal rate, the lockout time, and the total maximum hourly dose (Fig. 9-4).

Basal rate is the amount of medication that is infused continuously each hour. *PCA dose* is the amount of medication infused when the patient activates the button control. *Lockout time* or *delay*—a feature that prevents overdosage—is the interval during which the patient cannot initiate another dose after giving a self-dose. *Total hourly dose* is the maximum amount of medication the patient can receive in an hour. The physician or healthcare provider writes all this information on an order form.

Figure 9-5 shows a narcotic PCA medication record. Morphine concentration is 1 mg/mL. The pharmacy dispenses a 100-mL NS bag with 100 mL morphine. The patient continuously receives 0.5 mg by infusion pump and can give 1 mg by pressing the PCA button. Eight minutes must elapse before another PCA dose can be delivered. Note that at 12 noon, the nurse charted that the patient made three attempts but received only two injections. This indicates that 8 minutes had not elapsed before one of the attempts.

The nurse's responsibility is to assess the patient every hour, noting how the patient scores his or her pain, the number of PCA attempts, and the total hourly dose received, as well as the cumulative dose, the patient's level of consciousness, side effects, and respirations.

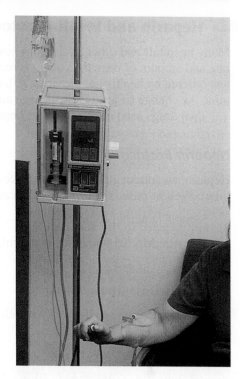

FIGURE 9-4

Patient-controlled analgesia allows the client to self-administer medication, as necessary, to control pain. (From Roach, S. S. [2004]. *Introductory clinical pharmacology* [7th ed.]. Philadelphia: Lippincott Williams & Wilkins, p. 173.)

AVERY MEDICAL CENTER
Narcotic PCA
Medication Administration Record

Check appropriate order: Dose: __1__ mg/mL
__X__ Morphine 1 mg/1 mL:50 mL   Lockout: __8__ min
____ Fentanyl. Concentration: ____ Volume: ____   1 hour limit: __8__ mg/mL
____ Demerol 10 mg/1 mL:50 mL   Basal _0.5_ mg/hr
____ Other: _____ Concentration ____ Volume: ____

Infusion started by: _____   RN
      (zero out prior shift volume with each new bag/syringe)
Settings confirmed by: _____   RN
Date/Time discoutinued: _____
Discontinued by: _____   RN
Total Amount Administered: _____
Waste returned to pharmacy: _____

Pharmacist: Witness: Witness:

Date	0600	0800	1000	1200	1400	1600
Number of attempts	3	2	2	3		
Number of injections	3	2	2	2		
Basal dose	0.5	0.5	0.5	0.5		
Total mL	3.5	4.5	4.5	2.5		
Cumulative mL	3.5	8	12.5	15		
Pain score	5	5	5	6		
Level of consciousness	1	1	1	1		
Respiratory rate (per minute)	16	20	16	22		
Nurse's initials	GP	GP	GP	GP		

Level of Consciousness: 1-alert, 2-drowsy, 3-sleeping, 4-confused, 5-difficult to arouse

Nurse's signature _____ Initial _____
Nurse's signature _____ Initial _____
Nurse's signature _____ Initial _____
Nurse's signature _____ Initial _____

FIGURE 9-5

Sample PCA medication record.

Heparin and Insulin Protocols

Many hospitals and other institutions now use protocols to give the nurse more freedom in determining the rate and amount of drug the patient is receiving. These protocols are based on a parameter, usually a lab test ordered by healthcare provider. After receiving the lab test results, the nurse uses the protocol to determine the change (if any) in the dosage amount.

Two drugs used in protocols are heparin and insulin.

Heparin Protocol

Heparin, an anticoagulant, is titrated according to the results of the lab test, PTT (partial thromboplastin time). Weight-based heparin protocol calculates the dose of heparin based on the patient's weight.

Sample heparin protocol:

Heparin drip: 25,000 units in 500 mL D5W

Bolus: 80 units/kg

Starting Dose: 18 units/kg/hr

Titrate according to the following chart:

PTT (seconds)	<45 seconds	45-48 seconds	49-66 seconds	67-70 seconds	71-109 seconds	110-130 seconds	>130 seconds
Bolus	Bolus with 40 units/kg	Bolus with 40 units/kg	No bolus	No bolus	No bolus	No bolus	No bolus
Rate adjustment	Increase rate by 3 units/kg/hr	Increase rate by 2 units/kg/hr	Increase rate by 1 unit/kg/hr	No change	No change	Decrease rate by 1 unit/kg/hr	Stop infusion for 1 hour. Decrease rate by 2 units/kg/hr
Next lab	PTT in 6 hours	PTT in 6 hours	PTT in 6 hours	PTT next AM	PTT next AM	PTT in 6 hours	PTT in 6 hours

Example

Example: patient weight is 70 kg.

1. Calculation for bolus dose: 80 units/kg

Multiply 80 units times 70 kg = 5600 units/kg.

2. Infusion rate

First calculate what the dose will be.

Starting dose is 18 units/kg/hr.

Multiply 18 times 70 kg = 1260 units/kg.

Now use the calculation similar to that on p. 238.

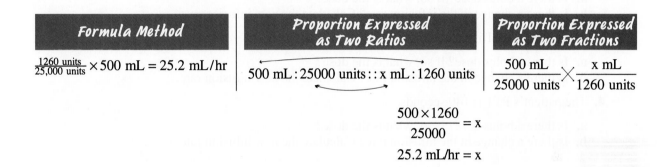

Formula Method	*Proportion Expressed as Two Ratios*	*Proportion Expressed as Two Fractions*
$\frac{1260 \text{ units}}{25{,}000 \text{ units}} \times 500 \text{ mL} = 25.2 \text{ mL/hr}$	$500 \text{ mL} : 25000 \text{ units} :: x \text{ mL} : 1260 \text{ units}$	$\frac{500 \text{ mL}}{25000 \text{ units}} \times \frac{x \text{ mL}}{1260 \text{ units}}$

$$\frac{500 \times 1260}{25000} = x$$

$$25.2 \text{ mL/hr} = x$$

Set the pump at 25 mL/hr.

3. The PTT result 6 hours after the infusion started is 50. According to the table, we increase the drip by 1 u/kg/hr.

First, calculate the dose.

1 unit times 70 kg = 70 units/kg

Then set up the same formula:

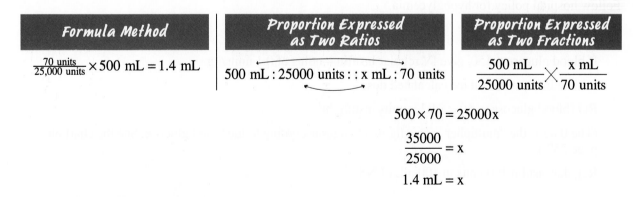

Formula Method	*Proportion Expressed as Two Ratios*	*Proportion Expressed as Two Fractions*
$\frac{70 \text{ units}}{25{,}000 \text{ units}} \times 500 \text{ mL} = 1.4 \text{ mL}$	$500 \text{ mL} : 25000 \text{ units} :: x \text{ mL} : 70 \text{ units}$	$\frac{500 \text{ mL}}{25000 \text{ units}} \times \frac{x \text{ mL}}{70 \text{ units}}$

$$500 \times 70 = 25000x$$

$$\frac{35000}{25000} = x$$

$$1.4 \text{ mL} = x$$

Increase the infusion rate by 1.4 mL

25.2 + 1.4 = 26.6 mL/hr. Set the pumps at 27 mL/hr.

Recheck the PTT in 6 hours, and titrate according to the result.

Use the chart on page 254 to solve the following problems. Use heparin 25,000 units in 500 mL as your IV solution. The patient's weight is 70 kg. Beginning infusion rate for each problem is 25.2 mL/hr. Answers appear at the end of the chapter.

1. The patient's PTT is 45 seconds.

   a. Is there a bolus dose? If so, what is the dose?
   b. Is there a change in the infusion rate? Calculate the new infusion rate.

2. The patient's PTT is 40 seconds.

   a. Is there a bolus dose? If so, what is the dose?
   b. Is there a change in the infusion rate? Calculate the new infusion rate.

3. The patient's PTT is 110 seconds.

   a. Is there a bolus dose? If so, what is the dose?
   b. Is there a change in the infusion rate? Calculate the new infusion rate.

4. The patient's PTT is 140 seconds.

   a. Is there a bolus dose? If so, what is the dose?
   b. Is there a change in the infusion rate? Calculate the new infusion rate.

Insulin Protocol (also called hypoglycemic protocol or hyperglycemic protocol)

Regular insulin can be given by continuous IV infusion. The rate is titrated according to the blood glucose. Several conditions must be considered before initiating an insulin protocol; for example, an elevated blood glucose, weight, and renal function. Always follow hospital or institutional policy regarding these variables. This section includes only the calculation of an insulin drip and the titration in infusion rate. (If the blood glucose falls below a certain level such as 70, the patient may need to receive an ampule of D50W. Follow hospital policy for hypoglycemia.)

Insulin protocol:

If blood glucose > 150, give IV regular insulin—bolus of 0.1 units/kg

Initiate infusion rate at the calculated dose:

BG (blood glucose) – 60 × 0.02 = units insulin/hr

(The 0.02 is the "multiplier." This figure changes according to the blood glucose. See the chart on page 257.)

Regular insulin 100 units in 100 mL of NS.

Example   Patient weight 70 kg. Blood glucose 200.

1. Calculate the bolus dose.

   0.1 units times 70 kg = 7 units of regular insulin IV

2. Calculate the infusion rate.

   (200 – 60) × 0.02 = 2.8 units

3. Now use the calculation similar to that on page 240.

Formula Method	Proportion Expressed as Two Ratios	Proportion Expressed as Two Fractions
$\frac{2.8 \text{ units}}{100 \text{ units}} \times 100 \text{ mL} = 2.8 \text{ mL/hr}$	$100 \text{ mL} : 100 \text{ units} :: x \text{ mL} : 2.8 \text{ units}$	$\frac{100 \text{ mL}}{100 \text{ units}} = \frac{x \text{ mL}}{2.8 \text{ units}}$

$$100 \text{ mL} \times 2.8 = 100x$$

$$2.8 \text{ mL} = x$$

Set the pump at 2.8 mL/hr or 3mL/hr.

Recheck the blood glucose in 1 hour and titrate.

Sample insulin protocol titration chart:

Blood Glucose Result	Rate/Multiplier Change
80-110	Continue same rate. No change in rate or multiplier.
>110 and <150	Continue same rate. Recheck blood glucose in 1 hour and if >110, increase multiplier by 0.01 and calculate new infusion rate.
>150	Increase multiplier by 0.01 and calculate new infusion rate.

SELF-TEST 6

Use regular insulin 100 units in 100 mL NS. Patient weight of 70 kg. Use initial formula: BG (blood glucose) − 60 × 0.02 = units insulin/hr. Use the above chart for changes.

1. Blood glucose is 300.

   a. What is the infusion rate?
   b. Is there a change in the formula? If so, what is the new formula?

2. Blood glucose is 350.

   a. Use the new formula from question 1b. What is the infusion rate?
   b. Is there a change in the formula? If so, what is the new formula?

3. Blood glucose is 140. Rechecked in 1 hour and remains 140.

   a. Use the new formula from question 2b. What is the infusion rate?
   b. Is there a change in the formula? If so, what is the new formula?

4. Blood glucose is 100.

   a. Use the new formula from question 3b. What is the infusion rate?
   b. Is there a change in the formula? If so, what is the new formula?

SELF-TEST 7 Infusion Problems

Solve these problems. Answers are given at the end of the chapter.

1. Order: start Normadyne (labetalol) 0.5 mg/min on pump
   Supply: infusion pump, standard solution of 200 mg in 200 mL D5W
   What is the pump setting?

2. Order: aminophylline 250 mg in 250 mL D5W at 75 mg/hr IV
   Supply: infusion pump, vial of aminophylline labeled 250 mg/10 mL

   a. How much drug is needed?
   b. What is the pump setting?

3. Order: Bretylol (bretylium) 2 g in 500 mL D5W at 4 mg/min IV
   Supply: infusion pump, standard solution of 2 g in 500 mL D5W
   What is the pump setting?

4. Order: Zovirax (acyclovir) 400 mg in 100 mL D5W over 2 hr
   Supply: infusion pump, 500-mg vials of Zovirax (acyclovir) with 10 mL diluent; makes
               50 mg/mL

   a. How much drug is needed?
   b. What is the pump setting?

5. Order: Abbokinase (urokinase) 5000 units/hr over 5 hr IV
   Supply: infusion pump, vials of 5000 units
   Directions: Dissolve Abbokinase (urokinase) in 1 mL sterile water. Add to 250 mL D5W.

   a. How much drug is needed?
   b. What is the pump setting?

6. Order: Magnesium Sulfate 4 g in 100 mL D5W to infuse over 30 min IV
   Supply: infusion pump, 50% solution of Magnesium Sulfate

   a. How much drug is needed?
   b. What is the pump setting?

7. Order: nitroglycerin 80 mcg/min IV
   Supply: infusion pump, standard solution of 50 mg in 250 mL D5W
   What is the pump setting?

8. Order: Dobutrex (dobutamine) 6 mcg/kg/min IV
   Supply: infusion pump, solution 500 mg/250 mL D5W; weight, 180 lb
   Change pounds to kilograms. What is the pump setting?

9. Order: Pitocin (oxytocin) 2 milliunits/min IV
   Supply: infusion pump, solution of 9 units in 150 mL NS
   What is the pump setting?

10. Hgt, 60″; wt, 110 lb; BSA, 1.55 m^2
    Order: Platinol (cisplatin) 124 mg (80 mg/m^2) in 1 L NS to infuse over 4 hr

    a. Is dose correct?
    b. How should the pump be set?

CRITICAL THINKING: TEST YOUR CLINICAL SAVVY

A 65-year-old NIDDM patient with a 10-year history of congestive heart failure is admitted to the intensive care unit with chest pain of more than 24 hours. The patient is receiving heparin, insulin, calcium gluconate, and potassium chloride, all intravenously.

a. Why would an infusion pump be needed with these medications?
b. Why would medications that are based on body weight require the use of a pump? Why would medications based on BSA require an infusion pump?
c. Can any of these medications be regulated with standard roller clamp tubing? What would be the advantage? What would be the contraindication?
d. What other information would you need to calculate the drip rates of these medications?
e. Why would it be necessary to calculate how long each infusion will last?

Putting it Together

Mrs. R is a 79 year old female with dyspnea without chest pain, fever, chills or sweats. No evidence for bleeding. Admitted through the ER with BP 82/60, afebrile, Sinus Tachycardia at 110/minute. She underwent emergency dialysis and developed worsening dyspnea and was transferred to the ICU. BP on admission to ICU was 70/30, tachypneic on 100% nonrebreather mask. No c/o chest discomfort or abdominal pain. Dyspnea worsened and patient became bradycardic and agonal respirations developed. A Code Blue was called and the patient was resuscitated after intubation. Spontaneous pulse and atrial fibrillation was noted.

Past Medical History: cardiomegaly, severe cardiomyopathy, chronic atrial fibrillation, unstable angina, hypertension, chronic kidney disease with hemodialysis, TIA in 3/07.

Allergies: calcium channel blockers

Current Vital Signs: pulse 150/minute, blood pressure is 90/40, RR 18 via the ventilator. Afebrile. Weight: 90 kg

Medication Orders

Zosyn (piperacillin/tazobactam) *antibiotic* 0.75 G IV in 50 mL q 8h
Protonix (pantoprazole) *antiulcer* 40 mg IV q 12 h. dilute in 10 mL NS and give slow IV push.
Neo-Synephrine (phenylephrine) *vasopressor* drip 30 mg in 500 mL D5W
   100 mcg/min titrate for SBP > 90
Levophed (norepinephrine) *vasopressor* in 4 mg in 500 mL D5W
   Titrate SBP >90 start at 0.5 mcg/min
½ NS 1000 mL at 150 mL/hr
Heparin (*anticoagulant*) 12 units/kg/hr. no loading dose. IV solution 25000 units in 500 mL D5W
   Titrate to keep PTT 49-70
Aspirin (*antiplatelet*) 81 mg PO/N/G daily
Lanoxin (digoxin) *cardiac glycoside* 0.25 mg IV daily
Diprivan (propofol) *sedative* 10 mg/mL
   Titrate 5-50 mcg/kg/min for sedation

(continued)

Putting it Together

Calculations

1. Calculate how many mcg/mL of Neo-synephrine.

2. Calculate the rate on the infusion pump of Neo-synephrine 100 mcg/min.

3. Calculate how many mcg/mL of Levophed.

4. Calculate the rate on the infusion pump of Levophed 0.5 mcg/min.

5. Calculate the dose of heparin.

6. Calculate the rate on the infusion pump of the heparin dose. When is the next PTT due?

7. Diprivan is mixed in 100 mL. How many mg are mixed to equal 10 mg/mL?

8. Calculate the rate on the infusion pump of Diprivan-calculate using the range 5–50 mcg/kg/min.

Critical Thinking Questions

1. Do any of the patient's medical conditions warrant changes in the medication orders?

2. Why would two vasopressors be given together?

3. What is the reason for giving the patient Diprivan?

4. What medication may help atrial fibrillation yet be contraindicated in this patient?

5. What is a possible reason for the sinus tachycardia of 150/minute?

6. What is the reason for giving a drug slow IV push, such as the Protonix?

Answers in Appendix B.

PROFICIENCY TEST 1 **Special IV Calculations**

Name: _____

Solve these problems. Answers are given in Appendix A.

1. Order: regular insulin 15 units/hr IV
    Supply: infusion pump, standard solution 125 units in 250 mL NS
    What is the pump setting?

2. Order: heparin sodium 1500 units/hr IV
    Supply: infusion pump, standard solution 25,000 units in 500 mL D5W IV
    What is the pump setting?

3. Order: Bretylol (bretylium) 2 g in 500 mL D5W at 2 mg/min IV
    Supply: infusion pump, standard solution of 2 g in 500 mL D5W
    What is the pump setting?

4. Order: Cardizem (diltiazem) 125 mg in 100 mL D5W at 5 mg/hr IV
    Supply: infusion pump, vial of Cardizem (diltiazem) labeled 5 mg/mL

    a. What is the pump setting?
    b. How much drug is needed?

5. Order: lidocaine 4 mg/min IV
    Supply: infusion pump, standard solution of 2 g in 500 mL D5W
    What is the pump setting?

6. Order: KCl 40 mEq/L at 10 mEq/hr IV
    Supply: infusion pump, vial of KCl labeled 20 mEq/10 mL in D5W 1000 mL

    a. How much KCl should be added?
    b. What is the pump setting?

7. Order: Pronestyl (procainamide) 1 mg/min IV
    Supply: infusion pump, standard solution of 2 g in 500 mL D5W
    What is the pump setting?

8. Order: Fungizone (amphotericin) B 50 mg in 500 mL D5W over 6 hr IV
    Supply: infusion pump, vial of 50 mg

    a. How should the drug be added to the IV?
    b. What is the pump setting?

9. Order: Pitressin (vasopressin) 18 units/hr IV, solution 200 units in 500 mL D5W
    Supply: infusion pump, vial of Pitressin (vasopressin) labeled 20 units/mL

    a. How much drug is needed?
    b. What is the pump setting?

10. Order: Dobutrex (dobutamine) 250 mcg/min IV
    Supply: infusion pump, solution of 500 mg in 500 mL D5W
    What is the pump setting?

11. Order: renal dose Intropin (dopamine) 2.5 mcg/kg/min
    Supply: infusion pump, solution 400 mg in 250 mL D5W; wgt, 60 kg
    What is the pump setting?

(continued)

12. Order: Pitocin (oxytocin) 2 milliunits/min IV
    Supply: infusion pump, solution of 9 units in 150 mL NS
    What is the pump setting?

13. Hgt, 5′3″; wgt, 143 lb; BSA, 1.7 m²
    Order: Ara-C 170 mg (100 mg/m²) in 1 L D5W over 24 hr

    a. Is dose correct?
    b. How should the pump be set?

14. Order: Nipride (nitroprusside) 5 mcg/kg/mm IV
    Supply: patient weight = 90 kg; Nipride (nitroprusside) 50 mg in 250 mL D5W, infusion
                 pump
    What is the pump setting?

15. Order: epinephrine 2 mcg/min
    Supply: epinephrine 4 mg in 250 mL D5W, infusion pump
    What is the pump setting?

16. Patient's PTT is 45 seconds. Use the heparin protocol chart on page 254. Patient's weight is
    90 kg. Heparin 25,000 units in 500 mL. Rate is currently 32 mL/hr.

    a. Is there a bolus dose? If so, what is the dose?
    b. Is there a change in the infusion rate? Calculate the new infusion rate.

17. Patient's PTT is 40 seconds. Use the heparin protocol chart on page 254. Patient's weight is
    90 kg. Heparin 25,000 units in 500 mL. Rate is currently 32 mL/hr.

    a. Is there a bolus dose? If so, what is the dose?
    b. Is there a change in the infusion rate? Calculate the new infusion rate.

18. Patient's PTT is 110 seconds. Use the heparin protocol chart on page 254. Patient's weight is
    90 kg. Heparin 25,000 units in 500 mL. Rate is currently 32 mL/hr.

    a. Is there a bolus dose? If so, what is the dose?
    b. Is there a change in the infusion rate? Calculate the new infusion rate.

19. Use regular insulin 100 units in 100 mL NS. Patient weight of 70 kg. BG (blood glucose)
    $- 60 \times 0.02 =$ units insulin/hr. Use the insulin protocol chart on p. 257 for changes.

    Patient's blood glucose is 120. Repeat blood glucose in 1 hour is 125.

    a. What is the infusion rate?
    b. Is there a change in the formula? If so, what is the new formula?

20. Use regular insulin 100 units in 100 mL NS. Patient weight of 70 kg. BG (blood glucose)
    $- 60 \times 0.02 =$ units insulin/hr. Use the chart on p. 257 for changes.

    a. What is the infusion rate?
    b. Is there a change in the formula? If so, what is the new formula?

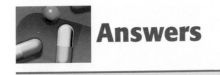

Answers

Self-Test 1 Infusion Rates

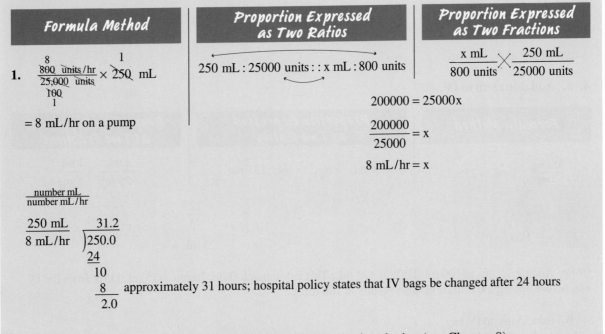

Formula Method	Proportion Expressed as Two Ratios	Proportion Expressed as Two Fractions

1. $\dfrac{\overset{8}{\cancel{800}}\ \text{units/hr}}{\underset{\underset{1}{100}}{\cancel{25,000}}\ \text{units}} \times \overset{1}{\cancel{250}}\ \text{mL}$

$250\ \text{mL} : 25000\ \text{units} :: x\ \text{mL} : 800\ \text{units}$

$\dfrac{x\ \text{mL}}{800\ \text{units}} \times \dfrac{250\ \text{mL}}{25000\ \text{units}}$

$= 8\ \text{mL/hr on a pump}$

$200000 = 25000x$

$\dfrac{200000}{25000} = x$

$8\ \text{mL/hr} = x$

$\dfrac{\text{number mL}}{\text{number mL/hr}}$

$\dfrac{250\ \text{mL}}{8\ \text{mL/hr}}$

$\begin{array}{r} 31.2 \\ 8\,\overline{)250.0} \\ \underline{24} \\ 10 \\ \underline{8} \\ 2.0 \end{array}$ approximately 31 hours; hospital policy states that IV bags be changed after 24 hours

2. Add 500 mg acyclovir to 100 mL D5W using a reconstitution device (see Chapter 8).

$\dfrac{\text{number mL}}{\text{number hr}} = \text{mL/hr}$

$\dfrac{100\ \text{mL}}{1\ \text{hr}}$ No math is necessary. Set the pump at 100 mL/hr.

3. a. Add amicar to IV.

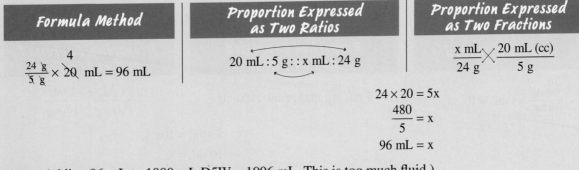

Formula Method	Proportion Expressed as Two Ratios	Proportion Expressed as Two Fractions

$\dfrac{24\ \cancel{g}}{\underset{1}{\cancel{5}}\ \cancel{g}} \times \overset{4}{\cancel{20}}\ \text{mL} = 96\ \text{mL}$

$20\ \text{mL} : 5\ \text{g} :: x\ \text{mL} : 24\ \text{g}$

$\dfrac{x\ \text{mL}}{24\ \text{g}} \times \dfrac{20\ \text{mL (cc)}}{5\ \text{g}}$

$24 \times 20 = 5x$

$\dfrac{480}{5} = x$

$96\ \text{mL} = x$

(*Note:* Adding 96 mL to 1000 mL D5W = 1096 mL. This is too much fluid.)

Use five vials. Empty four completely.
Take 16 mL from the last vial.
20 mL × 4 vials = 80 mL + 16 mL = 96 mL
Remove 96 mL D5W from the IV bag before adding the amicar. This results in 1000 mL.

b. $\dfrac{\text{number mL}}{\text{number hr}} = \text{mL/hr}$

$$\dfrac{1000 \text{ mL}}{24 \text{ hr}} \quad 24 \overline{\smash{\big)}\,1000.0} \quad \begin{array}{r} 41.6 \\ \end{array}$$

$$\begin{array}{r} \underline{96} \\ 40 \\ \underline{24} \\ 16.0 \\ \underline{14.4} \end{array}$$

Set pump at 42 mL/hr.

4. a. Add diltiazem to IV.

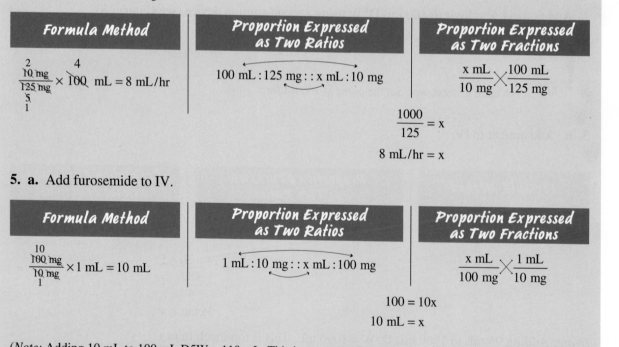

Formula Method	Proportion Expressed as Two Ratios	Proportion Expressed as Two Fractions
$\dfrac{\overset{25}{\cancel{125}\text{ mg}}}{\cancel{5}\text{ mg}} \times 1 \text{ mL} = 25 \text{ mL}$	$1 \text{ mL} : 5 \text{ mg} :: x \text{ mL} : 125 \text{ mg}$	$\dfrac{x \text{ mL}}{125 \text{ mg}} \times \dfrac{1 \text{ mL}}{5 \text{ mg}}$

$$\dfrac{125}{5} = x$$

$$25 \text{ mL} = x$$

(*Note:* Adding 25 mL to 100 mL D5W = 125 mL. This is too much fluid. Remove 25 mL D5W from the IV bag before adding the diltiazem. This results in 100 mL.)

b. Add 25 mL to IV bag.

Formula Method	Proportion Expressed as Two Ratios	Proportion Expressed as Two Fractions
$\dfrac{\overset{2}{\cancel{10}\text{ mg}}}{\underset{1}{\cancel{\underset{5}{125}\text{ mg}}}} \times \overset{4}{\cancel{100}} \text{ mL} = 8 \text{ mL/hr}$	$100 \text{ mL} : 125 \text{ mg} :: x \text{ mL} : 10 \text{ mg}$	$\dfrac{x \text{ mL}}{10 \text{ mg}} \times \dfrac{100 \text{ mL}}{125 \text{ mg}}$

$$\dfrac{1000}{125} = x$$

$$8 \text{ mL/hr} = x$$

5. a. Add furosemide to IV.

Formula Method	Proportion Expressed as Two Ratios	Proportion Expressed as Two Fractions
$\dfrac{\overset{10}{\cancel{100}\text{ mg}}}{\underset{1}{\cancel{10}\text{ mg}}} \times 1 \text{ mL} = 10 \text{ mL}$	$1 \text{ mL} : 10 \text{ mg} :: x \text{ mL} : 100 \text{ mg}$	$\dfrac{x \text{ mL}}{100 \text{ mg}} \times \dfrac{1 \text{ mL}}{10 \text{ mg}}$

$$100 = 10x$$

$$10 \text{ mL} = x$$

(*Note:* Adding 10 mL to 100 mL D5W = 110 mL. This is too much fluid. Remove 10 mL D5W from the IV bag before adding the furosemide. This results in 100 mL.)

Add 10 mL to the IV bag.

b. Because the solution is 100 mg/100 mL (1:1) and the order reads 4 mg/hr, the pump should be set at 4 mL/hr.

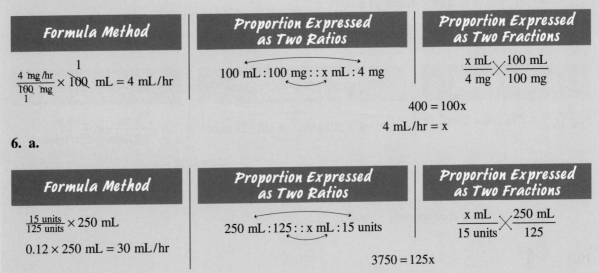

Formula Method	Proportion Expressed as Two Ratios	Proportion Expressed as Two Fractions
$\frac{4 \ \cancel{mg}/hr}{\underset{1}{\cancel{100} \ \cancel{mg}}} \times \overset{1}{\cancel{100}} \ mL = 4 \ mL/hr$	$100 \ mL : 100 \ mg :: x \ mL : 4 \ mg$	$\frac{x \ mL}{4 \ mg} \times \frac{100 \ mL}{100 \ mg}$
		$400 = 100x$
		$4 \ mL/hr = x$

6. a.

Formula Method	Proportion Expressed as Two Ratios	Proportion Expressed as Two Fractions
$\frac{15 \ units}{125 \ units} \times 250 \ mL$ $0.12 \times 250 \ mL = 30 \ mL/hr$	$250 \ mL : 125 :: x \ mL : 15 \ units$	$\frac{x \ mL}{15 \ units} \times \frac{250 \ mL}{125}$
		$3750 = 125x$
		$30 \ mL/hr = x$

b. The total volume of medication is 125 units and the client receives 15 units/hr.

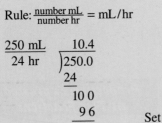

$$\frac{125}{15} \quad \overset{8.33}{\overline{)125.00}} = \text{approximately 8 hours}$$
$$\underline{120}$$
$$5.0$$
$$\underline{4.5}$$
$$50$$

7. Nitroglycerin is prepared by the pharmacy as a standard solution of 50 mg in 250 mL/hr. We only need to calculate mL/hr.

Rule: $\frac{\text{number mL}}{\text{number hr}} = mL/hr$

$$\frac{250 \ mL}{24 \ hr} \quad \overset{10.4}{\overline{)250.0}}$$
$$\underline{24}$$
$$10 \ 0$$
$$\underline{9 \ 6}$$

Set pump at 10 mL/hr.

8. a.

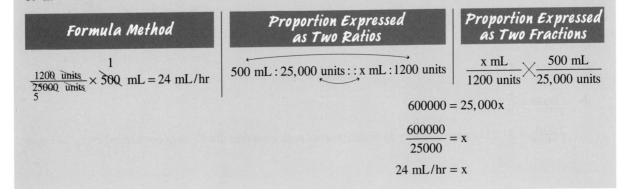

Formula Method	Proportion Expressed as Two Ratios	Proportion Expressed as Two Fractions
$\frac{1200 \ \cancel{units}}{\underset{5}{\cancel{25000} \ \cancel{units}}} \times \overset{1}{\cancel{500}} \ mL = 24 \ mL/hr$	$500 \ mL : 25,000 \ units :: x \ mL : 1200 \ units$	$\frac{x \ mL}{1200 \ units} \times \frac{500 \ mL}{25,000 \ units}$
		$600000 = 25,000x$
		$\frac{600000}{25000} = x$
		$24 \ mL/hr = x$

b. Rule: $\frac{\text{number mL}}{\text{number mL/hr}}$

$\frac{500 \text{ mL}}{24 \text{ mL/hr}} = 20.8$ or approximately 21 hours

9. a.

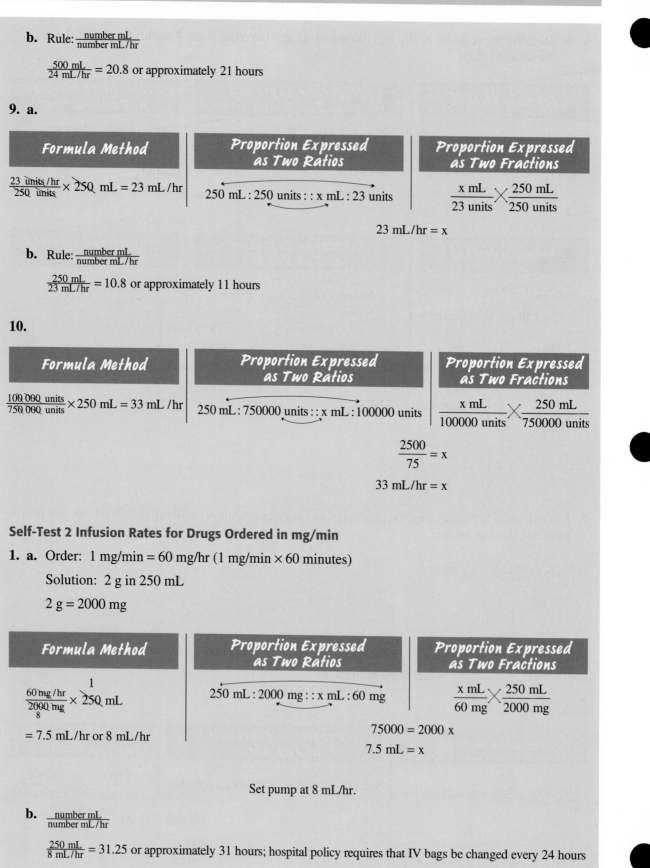

Formula Method	Proportion Expressed as Two Ratios	Proportion Expressed as Two Fractions
$\frac{23 \text{ units/hr}}{250 \text{ units}} \times 250 \text{ mL} = 23 \text{ mL/hr}$	250 mL : 250 units : : x mL : 23 units	$\frac{x \text{ mL}}{23 \text{ units}} \times \frac{250 \text{ mL}}{250 \text{ units}}$

23 mL/hr = x

b. Rule: $\frac{\text{number mL}}{\text{number mL/hr}}$

$\frac{250 \text{ mL}}{23 \text{ mL/hr}} = 10.8$ or approximately 11 hours

10.

Formula Method	Proportion Expressed as Two Ratios	Proportion Expressed as Two Fractions
$\frac{100,000 \text{ units}}{750,000 \text{ units}} \times 250 \text{ mL} = 33 \text{ mL/hr}$	250 mL : 750000 units : : x mL : 100000 units	$\frac{x \text{ mL}}{100000 \text{ units}} \times \frac{250 \text{ mL}}{750000 \text{ units}}$

$\frac{2500}{75} = x$

33 mL/hr = x

Self-Test 2 Infusion Rates for Drugs Ordered in mg/min

1. a. Order: 1 mg/min = 60 mg/hr (1 mg/min × 60 minutes)

Solution: 2 g in 250 mL

2 g = 2000 mg

Formula Method	Proportion Expressed as Two Ratios	Proportion Expressed as Two Fractions
$\frac{60 \text{ mg/hr}}{\underset{8}{2000 \text{ mg}}} \times \overset{1}{250} \text{ mL}$	250 mL : 2000 mg : : x mL : 60 mg	$\frac{x \text{ mL}}{60 \text{ mg}} \times \frac{250 \text{ mL}}{2000 \text{ mg}}$
= 7.5 mL/hr or 8 mL/hr		

75000 = 2000 x

7.5 mL = x

Set pump at 8 mL/hr.

b. $\frac{\text{number mL}}{\text{number mL/hr}}$

$\frac{250 \text{ mL}}{8 \text{ mL/hr}} = 31.25$ or approximately 31 hours; hospital policy requires that IV bags be changed every 24 hours

2. a. Order: 3 mg/min = 180 mg/hr (3 mg/min × 60 minutes)

   Solution: 1 g in 250 mL

   1 g = 1000 mg

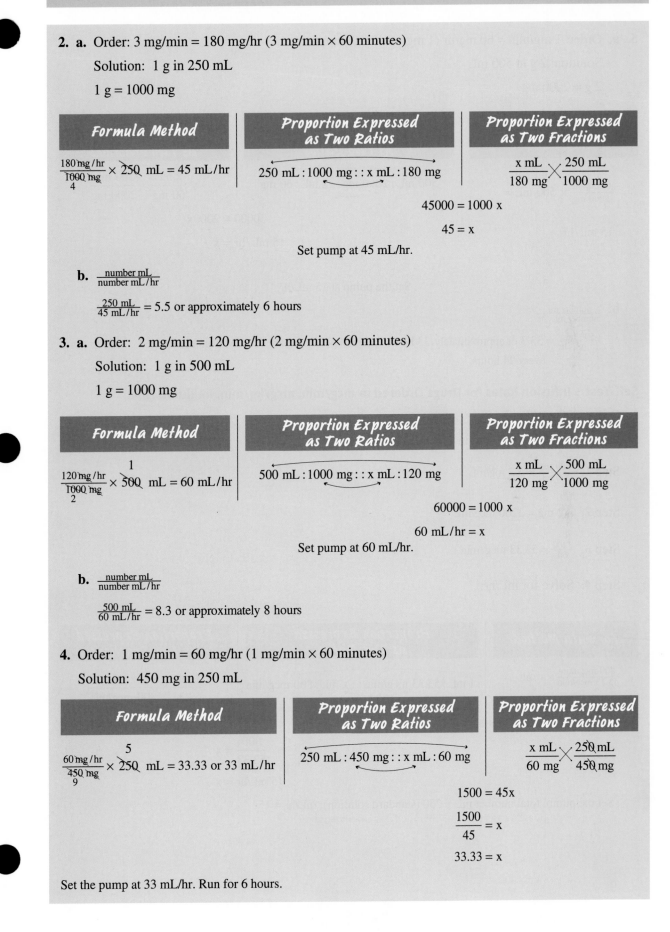

Formula Method	Proportion Expressed as Two Ratios	Proportion Expressed as Two Fractions
$\dfrac{180 \text{ mg/hr}}{\underset{4}{1000 \text{ mg}}} \times \overset{}{250} \text{ mL} = 45 \text{ mL/hr}$	250 mL : 1000 mg : : x mL : 180 mg	$\dfrac{\text{x mL}}{180 \text{ mg}} \times \dfrac{250 \text{ mL}}{1000 \text{ mg}}$

45000 = 1000 x

45 = x

Set pump at 45 mL/hr.

b. $\dfrac{\text{number mL}}{\text{number mL/hr}}$

   $\dfrac{250 \text{ mL}}{45 \text{ mL/hr}} = 5.5$ or approximately 6 hours

3. a. Order: 2 mg/min = 120 mg/hr (2 mg/min × 60 minutes)

   Solution: 1 g in 500 mL

   1 g = 1000 mg

Formula Method	Proportion Expressed as Two Ratios	Proportion Expressed as Two Fractions
$\dfrac{120 \text{ mg/hr}}{\underset{2}{1000 \text{ mg}}} \times \overset{1}{500} \text{ mL} = 60 \text{ mL/hr}$	500 mL : 1000 mg : : x mL : 120 mg	$\dfrac{\text{x mL}}{120 \text{ mg}} \times \dfrac{500 \text{ mL}}{1000 \text{ mg}}$

60000 = 1000 x

60 mL/hr = x

Set pump at 60 mL/hr.

b. $\dfrac{\text{number mL}}{\text{number mL/hr}}$

   $\dfrac{500 \text{ mL}}{60 \text{ mL/hr}} = 8.3$ or approximately 8 hours

4. Order: 1 mg/min = 60 mg/hr (1 mg/min × 60 minutes)

   Solution: 450 mg in 250 mL

Formula Method	Proportion Expressed as Two Ratios	Proportion Expressed as Two Fractions
$\dfrac{60 \text{ mg/hr}}{\underset{9}{450 \text{ mg}}} \times \overset{5}{250} \text{ mL} = 33.33 \text{ or } 33 \text{ mL/hr}$	250 mL : 450 mg : : x mL : 60 mg	$\dfrac{\text{x mL}}{60 \text{ mg}} \times \dfrac{250 \text{ mL}}{450 \text{ mg}}$

1500 = 45x

$\dfrac{1500}{45} = x$

33.33 = x

Set the pump at 33 mL/hr. Run for 6 hours.

5. a. Order: 1 mg/min = 60 mg/hr (1 mg/min × 60 minutes)

Solution: 2 g in 500 mL

2 g = 2000 mg

Formula Method	Proportion Expressed as Two Ratios	Proportion Expressed as Two Fractions
$\frac{60 \text{ mg/hr}}{\underset{4}{\cancel{2000}} \text{ mg}} \times \overset{1}{\cancel{500}} \text{ mL} =$ 15 mL/hr	500 mL : 2000 mg : : x mL : 60 mg	$\frac{x \text{ mL}}{60 \text{ mg}} \times \frac{500 \text{ mL}}{2000 \text{ mg}}$ $30000 = 2000x$ $15 \text{ mL/hr} = x$

Set the pump at 15 mL/hr.

b. $\frac{\text{number mL}}{\text{number mL/hr}}$

$\frac{500 \text{ mL}}{15 \text{ mL/hr}}$ = 33.3 or approximately 33 hours; hospital policy requires that IV bags be changed every 24 hours

Self-Test 3 Infusion Rates for Drugs Ordered in mcg/min, mcg/kg/min, milliunits/min

1. Order: 800 mcg/min

Standard solution: 800 mg in 250 mL D5W

Step 1. $\frac{800 \text{ mg}}{250 \text{ mL}}$ = 3.2 mg/mL

Step 2. 3.2 mg = 3200 mcg/mL

Step 3. $\frac{3200}{60}$ = 53.33 mcg/min

Step 4. Solve for mL/hr:

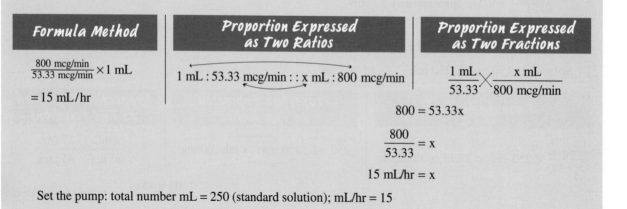

Formula Method	Proportion Expressed as Two Ratios	Proportion Expressed as Two Fractions
$\frac{800 \text{ mcg/min}}{53.33 \text{ mcg/min}} \times 1 \text{ mL}$ = 15 mL/hr	1 mL : 53.33 mcg/min : : x mL : 800 mcg/min	$\frac{1 \text{ mL}}{53.33} \times \frac{x \text{ mL}}{800 \text{ mcg/min}}$ $800 = 53.33x$ $\frac{800}{53.33} = x$ $15 \text{ mL/hr} = x$

Set the pump: total number mL = 250 (standard solution); mL/hr = 15

2. Order: 12 mcg/min

Standard solution: 4 mg in 250 mL D5W

Step 1. $\frac{4 \text{ mg}}{250 \text{ mL}} = 0.016$ mg/mL

Step 2. 0.016 mg = 16 mcg/mL

Step 3. $\frac{16 \text{ mcg}}{60 \text{ min}} = 0.27$ mcg/min

Step 4. Solve for mL/hr:

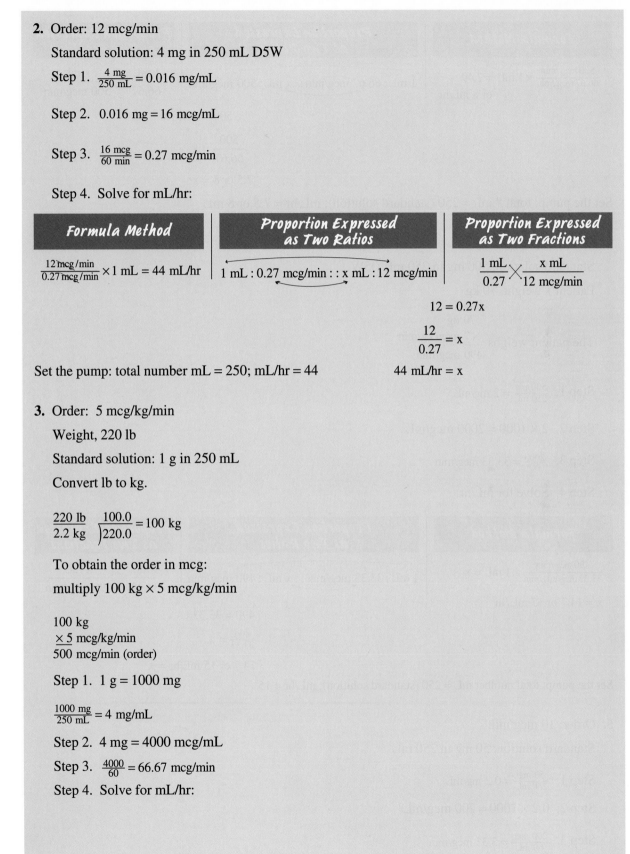

Formula Method	Proportion Expressed as Two Ratios	Proportion Expressed as Two Fractions
$\frac{12 \text{ mcg/min}}{0.27 \text{ mcg/min}} \times 1 \text{ mL} = 44 \text{ mL/hr}$	1 mL : 0.27 mcg/min : : x mL : 12 mcg/min	$\frac{1 \text{ mL}}{0.27} \times \frac{x \text{ mL}}{12 \text{ mcg/min}}$

$$12 = 0.27x$$

$$\frac{12}{0.27} = x$$

Set the pump: total number mL = 250; mL/hr = 44   44 mL/hr = x

3. Order: 5 mcg/kg/min

Weight, 220 lb

Standard solution: 1 g in 250 mL

Convert lb to kg.

$$\frac{220 \text{ lb}}{2.2 \text{ kg}} \quad 2.2 \overline{)\begin{array}{c} 100.0 \\ 220.0 \end{array}} = 100 \text{ kg}$$

To obtain the order in mcg:

multiply 100 kg × 5 mcg/kg/min

100 kg
× 5 mcg/kg/min
500 mcg/min (order)

Step 1. 1 g = 1000 mg

$\frac{1000 \text{ mg}}{250 \text{ mL}} = 4$ mg/mL

Step 2. 4 mg = 4000 mcg/mL

Step 3. $\frac{4000}{60} = 66.67$ mcg/min

Step 4. Solve for mL/hr:

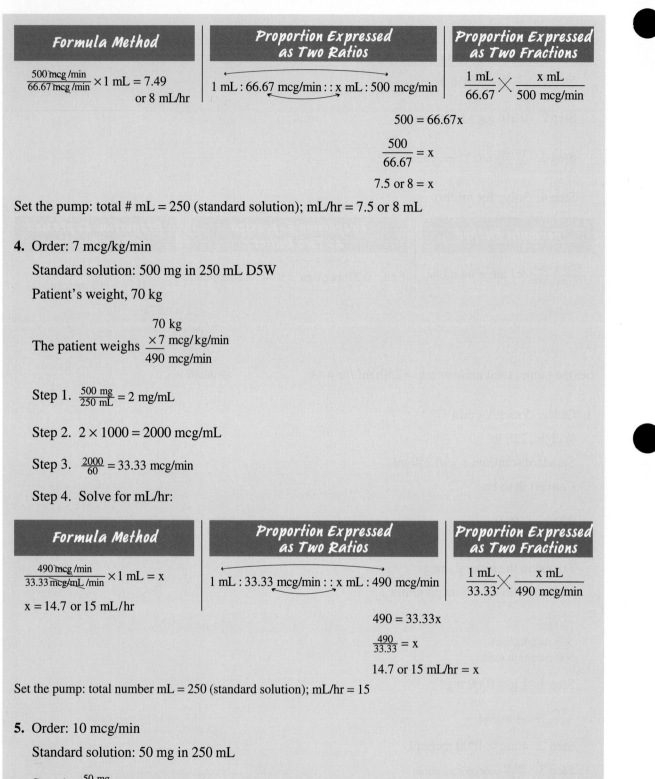

Formula Method	Proportion Expressed as Two Ratios	Proportion Expressed as Two Fractions
$\frac{500\text{ mcg/min}}{66.67\text{ mcg/min}} \times 1 \text{ mL} = 7.49$ or 8 mL/hr	1 mL : 66.67 mcg/min : : x mL : 500 mcg/min	$\frac{1 \text{ mL}}{66.67} \times \frac{\text{x mL}}{500 \text{ mcg/min}}$

$$500 = 66.67x$$

$$\frac{500}{66.67} = x$$

$$7.5 \text{ or } 8 = x$$

Set the pump: total # mL = 250 (standard solution); mL/hr = 7.5 or 8 mL

4. Order: 7 mcg/kg/min

Standard solution: 500 mg in 250 mL D5W

Patient's weight, 70 kg

The patient weighs $\begin{array}{r} 70 \text{ kg} \\ \times 7 \text{ mcg/kg/min} \\ \hline 490 \text{ mcg/min} \end{array}$

Step 1. $\frac{500 \text{ mg}}{250 \text{ mL}} = 2 \text{ mg/mL}$

Step 2. $2 \times 1000 = 2000 \text{ mcg/mL}$

Step 3. $\frac{2000}{60} = 33.33 \text{ mcg/min}$

Step 4. Solve for mL/hr:

Formula Method	Proportion Expressed as Two Ratios	Proportion Expressed as Two Fractions
$\frac{490\text{ mcg/min}}{33.33\text{ mcg/mL/min}} \times 1 \text{ mL} = x$ $x = 14.7$ or 15 mL/hr	1 mL : 33.33 mcg/min : : x mL : 490 mcg/min	$\frac{1 \text{ mL}}{33.33} \times \frac{\text{x mL}}{490 \text{ mcg/min}}$

$$490 = 33.33x$$

$$\frac{490}{33.33} = x$$

$$14.7 \text{ or } 15 \text{ mL/hr} = x$$

Set the pump: total number mL = 250 (standard solution); mL/hr = 15

5. Order: 10 mcg/min

Standard solution: 50 mg in 250 mL

Step 1. $\frac{50 \text{ mg}}{250 \text{ mL}} = 0.2 \text{ mg/mL}$

Step 2. $0.2 \times 1000 = 200 \text{ mcg/mL}$

Step 3. $\frac{200 \text{ mcg}}{60 \text{ mL}} = 3.33 \text{ mcg/min}$

Step 4. Solve for mL/hr:

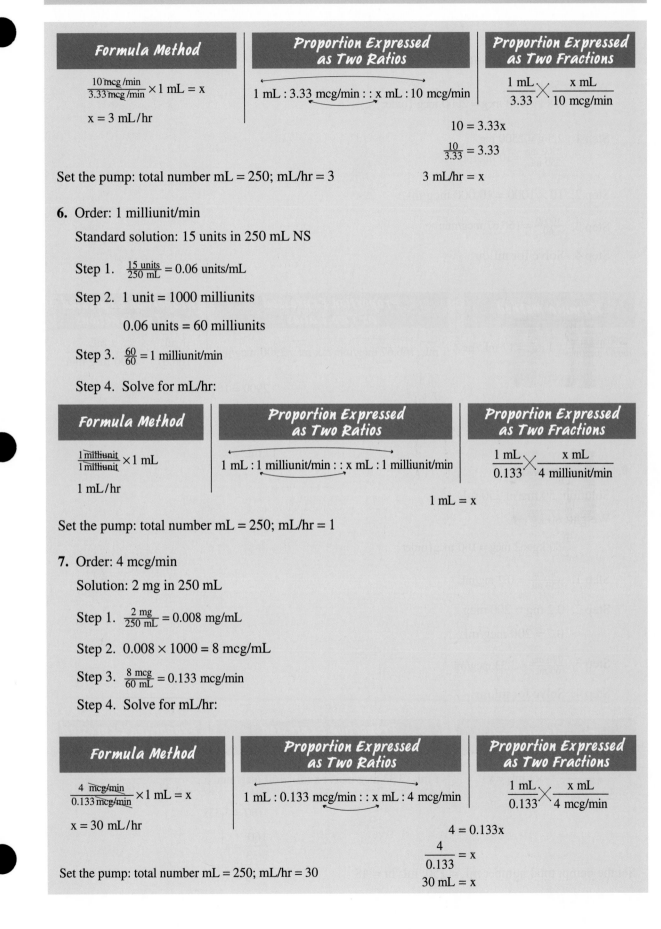

Formula Method	Proportion Expressed as Two Ratios	Proportion Expressed as Two Fractions
$\frac{10 \text{ mcg/min}}{3.33 \text{ mcg/min}} \times 1 \text{ mL} = x$ $x = 3 \text{ mL/hr}$	1 mL : 3.33 mcg/min : : x mL : 10 mcg/min	$\frac{1 \text{ mL}}{3.33} \times \frac{x \text{ mL}}{10 \text{ mcg/min}}$ $10 = 3.33x$ $\frac{10}{3.33} = 3.33$

Set the pump: total number mL = 250; mL/hr = 3   3 mL/hr = x

6. Order: 1 milliunit/min

Standard solution: 15 units in 250 mL NS

Step 1. $\frac{15 \text{ units}}{250 \text{ mL}} = 0.06 \text{ units/mL}$

Step 2. 1 unit = 1000 milliunits

   0.06 units = 60 milliunits

Step 3. $\frac{60}{60} = 1 \text{ milliunit/min}$

Step 4. Solve for mL/hr:

Formula Method	Proportion Expressed as Two Ratios	Proportion Expressed as Two Fractions
$\frac{1 \text{ milliunit}}{1 \text{ milliunit}} \times 1 \text{ mL}$ 1 mL/hr	1 mL : 1 milliunit/min : : x mL : 1 milliunit/min	$\frac{1 \text{ mL}}{0.133} \times \frac{x \text{ mL}}{4 \text{ milliunit/min}}$ 1 mL = x

Set the pump: total number mL = 250; mL/hr = 1

7. Order: 4 mcg/min

Solution: 2 mg in 250 mL

Step 1. $\frac{2 \text{ mg}}{250 \text{ mL}} = 0.008 \text{ mg/mL}$

Step 2. $0.008 \times 1000 = 8 \text{ mcg/mL}$

Step 3. $\frac{8 \text{ mcg}}{60 \text{ mL}} = 0.133 \text{ mcg/min}$

Step 4. Solve for mL/hr:

Formula Method	Proportion Expressed as Two Ratios	Proportion Expressed as Two Fractions
$\frac{4 \text{ mcg/min}}{0.133 \text{ mcg/min}} \times 1 \text{ mL} = x$ $x = 30 \text{ mL/hr}$	1 mL : 0.133 mcg/min : : x mL : 4 mcg/min	$\frac{1 \text{ mL}}{0.133} \times \frac{x \text{ mL}}{4 \text{ mcg/min}}$ $4 = 0.133x$ $\frac{4}{0.133} = x$

Set the pump: total number mL = 250; mL/hr = 30   30 mL = x

8. Order: 50 mcg/kg/min

Solution: 2.5 g in 250 mL

Weight: 58 kg

$$58 \text{ kg} \times 50 \text{ mcg} = 2900 \text{ mcg (order)}$$

Step 1. 2.5 g = 2500 mg
$$\frac{2500 \text{ mg}}{250 \text{ mL}} = 10 \text{ mg/mL}$$

Step 2. $10 \times 1000 = 10{,}000 \text{ mcg/mL}$

Step 3. $\frac{10000}{60} = 166.67 \text{ mcg/min}$

Step 4. Solve for mL/hr:

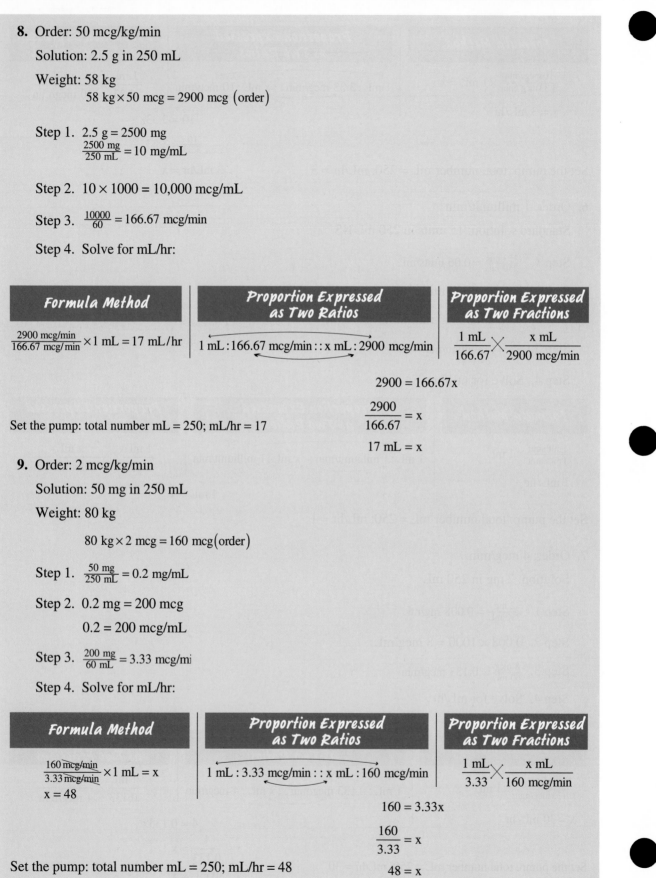

Formula Method	Proportion Expressed as Two Ratios	Proportion Expressed as Two Fractions
$\frac{2900 \text{ mcg/min}}{166.67 \text{ mcg/min}} \times 1 \text{ mL} = 17 \text{ mL/hr}$	$1 \text{ mL} : 166.67 \text{ mcg/min} :: x \text{ mL} : 2900 \text{ mcg/min}$	$\frac{1 \text{ mL}}{166.67} \times \frac{x \text{ mL}}{2900 \text{ mcg/min}}$

$$2900 = 166.67x$$

$$\frac{2900}{166.67} = x$$

$$17 \text{ mL} = x$$

Set the pump: total number mL = 250; mL/hr = 17

9. Order: 2 mcg/kg/min

Solution: 50 mg in 250 mL

Weight: 80 kg

$$80 \text{ kg} \times 2 \text{ mcg} = 160 \text{ mcg (order)}$$

Step 1. $\frac{50 \text{ mg}}{250 \text{ mL}} = 0.2 \text{ mg/mL}$

Step 2. 0.2 mg = 200 mcg
$$0.2 = 200 \text{ mcg/mL}$$

Step 3. $\frac{200 \text{ mg}}{60 \text{ mL}} = 3.33 \text{ mcg/mi}$

Step 4. Solve for mL/hr:

Formula Method	Proportion Expressed as Two Ratios	Proportion Expressed as Two Fractions
$\frac{160 \text{ mcg/min}}{3.33 \text{ mcg/min}} \times 1 \text{ mL} = x$ $x = 48$	$1 \text{ mL} : 3.33 \text{ mcg/min} :: x \text{ mL} : 160 \text{ mcg/min}$	$\frac{1 \text{ mL}}{3.33} \times \frac{x \text{ mL}}{160 \text{ mcg/min}}$

$$160 = 3.33x$$

$$\frac{160}{3.33} = x$$

$$48 = x$$

Set the pump: total number mL = 250; mL/hr = 48

10. Order: 200 mcg/min

Solution: 0.1 g in 100 mL

100 mg in 100 mL

Step 1. $\frac{100 \text{ mg}}{100 \text{ mL}} = 1$ mg/mL

Step 2. 1 mg = 1000 mcg

1000 mcg/1 mL

Step 3. $\frac{1000 \text{ mg}}{60} = 16.67$ mcg/min

Step 4. Solve for mL/hr:

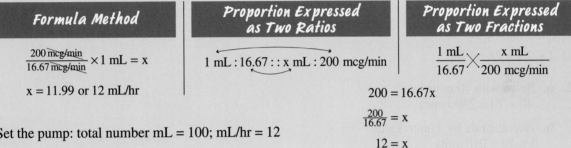

Formula Method	Proportion Expressed as Two Ratios	Proportion Expressed as Two Fractions
$\frac{200 \text{ mcg/min}}{16.67 \text{ mcg/min}} \times 1$ mL = x	1 mL : 16.67 : : x mL : 200 mcg/min	$\frac{1 \text{ mL}}{16.67} \times \frac{x \text{ mL}}{200 \text{ mcg/min}}$
x = 11.99 or 12 mL/hr		200 = 16.67x
		$\frac{200}{16.67} = x$
		12 = x

Set the pump: total number mL = 100; mL/hr = 12

Self-Test 4 Use of Nomogram

1. **a.** Dose is correct; 20 mg/m^2 × 1.96 = 39 mg

   b. Order calls for 250 mL over ½ hour, but pump is set in mL/hr. Double 250 mL.

   Setting: total number mL = 250; mL/hr = 500.

   The pump will deliver 250 mL in ½ hour.

2. **a.** Correct; 130 mg/m^2 × 1.77 = 230 mg

   b. Pour two 100-mg tabs and three 10-mg tabs.

3. **a.** Correct; 40 mg/m^2 × 2 = 80 mg

   b. Rapidly flowing IV is the primary line. Set the secondary pump: total number mL, 80; mL/hr, 80 (see Chapter 8 for IVPB).

4. **a.** Correct; 200 mg/m^2 × 2 = 400 mg

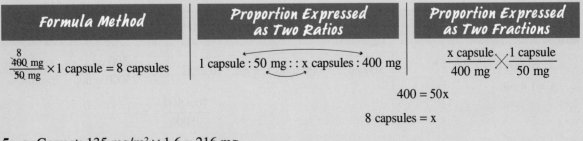

Formula Method	Proportion Expressed as Two Ratios	Proportion Expressed as Two Fractions
$\frac{8}{\frac{400 \text{ mg}}{50 \text{ mg}}} \times 1$ capsule = 8 capsules	1 capsule : 50 mg : : x capsules : 400 mg	$\frac{x \text{ capsule}}{400 \text{ mg}} \times \frac{1 \text{ capsule}}{50 \text{ mg}}$
		400 = 50x
		8 capsules = x

5. **a.** Correct; 135 mg/m^2 × 1.6 = 216 mg

   b. ½ L = 500 mL over 3 hr; $\frac{500}{3}$ $\overset{166.6}{\overline{)500}} = 167$

Set the pump: total number mL = 500; mL/hr = 167

Self-Test 5

1. **a.** Bolus with 40 units/kg
$40 \times 70 = 2800$ units

   b. increase rate by 2 units/kg per hour
$2 \times 70 = 140$ units

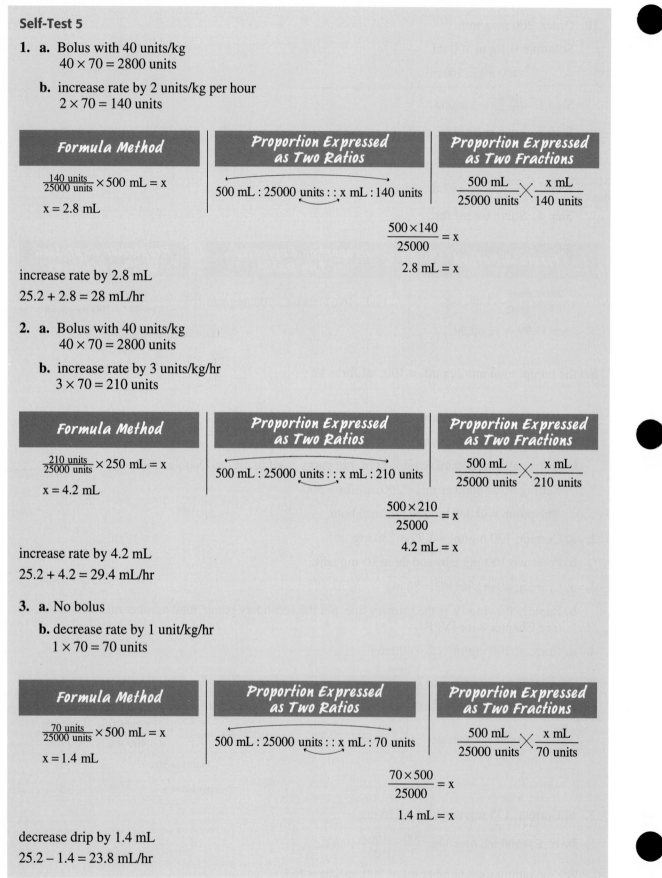

Formula Method	**Proportion Expressed as Two Ratios**	**Proportion Expressed as Two Fractions**
$\frac{140 \text{ units}}{25000 \text{ units}} \times 500 \text{ mL} = x$	500 mL : 25000 units : : x mL : 140 units	$\frac{500 \text{ mL}}{25000 \text{ units}} \times \frac{x \text{ mL}}{140 \text{ units}}$
$x = 2.8$ mL		$\frac{500 \times 140}{25000} = x$
		$2.8 \text{ mL} = x$

increase rate by 2.8 mL
$25.2 + 2.8 = 28$ mL/hr

2. **a.** Bolus with 40 units/kg
$40 \times 70 = 2800$ units

   b. increase rate by 3 units/kg/hr
$3 \times 70 = 210$ units

Formula Method	**Proportion Expressed as Two Ratios**	**Proportion Expressed as Two Fractions**
$\frac{210 \text{ units}}{25000 \text{ units}} \times 250 \text{ mL} = x$	500 mL : 25000 units : : x mL : 210 units	$\frac{500 \text{ mL}}{25000 \text{ units}} \times \frac{x \text{ mL}}{210 \text{ units}}$
$x = 4.2$ mL		$\frac{500 \times 210}{25000} = x$
		$4.2 \text{ mL} = x$

increase rate by 4.2 mL
$25.2 + 4.2 = 29.4$ mL/hr

3. **a.** No bolus

   b. decrease rate by 1 unit/kg/hr
$1 \times 70 = 70$ units

Formula Method	**Proportion Expressed as Two Ratios**	**Proportion Expressed as Two Fractions**
$\frac{70 \text{ units}}{25000 \text{ units}} \times 500 \text{ mL} = x$	500 mL : 25000 units : : x mL : 70 units	$\frac{500 \text{ mL}}{25000 \text{ units}} \times \frac{x \text{ mL}}{70 \text{ units}}$
$x = 1.4$ mL		$\frac{70 \times 500}{25000} = x$
		$1.4 \text{ mL} = x$

decrease drip by 1.4 mL
$25.2 - 1.4 = 23.8$ mL/hr

4. a. No bolus

b. Stop infusion for 1 hour
decrease rate by 2 units/kg/hr
$2 \times 70 = 140$ units

Formula Method	Proportion Expressed as Two Ratios	Proportion Expressed as Two Fractions
$\frac{140 \text{ units}}{25000 \text{ units}} \times 500 \text{ mL} = x$ $x = 2.8 \text{ mL}$	500 mL : 25000 units : : x mL : 140 units	$\frac{500 \text{ mL}}{25000 \text{ units}} \times \frac{x \text{ mL}}{140 \text{ units}}$ $\frac{500 \times 140}{25000} = x$ $2.8 \text{ mL} = x$

decrease rate by 2.8 mL
$25.2 - 2.8 = 22.4$ mL/hr

Self-Test 6

1. a. $(300 - 60) \times 0.02 = 4.8$ units

Formula Method	Proportion Expressed as Two Ratios	Proportion Expressed as Two Fractions
$\frac{4.8 \text{ units}}{100 \text{ units}} \times 100 \text{ mL} = x$ $x = 4.8 \text{ mL/hr}$	100 units : 100 mL : : x mL : 4.8 units	$\frac{100 \text{ mL}}{100 \text{ units}} \times \frac{x \text{ mL}}{4.8 \text{ units}}$ $\frac{4.8 \times 100}{100} = x$ $4.8 \text{ mL/hr} = x$

b. yes. $(BG - 60) \times 0.03$

2. a. $(350 - 60) \times 0.03 = 8.7$ units

Formula Method	Proportion Expressed as Two Ratios	Proportion Expressed as Two Fractions
$\frac{8.7 \text{ units}}{100 \text{ units}} \times 100 \text{ mL} = x$ $x = 8.7 \text{ mL}$	100 units : 100 mL : : x mL : 8.7 units	$\frac{100 \text{ mL}}{100 \text{ units}} \times \frac{x \text{ mL}}{8.7 \text{ units}}$ $\frac{8.7 \times 100}{100} = x$ $8.7 \text{ mL/hr} = x$

b. yes. $(BG - 60) \times 0.04$

3. a. Continue same rate 4.8 mL/hr

b. yes. $(BG - 60) \times 0.05$

4. a. Continue same rate 4.8 mL/hr

b. no. remains $(BG - 60) \times 0.05$

Self-Test 7 Infusion Problems

1. A pump is needed. This is set in mL/hr. The order calls for 0.5 mg/min. Because there are 60 minutes in an hour, multiply 0.5 mg × 60 = 30 mg/hr. The standard solution is 200 mg in 200 mL. This is a 1:1 solution, so 30 mg/hr = 30 mL/hr. You can also solve using the three methods:

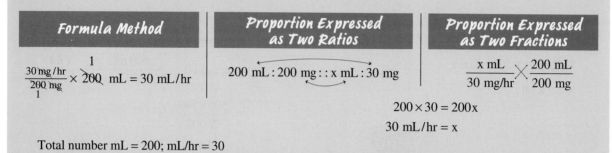

Formula Method	Proportion Expressed as Two Ratios	Proportion Expressed as Two Fractions
$\frac{30 \text{ mg/hr}}{\frac{200 \text{ mg}}{1}} \times \overset{1}{200} \text{ mL} = 30 \text{ mL/hr}$	200 mL : 200 mg :: x mL : 30 mg	$\frac{x \text{ mL}}{30 \text{ mg/hr}} \times \frac{200 \text{ mL}}{200 \text{ mg}}$ $200 \times 30 = 200x$ $30 \text{ mL/hr} = x$

Total number mL = 200; mL/hr = 30

2. Aminophylline comes 250 mg/10 mL. Remove 10 mL from the IV bag and add 10 mL drug. Order is 75 mg/hr. You have 250 mg in 250 mL (a 1:1 solution); therefore, set the pump at 75 mL/hr. You can also solve using the three methods:

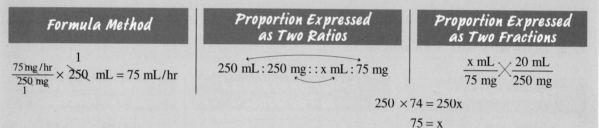

Formula Method	Proportion Expressed as Two Ratios	Proportion Expressed as Two Fractions
$\frac{75 \text{ mg/hr}}{\frac{250 \text{ mg}}{1}} \times \overset{1}{250} \text{ mL} = 75 \text{ mL/hr}$	250 mL : 250 mg :: x mL : 75 mg	$\frac{x \text{ mL}}{75 \text{ mg}} \times \frac{20 \text{ mL}}{250 \text{ mg}}$ $250 \times 74 = 250x$ $75 = x$

Total number mL = 250; mL/hr = 75

3. 2 g = 2000 mg

A pump is needed and is set in mL/hr. Order calls for 4 mg/min. There are 60 minutes in an hour: 60 × 4 = 240 mg/hr

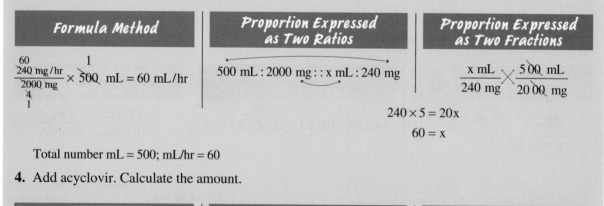

Formula Method	Proportion Expressed as Two Ratios	Proportion Expressed as Two Fractions
$\frac{\overset{60}{240 \text{ mg/hr}}}{\underset{\overset{4}{1}}{2000 \text{ mg}}} \times \overset{1}{500} \text{ mL} = 60 \text{ mL/hr}$	500 mL : 2000 mg :: x mL : 240 mg	$\frac{x \text{ mL}}{240 \text{ mg}} \times \frac{5\,00 \text{ mL}}{20\,00 \text{ mg}}$ $240 \times 5 = 20x$ $60 = x$

Total number mL = 500; mL/hr = 60

4. Add acyclovir. Calculate the amount.

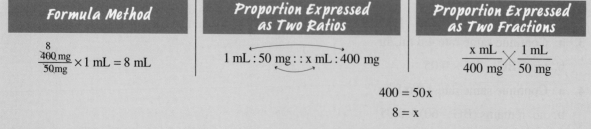

Formula Method	Proportion Expressed as Two Ratios	Proportion Expressed as Two Fractions
$\frac{\overset{8}{400 \text{ mg}}}{50 \text{mg}} \times 1 \text{ mL} = 8 \text{ mL}$	1 mL : 50 mg :: x mL : 400 mg	$\frac{x \text{ mL}}{400 \text{ mg}} \times \frac{1 \text{ mL}}{50 \text{ mg}}$ $400 = 50x$ $8 = x$

Remove 8 mL fluid from the IV bag and add 8 mL of drug. 8 mL × 50 mg/mL = 400 mg. This is now 400 mg/100 mL.

$$\frac{number\ mL}{number\ hr} = mL/hr$$

$$\frac{\overset{50}{\cancel{100}}\ mL}{\underset{1}{\cancel{2}}\ hr} = 50\ mL/hr\ on\ a\ pump$$

Total number mL = 100; mL/hr = 50

5. 5000 units/hr × 5 hr = 25,000 units in 250 mL D5W. Need five vials. Dissolve each with 1 mL sterile water. Remove 5 mL from the IV bag and add the 5 mL of urokinase.

Calculate the mL/hr:

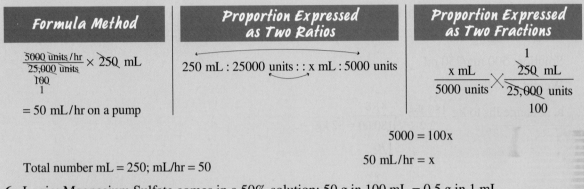

Formula Method	Proportion Expressed as Two Ratios	Proportion Expressed as Two Fractions
$\dfrac{\overset{}{\cancel{5000\ units/hr}}}{\underset{\underset{1}{100}}{\cancel{25,000\ units}}} \times \cancel{250}\ mL$ $= 50\ mL/hr\ on\ a\ pump$	250 mL : 25000 units : : x mL : 5000 units	$\dfrac{x\ mL}{5000\ units} \times \dfrac{\overset{1}{\cancel{250}}\ mL}{\underset{100}{\cancel{25,000}}\ units}$

$$5000 = 100x$$
$$50\ mL/hr = x$$

Total number mL = 250; mL/hr = 50

6. Logic: Magnesium Sulfate comes in a 50% solution; 50 g in 100 mL = 0.5 g in 1 mL

Calculate the mL/hr:

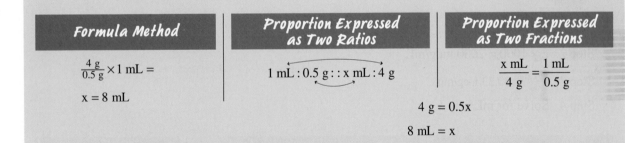

Formula Method	Proportion Expressed as Two Ratios	Proportion Expressed as Two Fractions
$\dfrac{4\ g}{0.5\ g} \times 1\ mL =$ $x = 8\ mL$	1 mL : 0.5 g : : x mL : 4 g	$\dfrac{x\ mL}{4\ g} = \dfrac{1\ mL}{0.5\ g}$

$$4\ g = 0.5x$$
$$8\ mL = x$$

Add 8 mL MgSO$_4$ to 100 mL D5W. Infuse over 30 minutes. The pump is set in mL/hr (60 minutes).

$$\frac{60\ minutes}{30\ minutes} = 2$$

Multiply 100 mL × 2 = 200 mL/hr

Total number mL = 100 mL

7. Order: 80 mcg/min

Supply: 50 mg in 250 mL

Step 1. $\frac{50\ mg}{250\ mL} = 0.2\ mg/mL$

Step 2. $0.2 \times 1000 = 200\ mcg/mL$

Step 3. $\frac{200}{60} = 3.33\ mcg/min$

Step 4. Solve for mL/hr:

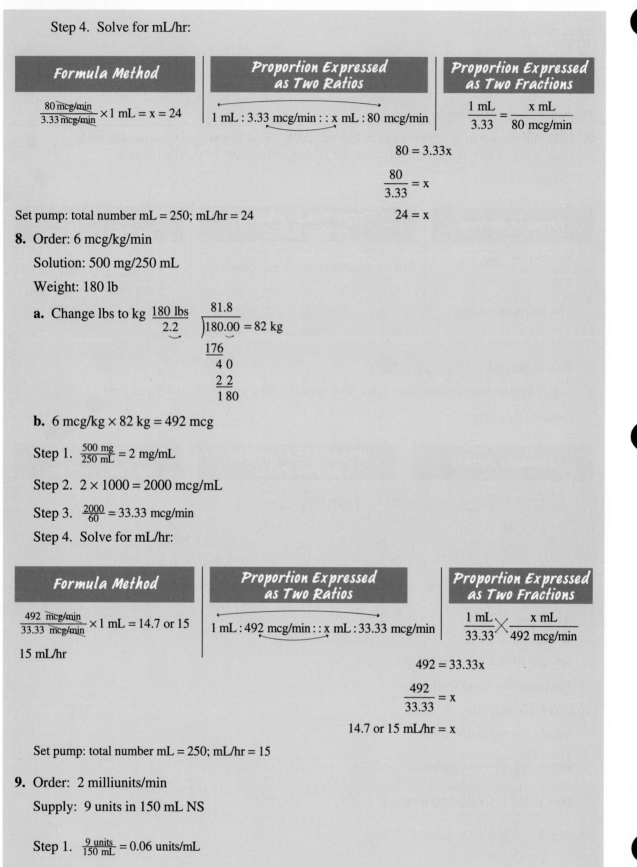

Formula Method	Proportion Expressed as Two Ratios	Proportion Expressed as Two Fractions
$\dfrac{80 \text{ mcg/min}}{3.33 \text{ mcg/min}} \times 1 \text{ mL} = x = 24$	$1 \text{ mL} : 3.33 \text{ mcg/min} :: x \text{ mL} : 80 \text{ mcg/min}$	$\dfrac{1 \text{ mL}}{3.33} = \dfrac{x \text{ mL}}{80 \text{ mcg/min}}$

$$80 = 3.33x$$

$$\frac{80}{3.33} = x$$

Set pump: total number mL = 250; mL/hr = 24 $24 = x$

8. Order: 6 mcg/kg/min

Solution: 500 mg/250 mL

Weight: 180 lb

a. Change lbs to kg $\dfrac{180 \text{ lbs}}{2.2}$ $2.2 \overline{)180.00} = 82 \text{ kg}$ $\begin{array}{r} 81.8 \\ \hline 180.00 \\ 176 \\ \hline 4\,0 \\ 2\,2 \\ \hline 1\,80 \end{array}$

b. 6 mcg/kg × 82 kg = 492 mcg

Step 1. $\dfrac{500 \text{ mg}}{250 \text{ mL}} = 2 \text{ mg/mL}$

Step 2. 2 × 1000 = 2000 mcg/mL

Step 3. $\dfrac{2000}{60} = 33.33 \text{ mcg/min}$

Step 4. Solve for mL/hr:

Formula Method	Proportion Expressed as Two Ratios	Proportion Expressed as Two Fractions
$\dfrac{492 \text{ mcg/min}}{33.33 \text{ mcg/min}} \times 1 \text{ mL} = 14.7 \text{ or } 15$ 15 mL/hr	$1 \text{ mL} : 492 \text{ mcg/min} :: x \text{ mL} : 33.33 \text{ mcg/min}$	$\dfrac{1 \text{ mL}}{33.33} \times \dfrac{x \text{ mL}}{492 \text{ mcg/min}}$

$$492 = 33.33x$$

$$\frac{492}{33.33} = x$$

$$14.7 \text{ or } 15 \text{ mL/hr} = x$$

Set pump: total number mL = 250; mL/hr = 15

9. Order: 2 milliunits/min

Supply: 9 units in 150 mL NS

Step 1. $\dfrac{9 \text{ units}}{150 \text{ mL}} = 0.06 \text{ units/mL}$

Step 2. 1 unit = 1000 milliunits
0.06 × 1000 = 60 milliunits/mL

Step 3. $\frac{60}{60}$ = 1 milliunit/mL

Step 4. Solve for mL/hr:

Formula Method	Proportion Expressed as Two Ratios	Proportion Expressed as Two Fractions
$\frac{2 \text{ milliunits/min}}{1 \text{ milliunit/min}} \times 1 \text{ mL}$	1 mL : 1 milliunit : : x mL : 2 milliunits	$\dfrac{1 \text{ mL}}{1 \text{ milliunit}} \times \dfrac{x \text{ mL}}{2 \text{ milliunits}}$

$$2 = x$$

Set pump: total number mL = 150 mL; mL/hr = 2

10. **a.** Correct; 1.55 BSA × 80 mg = 124 mg

   b. 1 L = 1000 mL

$$\frac{\text{number mL}}{\text{number hr}} = \frac{\overset{250}{\cancel{1000} \text{ mL}}}{\underset{1}{\cancel{4} \text{ hr}}} = 250 \text{ mL/hr}$$

Set the pump: total number mL = 1000; mL/hr = 250

CHAPTER 10

Dosage Problems for Infants and Children

LEARNING OBJECTIVES

1. Dosage based on mg/kg body weight; body surface area

2. Converting ounces to pounds

3. Converting pounds to kilograms

4. Determining a safe dose

5. mg/kg body weight calculations

6. BSA calculations

7. Calculating oral and parenteral doses

In previous chapters we discussed calculations for adult medications administered orally and parenterally. This chapter considers dosage for infants and children. Wide variations in age, weight, growth, and development within this group require special care in computation. Because pediatric doses are lower than adult doses and are narrower in dosage range, a slight error can result in serious harm.

Before preparing and administering a pediatric medication, the nurse determines that the dose is safe for the child. Safe means that the amount ordered is neither an overdose (which can produce toxic effects) nor an underdose (which may lead to therapeutic failure). If you notice a discrepancy in the dose, consult the physician or healthcare provider who ordered the drug.

Children's medications are usually given either by mouth in a liquid form or intravenously. This chapter also includes subcutaneous and IM injections, which are used primarily for immunizations. Pediatric injections are calculated to the nearest hundredth and are often administered using a 1-mL precision (formerly called tuberculin) syringe. For pediatric IV therapy, microdrip, Buretrols, other volume control sets or infusion pumps are used. In the pediatric setting, you often find infusion pumps that can be set in tenths or hundredths. Most institutions have guidelines for pediatric infusions; if no guidelines are available, consult a reliable pediatric reference. Adult guidelines are not safe for children.

Chapter 13 gives a brief overview of pediatric medication administration. For more information related to this topic, such as needle size and injection sites, check pediatric nursing textbooks. Always follow institutional policy. Administering liquid medication to an infant or toddler often requires gently holding the child and using a syringe or dropper (Fig. 10-1A). School age children often need to be involved in decision-making when administering medication (Fig. 10-1B).

Because pediatric doses must be accurate, it's advisable to use a calculator. The nurse still bears the responsibility, however, of knowing what numbers to enter into the calculator so as to calculate the correct amount. To be safe, double- or triple-check your answer.

Recall these equivalents and abbreviations as you begin this chapter:

1 g = 1000 mg	16 oz = 1 lb
1 kg = 2.2 lb	microdrip = 60 gtt/mL
1 mg = 1000 mcg	> = greater than
1 tsp = 5 mL	< = less than
1 oz = 30 mL	q4° = every four hours

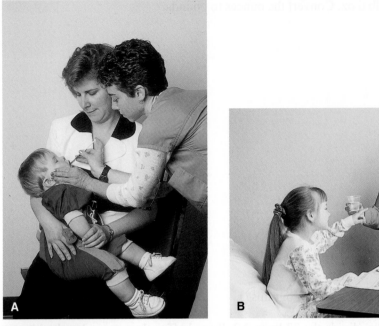

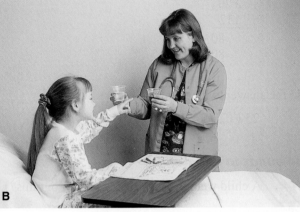

FIGURE 10-1

(A) Administration of liquid medication to infants and toddlers requires gently holding the child and administering with a syringe or dropper. **(B)** Administration of liquid medication to school age children involves giving them choices, for example what type of liquid to mix a medication that is distasteful. (Used with permission from Pillitteri, A. [2007]. *Maternal and Child Health Nursing* [5th ed.]. Philadelphia: Lippincott Williams & Wilkins, pp. 1145 and 1080.)

Dosage Based on mg/kg and Body Surface Area

The dose of most pediatric drugs is based on mg/kg body weight or BSA in meters squared. This section shows you how to convert pounds to kilograms, how to use a nomogram to calculate BSA, how to estimate the safety of a dose, and, finally, how to determine the dose. To ensure accuracy, use a calculator.

Converting Ounces to Pounds

Example An infant weighs 20 lb 12 oz. Convert the ounces to pounds.

Step 1. Because there are 16 oz in 1 lb, divide the 12 oz by 16. You should get a decimal.

$$
\begin{array}{r}
0.75 \\
16\overline{)12.00} \\
\underline{11\ 2} \\
80 \\
\underline{80} \\
0
\end{array}
$$

Step 2. Add the answer to the pounds to get the total number of pounds.

$$20 + 0.75 = 20.75 \text{ lb}$$

Example   An infant weighs 25 lb 6 oz. Convert the ounces to pounds.

Step 1.   Divide 6 by 16.

$$
\begin{array}{r}
0.375 \\
16\overline{)6.0} \\
\underline{4\,8} \\
1\,20 \\
\underline{1\,12} \\
80 \\
\underline{80} \\
0
\end{array}
$$

Step 2.   Add the answer to the pounds.

$$25 + 0.375 = 25.375 \text{ lb}$$

Converting Pounds to Kilograms

Example   A child weighs 33 lb. How many kilograms?

Step 1.   Because there are 2.2 lb per 1 kg, divide the 33 lb by 2.2. Round off to the nearest hundredth.

$$
\dfrac{33}{2.2}\begin{array}{r}
15 \\
\overline{)33.0} \\
\underline{22} \\
11\,0 \\
\underline{11\,0} \\
0
\end{array}
$$

The child weighs 15 kg.

Example   An infant weighs 18 lb 12 oz. How many kilograms?

Step 1.   Convert ounces to pounds first.

$$
\dfrac{12}{16}\begin{array}{r}
0.75 \\
\overline{)12.0} \\
\underline{11\,2} \\
80 \\
\underline{80} \\
0
\end{array}
$$

Step 2.   Add the answer to the pounds.

$$18 + 0.75 = 18.75 \text{ lb}$$

Step 3.   Convert to kilograms. Round off to the nearest hundredth.

$$
\dfrac{18.75}{2.2}\begin{array}{r}
8.522 \\
\overline{)18.75} \\
\underline{17\,6} \\
1\,15 \\
\underline{1\,10} \\
50 \\
\underline{44} \\
60 \\
44
\end{array}
$$

The infant weighs 8.52 kg.

SELF-TEST 1 Converting Pounds to Kilograms

Convert pounds to kilograms. Use a calculator. Round the final answer to the nearest hundredths place. Answers appear at the end of the chapter.

1. 30 lb = _____ kg   6. 4 lb 5 oz = _____ kg

2. 15 lb 5 oz = _____ kg   7. 75 lb = _____ kg

3. 7¼ lb = _____ kg   8. 12 lb 3 oz = _____ kg

4. 22 lb = _____ kg   9. 66 lb = _____ kg

5. 54 lb 8 oz = _____ kg   10. 10½ lb = _____ kg

Steps and Rule–mg/kg Body Weight

Example   Augmentin (amoxicillin) 150 mg po q8h is ordered for a child weighing 33 lb. Figure 10-2 shows the label for Augmentin (amoxicillin), which comes as a dry powder. The accompanying prescribing information states that children ≤ 40 kg receive 6.7 to 13.3 mg/kg q8h.

We need to convert 33 lb to kg, calculate the low and high safe dose, determine whether the dose ordered is within the safe range, and prepare the dose. These are the steps:

STEP 1. Convert lb to kg, dividing by 2.2.

STEP 2. Determine the safe dose range in milligrams per kilograms. Using a reference, determine the safe dose range in milligrams per kilogram.

STEP 3. Decide whether the ordered dose is safe by comparing the order with the safe dose range listed in the reference.

STEP 4. Calculate the dose needed.

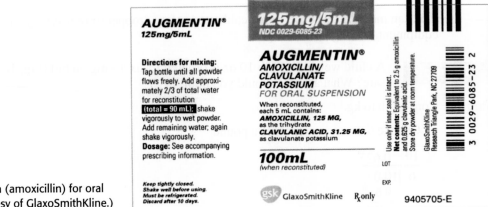

FIGURE 10-2

Label for Augmentin (amoxicillin) for oral suspension. (Courtesy of GlaxoSmithKline.)

Step 1. Convert lb to kg. Divide the number of pounds by 2.2.

$$2.2\overline{)33.0}$$ = 15.

The child weighs 15 kg.

Step 2. Determine the safe dose range. The literature states that the dose should range from 6.7 to 12.3 mg/kg q8h.

Low Dose	*High Dose*
6.7 mg	13.3 mg
× 15 kg	× 15 kg
100.5	199.5 = 200 mg

Step 3. Is the dose safe? The safe range is 100 to 200 mg q8h. The dose ordered (150 mg q8h) is indeed safe because it falls within the 100- to 200-mg range.

Step 4. Calculate the dose.

The label states that 90 mL water should be added gradually (see Fig. 10-2) to make a concentration of 125 mg/5 mL.

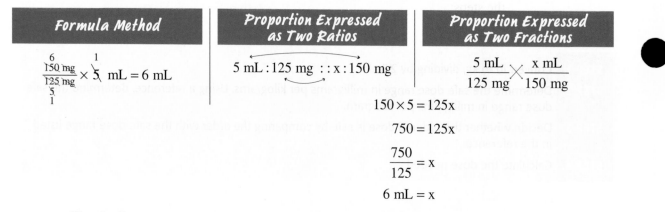

Formula Method	**Proportion Expressed as Two Ratios**	**Proportion Expressed as Two Fractions**
$$\frac{\overset{6}{\cancel{150\ mg}}}{\underset{5}{\cancel{125\ mg}}} \times \overset{1}{\cancel{5}} \ mL = 6\ mL$$	5 mL : 125 mg : : x : 150 mg	$$\frac{5\ mL}{125\ mg} \times \frac{x\ mL}{150\ mg}$$
	$$150 \times 5 = 125x$$	
	$$750 = 125x$$	
	$$\frac{750}{125} = x$$	
	$$6\ mL = x$$	

Give 6 mL.

You can measure this dose with a calibrated safety dropper or oral syringe. For examples of this equipment, see Figure 10-3.

Example   A child weighing 16 lb 10 oz is ordered Lasix 15 mg po bid (Fig. 10-4). Is the dose safe? What amount should you pour?

Step 1. Convert lb to kg.

a. Change the ounces to part of a pound.

$$6\overline{)10.0}$$ = 0.625

$$\begin{array}{r} 0.625 \\ 6\overline{)10.0} \\ \underline{9\ 6} \\ 40 \\ \underline{32} \\ 80 \\ \underline{80} \\ 0 \end{array}$$

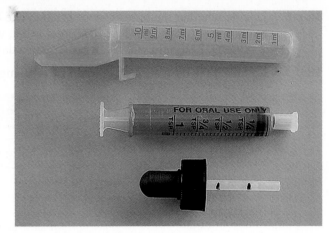

FIGURE 10-3

Examples of equipment used to obtain pediatric doses: (*top*) a medication spoon calculated in mL and teaspoons; (*center*) an oral syringe calculated in teaspoons; (*bottom*) a safety dropper calibrated in mL.

The child's weight is 16 + 0.625 = 16.625 lb.

b. Change pounds to kilograms. Round off to the nearest hundredth.

$$
\begin{array}{r}
7.556 \\
2.2 \overline{\smash{\big)}\ 16.625} \\
\underline{15\ 4} \\
1\ 22 \\
\underline{1\ 10} \\
125 \\
\underline{110} \\
150 \\
\underline{110} \\
\end{array}
$$

The child weighs 7.56 kg.

Step 2. Determine the safe dose range in mg/kg. The package insert states: The initial dose of oral Lasix (furosemide) in infants and children is 2 mg/kg body weight, given as a single dose. If the diuretic response is not satisfactory after the initial dose, dosage may be increased by 1 or 2 mg/kg no sooner than 6 to 8 hours after the previous dose. Doses greater than 6 mg/kg body weight are not recommended.

Single Dose	*High Range*
7.56 kg	7.56 kg
× 2 mg	× 6
15.12 mg/day	45.36 mg/day

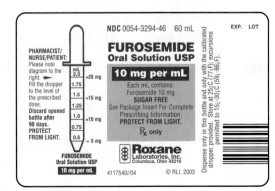

FIGURE 10-4

Label for Lasix (furosemide). (Used with permission of Roxane Laboratories, Inc.)

Step 3. Decide whether the ordered dose is safe. The order is 15 mg po bid. The 15 mg meets the requirement for a single dose. The order is bid, which means twice in a day; you calculate 15 mg × 2 = 30 mg. The child will receive 30 mg in a day. The high range is 45 mg, so the dose is safe.

Step 4. Calculate the dose needed. The supply is 10 mg/mL (Fig. 10-4).

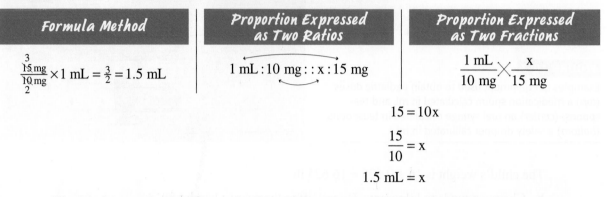

Formula Method	*Proportion Expressed as Two Ratios*	*Proportion Expressed as Two Fractions*
$\dfrac{\overset{3}{\cancel{15\,mg}}}{\underset{2}{\cancel{10\,mg}}} \times 1\ mL = \dfrac{3}{2} = 1.5\ mL$	$1\ mL : 10\ mg :: x : 15\ mg$	$\dfrac{1\ mL}{10\ mg} \times \dfrac{x}{15\ mg}$

$$15 = 10x$$

$$\frac{15}{10} = x$$

$$1.5\ mL = x$$

The label states that Lasix comes with a calibrated safety dropper. You can use the dropper to obtain the dose of 1.5 mL.

Example Lanoxin (digoxin) 37.5 mcg po × 1 is ordered for a premature infant weighing 1500 g. Is the dose safe? What amount should be given?

Step 1. Convert grams to kilograms (1000 grams = 1 kg).

$$\frac{1500}{1000} = 1.5\ kg$$

Step 2. Determine the safe dose range in mg/kg.

The *Nursing Drug Guide* states that the loading dose (oral) for the premature infant is 20 to 30 mcg/kg.

a. Convert mcg to mg (1000 mcg = 1 mg).

$$\frac{20\ mcg}{1000} = 0.02\ mg$$

$$\frac{30\ mcg}{1000} = 0.03\ mg$$

b.

Low Dose	*High Dose*
1.5 kg	1.5 kg
×0.02 mg	× 0.03 mg
0.03 mg	0.045 mg

Step 3. The ordered dose is 37.5 mcg. Convert to mg.

$$\frac{37.5\ mcg}{1000} = 0.0375\ mg$$

The dosage ordered is safe.

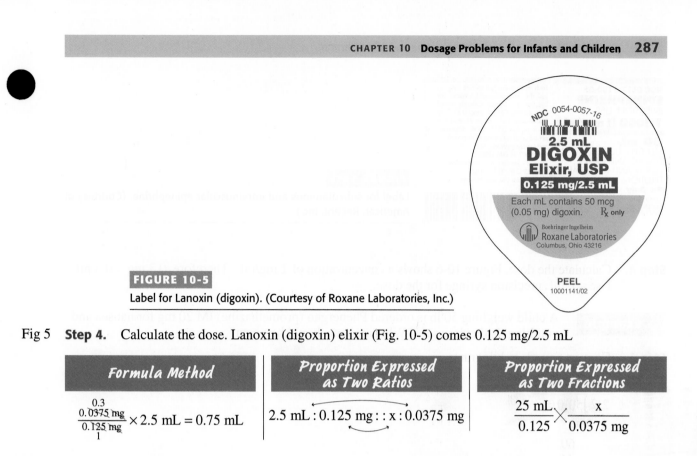

FIGURE 10-5
Label for Lanoxin (digoxin). (Courtesy of Roxane Laboratories, Inc.)

Fig 5   **Step 4.**   Calculate the dose. Lanoxin (digoxin) elixir (Fig. 10-5) comes 0.125 mg/2.5 mL

Formula Method	Proportion Expressed as Two Ratios	Proportion Expressed as Two Fractions
$\dfrac{\overset{0.3}{\cancel{0.0375}\text{ mg}}}{\underset{1}{\cancel{0.125}\text{ mg}}} \times 2.5\text{ mL} = 0.75\text{ mL}$	$2.5\text{ mL} : 0.125\text{ mg} :: x : 0.0375\text{ mg}$	$\dfrac{25\text{ mL}}{0.125} \times \dfrac{x}{0.0375\text{ mg}}$

$$2.5 \times 0.0375 = 0.125x$$

$$\frac{0.09375}{0.125} = x$$

$$0.75\text{ mL} = x$$

Use a calibrated safety dropper or oral syringe (1 mL) to draw up 0.75 mL.

Example   A child weighing 66 lb is prescribed epinephrine subcutaneous injection for an allergic reaction. The dosage prescribed is 0.3 mg. Is the dose safe? What amount should be given?

Step 1.   Convert pounds to kilograms.

$$\frac{66}{2.2} \quad 2.2\overline{)66.0}\ \ {\overset{3\,0.}{}}$$
$$\underline{66}$$
$$0$$

The child weighs 30 kg.

Step 2.   Determine the safe dose range in mg/kg.

The *Nursing Drug Guide* states 0.01 mg/kg subcutaneous every 20 minutes. Do not exceed 0.5 mg in a single dose.

Step 3.   The ordered dose is 0.3 mg.

$$30\text{ kg}$$
$$\underline{\times\ 0.01\text{ mg/kg}}$$
$$0.3\text{ mg}$$

The dosage is safe.

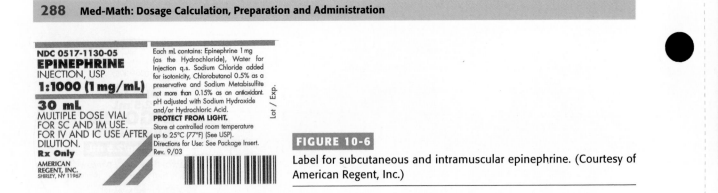

FIGURE 10-6

Label for subcutaneous and intramuscular epinephrine. (Courtesy of American Regent, Inc.)

Step 4.   Calculate the dose. Figure 10-6 shows a concentration of 1 mg/mL. Therefore, 0.3 mg = 0.3 mL. Use a 1-mL precision syringe for the dose.

Example   A child weighing 50 lb is ordered Phenergan (promethazine) IM 20 mg for nausea and vomiting. Is the dose safe? What amount should be given?

Step 1.   Convert pounds to kilograms.

$$
\begin{array}{r}
22.727 \\
2.2\overline{)50.00} \\
44 \\
\hline
60 \\
44 \\
\hline
16\,0 \\
15\,4 \\
\hline
60 \\
44 \\
\hline
160
\end{array}
$$

The child weighs 22.73 kg.

Step 2.   Determine the safe dosage range. The *Nursing Drug Guide* states 1 mg/kg IM q4–6h as needed. The safe dosage range is 10 to 25 mg.

Step 3.   The ordered dose is 20 mg.

22.73 kg

×   1 mg/kg

22.73 mg

A total of 22.73 mg is the calculated dose; however, the ordered dose is within the safe range and can be used.

Step 4.   Calculate the dose.

Promethazine is available 25 mg/mL (Fig. 10-7).

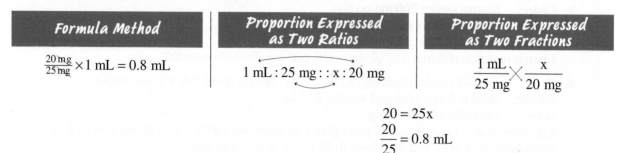

Formula Method	Proportion Expressed as Two Ratios	Proportion Expressed as Two Fractions
$\dfrac{20\,\text{mg}}{25\,\text{mg}} \times 1\,\text{mL} = 0.8\,\text{mL}$	$1\,\text{mL} : 25\,\text{mg} :: x : 20\,\text{mg}$	$\dfrac{1\,\text{mL}}{25\,\text{mg}} \times \dfrac{x}{20\,\text{mg}}$

$$20 = 25x$$
$$\frac{20}{25} = 0.8\,\text{mL}$$

Use a 1-mL precision syringe to draw up and administer the dose.

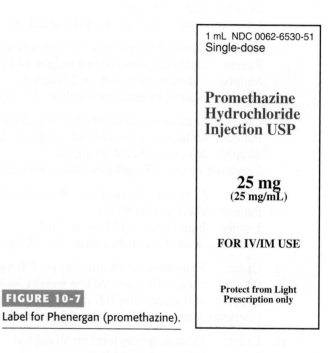

1 mL NDC 0062-6530-51
Single-dose

Promethazine
Hydrochloride
Injection USP

25 mg
(25 mg/mL)

FOR IV/IM USE

Protect from Light
Prescription only

FIGURE 10-7
Label for Phenergan (promethazine).

SELF TEST 2   **Dosage Calculations**

In these practice problems, determine whether the doses are safe and calculate the amount needed. Answers appear at the end of the chapter.

1. Order: Amoxil (amoxicillin) 60 mg po q8h
   Patient: child weighing 20 lb
   Supply: Amoxil (amoxicillin) 125 mg/5 mL; label states 20 to 40 mg/kg/day in divided doses q8h

2. Order: Augmentin (amoxicillin) 175 mg po q8h
   Patient: child weighing 29 lb
   Supply: Literature states 40 mg/kg/day in divided doses; bottle of 125 mg/5 mL

(continued)

3. Order: ferrous sulfate 200 mg po tid
   Patient: child is 9 years old and weighs 30 kg
   Supply: bottle of 125 mg/5 mL
   Literature states: children 6 to 12 years old, 600 mg divided doses tid

4. Order: Tylenol (acetaminophen) 80 mg po q4° prn for temp 100.9°F and above
   Patient: child is 6 years old and weighs 20.5 kg
   Supply: chewable tablets 80 mg
   Literature states: for child 6 to 8 years give four chewable tablets. May repeat four or five times daily. Not to exceed five doses in 24 hours. Is the dose safe?

5. Order: Valium (diazepam) 1 mg IM q3–4h prn
   Patient: infant 30 days old
   Supply: vial 5 mg/1 mL
   Literature states: child < 6 mo IM 1 to 2.5 mg tid or qid

6. Order: Demerol (meperidine) 15 mg subcutaneous q3–4h for relief of pain
   Patient: child is 3 years old and weighs 14 kg
   Supply: injection 10 mg/mL or 25 mg/mL
   Literature states Demerol (meperidine) 1.1 mg/kg/dose q3–4h not to exceed 100 mg/dose

7. Order: Dramamine (dimenhydrinate) 25 mg IM q6h as needed
   Patient: child is 10 years old and weighs 30 kg
   Supply: injection labeled 50 mg/mL
   Literature states 1.25 mg/kg qid not to exceed 300 mg/day

8. Order: Cloxapen (cloxacillin) 250 mg po q6h
   Patient: child weighs 48 lbs
   Supply: liquid labeled 125 mg in 5 mL
   Literature states for children more than 20 kg, the dose should be 250 to 500 mg q6h.

9. Order: Zithromax (azithromycin) po 300 mg × 1 dose
   Patient: child is 10 years old and weighs 30 kg
   Supply: oral suspension 100 mg/5 mL in 15-mL bottle
   Literature states for children 2 to 15 years, 10 mg/kg (not more than 500 mg/dose) on day 1.

10. Order: Dilantin (phenytoin) po 60 mg bid
    Patient: infant weighs 12 lb 8 oz
    Supply: Dilantin (phenytoin) suspension 30 mg/5 mL
    Literature states 4 to 8 mg/kg/day divided into two doses. Maximum dose is 300 mg/day.

Determining BSA in m²

A second method to determine pediatric dosage is to calculate BSA (body surface area) in meters squared (m²) using a chart called a nomogram (Fig. 10-8). Height is marked in the left column, weight in the right column. A line is drawn between these two marks. The point at which the line intersects the middle column indicates BSA in m².

There are several mathematical formulas to calculate body surface area. One often used is:

$$\sqrt{\frac{weight(kg) \times height(cm)}{3600}} = \text{BSA}$$

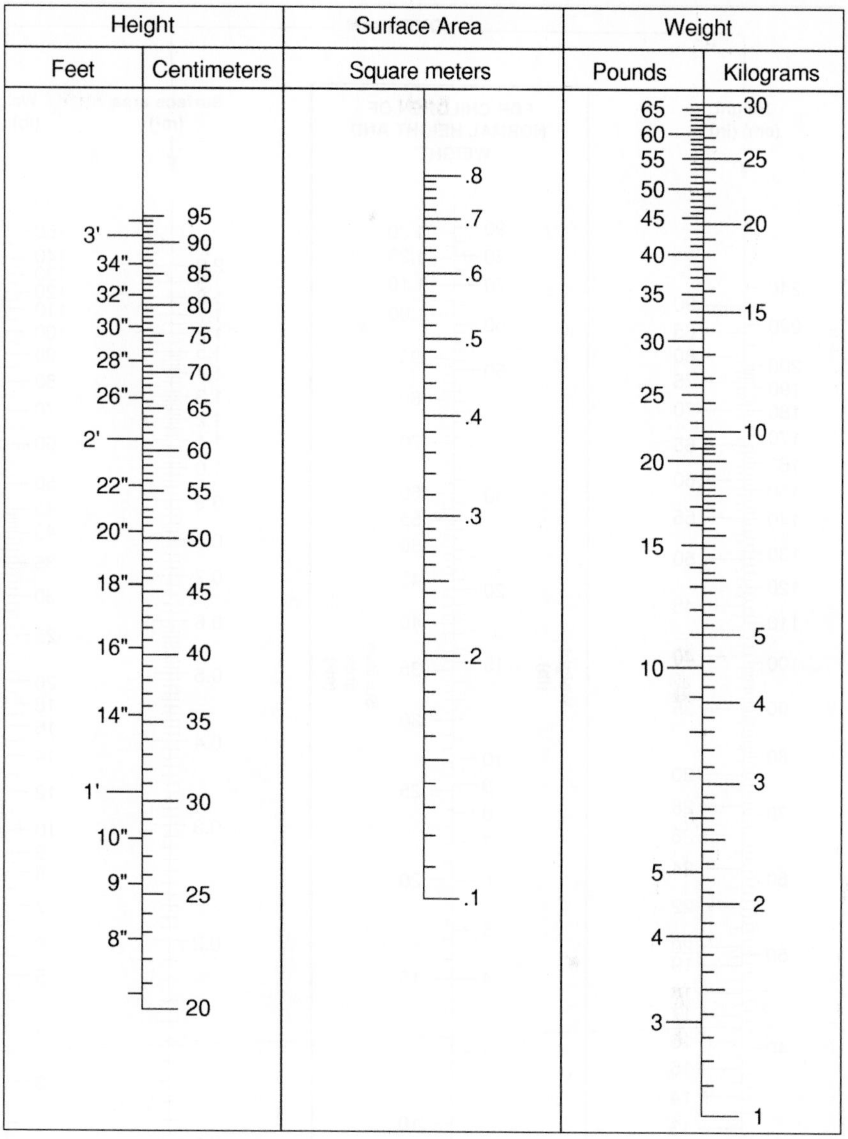

Height		Surface Area	Weight	
Feet	Centimeters	Square meters	Pounds	Kilograms

Height — Feet: 3', 34", 32", 30", 28", 26", 2', 22", 20", 18", 16", 14", 1', 10", 9", 8"

Height — Centimeters: 95, 90, 85, 80, 75, 70, 65, 60, 55, 50, 45, 40, 35, 30, 25, 20

Surface Area — Square meters: .8, .7, .6, .5, .4, .3, .2, .1

Weight — Pounds: 65, 60, 55, 50, 45, 40, 35, 30, 25, 20, 15, 10, 5, 4, 3

Weight — Kilograms: 30, 25, 20, 15, 10, 5, 4, 3, 2, 1

FIGURE 10-8

Nomogram for infants and toddlers.

Average BSA for children and infants:

9 year old: 1.07 m^2

10 year old: 1.14 m^2

12-13 year old: 1.33 m^2

Neonate: 0.25 m^2

2 year old: 0.5 m^2

Because of differences in growth, charts used for infants and young children are different than those for older children and adults. If a child weighs more than 65 lb or is more than 3 ft tall, use the adult nomogram (Fig. 10-9).

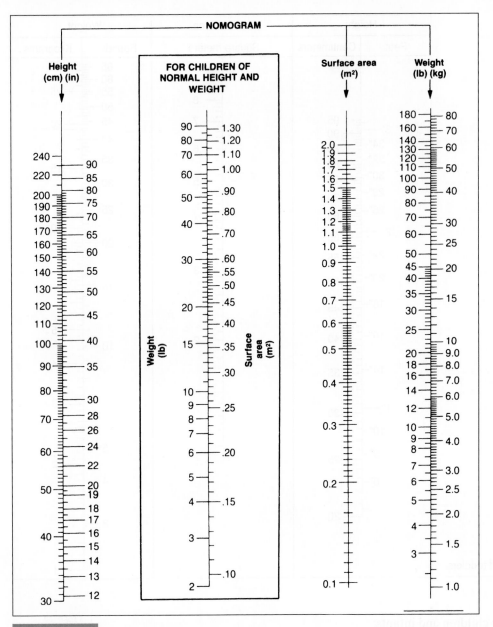

Nomogram for adults and children. To determine the surface area, draw a straight line between the point representing the patient's height on the left vertical scale to the point representing the patient's weight on the right vertical scale. The point at which this line intersects the middle vertical scale represents the surface area in square meters.

Example

1. An infant with a height of 12 in weighing 15 lb has a BSA of 0.19 m².
2. A child 4'2" weighing 130 lb has a BSA of 1.55 m².

BSA is used mainly in calculating chemotherapy dosages. Determining BSA can be done with a special calculator or using the internet. One useful website for calculating BSA is www.halls.md/body-surface-area/bsa.htm.

SELF TEST 3 Determining BSA

Convert height and weight to BSA in m² using Figure 10-8 or 10-9. Answers appear at the end of this chapter.

Height	Weight	BSA in m²
1. 36 in	26 lb	_____
2. 80 cm	13 kg	_____
3. 50 in	75 lb	_____
4. 17 in	9 lb	_____

STEPS AND RULE—m² MEDICATION ORDERS

STEP 1. Find the BSA in m².

STEP 2. Determine the safe dose using a reference.

STEP 3. Decide whether the ordered dose is safe.

STEP 4. Calculate the dose needed.

Example

A 2-year-old child weighing 27 lb 12 oz; height, 35 in; is prescribed leucovorin calcium 5.5 mg po q6h × 72 hr.

Literature states dose of leucovorin for rescue after methotrexate therapy is 10 mg/m²/dose q6h × 72 hours.

Supply: 1 mg/mL reconstituted by the pharmacy

Step 1. Use Figure 10-8.

Height, 35 in; weight, 27 lb 12 oz (12 ounces = 0.75 or ¾ lb)

Make weight 27¾ lbs.

BSA = 0.55

Step 2. Safe dose is 10 mg/m²/dose q6h.

$$
\begin{array}{r}
10 \text{ mg} \\
\times\ 0.55 \text{ m}^2 \\
\hline
5.5 \text{ mg} = \text{safe dose q6h}
\end{array}
$$

Step 3. Order is 5.5 mg q6h. Dose is safe.

Step 4.

Formula Method	Proportion Expressed as Two Ratios	Proportion Expressed as Two Fractions
$\dfrac{5.5\,\text{mg}}{1\,\text{mg}} \times 1\,\text{mL} = 5.5\,\text{mL}$	1 mL : 1 mg : : x : 5.5 mg	$\dfrac{1\,\text{mL}}{1\,\text{mg}} \times \dfrac{\text{x}}{5.5\,\text{mg}}$

$$5.5 = x$$

Give 5.5 mL po q6h.

Example A 6-year-old child weighing 40 lb; height, 45 in; is prescribed methotrexate 7.5 mg po twice weekly.

Literature states methotrexate 7.5 to 30 mg/m^2/dose twice weekly

Supply: 2.5-mg tablets

Step 1: Use Figure 10-9.

Height, 45 in; weight, 40 lb

BSA = 0.75

Step 2. Safe dose is 7.5 to 30 mg/m^2/dose twice weekly

7.5 kg	30 mg
$\times\, 0.75\,\text{m}^2$	$\times\, 0.55\,\text{m}^2$
5.625 mg	16.5 mg

Step 3: Order is 7.5 mg po twice weekly. Dose is safe.

Step 4:

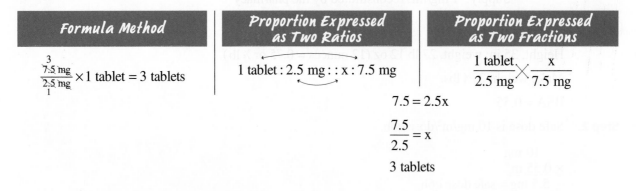

Formula Method	Proportion Expressed as Two Ratios	Proportion Expressed as Two Fractions
$\dfrac{\overset{3}{7.5\,\text{mg}}}{\underset{1}{2.5\,\text{mg}}} \times 1\,\text{tablet} = 3\,\text{tablets}$	1 tablet : 2.5 mg : : x : 7.5 mg	$\dfrac{1\,\text{tablet}}{2.5\,\text{mg}} \times \dfrac{\text{x}}{7.5\,\text{mg}}$

$$7.5 = 2.5x$$

$$\frac{7.5}{2.5} = x$$

3 tablets

Give 3 tablets po twice weekly.

SELF TEST 4 **Use of the Nomogram**

In these problems, determine whether the dose is safe, using the nomogram in Figure 10-8 or 10-9 and calculating. Answers appear at the end of the chapter.

1. **Child:** 8 years; height, 50 in; weight, 55 lb
   Order: Tambocor (flecainide) 50 mg po q8h
   Literature: dose 100 to 200 mg/m^2/24 hours divided q8–12h
   Supply: 50-mg tablets

2. **Child:** 12 years; height, 59 in; weight, 88 lb
   Order: methotrexate 12.5 mg po q week
   Literature: 10 mg/m^2/dose as needed weekly to control fever and joint inflammation in rheumatoid arthritis
   Supply: 2.5-mg tablets

3. **Infant:** 12 months; height, 30 in; weight, 22 lb 8 oz
   Order: Deltasone (prednisone) 5 mg po q12h
   Literature: immunosuppressive dose 6–30 mg/m^2/24 hours
   Supply: 5 mg/5 mL syrup

4. **Child:** 10 years; height, 50 in; weight, 35 kg
   Order: Marinol (dronabinol) po 5 mg × 1
   Literature: dose 5 mg/m^2 1 to 3 hours before chemotherapy
   Supply: 2.5 mg capsules

5. **Child:** 12 years; height, 60 in; weight, 100 lb
   Order: Quinaglute (quinidine) po 250 mg/dose
   Literature: dose 900 mg/m^2/day in 5 divided doses
   Supply: 200-mg, 300-mg tablets

Administering Intravenous Medications

IV medications are administered when a child cannot maintain an oral fluid intake, has fluid electrolyte imbalances, or requires IV medication. Dosages for IV medications are calculated in mg/kg.

IVP (IV push) medications are calculated according to weight and are then administered, using the correct dilution and administration time. This information is in a drug handbook or hospital policy. Continuous IV medications are also calculated according to weight and are then infused through an infusion pump.

IVPB medications are administered in small amounts of diluent. Consult a pediatric reference or institutional manual to determine the minimum and maximum safe amount of diluent. Drugs for IVPB must be initially diluted following the manufacturer's directions. Once you make the initial dilution, withdraw from the vial the amount of drug required to obtain the dose.

Buretrols or other volume control units are used to administer IV fluids (Fig. 10-10). Buretrols are calibrated; they hold only 100 to 150 mL at a time, thus reducing the possibility of fluid overload. In the pediatric setting, Buretrols are usually filled with only one hour's worth of IV fluid, so the nurse is responsible for checking the IV every hour to make sure the child is not receiving too much or too little of fluid or medication. Drugs for IVPB that have been diluted can be added to a Buretrol (Fig. 10-11).

For smaller children and infants requiring IVPB medications, the medication is usually added to only 10-20 mL in the Buretrol. This amount of fluid will fill the tubing from the Buretrol to the patient. When the Buretrol is empty of the IV medication, most of the drug will still be in the tubing. For this reason, you need to add an IV flush of 20 mL to the Buretrol after the medication is infused, to ensure that the patient receives the drug.

Infusion pumps provide a second safeguard (Fig. 10-12). To ensure that pediatric patients receive accurate dosing, you can set infusion pump rates in tenths and hundredths. In neonatal areas, syringe pumps can deliver IV fluid ranging from 1 to 60 mL.

This section considers the calculation of pediatric doses for IV and IVPB administration.

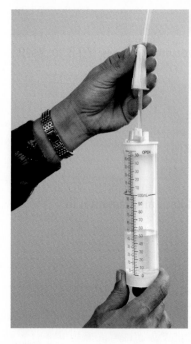

FIGURE 10-10

Volume control infusion device (Buretrol). (Used with permission from Taylor, C. [2008]. *Fundamentals of nursing* [6th ed.]. Philadelphia: Lippincott, Williams, and Wilkins, p. 853.)

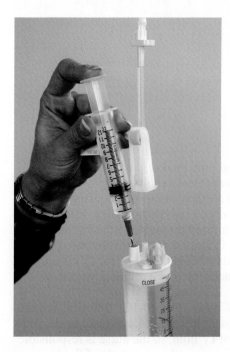

FIGURE 10-11

Adding medication to a volume control infusion device (Buretrol). (Used with permission from Taylor, C. [2008]. *Fundamentals of nursing* [6th ed.]. Philadelphia: Lippincott, Williams, and Wilkins, p. 854.)

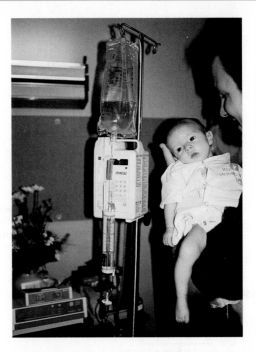

FIGURE 10-12

An infusion pump with a volume control unit. (With permission from Pillitteri, A. [2002]. *Maternal and child health nursing* [4th ed.]. Philadelphia: Lippincott Williams & Wilkins, p. 1106.)

	STEPS TO SOLVING PARENTERAL PEDIATRIC MEDICATIONS IVP
STEP 1.	Convert lb to kg.
STEP 2.	Determine the safe dose range in mg/kg using a drug reference.
STEP 3.	Decide whether the ordered dose is safe by comparing the order with the safe dosage range listed in the reference.
STEP 4.	Calculate the dose needed.
STEP 5.	Check the reference for diluent and duration for administration.

(To determine how fast to push the medication, you can take the volume calculated and divide by the minutes. Then take that number and divide by 4; the answer tells you approximately how much to push every 15 seconds. Or you can divide that number by 6, and the answer is approximately how much to push every 10 seconds. The important point is to push the drug slowly over the time period required and to monitor the IV infusion site.)

Example   Child: 5 years; weight, 44 lb

Order: Tagamet (famotidine) 5 mg IV bid

Literature: 0.25 mg/kg q12h IV up to 40 mg/day

Dilute with 5 or 10 mL with 5% dextrose or 0.9% sodium chloride and injected over at least 2 minutes.

Supply: See label (Fig. 10-13).

Step 1. Convert pounds to kg.

$$\frac{44}{2.2} \quad 2.2\overline{)44.0} \quad \frac{20.}{} $$
$$\underline{44}$$
$$0$$

The child weighs 20 kg.

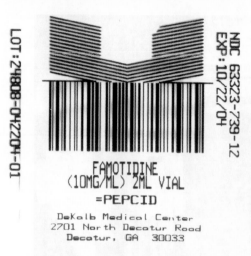

FIGURE 10-13

Famotidine. (Courtesy of DeKalb Medical Center, Decatur, GA.)

Step 2. Determine the safe dose.

$$
\begin{array}{r}
20 \text{ kg} \\
\times 0.25 \text{ mg/kg} \\
\hline
5 \text{ mg}
\end{array}
$$

Step 3. The dose is safe. It meets the mg/kg rule and does not exceed 40 mg/day.

5 mg bid = total 10 mg/day

Step 4. Calculate the dose.

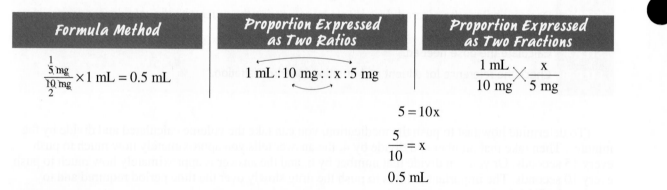

Formula Method	Proportion Expressed as Two Ratios	Proportion Expressed as Two Fractions
$\dfrac{\overset{1}{\cancel{5}}\text{ mg}}{\underset{2}{\cancel{10}}\text{ mg}} \times 1 \text{ mL} = 0.5 \text{ mL}$	$1 \text{ mL} : 10 \text{ mg} :: x : 5 \text{ mg}$	$\dfrac{1 \text{ mL}}{10 \text{ mg}} \times \dfrac{x}{5 \text{ mg}}$

$$5 = 10x$$

$$\frac{5}{10} = x$$

$$0.5 \text{ mL}$$

Step 5. Dilute with 5 or 10 mL suggested diluent. Inject over 2 minutes.

Example Child: 10 years; weight, 40 kg.

Order: Lasix (furosemide) 40 mg IV bid

Literature: 1 mg/kg q12h IV, no more than 6 mg/kg/day

Inject directly or into tubing of actively running IV; inject slowly over 1 to 2 minutes.

Supply: See label (Fig. 10-14).

Step 1.   Weight is in kg: 40 kg

Step 2.   1 mg/kg

40 kg = 40 mg

Step 3.   40 mg bid would be a total of 80 mg

Maximum dose: 6 mg/kg/day

40 kg × 6 = 240 mg

The dosage is safe.

FIGURE 10-14

Furosemide. (Courtesy of DeKalb Medical Center, Decatur, GA.)

Step 4.   Calculate the dose needed.

Formula Method	Proportion Expressed as Two Ratios	Proportion Expressed as Two Fractions
$\dfrac{\overset{4}{40}\ \text{mg}}{\underset{1}{10}\ \text{mg}} \times 1\ \text{mL} = 4\ \text{mL}$	1 mL : 10 mg : : x : 40 mg	$\dfrac{1\ \text{mL}}{10\ \text{mg}} \times \dfrac{x}{40\ \text{mg}}$

$$40 = 10x$$
$$\frac{40}{10} = x$$
$$4\ \text{mL}$$

Step 5.   Check the reference for diluent and duration for administration. To inject 4 mL over 2 minutes, you can push about ½ mL every 15 seconds.

STEPS TO SOLVE PARENTERAL PEDIATRIC MEDICATIONS IVPB

1. Decide whether the dose is safe; check a pediatric reference.
2. Decide whether the dilution ordered meets the minimum pediatric safety standard.
3. Prepare the medication according to directions.
4. Draw up the dose and dilute further as needed.
5. Set the pump in mL/hr. If the infusion time is 30 minutes, set the pump for double the amount because the pump delivers mL/hr.

   Example   The order is 10 mL over 30 minutes. Set the pump for 20 mL/hr. It will deliver 10 mL in 30 minutes.

6. When the IV is completed, add a flush of 20 mL to the Buretrol to clear the tubing of the medication. Be sure to chart the flush as fluid intake. Follow institutional requirements regarding IV flush.

Example

Child: 4 years; weight, 17 kg

Order: Fortaz (ceftazidime) 280 mg IV q8h in 10 mL D5½NS

Literature: Safe dose 30 to 50 mg/kg/day
Concentration for IV use: 50 mg/mL over 30 minutes

Supply: 1 g powder. Directions: Dilute with 10 mL sterile water for injection to make 95 mg/mL; stable for 7 days if refrigerated (Fig. 10-15).

1. Safe dose is 30 to 50 mg/kg/day.

Low Dose	*High Dose*
30 mg	50 mg
× 17 mg	× 17 mg
510 mg/day	850 mg/day

   Order is 280 mg q8h (three doses).

   280 mg × 3 = 840 mg

   Dose falls within the range and is safe.

2. Minimum safe dilution is 50 mg/mL. Dose is 280 mg.

   5.6 = 6 mL, the minimum dilution. The order of 10 mL is safe because it is more than the minimum.

   $$50\overline{)280.}$$
   $$\underline{250}$$
   $$300$$
   $$\underline{300}$$

3. Dilute 1 g with 10 mL sterile water to make 95 mg/mL.

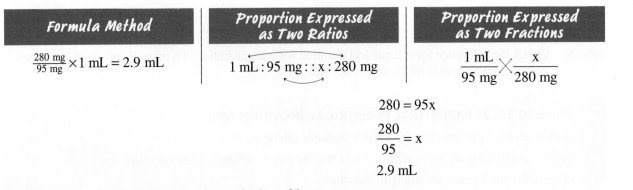

Formula Method	**Proportion Expressed as Two Ratios**	**Proportion Expressed as Two Fractions**
$\frac{280 \text{ mg}}{95 \text{ mg}} \times 1 \text{ mL} = 2.9 \text{ mL}$	1 mL : 95 mg : : x : 280 mg	$\frac{1 \text{ mL}}{95 \text{ mg}} \times \frac{\text{x}}{280 \text{ mg}}$

$$280 = 95x$$
$$\frac{280}{95} = x$$
$$2.9 \text{ mL}$$

Withdraw 2.9 mL; label the vial and store in the refrigerator.

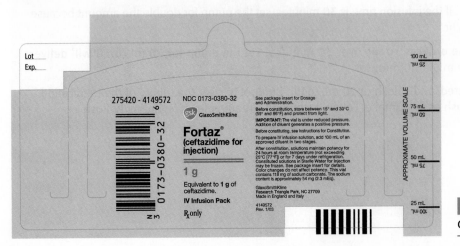

Lot
Exp.

275420 - 4149572

NDC 0173-0380-32

gsk GlaxoSmithKline

Fortaz®
(ceftazidime for injection)

1 g

Equivalent to **1 g** of ceftazidime.

IV Infusion Pack

℞ only

See package insert for Dosage and Administration.

Before constitution, store between 15° and 30°C (59° and 86°F) and protect from light.

IMPORTANT: The vial is under reduced pressure. Addition of diluent generates a positive pressure.

Before constituting, see Instructions for Constitution.

To prepare IV infusion solution, add 100 mL of an approved diluent in two stages.

After constitution, solutions maintain potency for 24 hours at room temperature (not exceeding 25°C (77°F)) or for 7 days under refrigeration. Constituted solutions in Sterile Water for Injection may be frozen. See package insert for details. Color changes do not affect potency. This vial contains 118 mg of sodium carbonate. The sodium content is approximately 54 mg (2.3 mEq).

GlaxoSmithKline
Research Triangle Park, NC 27709
Made in England and Italy

4149572
Rev. 1/03

APPROXIMATE VOLUME SCALE

100 mL / 25 mL
75 mL / 50 mL
50 mL / 75 mL
25 mL / 100 mL

FIGURE 10-15

Courtesy of GlaxoSmithKline.

4. Run about 5 mL D5½NS into the Buretrol. Add the 2.9 mL drug. Add more D5½NS to make 10 mL.

5. Set the pump at 20. This is 20 mL/hr. The pump will deliver 10 mL in 30 minutes.

6. When the IV is completed, add a 20-mL flush of D5½NS to clear the IV tubing of medication.

Example Infant: 4.3 kg

Order: ampicillin 100 mg IV q6h in 10 mL D5½NS

Literature: The safe dose is 75 to 200 mg/kg/24 hours given q6 to 8h IV.

Concentration for IV use: 50 mg/mL over 10 to 30 minutes

Supply: Vial of powder labeled 500 mg. Directions: Add 1.8 mL sterile water for injection to make 250 mg/mL; use within 1 hour.

1. Safe dose is 75 to 200 mg/kg/24 hours given q6–8h.

Low Dose	*High Dose*
75 mg	200 mg
× 4.3 kg	× 4.3 kg
322.5 mg/24 hr	860 mg/24 hr

Order is 100 mg q6h (four doses).

100 mg × 4 doses = 400 mg.

This is within the range. The dose is safe.

2. Minimum safe dilution is 50 mg/mL (Table 10-1). Dose is 100 mg.

$$50\overline{)100}\quad 2 \text{ mL is the minimum dilution; 10 mL is safe.}$$

TABLE 10-1 Sample of a Dilution Table for Pediatric Antibiotics

Antibiotic	Recommended Final Concentration IV	Recommendation Duration of IV
Ampicillin	50 mg/mL	10–30 min
Fortaz (ceftazidime)	50 mg/mL	10–30 min
Cleocin (clindamycin)	6–12 mg/mL	15–30 min
Garamycin (gentamicin)	2 mg/mL	15–30 min
Penicillin G	Infants: 50,000 units/mL Large child: 100,000 units/mL	10–30 min
Nebupent (pentamidine)	2.5 mg/mL	1 hr

3.   Add 1.8 mL sterile water for injection to 500 mg powder to make 250 mg/mL.

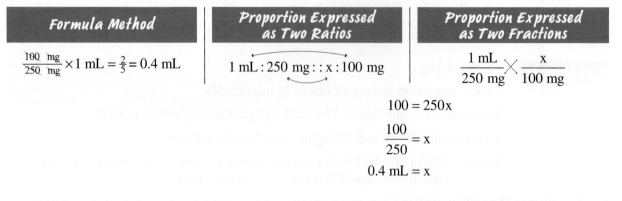

Formula Method	*Proportion Expressed as Two Ratios*	*Proportion Expressed as Two Fractions*
$\frac{100\ \text{mg}}{250\ \text{mg}} \times 1\ \text{mL} = \frac{2}{5} = 0.4\ \text{mL}$	$1\ \text{mL} : 250\ \text{mg} :: x : 100\ \text{mg}$	$\dfrac{1\ \text{mL}}{250\ \text{mg}} \times \dfrac{x}{100\ \text{mg}}$

$$100 = 250x$$
$$\frac{100}{250} = x$$
$$0.4\ \text{mL} = x$$

Withdraw 0.4 mL from the vial. Discard the remainder (directions say to use within 1 hour).

4.   Add about 5 mL D5½NS to the Buretrol. Add 0.4 mL drug. Add more D5½NS to make 10 mL.

5.   Set the pump at 20. This means 20 mL/hr. The pump will deliver 10 mL in 30 minutes.

6.   When the IV is finished, add a 20-mL flush of D5½NS to the Buretrol to clear the tubing of medication.

Example

Child: 3 years; weight, 15 kg

Order: Rocephin 600 mg IV q12h in 30 mL D5½NS

Literature: safe dose up to 100 mg/kg/day in 2 divided doses

Concentration for IV use: 50 mg/mL over 30 minutes

Supply: 1 g powder. Directions: Dilute with 9.6 mL sterile water for injection to make 100 mg/mL; stable for 7 days if refrigerated (Fig. 10-16).

1.   Safe dose is up to 100 mg/kg/day.

$$\begin{array}{r} 100 \\ \times\ \ 15 \\ \hline 1500\ \text{mg/day} \end{array}$$ or 750 mg/day

Order is 600 mg q12h (two doses).

600 mg x 2 = 1200 mg

The dose falls within the range and therefore is safe.

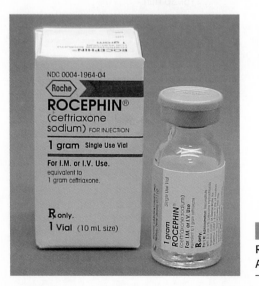

2. Minimum safe dilution is 150 mg/mL. The dose is 600 mg.

   600 mg divided by 150 mg gives us 4 mL as a minimal dilution

   The order of 10 mL is safe, because it is more than the minimum.

3. Dilute 1 g with 9.6 mL sterile water to make 100 mg/mL.

Formula Method	Proportion Expressed as Two Ratios	Proportion Expressed as Two Fractions
$\dfrac{600 \text{ mg}}{100 \text{ mg}} \times 1 \text{ mL} = x$ 6 mL	1 mL : 100 mg : : x : 600 mg	$\dfrac{1 \text{ mL}}{100 \text{ mg}} \times \dfrac{x}{600 \text{ mg}}$ $600 = 100x$ $\dfrac{600}{100} = 6 \text{ mL}$

Withdraw 6 mL; label the vial and store in the refrigerator.

4. Run about 5 mL D5½NS into the Buretrol. Add the 6 mL drug. Add more D5½NS to make 20 mL.

5. Set the pump at 40, which means 40 mL/hr. The pump will deliver 20 mL in 30 minutes.

6. When the IV is completed, add a 20-mL flush of D5½NS to clear the medication from the tubing.

General Guidelines for Continuous IV Medications

1. Calculate continuous IV medications for children and infants by using the methods and formulas used in Chapter 9.
2. Base continuous IV dosages on weight in kilograms.
3. Always use an infusion pump and/or volume control sets.
4. Use small bags of fluid to prevent fluid overload.
5. Follow institutional requirements for continuous IV infusions.
6. To determine the safe dosage range consult a pediatric text or drug reference.

SELF TEST 5   Parenteral Medication Calculations

In these practice problems, determine whether the dose is safe, calculate the amount needed, and state how the order should be administered. Answers appear at the end of this chapter. Follow the steps used in the examples.

1. Infant: 6 months; weight, 8 kg
   Order: Ceftin (cefuroxime) 200 mg IV q6h in 10 mL D5½NS
   Literature: The safe dose is 50 to 100 mg/kg/24h given q6–8h
                Concentration for IV use: 50 mg/mL over 30 minutes
   Supply: 750-mg vial of powder. Directions: Dilute with 8 mL sterile water for injection
                to make 90 mg/mL; stable for 3 days if refrigerated.

(continued)

2. Child: 3 years; weight, 15 kg
   Order: Bactrim (as TMP/SMX) 75 mg IV q12h in 75 mL D5W over 1 hr
   Literature: Safe dose for a child is 8 to 10 mg/kg/24h given q12h
                Concentration for IV use: 1 mL in 15 to 25 mL (supply is a liquid)
   Supply: Vial labeled 80 mg/5 mL

3. Child: 12 years; weight, 40 kg
   Order: Nebcin (tobramycin) 100 mg IV q8h in 50 mL D5½NS
   Literature: The safe dose is 3 to 5 mg/kg/24h given q8h
                Concentration for IV use: 2 mg/mL over 15 to 30 minutes
   Supply: vial 80 mg/2 mL

4. Child: 5 years; weight, 18 kg
   Order: Claforan (cefotaxime) 900 mg IV q6h in 25 mL D5½NS
   Literature: The safe dose is 50 to 200 mg/kg/24h given q6h
                Concentration for IV use: 50 mg/mL; give over 30 minutes
   Supply: 1 g powder. Directions: Dilute with 10 mL sterile water for injection to make
                95 mg/mL; stable in the refrigerator 10 days.

5. Infant: 3 months; weight, 6 kg
   Order: Unipen (nafcillin) 150 mg IV q8h in 10 mL D5½NS
   Literature: The safe dose is 100 to 200 mg/kg/24h given q6h
                Concentration for IV use: 6 mg/mL over 30 to 60 minutes
   Supply: 500-mg vial of powder. Directions: Add 1.7 mL sterile water for injection to
                make 500 mg/2 mL; stable for 48 hr if refrigerated.

6. Child: 8 years; weight, 30 kg
   Order: morphine 2.5 mg IV q4h
   Literature: 0.05 to 0.1 mg/kg/q4h IV. Dilute 2 to 10 mg in at least 5 mL NS. Administer
                over 4 to 5 minutes.
   Supply: morphine injection 1 mg/mL

7. Child: 6 years; weight, 25 kg
   Order: Decadron (dexamethasone) 4 mg IV bid
   Literature: 0.08 to 0.3 mg/kg/day divided q6–12h. Give undiluted IVP over 30 seconds or less.
   Supply: Decadron 4 mg/mL injection

8. Child: 12 years; weight, 45 kg
   Order: Benadryl (diphenhydramine) 25 mg IV q4–6h
   Literature: 12.5 to 25 mg IV q4–6 h; maximum dose, 300 mg/24 hr
                Give undiluted IVP over 1 minute.
   Supply: 50 mg/mL injection

9. Infant: 15 lb
   Order: Lanoxin (digoxin) maintenance dose IV 50 mcg/day
   Literature: 6 to 7.5 mcg/kg/day. Give undiluted or diluted in 4 mL D5W or NS over
                5 minutes.
   Supply: 0.1 mg/mL injection

10. Child: 9 years; weight, 80 lb
    Order: SoluMedrol (methylprednisolone) IV 60 mg bid
    Literature: 0.5 to 1.7 mg/kg/day divided q12h. Give each 500 mg over 2 to 3 minutes.
    Supply: SoluMedrol 40 mg/mL

CRITICAL THINKING: TEST YOUR CLINICAL SAVVY

You are working in a pediatric unit and taking care of 5-year-old Georgia Smith. Although she usually has a sweet disposition, she has her moments when she will not do anything she doesn't want to do. She is receiving IV fluids continuously and is ordered an oral medication three times a day that has an aftertaste. Each time the medication is brought to her, she refuses to take it.

a. What are techniques to help her take the medication?
b. Are there other alternatives you could use regarding the medication? How would you implement any of these alternatives?
c. Are there strategies to suggest to the family to promote easier compliance?
d. Besides reducing the possibility of fluid overload, what are some other reasons IV infusion pumps are used with children?

Another patient, 14-year-old Sean McBrady, is unable to swallow pills.

a. What are some alternatives to the medication?
b. Are there contraindications to any of the medication alternatives?
c. What are some ways to get children to swallow pills?
d. What would you suggest to the family to promote easier administration?

Putting it Together

Andy Bee is a 7 year old admitted to the ER with a 6 hour history of wheezing. The mother reports a history of "flu-like" symptoms for 48 hours. He has not had any solid food for 2 days and had minimal fluid intake.

Past Medical History: premature birth at 32 weeks. The child was on a ventilator for 1 week post partum. Small birth weight. Asthma.

Allergies: Penicillin, causing rash and hives.

Current Vital Signs: Blood pressure is 110/80, pulse 120–140/minute, respirations 29/minute, oxygen saturation 95%, temp 101.8. Weight 30 kg.

Medication Orders

Solu-Medrol (methylprednisolone) *corticosteroid, glucocorticoid* 20 mg IVP x 1 then 10 mg every 6 hours

Proventil (albuterol) *bronchodilator* 0.6 mL in 3 mL NS per nebulizer every 20 minutes x 3

Tylenol (acetaminophen) *antipyretic* liquid 400 mg PO for temp >101 prn q 4 hours.

NS 10 mL/kg/hr for 1 hour, then 100 mL/hr

Mortin (ibuprofen) *anti-inflammatory* 5 mg/kg PO q 6h prn for continued temp >101 if not relieved by Tylenol

Fortaz (ceftazidime) *antiinfective* 2 g IVPB q 8h in 50 mL D5½ NS

Lanoxin (digoxin) *cardiac glycoside* 0.72 mg/m^2 PO every day.

Augmentin (amoxicillin/clavulanate) *antiinfective* 150 mg PO q 8h.

Phenergan (promethazine) *antiemetic* 1 mg/kg IM prn q 4–6h for nausea

(continued)

Putting it Together

Calculations

1. Calculate how many mL of Solu-Medrol to give. Available Solu-Medrol vial that yields 20 mg/mL.
   a. One time dose of 20 mg.
   b. Scheduled dose 10 mg every six hours.

2. Calculate how many mL and how many teaspoons of Tylenol elixir to give.
   Available: liquid Tylenol 160 mg/5 mL.
   a. Conversion to mL.
   b. Conversion to tsp.

3. Calculate how many mg of Motrin to give and how many mL to administer. Available: 100 mg/5 mL

4. Calculate how many mL of Fortaz to prepare. Calculate the infusion rate. Available: 2 gram vial of powder. Dilute initially with 10 mL sterile water for injection. Infuse 50 mg/mL over 15–30 minutes.

5. Calculate the dose of Digoxin. BSA is 0.9 square meter.

6. Calculate the dose of Augmentin. Available 125 mg/mL.

7. Calculate how many mg of Phenergan. Is the dose safe? Literature states safe dose 10–25 mg.

8. Calculate the amount of NS to infuse the first hour.

Critical Thinking Questions

1. Should any medication(s) be held and if so why?

2. What medication(s) should be questioned and why?

3. What route of medication may be difficult for this patient? What are some alternatives to medication administration for this patient?

4. Is the amount of NS to infuse abnormally high for this patient? Why or why not?

Answers in Appendix B.

PROFICIENCY TEST 1   **Infants and Children Dosage Problems**

Name: _____

Here is a mix of oral and parenteral pediatric orders. For each problem, determine the safe dose and calculate the amount to give. Answers are given in Appendix A.

1. Newborn: weight, 4 kg
   Order: vitamin K 1 mg IM × 1 dose
   Literature: Prophylaxis and treatment: 0.5 to 1 mg/dose IM, subcutaneous, IV × 1
   Supply: vial 10 mg/mL

2. Infant: 1 yr; 10 kg
   Order: Augmentin (amoxicillin/clavulanate) 125 mg po q8h
   Literature: Safe dose Augmentin (amoxicillin/clavulanate): 20 to 40 mg/kg/24 hours given q8h po
   Supply: 125 mg/5 mL

3. Infant: 10 mo; 10 kg
   Order: benzathine penicillin 500,000 units IM × 1 dose
   Literature: Safe dose 50,000 units/kg × 1 IM. Maximum, 2.4 milliunits
   Supply: vial labeled 600,000 units/mL

4. Infant: 3.6 kg
   Order: gentamicin 9 mg IV q8h in 10 mL D5½NS
   Literature: Safe dose is 2.5 mg/kg/dose q8h
   Concentration for IV 2 mg/mL given over 15 to 30 min
   Supply: vial 40 mg/mL

5. Infant: 6.7 kg
   Order: Colace Syrup (docusate) 10 mg po bid
   Literature: Infants and children under 3: 10 to 40 mg/day
   Supply: 20 mg/5 mL

6. Infant: 5.5 kg
   Order: vancomycin 54 mg IV q8h in 12 mL D5½NS
   Literature: Safe dose is 10 mg/kg q8h IV
   Concentration for IV 5 mg/mL; infuse over 1 hour
   Supply: 500 mg powder
   Directions: Add 10 mL sterile water for injection to give 50 mg/mL; stable in the refrigerator 14 days.

7. Infant: 6.7 kg
   Order: chloral hydrate 350 mg po prior to electroencephalogram
   Literature: Hypnotic for children: 25 to 50 mg/kg/dose po not to exceed 100 mg/kg.
   Supply: 500 mg/5 mL

8. Child: 12 years; height, 60 in; weight, 40 kg; BSA, 1.32
   Order: methotrexate 10 mg po 1–2×/week
   Literature: 7.5–30 mg/m² 1–2×/week
   Supply: 2.5-mg tablet

9. Child: 8 yr; 24 kg
   Order: Fortaz (ceftazidime) 2 g IVPB q8h in 50 mL D5½NS
   Literature: Safe dose is 2 to 6 g/24 hours given q8–12h IV
   Concentration for IV 50 mg/mL over 15 to 30 minutes
   Supply: 2-g vial of powder
   Dilute initially with 10 mL sterile water for injection.

10. Child: 35 lb
    Order: Demerol (meperidine) HCl 20 mg IV stat
    Literature: Children: usual dose 1 to 1.5 mg/kg/dose q 3–4h prn. Maximum dose, 100 mg.
    Supply: 50 mg/mL

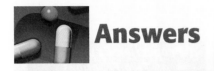

Answers

Self-Test 1 Converting Pounds to Kilograms

1. 13.64 kg (calculator)

2. $\dfrac{5 \text{ oz}}{16 \text{ oz}} = 0.3125 \text{ lb}$ (calculator)

Weight = 15.3125 lb
Change to kilograms.

$\dfrac{15.3125}{2.2} = 6.96 \text{ kg}$ (calculator)

3. ¼ lb = 0.25 lb
Weight = 7.25 lb
Change to kilograms.

$\dfrac{7.25}{2.2} = 3.3 \text{ kg}$ (calculator)

4. 10 kg (calculator)

5. $\dfrac{8 \text{ oz}}{16} = 0.5 \text{ lb}$

Weight = 54.5 lb.
Change to kilograms.

$\dfrac{54.5 \text{ lb}}{2.2} = 24.77 \text{ kg}$

6. $\dfrac{5 \text{ oz}}{16} = 0.3125 \text{ lb}$

Weight = 4.3125 lb.

$\dfrac{4.3125}{2.2} = 1.96 \text{ kg}$ (calculator)

7. $\dfrac{75 \text{ lb}}{2.2} = 34.09 \text{ kg}$ (calculator)

8. $\dfrac{3 \text{ oz}}{16} = 0.1875 \text{ lb}$

Weight = 12.1875 lb.

$\dfrac{12.1875}{2.2} = 5.54 \text{ kg}$

9. $\dfrac{66 \text{ lb}}{2.2} = 30 \text{ kg}$

10. ½ lb = 0.5 lb
Weight = 10.5 lb.
$\dfrac{10.5}{2.2} = 4.77 \text{ kg}$

Self-Test 2 Dosage Calculations

1. Step 1. $\dfrac{20}{2.2} = 9.09 \text{ kg}$

Step 2. Low dose $\quad$ 9.09 kg

$\underline{\times \ 20 \text{ mg}}$

181.8 mg/day

High dose $\quad$ 9.09 kg

$\underline{\times \ 40 \text{ mg}}$

363.6 mg/day

Step 3. 60 mg × 3 doses = 180 mg/day
The order is safe, although on the low side.

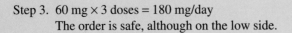

Step 4.

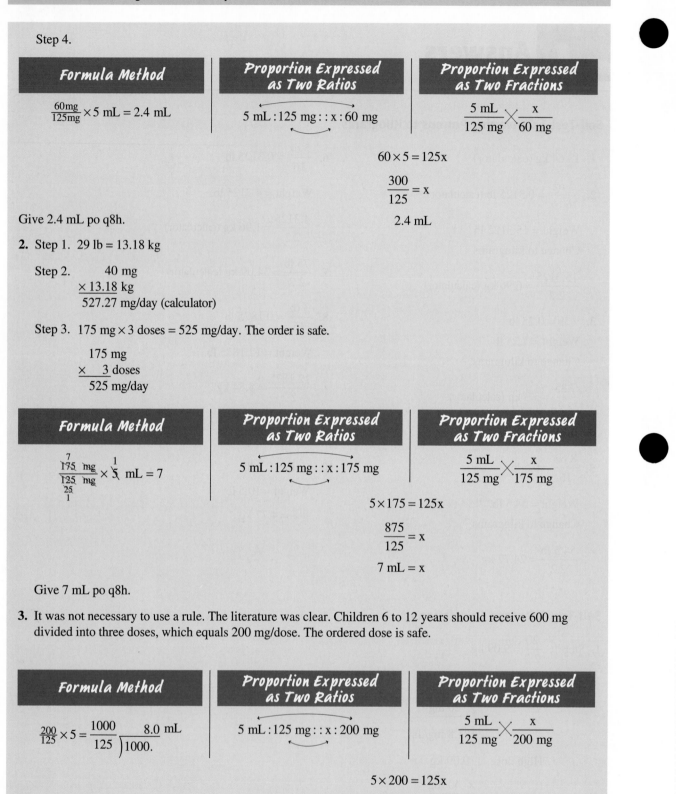

Formula Method	Proportion Expressed as Two Ratios	Proportion Expressed as Two Fractions
$\frac{60mg}{125mg} \times 5\ mL = 2.4\ mL$	$5\ mL : 125\ mg :: x : 60\ mg$	$\frac{5\ mL}{125\ mg} \times \frac{x}{60\ mg}$

$$60 \times 5 = 125x$$

$$\frac{300}{125} = x$$

Give 2.4 mL po q8h.

2.4 mL

2. Step 1. 29 lb = 13.18 kg

Step 2.   40 mg
          $\times$ 13.18 kg
           527.27 mg/day (calculator)

Step 3. 175 mg $\times$ 3 doses = 525 mg/day. The order is safe.

           175 mg
       $\times$ 3 doses
           525 mg/day

Formula Method	Proportion Expressed as Two Ratios	Proportion Expressed as Two Fractions
$\frac{\overset{7}{\cancel{175}}\ \text{mg}}{\underset{\underset{1}{25}}{\cancel{125}}\ \text{mg}} \times \overset{1}{\cancel{5}}\ mL = 7$	$5\ mL : 125\ mg :: x : 175\ mg$	$\frac{5\ mL}{125\ mg} \times \frac{x}{175\ mg}$

$$5 \times 175 = 125x$$

$$\frac{875}{125} = x$$

$$7\ mL = x$$

Give 7 mL po q8h.

3. It was not necessary to use a rule. The literature was clear. Children 6 to 12 years should receive 600 mg divided into three doses, which equals 200 mg/dose. The ordered dose is safe.

Formula Method	Proportion Expressed as Two Ratios	Proportion Expressed as Two Fractions
$\frac{200}{125} \times 5 = \frac{1000}{125}\ \overset{8.0\ mL}{\overline{)1000.}}$	$5\ mL : 125\ mg :: x : 200\ mg$	$\frac{5\ mL}{125\ mg} \times \frac{x}{200\ mg}$

$$5 \times 200 = 125x$$

$$\frac{1000}{125} = x$$

Give 8 mL po tid.

8 mL = x

4. Tylenol 80 mg seems low. Literature says a child of 6 years should receive four chewable tablets. This would be 320 mg. Check with the physician or healthcare provider.

5. The literature states that children under 6 months can receive 1 to 2.5 mg IM three to four times a day. The individual dose for the infant is 1 mg. This is safe, but the physician wrote q3–4h prn for the time. This would allow six to eight doses per 24 hours. The nurse can give the first dose but should clarify the times with the physician or healthcare provider.

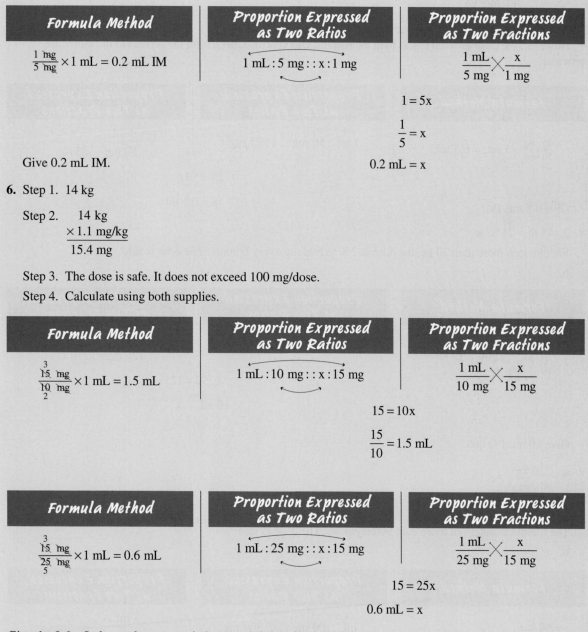

Formula Method	Proportion Expressed as Two Ratios	Proportion Expressed as Two Fractions
$\dfrac{1 \text{ mg}}{5 \text{ mg}} \times 1 \text{ mL} = 0.2 \text{ mL IM}$	$1 \text{ mL} : 5 \text{ mg} :: x : 1 \text{ mg}$	$\dfrac{1 \text{ mL}}{5 \text{ mg}} \times \dfrac{x}{1 \text{ mg}}$
		$1 = 5x$
		$\dfrac{1}{5} = x$
Give 0.2 mL IM.		$0.2 \text{ mL} = x$

6. Step 1. 14 kg

   Step 2.   14 kg
   $\underline{\times 1.1 \text{ mg/kg}}$
   15.4 mg

   Step 3. The dose is safe. It does not exceed 100 mg/dose.

   Step 4. Calculate using both supplies.

Formula Method	Proportion Expressed as Two Ratios	Proportion Expressed as Two Fractions
$\dfrac{\overset{3}{\cancel{15}} \text{ mg}}{\underset{2}{\cancel{10}} \text{ mg}} \times 1 \text{ mL} = 1.5 \text{ mL}$	$1 \text{ mL} : 10 \text{ mg} :: x : 15 \text{ mg}$	$\dfrac{1 \text{ mL}}{10 \text{ mg}} \times \dfrac{x}{15 \text{ mg}}$
		$15 = 10x$
		$\dfrac{15}{10} = 1.5 \text{ mL}$

Formula Method	Proportion Expressed as Two Ratios	Proportion Expressed as Two Fractions
$\dfrac{\overset{3}{\cancel{15}} \text{ mg}}{\underset{5}{\cancel{25}} \text{ mg}} \times 1 \text{ mL} = 0.6 \text{ mL}$	$1 \text{ mL} : 25 \text{ mg} :: x : 15 \text{ mg}$	$\dfrac{1 \text{ mL}}{25 \text{ mg}} \times \dfrac{x}{15 \text{ mg}}$
		$15 = 25x$
		$0.6 \text{ mL} = x$

Give the 0.6-mL dose subcutaneously because it is less liquid to inject.

7. Step 1. 30 kg

Step 2. $\begin{array}{r} 30 \text{ kg} \\ \times 1.25 \text{ mg/kg} \\ \hline 37.5 \text{ mg} \end{array}$

Step 3. $\begin{array}{r} 25 \\ \times\ 4 \ \ (\text{q6h}) \\ \hline 100 \ \ \text{mg/day} \end{array}$

The dose does not exceed 300 mg/day.

However, the dose ordered is less than the recommended dose. Check with the physician or healthcare provider.

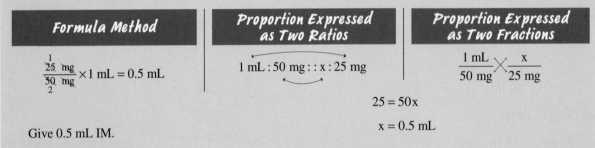

Give 0.5 mL IM.

8. a. 48 lb = 21.82 kg

For children more than 20 kg, the dose is 250 to 500 mg every 6 hours. The dose is safe.

b.

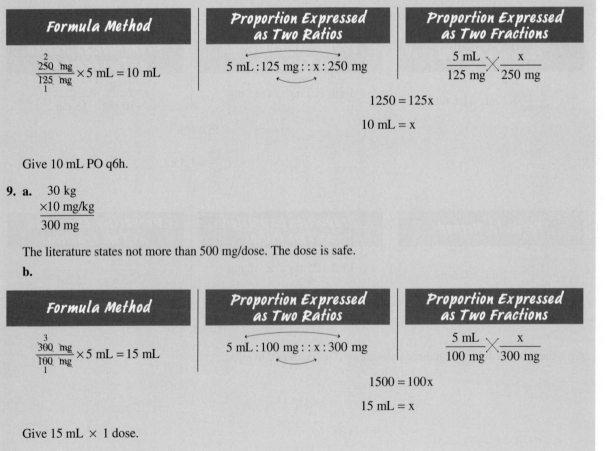

Give 10 mL PO q6h.

9. a. $\begin{array}{r} 30 \text{ kg} \\ \times 10 \text{ mg/kg} \\ \hline 300 \text{ mg} \end{array}$

The literature states not more than 500 mg/dose. The dose is safe.

b.

Give 15 mL × 1 dose.

10. a. $\frac{8 \text{ oz}}{16} = 0.5$ lb

$\frac{12.5 \text{ lb}}{2.2} = 5.68$ kg

$$
\begin{array}{rr}
5.68 \text{ kg} & 5.68 \text{ kg} \\
\times \quad 4 \text{ mg/kg} & \times \quad 8 \text{ mg/kg} \\
\hline
22.72 \text{ mg} & 45.44 \text{ mg}
\end{array}
$$

The dose (60 mg) is too high. Check with the physician.

Self-Test 3 Determining BSA

1. 0.54 m^2

2. 0.51 m^2

3. 1.1 m^2 (adult nomogram)

4. 0.255 m^2

Self-Test 4 Use of the Nomogram

1. Step 1. Find the BSA in m^2 = 0.94.

Step 2. Determine safe dose.

$$
\begin{array}{cc}
\textit{Low Dose} & \textit{High Dose} \\
100 \text{ mg} & 200 \text{ mg} \\
\times\, 0.94 & \times\, 0.94 \\
\hline
94 \text{ mg} & 188 \text{ mg}
\end{array}
$$

The safe dose is 94 to 188 mg over 24 hr.

Step 3. Is the order safe?

50 mg q8h = 50 mg × 3 = 150 mg/24 hr

The dose is safe.

Step 4. Order is 50 mg; supply is 50 mg. Give 1 tablet q8h.

2. Step 1. Find the BSA in m^2 = 1.29.

Step 2. The safe dose is

$$
\begin{array}{r}
10 \text{ mg} \\
\times\, 1.29 \\
\hline
12.9 \text{ mg}
\end{array}
$$

Step 3. Is the order safe? Yes; 12.5 mg is below the maximum.

Step 4.

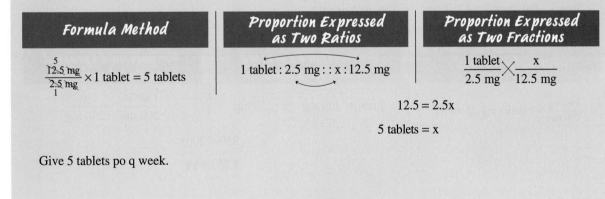

Formula Method	Proportion Expressed as Two Ratios	Proportion Expressed as Two Fractions
$\dfrac{\overset{5}{\cancel{12.5 \text{ mg}}}}{\underset{1}{\cancel{2.5 \text{ mg}}}} \times 1$ tablet = 5 tablets	1 tablet : 2.5 mg : : x : 12.5 mg	$\dfrac{1 \text{ tablet}}{2.5 \text{ mg}} \times \dfrac{x}{12.5 \text{ mg}}$

12.5 = 2.5x

5 tablets = x

Give 5 tablets po q week.

3. Step 1. Find the BSA in m² = 0.46.

Step 2. The safe dose is 6.30 mg/m²/24 hr.

Low Dose	*High Dose*
6 mg	30 mg
× 0.46	× 0.46
2.76 mg	13.8 mg

The safe dose is 2.8 mg to 13.8 mg over 24 hr.

Step 3. Order is 5 mg × 12 hr = 10 mg. The dose is safe.

Step 4. Order is 5 mg; supply is 5 mg/5 mL. Give 5 mL PO q12h.

4. Step 1. Find the BSA in m² = 1.1

Step 2. Determine the safe dose.

$$5 \text{ mg} \times 1.1 = 5.5 \text{ mg}$$

Step 3. Is the order safe?

Yes. The order is 5 mg.

Step 4.

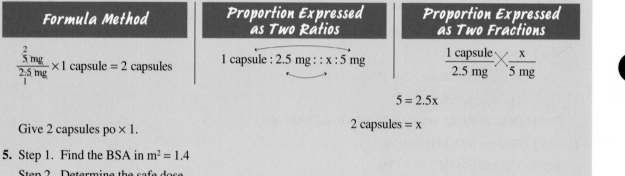

Formula Method	**Proportion Expressed as Two Ratios**	**Proportion Expressed as Two Fractions**
$\dfrac{\overset{2}{5} \text{ mg}}{\underset{1}{2.5} \text{ mg}} \times 1 \text{ capsule} = 2 \text{ capsules}$	1 capsule : 2.5 mg : : x : 5 mg	$\dfrac{1 \text{ capsule}}{2.5 \text{ mg}} \times \dfrac{\text{x}}{5 \text{ mg}}$

$$5 = 2.5x$$
$$2 \text{ capsules} = x$$

Give 2 capsules po × 1.

5. Step 1. Find the BSA in m² = 1.4

Step 2. Determine the safe dose.

$$900 \text{ mg} \times 1.4 = 1260 \text{ mg/day}$$

Step 3. 250 mg × 5 = 1250 mg/day. The order is safe.

Step 4. Calculate using both dosage supplies.

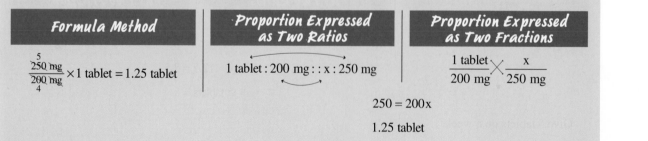

Formula Method	**Proportion Expressed as Two Ratios**	**Proportion Expressed as Two Fractions**
$\dfrac{\overset{5}{250} \text{ mg}}{\underset{4}{200} \text{ mg}} \times 1 \text{ tablet} = 1.25 \text{ tablet}$	1 tablet : 200 mg : : x : 250 mg	$\dfrac{1 \text{ tablet}}{200 \text{ mg}} \times \dfrac{\text{x}}{250 \text{ mg}}$

$$250 = 200x$$
$$1.25 \text{ tablet}$$

Formula Method	Proportion Expressed as Two Ratios	Proportion Expressed as Two Fractions
$\dfrac{\overset{5}{\cancel{250\ mg}}}{\underset{6}{\cancel{300\ mg}}} \times 1\ \text{tablet} = 0.83\ \text{tablet}$	1 tablet : 300 mg : : x : 250 mg	$\dfrac{1\ \text{tablet}}{300\ mg} = \dfrac{x}{250\ mg}$

$250 = 300x$

Use the 200-mg tablets to give 1.25 tablets.

0.83 tablet

Self-Test 5 Parenteral Medication Calculations

1. Step 1. The safe dose is 50 to 100 mg/kg/24 h.

Low Dose	*High Dose*
50 mg	100 mg
× 8 kg	× 8 kg
400 mg/24 hr	800 mg/24 hr

Order is 200 mg q6h (4 doses).

200 mg × 4 = 800 mg/24 h. Dose is safe.

Step 2. Minimum safe dilution is 50 mg/mL.

$$50\overline{)200\ mg}$$ $\dfrac{4\ mL}{}$ is the minimum dilution

A total of 10 mL is safe.

Step 3. Dilute 750 mg with 8 mL sterile water to make 90 mg/mL.

Formula Method	Proportion Expressed as Two Ratios	Proportion Expressed as Two Fractions
$\dfrac{200\ mg}{90\ mg} \times 1\ mL = 2.2\ mL$ (calculator)	1 mL : 90 mg : : x : 200 mg	$\dfrac{1\ mL}{90\ mg} \diagup \dfrac{x}{200\ mg}$

$200 = 90x$

2.2 mL

Withdraw 2.2 mL of the drug into a syringe. Label the remainder and store in the refrigerator.

Step 4. Add about 5 mL D5½NS to the Buretrol.

Add the 2.2 mL of drug. Add more D5¼NS to make 10 mL.

Step 5. Set the pump at 20. This means 20 mL/hr. The pump will deliver 10 mL in 30 minutes.

Step 6. When the IV is finished, add a 20-mL flush of D5½NS to clear the tubing of medication.

2. Step 1. The safe dose is 8 to 10 mg/kg/24 hours given q12h.

Low Dose	*High Dose*
8 mg	10 mg
× 15 kg	× 15 kg
120 mg/24 hr	150 mg/24 hr

Order is 75 mg q12h (two doses) = 150 mg/24h. The dose is safe.

Step 2. The minimum safe dilution is 1 mL in 15 to 25 mL. The drug comes as a liquid, 80 mg/5 mL.

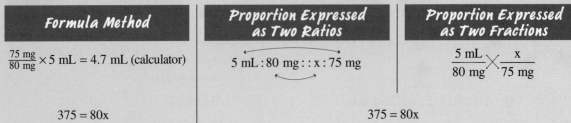

Formula Method	Proportion Expressed as Two Ratios	Proportion Expressed as Two Fractions
$\frac{75 \text{ mg}}{80 \text{ mg}} \times 5 \text{ mL} = 4.7 \text{ mL}$ (calculator)	5 mL : 80 mg : : x : 75 mg	$\dfrac{5 \text{ mL}}{80 \text{ mg}} \times \dfrac{\text{x}}{75 \text{ mg}}$
	375 = 80x 4.7 mL	375 = 80x 4.7 mL

Step 3. 75 mL D5W is a safe concentration (more than 70.5 mL).

Step 4. Draw up 4.7 mL drug into a syringe. Discard the remainder.

Step 5. Add about 50 mL D5W to the Buretrol. Add the 4.7 mL medication. Now add D5W until 75 mL is reached. Order is to administer over 1 hr. Set the pump at 75.

Step 6. When the IV is completed, add a 20-mL flush of D5W to clear the tubing of medication.

3. Step 1. The safe dose range is 3 to 5 mg/kg/24h given q8h.

Low Dose	*High Dose*
3 mg	5 mg
× 40 kg	× 40 kg
120 mg/24 hr	200 mg/24 hr

Order is 100 mg q8h (3 doses).

100 mg × 3 = 300 mg. Dose is not safe. Contact the physician or healthcare provider.

4. Step 1. The safe dose is 50 to 200 mg/kg/24h given q6h.

Low Dose	*High Dose*
50 mg	200 mg
× 18 kg	× 18 kg
900 mg/24 hr	3600 mg/24 hour

The order is 900 mg q6h (4 doses).

900 mg × 4 = 3600 mg/24 hours

The dose is safe.

Step 2. The minimum safe dilution is 50 mg/mL.

$$50 \text{ mg} \overline{)900 \text{ mg}}^{\,18}$$

18 mL is the minimum safe dilution.

25 mL is safe.

Step 3. 1-g powder.

Dilute with 10 mL to make 95 mg/mL.

Formula Method	Proportion Expressed as Two Ratios	Proportion Expressed as Two Fractions
$\frac{900 \text{ mg}}{95 \text{ mg}} \times 1 \text{ mL} = 9.5 \text{ mL drug}$	$1 \text{ mL} : 95 \text{ mg} :: x : 900 \text{ mg}$	$\frac{1 \text{ mL}}{95 \text{ mg}} \times \frac{x}{900 \text{ mg}}$

$$900 = 95x$$

$$9.5 \text{ mL}$$

Draw up the 9.5 mL in a syringe.

Discard the remainder; the amount is too small to keep.

Step 4. Add about 10 mL of D5½NS to the Buretrol. Add the 9.5 mL medication. Add D5½NS to make a total of 25 mL.

Step 5. Set the pump at 50. The pump will deliver 25 mL in 30 min.

Step 6. When the IV is finished, add a flush of 20 mL D5½NS to clear the tubing of medication.

5. Step 1. The safe dose is 100 to 200 mg/kg/24h.

Low Dose	High Dose
100 mg	200 mg
× 6 kg	× 6 kg
600 mg/24 hours	1200 mg/24 hours

Order is 150 mg q8h (three doses) = 450 mg/24 hours

The dose is below range and is q8h. The literature states q6h.

Step 2. The minimum safe dilution is 6 mg/mL.

The order is 150 mg.

$$6\overline{)150}\overset{25}{} = 25 \text{ mL}$$

The dilution of 10 mL does not meet concentration requirements. It should be 25 mL. Consult with the physician or healthcare provider regarding the dose, times of administration, and dilution.

6. Step 1. 30 kg

Step 2. Determine the safe dose.

Low Dose	High Dose
0.05 mg	0.1 mg
× 30 kg	× 30 kg
1.5 mg	3 mg

Step 3. The dose is safe.

Step 4. Supply: 1 mg = 1 mL

2.5 mg = 2.5 mL

Step 5. Dilute in at least 5 mL NS and administer over 4 to 5 minutes.

7. Step 1. 25 kg

Step 2. Determine the safe dose.

Low Dose	*High Dose*
0.08 mg	0.3 mg
× 25 kg	× 25 kg
2 mg/day	7.5 mg/day

Step 3. The dose is slightly high. Consult the physician or healthcare provider. 4 mg bid = 8 mg/day.

Step 4. Supply is 4 mg/mL. Give 1 mL after notifying physician of higher dose.

Step 5. Give 1 mL undiluted over 30 seconds or less.

8. Step 1. 45 kg

Step 2. Determine the safe dose.

Ordered dose (25 mg) is within 12.5–25-mg range.

Step 3. The dose is safe.

q4h: 25 mg × 6 hours = 150 mg

q6h: 25 mg × 4 hours = 100 mg

It does not exceed 300 mg/24 hr.

Step 4.

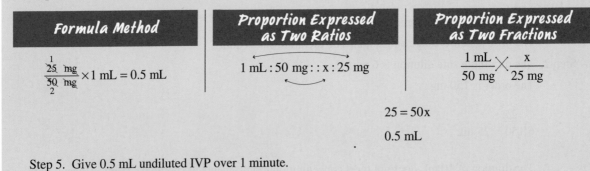

Formula Method	**Proportion Expressed as Two Ratios**	**Proportion Expressed as Two Fractions**
$\dfrac{\overset{1}{\cancel{25}} \text{ mg}}{\underset{2}{\cancel{50}} \text{ mg}} \times 1 \text{ mL} = 0.5 \text{ mL}$	1 mL : 50 mg : : x : 25 mg	$\dfrac{1 \text{ mL}}{50 \text{ mg}} \times \dfrac{x}{25 \text{ mg}}$
	25 = 50x	
	0.5 mL	

Step 5. Give 0.5 mL undiluted IVP over 1 minute.

9. Step 1. $\frac{15}{2.2} = 6.82$ kg

Step 2. Determine the safe dose.

Low Dose	*High Dose*
6 mcg/kg	7.5 mcg/kg
× 6.82 kg	× 6.82 kg
40.92 mcg/day	51.15 mcg/day

Step 3. The dose is safe (50 mcg/day).

Step 4. Calculate the dose.

0.1 mg = 100 mcg/1 mL

Formula Method	**Proportion Expressed as Two Ratios**	**Proportion Expressed as Two Fractions**
$\dfrac{\overset{1}{\cancel{50}}\ \cancel{mcg}}{\underset{2}{\cancel{100}}\ \cancel{mcg}} \times 1\ mL = 0.5\ mL$	$1\ mL : 100\ mcg :: x : 50\ mg$	$\dfrac{1\ mL}{100\ mcg} \times \dfrac{x}{50\ mcg}$

$$50 = 100x$$

$$0.5\ mL = x$$

Step 5. Give 0.5 mL undiluted or diluted in 4 mL D5W or NS over 5 minutes.

10. Step 1. $\dfrac{80\ lb}{2.2} = 36.36\ kg$

Step 2. Determine the safe dose.

Low Dose	*High Dose*
0.5 mg/kg	1.7 mg/kg
× 36.36 kg	× 36.36 kg
18.18 mg/day	61.81 mg/day

Step 3. 60 mg bid = 60 mg × 2 = 120 mg/day

The dose is too high. Contact the physician or healthcare provider.

Dimensional Analysis

LEARNING OBJECTI

1. Using dimensional analysis

2. Oral medication (solid and liquid) calculations

3. Parenteral medication calculations

4. Insulin

5. Equivalency conversion calculations

6. Weight based calculations, calculations

7. Reconstitution of medicatio

8. Intravenous fluids

9. Advanced intravenous calculations
   mL/hr
   mg/hr or units/hr
   mL/hr for drugs ordered in r
       mcg/min
   mL/hr for drugs ordered in
       mcg/kg/min
   Heparin and insulin protoco

A fourth method of dosage calculation is called dimensional analysis. This method is used extensively in mathematics and science, especially chemistry calculations. Students often say that once you master dimensional analysis, you tend to use it all the time, because it is simpler and more accurate than the other methods.

The dimensional analysis method uses terminology similar to that of other calculation methods. There are several ways to set up the dimensional analysis equation. As elsewhere in this book, the problems below start with a desired dose, using a supply or "available" amount. First you set up the entire equation with a numerator and a denominator, and then you solve the equation.

After learning dimensional analysis, you may want to go back to the other chapters and solve the problems in the proficiency tests using this new method. The answers to the proficiency tests in this chapter are worked in dimensional analysis as well as in the formula and proportion methods.

Oral Solid Medication Equation and Calculation

Start by calculating an equation for a simple oral solid medication:

Example   Order: Zyprexa (olanzapine) 7.5 mg po every day

Supply: Zyprexa 5-mg scored tablets (Fig. 11-1)

Write the desired dose first in the numerator:

7.5 mg

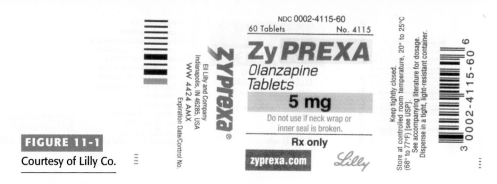

Then write the available dose as a fraction:

$$\frac{1 \text{ tablet}}{5 \text{ mg}}$$

Now combine both of these (note that the dimensional analysis set-up resembles a proportion expressed as two fractions).

$$\frac{7.5 \text{ mg}}{} \left| \frac{1 \text{ tablet}}{5 \text{ mg}} \right.$$

According to the basic rules of reducing fractions (review Chapter 1 if necessary), the two "mg" designations cancel each other. Reduce the numbers if possible. Divide both numbers by 5.

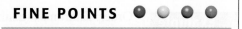

The setup should now look like this:

$$\frac{1.5}{} \left| \frac{1 \text{ tablet}}{1} \right.$$

> **FINE POINTS** ● ○ ● ●
>
> When reducing fractions, first attempt to divide the denominator evenly by the numerator.

Multiply the numerators, multiply the denominators, and then divide the product of the numerators by the product of the denominators. In this example, the numbers in the numerator are $1.5 \times 1 = 1.5$. The only number in the denominator is 1. Divide by 1 to get: 1.5 or $1\frac{1}{2}$ tablets.

$$\frac{1.5}{} \left| \frac{1 \text{ tablet}}{1} \right| \frac{1.5 \times 1}{1} = 1.5 \text{ or } 1\frac{1}{2} \text{ tablets}$$

Give $1\frac{1}{2}$ tablets po every day.

Example

Order: Depakote (divalproex) 500 mg po every day

Supply: See Figure 11-2.

The dose desired is 500 mg. The supply is 1 tablet = 250 mg.

The equation would look like

$$\frac{500 \text{ mg}}{} \left| \frac{1 \text{ tablet}}{250 \text{ mg}} \right.$$

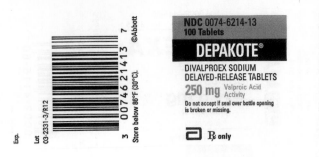

FIGURE 11-2

Courtesy of Abbott Laboratories.

Cancel the "mg." Reduce the fraction. Solve.

$$\frac{\overset{2}{\cancel{500}} \text{ mg}}{} \left| \frac{1 \text{ (tablet)}}{\underset{1}{\cancel{250}} \text{ mg}} \right. \qquad \frac{2 \times 1}{1} = 2 \text{ tablets}$$

Give 2 tablets po every day.

> ### FINE POINTS ● ○ ● ●
>
> Drawing a "circle" around the desired measurement system helps you know what you are solving for. This reminder is especially helpful when the equation becomes more complex.

Oral Liquid Medication Equation and Calculation

Follow the same basic rules of setting up the equation, using either the liquid medication available or the supply dose.

Example

Order: Zithromax (azithromycin) 150 mg po every day × 4 days

Supply: See Figure 11-3.

The equation is

$$\frac{150 \text{ mg}}{} \left| \frac{5 \text{ (mL)}}{200 \text{ mg}} \right.$$

Cancel the "mg." Reduce the fraction by dividing both numbers by 50. Continue the equation by multiplying the numerators and/or multiplying the denominators. Solve.

$$\frac{\overset{3}{\cancel{150}} \text{ mg}}{} \left| \frac{5 \text{ (mL)}}{\underset{4}{\cancel{200}} \text{ mg}} \right| \frac{3 \times 5}{4} = \frac{15}{4} = 3.75 \text{ mL}$$

Give 3.75 mL po every day × 4 days.

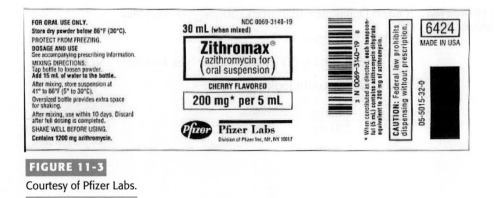

FIGURE 11-3

Courtesy of Pfizer Labs.

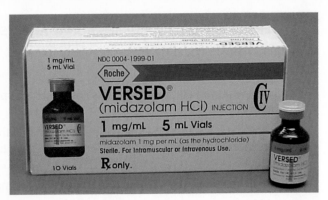

Parenteral Liquid Medication Equation and Calculation

Follow the same rules as with oral liquid.

Example   Order: Versed (midazolam) 2.5 mg IV q3–4h prn

Supply: See Figure 11-4.

The equation is

$$\frac{2.5\ \text{mg}\ \left|\ 1\ \text{mL}\right.}{\left|\ 1\ \text{mg}\right.}$$

Cancel the "mg." The fraction is already reduced. Solve.

$$\frac{2.5\ \cancel{\text{mg}}\ \left|\ 1\ \text{mL}\right.\ \left|\ 2.5 \times 1\right.}{\left|\ 1\ \cancel{\text{mg}}\right.\ \left|\ 1\right.} = 2.5\ \text{or}\ 2\tfrac{1}{2}\ \text{mL}$$

Give 2½ mL IV q3–4h prn. Follow dilution and administration guidelines.

Insulin Equation and Calculation

Follow the same basic set-up. The equation is the answer.

Example   Order: regular insulin 10 units subcutaneous now

Supply: See Figure 11-5.

The equation is

$$\frac{10\ \text{units}\ \left|\right.}{\left|\right.} = 10\ \text{units}$$

Use an insulin syringe.

Give 10 units subcutaneous.

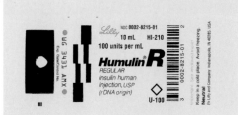

FIGURE 11-5

Courtesy of Eli Lilly Co.

STEPS TO SETTING UP A DIMENSIONAL ANALYSIS PROBLEM

1. Identify the desired dose. Place it in the numerator.
2. Identify the supply or available dose.
3. Identify what you are solving for (this is stated in the problem). Draw a "circle" around this measurement system.
4. Combine steps 1 and 2. Set up the problem so that the measurement systems that you do not need for the answer will cancel each other. This should leave the measurement system desired on the top of the equation.
5. If possible, reduce the fraction. Cancel out any like measurement systems.
6. Multiply the numbers in the numerator. Multiply the numbers in the denominator.
7. Divide the numerator by the denominator.

SELF-TEST 1   Calculation of Medications

Solve these problems using dimensional analysis. Answers are given at the end of the chapter. The answers show how to set up the problem and how to solve it.

1. Order: Xanax (alprazolam) 0.5 mg po bid
   Supply: Xanax (alprazolam) 0.25-mg tablets

2. Order: penicillin 800,000 units po q4h × 10 days
   Supply: 1 tablet equals 400,000 units

3. Order: Zithromax (azithromycin) 400 mg po every day × 4 days
   Supply: Zithromax (azithromycin) 200 mg/5 mL

4. Order: Deltasone (prednisone) 10 mg po tid
   Supply: tablets labeled 2.5 mg

5. Order: Lasix (furosemide) 60 mg po every day
   Supply: scored tablets labeled 40 mg

6. Order: Demerol (meperidine) 75 mg IV q4–6h prn
   Supply: Demerol (meperidine) 50 mg/mL

7. Order: Lanoxin (digoxin) 0.5 mg IV q4h × 3 doses
   Supply: Lanoxin (digoxin) 0.25 mg/mL

8. Order: heparin 1500 units subcutaneous bid
   Supply: heparin 5000 units/mL

9. Order: morphine 15 mg IV q4h prn
   Supply: morphine 10 mg/mL

10. Order: Solu Medrol (methylprednisolone) 80 mg IV every day
    Supply: Solu Medrol (methylprednisolone) 125 mg/2 mL

Dimensional Analysis Method With Equivalency Conversions

If the dosage desired and the dosage available are not in the same measurement system, an additional step is necessary. By using a conversion factor, you can convert the equation so that it contains only one measurement system.

Conversion factor, a term used in dimensional analysis, means the equivalents necessary to convert between systems of measurement. A conversion factor is a ratio of units that equals 1.

Example

Metric conversion factors

$$\frac{1 \text{ g}}{1000 \text{ mg}} \quad \text{or} \quad \frac{1000 \text{ mg}}{1 \text{ g}}$$

$$\frac{1 \text{ mg}}{1000 \text{ mcg}} \quad \text{or} \quad \frac{1000 \text{ mcg}}{1 \text{ mg}}$$

Each of these equals 1.

Metric apothecary conversion factors

$$\frac{60 \text{ mg (or 65 mg with aspirin and Tylenol)}}{1 \text{ gr}} \quad \text{or} \quad \frac{1 \text{ gr}}{60 \text{ mg (or 65 mg)}}$$

Each of these equal 1.

Metric/household conversion factors

$$\frac{1 \text{ tbsp}}{15 \text{ mL}} \quad \text{or} \quad \frac{15 \text{ mL}}{1 \text{ tbsp}}$$

$$\frac{1 \text{ tsp}}{5 \text{ mL}} \quad \text{or} \quad \frac{5 \text{ mL}}{1 \text{ tsp}}$$

$$\frac{1 \text{ kg}}{2.2 \text{ lb}} \quad \text{or} \quad \frac{2.2 \text{ lb}}{1 \text{ kg}}$$

$$\frac{16 \text{ oz}}{1 \text{ lb}} \quad \text{or} \quad \frac{1 \text{ lb}}{16 \text{ oz}}$$

Each of these equal 1.

Example

Order: Synthroid (levothyroxine) 150 mcg po every day

Supply: See Figure 11-6. Use 0.075 mg for this example.

$$\frac{150 \text{ mcg}}{} \left| \frac{1 \text{ tablet}}{0.075 \text{ mg}} \right.$$

Add a conversion factor to state the answer in mcg. 1 mg = 1000 mcg, so you include this conversion factor.

$$\frac{150 \text{ mcg}}{} \left| \frac{1 \text{ tablet}}{0.075 \text{ mg}} \right| \frac{1 \text{ mg}}{1000 \text{ mcg}}$$

Solve the problem in the same way as previous dimensional analysis examples. Cancel the measurement systems. Then reduce the fraction (dividing 50 into both 150 and 1000).

$$\frac{\overset{3}{150} \text{ mcg}}{} \left| \frac{1 \text{ tablet}}{0.075 \text{ mg}} \right| \frac{1 \text{ mg}}{\underset{20}{1000} \text{ mcg}} \left| \frac{3 \times 1 \times 1}{0.075 \times 20} \right. = \frac{3}{1.5} = 2 \text{ or 2 tablets}$$

Give 2 tablets po every day.

NDC 0074-5182-19
1000 TABLETS

SYNTHROID®

(levothyroxine sodium tablets, USP)

75 mcg   (0.075 mg)

Tablet identification marking change adopted August, 2002.

00745 18219

SPECIMEN

Rx only

Do not accept if seal over bottle opening is broken or missing.

See full prescribing information for dosage and administration.

Each tablet contains 75 mcg (0.075 mg) levothyroxine sodium.

Dispense in a tight, light-resistant container as described in USP.

Store at 25°C (77°F); excursions permitted to 15°-30°C (59°-86°F). [See USP Controlled Room Temperature]. Protect from light and moisture.

©Abbott

Abbott Laboratories
North Chicago, IL 60064, U.S.A.

02-8660-R2

FIGURE 11-6

Courtesy of Abbott Laboratories.

Example

Order: Romazicon (flumazenil) 200 mcg IV over 15 seconds for reversal of anesthesia

Supply: See Figure 11-7.

$$\frac{200 \text{ mcg}}{} \left| \frac{5 \text{ mL}}{0.5 \text{ mg}} \right| \frac{1 \text{ mg}}{1000 \text{ mcg}}$$

Reduce and solve (dividing 200 into both 200 and 1000).

$$\frac{\overset{1}{\cancel{200}} \text{ mcg}}{} \left| \frac{5 \text{ mL}}{0.5 \text{ mg}} \right| \frac{1 \text{ mg}}{\underset{5}{\cancel{1000}} \text{ mcg}} \left| \frac{1 \times 5 \times 1}{0.5 \times 5} = \frac{5}{2.5} = 2 \text{ mL} \right.$$

Give 2 mL IV over 15 seconds. Follow institutional requirements for diluting and administering IV drugs.

Place the same units of measurement opposite each other (one in the numerator, the other one in the denominator) in the equation. In this example, the two units of "mg" are placed on opposite sides in the fraction and the two "mcg" are placed on opposite sides. The two "mg" cancel each other and the two "mcg" cancel each other, leaving "mL" as the remaining unit of measurement.

An advantage to dimensional analysis is that you can place any conversion factor within the equation. This helps to reduce errors that may occur because a conversion was not included in the calculation.

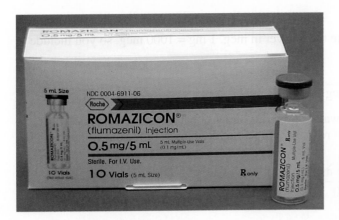

5 mL Size
NDC 0004-6911-06

Roche

ROMAZICON®

(flumazenil) Injection

0.5 mg/5 mL   5 mL Multiple-Use Vials (0.1 mg/mL)

Sterile. For I.V. Use.

10 Vials (5 mL Size)

10 Vials (5 mL Size)

R only

FIGURE 11-7

Reprinted with permission of Roche Laboratories, Inc. All rights reserved.

STEPS TO SETTING UP A DIMENSIONAL ANALYSIS PROBLEM

1. Identify the desired dose. Place it in the numerator.

2. Identify the supply or available dose.

3. Identify what you are solving for (this is stated in the problem). Draw a "circle" around this measurement system.

4. **Identify any conversions needed. Add the conversion factors to the equation. Add these to the equation so that like measurement systems will cancel each other.**

5. Combine steps 1 and 2. Set up the problem so that the measurement systems that you do not need for the answer will cancel each other. This should leave the measurement system desired on the top of the equation.

6. If possible, reduce the fraction. Cancel out any like measurement systems.

7. Multiply the numbers in the numerator. Multiply the numbers in the denominator.

8. Divide the numerator by the denominator.

SELF-TEST 2   Calculation of Medications Involving Equivalencies

Solve these problems using dimensional analysis. Answers are given at the end of the chapter. The answers show how to set up the problem and how to solve it.

1. Order: Motrin (ibuprofen) 0.8 g po bid
    Supply: 400-mg tablets

2. Order: Synthroid (levothyroxine) 0.3 mg po every day
    Supply: 300-mcg scored tablets

3. Order: codeine ½ gr po q4h prn
    Supply: 30-mg tablets

4. Order: Augmentin (amoxicillin/clavulunate acid) 500 mg
    Supply: Augmentin (amoxicillin/clavulunate acid) 250 mg/5 mL
    How many tsp?

5. Order: Tegretol (carbamazepine)100 mg po qid
    Supply: 100 mg/5 mL
    How many tsp?

6. Order: vitamin B12 1 mg IM every week
    Supply: 1000 mcg/mL

7. Order: ampicillin 500 mg IM q6h
    Supply: 1 g/mL

8. Order: epinephrine 0.4 mg subcutaneous × 1
    Supply: 1-mL ampule 1:1000 (Remember, 1:1000 = 1 g in 1000 mL)

9. Order: lidocaine 30 mg subcutaneous
    Supply: ampule labeled 2% (Remember, 2% = 2 g in 1000 mL)

10. Order: atropine gr 1/150 IM × 1
    Supply: atropine 0.4 mg/mL

Dimensional Analysis Method With Weight-Based Calculations

Medications that are calculated on the basis of weight will add a further step in the dimensional analysis method: the ordered dose must be multiplied by the weight or BSA.

Example

Order: Lasix (furosemide) 1 mg/kg IV bid for 12-year-old weighing 30 kg

Supply: See Figure 11-8.

Desired dose: 1 mg/kg

Set up the problem so that "kg" is in the denominator.

$$\frac{1 \text{ mg}}{\text{kg}}$$

Now add the supplied dose.

$$\frac{1 \text{ mg}}{\text{kg}} \bigg| \frac{1 \text{ mL}}{10 \text{ mg}}$$

Add the patient's weight in kg.

$$\frac{1 \text{ mg}}{\text{kg}} \bigg| \frac{1 \text{ mL}}{10 \text{ mg}} \bigg| \frac{30 \text{ kg}}{}$$

Proceed with the rest of the steps. Cancel out "mg" and "kg." Reduce the fraction. Multiply the numerators. Multiply the denominators. Divide the numerator by the denominator.

$$\frac{1 \text{ mg}}{\text{kg}} \bigg| \frac{1 \text{ mL}}{10 \text{ mg}} \bigg| \frac{\overset{3}{30} \text{ kg}}{1} \bigg| \frac{1 \times 1 \times 3}{1} = 3 \text{ mL}$$

Give 3 mL IV bid. Follow institutional requirements for diluting and administering IV drugs.

If the patient's weight is given in pounds, then use the conversion factor

$$\frac{1 \text{ kg}}{2.2 \text{ lb}}$$

to convert pounds to kilograms.

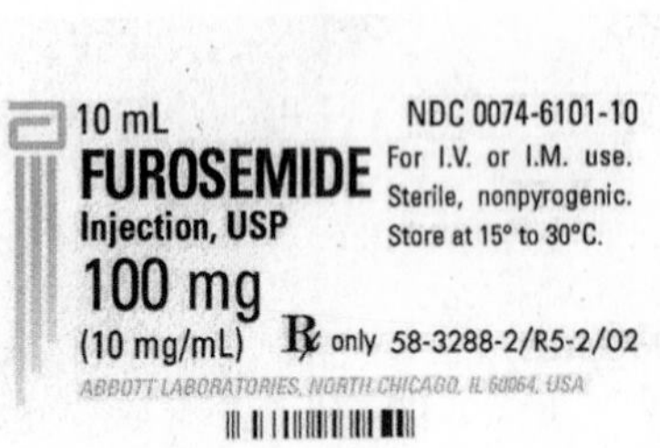

10 mL

FUROSEMIDE
Injection, USP

100 mg
(10 mg/mL)   ℞ only 58-3288-2/R5-2/02
ABBOTT LABORATORIES, NORTH CHICAGO, IL 60064, USA

NDC 0074-6101-10
For I.V. or I.M. use.
Sterile, nonpyrogenic.
Store at 15° to 30°C.

FIGURE 11-8
Courtesy of Abbott Laboratories.

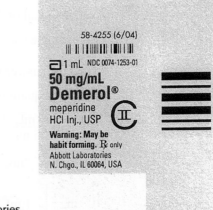

FIGURE 11-9
Courtesy of Abbott Laboratories.

Example

Order: Demerol (meperidine) 1.5 mg/kg IM q3–4h for pediatric patient weighing 75 lb

Supply: See Figure 11-9.

Set up the equation.

$$\frac{1.5 \text{ mg}}{\text{kg}} \left| \frac{1 \text{ mL}}{50 \text{ mg}} \right| \frac{75 \text{ lb}}{} \left| \frac{1 \text{ kg}}{2.2 \text{ lb}} \right.$$

Cancel "mg," "kg," and "lb." Reduce the fraction. Solve.

$$\frac{1.5 \text{ mg}}{\text{kg}} \left| \frac{1 \text{ mL}}{50 \text{ mg}} \right|^{3}_{2} \overset{3}{75} \text{ lb} \left| \frac{1 \text{ kg}}{2.2 \text{ lb}} \right| \frac{1.5 \times 1 \times 3 \times 1}{2 \times 2.2} = \frac{4.5}{4.4} = 1.02 \text{ or } 1 \text{ mL}$$

Give 1 mL IM q3–4h.

Calculation of Medications Based on BSA

Calculation of medications based on BSA is similar to setting up calculations for medications based on weight.

Example

Order: Zovirax (acyclovir) 500 mg/m² infused IV over 1 hour; BSA, 1.1 m²

Supply: reconstituted vial with concentration of 50 mg/mL

$$\frac{500 \text{ mg}}{\text{m}^2} \left| \frac{1 \text{ mL}}{50 \text{ mg}} \right| 1.1 \text{ m}^2$$

Cancel out the "mg" and the "m²." Reduce the fraction. Solve.

$$\overset{10}{\underset{}{500}} \text{ mg} \left| \frac{1 \text{ mL}}{\underset{1}{50} \text{ mg}} \right| 1.1 \text{ m}^2 \left| \frac{10 \times 1 \times 1.1}{1} = 11 \text{ mL} \right.$$

Give 11 mL IV over 1 hour.

If the weight-based medication is ordered in several doses, then add another step to the equation with the number of doses ordered. The solution will then be the amount of drug per dose.

Example

Order: Solu-Cortef (hydrocortisone) IM 10 mg/m²/day in 3 divided doses; BSA, 2.0 m²

Available: vial of 25 mg/mL

This example uses: $\dfrac{\text{day}}{3\text{ doses}}$

so that the answer will be the amount of drug for each dose.

Set up the equation.

$$\frac{10\text{ mg}}{\text{m}^2/\text{day}} \left| \frac{1\,\text{mL}}{25\text{ mg}} \right| 2.0\text{ m}^2 \left| \frac{\text{day}}{3\text{ doses}} \right.$$

Cancel "m²," "mg," "day." Reduce the fraction. Solve.

$$\frac{\cancel{10}^{\,2}\text{ mg}}{\cancel{\text{m}^2}/\cancel{\text{day}}} \left| \frac{1\,\text{mL}}{\cancel{25}_{\,5}\text{ mg}} \right| 2.0\,\cancel{\text{m}^2} \left| \frac{\cancel{\text{day}}}{3\,\text{doses}} \right| \frac{2\times1\times2}{5\times3} = \frac{4}{15} = 0.27\text{ mL/dose}$$

Give 0.27 mL IM per dose.

SELF-TEST 3   Calculation of Medications Using Weight or BSA

Solve these problems using dimensional analysis. Answers are given at the end of the chapter. The answers show how to set up the problem and how to solve it.

1. Order: Lasix (furosemide) 1 mg/kg IV; weight, 70 kg
   Supply: Lasix (furosemide) 10 mg/mL

2. Order: Augmentin (amoxicillin/clavulanate) 10 mg/kg po bid; weight, 30 kg
   Supply: Augmentin (amoxicillin/clavulanate) 125 mg/5 mL

3. Order: Keflex (cephalexin) 25 mg/kg/day in 4 divided doses; weight, 50 lb
   Supply: Keflex (cephalexin) 250 mg/5 mL
   How much per dose?

4. Order: Decadron (dexamethasone) 0.4 mg/kg/day in 4 divided doses; weight, 25 lb
   Supply: Decadron (dexamethasone) 4 mg/mL
   How much per dose?

5. Order: methotrexate 10 mg/m²/dose q week; BSA, 1.29 m²
   Supply: methotrexate 2.5-mg tablets

Dimensional Analysis Method With Reconstitution of Medications

These calculations are set up with the same method as parenteral calculations. Follow the reconstitution directions and use the result as the dosage available.

Example

Order: Rocephin 1 g IV q12h

Supply: Reconstitute with 9.6 mL sterile water to yield 100 mg/mL (Fig. 11-10).

Use the conversion factor of 1 g = 1000 mg.

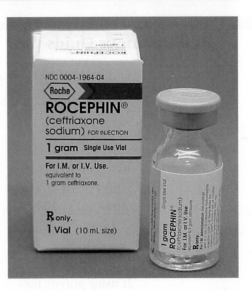

$$\frac{1 \text{ g}}{} \left| \frac{1 \text{ mL}}{100 \text{ mg}} \right| \frac{1000 \text{ mg}}{1 \text{ g}}$$

Cancel "mg" and "g." Reduce the fraction. Solve.

$$\frac{1 \cancel{\text{g}}}{} \left| \frac{1 \cancel{\text{mL}}}{\underset{1}{\cancel{100}} \cancel{\text{mg}}} \right| \frac{\overset{10}{\cancel{1000}} \cancel{\text{mg}}}{1 \cancel{\text{g}}} \right| \frac{1 \times 1 \times 10}{1 \times 1} = 10 \text{ mL}$$

Follow institutional requirements for dilution and administration of IV drugs.

SELF-TEST 4   Reconstitution

Solve these problems using dimensional analysis. Answers are given at the end of the chapter. The answers show how to set up the problem and how to solve it.

1. Order: Monocid (cefonicid) 0.5 g IM q12h
    Supply: 1-g vial of powder. Follow reconstitution directions to yield solution 250 mg/mL.

2. Order: penicillin 1 million units IM q6h
    Supply: 5-million-unit vial. Follow reconstitution directions to yield solution
              1 million units/mL.

3. Order: Ancef (cefazolin) 0.3 g IM
    Supply: 500 mg powder. Follow reconstitution directions to yield solution 225 mg/mL.

4. Order: Unasyn (ampicillin/sulbactam) 1500 mg IV q8h
    Supply: Unasyn (ampicillin/sulbactam) 1.5-g vial. Follow reconstitution directions to yield
              solution 1.5 g/5 mL.

5. Order: Fortaz (ceftazidime) 0.25 g
    Supply: Fortaz (ceftazidime) vial. Follow reconstitution directions to yield solution 500 mg/mL.

Dimensional Analysis Method With Calculation of Intravenous Fluids

Example

Order: D5W 1000 mL over 10 hr

To calculate mL/hr set up the equation:

$$\frac{1000 \text{ mL}}{10 \text{ hour}}$$

Reduce the fraction.

$$\frac{\overset{100}{\cancel{1000}} \text{ (mL)}}{\underset{1}{\cancel{10}} \text{ (hr)}} \Bigg| \frac{100}{1} = 100 \text{ mL/hr}$$

If an infusion pump is used, then the rate will be 100 mL/hr.

If using gravity flow tubing, then the equation will include the drop or tubing factor, and you must convert the "hour" to "minutes." To do this, use the conversion factor:

$$\frac{1 \text{ hour}}{60 \text{ minutes}}$$

Example

Order: D5W 1000 mL over 10 hr

Supply: Drop factor of 20 gtts/mL

$$\frac{1000 \text{ mL}}{10 \text{ hr}} \Bigg| \frac{20 \text{ gtts}}{\text{mL}} \Bigg| \frac{1 \text{ hr}}{60 \text{ min}}$$

Cancel the "mL" and the "hr." Reduce the fraction. Solve.

$$\frac{\overset{100}{\cancel{1000}} \text{ mL}}{\underset{1}{\cancel{10}} \text{ hr}} \Bigg| \frac{\overset{1}{\cancel{20}} \text{ (gtts)}}{\cancel{\text{mL}}} \Bigg| \frac{1 \text{ hr}}{\underset{3}{\cancel{60}} \text{ (min)}} \Bigg| \frac{100 \times 1 \times 1}{1 \times 3} = \frac{100}{3} = 33.3 \text{ or } 33 \text{ gtts/min}$$

SELF-TEST 5   **Basic IV Calculations and Drop Factors**

Solve these problems using dimensional analysis. Answers are given at the end of the chapter. The answers show how to set up the problem and how to solve it.

1. Order: D5½ NS 1000 mL over 8 hr
   How many mL/hr?

2. Order: D5W 500 mL over 5 hr
   How many mL/hr?

3. Order: NS 250 mL over 5 hr
   How many mL/hr?

4. Order: whole blood 500 mL over 4 hr
   How many mL/hr?

(continued)

SELF-TEST 5 **Basic IV Calculations and Drop Factors (Continued)**

5. Order: NS 250 mL over 2 hr; drop factor, 20 gtts/mL
   How many gtts/minute?

6. Order: D5W 100 mL over 30 min; drop factor, 15 gtts/mL
   How many gtts/minute?

7. Order: NS 500 mL over 4 hr; drop factor, 60 gtts/mL
   How many gtts/minute?

8. Order: D5W 300 mL over 90 minutes; drop factor 60 gtts/mL
   How many gtts/minute?

9. Order: NS 1000 mL over 8 hr; drop factor, 20 gtts/mL
   How many gtts/minute?

10. Order: ½ NS 500 mL over 4 hr; drop factor, 10 gtts/mL
    How many gtts/minute?

Dimensional Analysis Method With Advanced Intravenous Calculations

You can use the dimensional analysis method to calculate medications that are administered with continuous IV infusion. Infusion pumps are always used.

Calculating mL/hr

Example   Order: heparin 1200 units/hr per infusion pump

How many mL/hr? (Infusion pumps are set in mL/hr)

Supply: See Figure 11-11. Heparin 25,000 units in 500 mL ½ NS

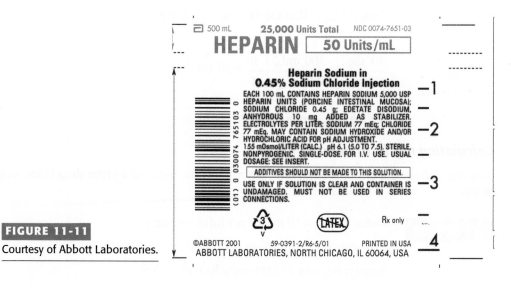

FIGURE 11-11
Courtesy of Abbott Laboratories.

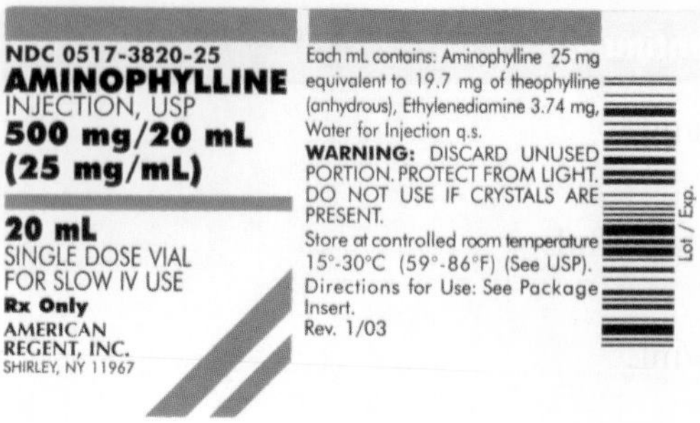

NDC 0517-3820-25
AMINOPHYLLINE
INJECTION, USP
500 mg/20 mL
(25 mg/mL)

20 mL
SINGLE DOSE VIAL
FOR SLOW IV USE
Rx Only
AMERICAN
REGENT, INC.
SHIRLEY, NY 11967

Each mL contains: Aminophylline 25 mg
equivalent to 19.7 mg of theophylline
(anhydrous), Ethylenediamine 3.74 mg,
Water for Injection q.s.
WARNING: DISCARD UNUSED
PORTION. PROTECT FROM LIGHT.
DO NOT USE IF CRYSTALS ARE
PRESENT.
Store at controlled room temperature
15°-30°C (59°-86°F) (See USP).
Directions for Use: See Package
Insert.
Rev. 1/03

FIGURE 11-12
Courtesy of American Regent, Inc.

Set up the equation.

$$\frac{1200 \text{ units}}{\text{hr}} \quad \frac{500 \text{ mL}}{25000 \text{ units}}$$

Cancel "units." Reduce the fraction. Solve.

$$\frac{1200 \text{ units}}{\text{hr}} \quad \frac{\overset{1}{500} \text{ mL}}{\underset{50}{25000} \text{ units}} \quad \frac{1200}{50} = 24 \text{ mL/hr}$$

Set pump at 24 mL/hr.

Example   Order: aminophylline 30 mg/hr per infusion pump

How many mL/hr?

Supply: See Figure 11-12. Aminophylline 500 mg/500 mL D5W

Set up the equation.

$$\frac{30 \text{ mg}}{\text{hr}} \quad \frac{500 \text{ mL}}{500 \text{ mg}}$$

Cancel "mg." Reduce the fraction. Solve.

$$\frac{30 \text{ mg}}{\text{hr}} \quad \frac{\overset{1}{500} \text{ mL}}{\underset{1}{500} \text{ mg}} \quad \frac{30}{1} = 30 \text{ mL/hr}$$

Set the infusion pump at 30 mL/hour.

Calculating mg/hr or units/hr

You can also use dimensional analysis to determine how much of a given drug is infusing per an infusion pump.

Example   Order: heparin 10 mL/hr per infusion pump

How many units infusing per hour?

Supply: heparin 25,000 units/500 mL ½ NS.

Set up the equation.

$$\frac{10 \text{ mL}}{\text{hr}} \quad \frac{25,000 \text{ units}}{500 \text{ mL}}$$

Cancel "mL." Reduce the fraction. Solve.

$$\frac{10 \ \cancel{mL}}{\cancel{hr}} \ \Bigg| \ \frac{\overset{50}{\cancel{25,000}} \ \text{\small(units)}}{\underset{1}{\cancel{500} \ \cancel{mL}}} \ \Bigg| \ \frac{10 \times 50}{1} = 500 \ \text{units/hr}$$

Example

Order: calcium gluconate 25 mL/hr

How many grams are infusing per hour?

Supply: calcium gluconate 1 g in 100 mL D5W.

Set up the equation.

$$\frac{25 \ mL}{hr} \ \Bigg| \ \frac{1 \ \text{\small(g)}}{100 \ mL}$$

Cancel "mL." Reduce the fraction. Solve.

$$\frac{\overset{1}{\cancel{25}} \ \cancel{mL}}{\cancel{hr}} \ \Bigg| \ \frac{1 \ \text{\small(g)}}{\underset{4}{\cancel{100}} \ \cancel{mL}} \ \Bigg| \ \frac{1}{4} = \frac{1}{4} \ \text{or} \ 0.25 \ \text{g/hr}$$

Calculating mL/hr for Drugs Ordered in mg or mcg/min

Vasoactive drugs are ordered in dosages per minute. Use the conversion factor: $\dfrac{60 \ \text{min}}{1 \ \text{hr}}$

Example

Order: Pronestyl (procainamide) 3 mg/min per infusion pump

How many mL/hr?

Available: See Figure 11-13. Procainamide 1 g/250 mL D5W

Set up the equation. Use the conversion factor $\dfrac{1 \ \text{g}}{1000 \ \text{mg}}$.

Use $\dfrac{60 \ \text{min}}{1 \ \text{hr}}$ because the order is in minutes but the answer will be in hours.

$$\frac{3 \ mg}{min} \ \Bigg| \ \frac{250 \ \text{\small(mL)}}{1 \ g} \ \Bigg| \ \frac{1 \ g}{1000 \ mg} \ \Bigg| \ \frac{60 \ min}{\text{\small(hr)}}$$

Cancel "mg," "g," and "min." Reduce the fraction. Solve.

$$\frac{3 \ \cancel{mg}}{\cancel{min}} \ \Bigg| \ \frac{\overset{1}{\cancel{250}} \ \text{\small(mL)}}{1 \ \cancel{g}} \ \Bigg| \ \frac{1 \ \cancel{g}}{\underset{4}{\cancel{1000}} \ \cancel{mg}} \ \Bigg| \ \frac{60 \ \cancel{min}}{\text{\small(hr)}} \ \Bigg| \ \frac{3 \times 1 \times 1 \times 60}{1 \times 4} = \frac{180}{4} = 45 \ \text{mL/hr}$$

Set the infusion pump at 45 mL/hr to deliver 3 mg/min.

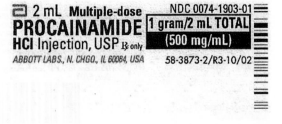

FIGURE 11-13
Courtesy of Abbott Laboratories.

Example

Order: nitroglycerine 30 mcg/min per infusion pump

How many mL/hr?

Supply: nitroglycerine 50 mg in 250 mL D5W

Set up the equation. Use the conversion factor: $\dfrac{1 \text{ mg}}{1000 \text{ mcg}}$.

$$\frac{30 \text{ mcg}}{\text{min}} \left| \frac{250 \text{ (mL)}}{50 \text{ mg}} \right| \frac{1 \text{ mg}}{1000 \text{ mcg}} \left| \frac{60 \text{ min}}{\text{(hr)}} \right.$$

Cancel "mcg," "mg," and "min." Reduce the fraction. Solve.

$$\frac{30 \text{ mcg}}{\text{min}} \left| \frac{\overset{1}{\cancel{250}} \text{ (mL)}}{\underset{10}{\cancel{50}} \text{ mg}} \right| \frac{1 \text{ mg}}{\underset{4}{\cancel{1000}} \text{ mcg}} \left| \frac{\overset{12}{\cancel{60}} \text{ min}}{\text{(hr)}} \right| \frac{30 \times 1 \times 1 \times 12}{10 \times 4} = \frac{360}{40} = 9 \text{ mL/hr}$$

Set the infusion pump at 9 mL/hr to deliver 30 mcg/minute.

Calculating mL/hr for Drugs Ordered in mcg/kg/min

Vasoactive drugs such as dobutamine, dopamine, nipride, and others are ordered in dosages per kilogram per minute. If needed, convert pounds to kilograms using the conversion factor: $\dfrac{1 \text{ kg}}{2.2 \text{ lb}}$. Then use the conversion factor: $\dfrac{60 \text{ min}}{1 \text{ hr}}$ to convert minutes to hours.

Example

Order: Infuse Intropin (dopamine) at 2 mcg/kg/min per infusion pump.

How many mL/hr?

Available: dopamine 800 mg/500 mL D5W; weight, 70 kg (Fig. 11-14). (Label represents a single dose; this will be mixed in 500 mL.)

Set up the equation. Use the conversion factor: $\dfrac{1 \text{ mg}}{1000 \text{ mcg}}$.

$$\frac{2 \text{ mcg}}{\text{kg/min}} \left| \frac{500 \text{ (mL)}}{800 \text{ mg}} \right| \frac{1 \text{ mg}}{1000 \text{ mcg}} \left| \frac{70 \text{ kg}}{} \right| \frac{60 \text{ min}}{\text{(hr)}}$$

Cancel "mcg," "mg," "kg," and "min." Reduce the fraction. Solve.

$$\frac{2 \text{ mcg}}{\text{kg/min}} \left| \frac{\overset{1}{\cancel{500}} \text{ (mL)}}{\cancel{800} \text{ mg}} \right| \frac{1 \text{ mg}}{\underset{2}{\cancel{1000}} \text{ mcg}} \left| \frac{70 \text{ kg}}{} \right| \frac{\cancel{60} \text{ min}}{\text{(hr)}} \left| \frac{2 \times 1 \times 1 \times 7 \times 6}{8 \times 2} \right.$$

$$= \frac{84}{16} = 5.25 \text{ or } 5 \text{ mL/hr}$$

Set the infusion pump at 5 mL/hr to deliver 2 mcg/kg/min for a 70-kg patient.

NDC 0517-1305-25
DOPamine HCl
INJECTION, USP
800 mg/5 mL
(160 mg/mL)

5 mL SINGLE DOSE VIAL
WARNING: NOT FOR DIRECT IV INJECTION
MUST BE DILUTED BEFORE USE
IV INFUSION ONLY
Rx Only
AMERICAN REGENT
LABORATORIES, INC.
SHIRLEY, NY 11967

PROTECT FROM LIGHT. Store at controlled room
temperature 15°-30°C (59°-86°F) (See USP).
DO NOT USE IF DARKER THAN SLIGHTLY YELLOW OR
DISCOLORED IN ANY OTHER WAY. AVOID CONTACT
WITH ALKALIES (INCLUDING SODIUM BICARBONATE)
OXIDIZING AGENTS OR IRON SALTS.
DISCARD UNUSED PORTION.
Directions for Use: See Package Insert.
Rev. 5/01

FIGURE 11-14

Courtesy of American Regent Laboratories, Inc.

Heparin and Insulin Intravenous Calculations

Heparin Protocol

Weight based heparin calculations will use a protocol such as the one in Chapter 9 (p. 254). One advantage to the dimensional analysis method is that two calculations will be combined into one equation (see step 2 below).

Sample heparin protocol:

Heparin drip: 25000 units in 500 mL

Bolus: 80 units/kg

Starting Dose: 18 units/kg/hr

Example Patient weight is 70 kg.

1. Calculation for bolus dose: 80 units/kg

   The dimensional analysis equation will look like:

   $$\frac{80\ \text{units}}{1\ \text{kg}} \left| 70\ \text{kg} \right.$$

   Cancel "kg". Multiply the numerators. Solve.

   $$\frac{80\ \cancel{\text{units}}}{1\ \cancel{\text{kg}}} \left| 70\ \cancel{\text{kg}} \right| \frac{80 \times 70}{} = 5600\ \text{units}$$

2. Infusion rate. The answer will be in mL/hr on an infusion pump.

   Heparin drip: 25000 units in 500 mL.

   Set up the equation:

   $$\frac{80\ \text{units}}{\text{kg/hr}} \left| \frac{500\ \text{mL}}{25000\ \text{units}} \right| 70\ \text{kg}$$

   Cancel "kg", "units". Reduce the fraction. Solve.

   $$\frac{18\ \cancel{\text{units}}}{\cancel{\text{kg}}\,/\text{hr}} \left| \frac{\overset{1}{\cancel{500}}\ \text{mL}}{\underset{50}{\cancel{25\,000}}\ \cancel{\text{units}}} \right| 70\ \cancel{\text{kg}} \left| \frac{18 \times 70}{50} = 25.2\ \text{mL/hr} \right.$$

3. The PTT result 6 hours after the infusion started is 50. According to the table, (p. 254) we increase the drip by 1 u/kg/hr.

   Set up the equation:

   $$\frac{1\ \text{unit}}{\text{kg/hr}} \left| \frac{500\ \text{mL}}{25000\ \text{units}} \right| 70\ \text{kg}$$

   Cancel "kg", "units". Reduce the fraction. Solve.

   $$\frac{1\ \cancel{\text{unit}}}{\cancel{\text{kg}}\,/\text{hr}} \left| \frac{\overset{1}{\cancel{500}}\ \text{mL}}{\underset{50}{\cancel{25000}}\ \cancel{\text{units}}} \right| 70\ \cancel{\text{kg}} \left| \frac{70}{50} = 1.4\ \text{mL} \right.$$

   Increase the drip by 1.4 mL: 25.2 + 1.4 = 26.6 mL/hr

   Repeat PTT in 6 hours and titrate per protocol

Insulin Protocol

Continuous insulin infusions based on blood sugar will use a protocol such as the one in Chapter 9 (page 257).

Sample insulin protocol:

If blood glucose > 150, give IV regular insulin—bolus of 0.1 units/kg

Initiate infusion rate at the calculated dose:

BG (blood glucose) − 60 × 0.02 = units insulin/hr

Example   Patient weight 70 kg. Blood glucose 200.

1. Calculate the bolus dose.

   The dimensional analysis equation will be:

   $$\frac{0.1 \text{ units} \mid 70 \text{ kg}}{1 \text{ kg} \mid}$$

   Cancel "kg". Multiply the numerators. Solve.

   $$\frac{0.1 \text{ units} \mid 70 \text{ kg}}{1 \text{ kg} \mid} \frac{0.1 \times 70}{} = 7 \text{ units regular insulin IV}$$

2. Calculate the infusion rate.

   Regular insulin 100 units in 100 mL of NS.

   Calculate the number of units:

   $(200 - 60) \times 0.02 = 2.8$ units/hr

   Then set up the equation. The answer will be in mL/hr on an infusion pump.

   $$\frac{2.8 \text{ units} \mid 100 \text{ mL}}{\text{hr} \mid 100 \text{ units}}$$

   Cancel "units". Reduce the fraction. Solve.

   $$\frac{2.8 \text{ units} \mid 100 \text{ mL} \mid 2.8 \text{ mL}}{\text{hr} \mid 100 \text{ units} \mid \text{hr}} = 2.8 \text{ mL/hr}$$

   Set the infusion pump at 2.8 mL/hr.

   Recheck the blood glucose in 1 hour and titrate according to the insulin protocol.

SELF-TEST 6 **Advanced IV Calculations**

Solve these problems using dimensional analysis. Answers are given at the end of the chapter. The answers show how to set up the problem and how to solve it.

1. Order: Infuse heparin at 1000 units/hr via infusion pump
   Supply: heparin 25,000 units in 250 mL D5W IV
   How many mL/hr?

2. Order: Infuse insulin at 20 units/hr via infusion pump
   Supply: insulin 125 units in 250 mL NS IV
   How many mL/hr?

3. Order: Infuse aminophylline at 50 mg/hr via infusion pump
   Supply: aminophylline 250 mg in 250 mL D5W
   How many mL/hr?

4. Order: Infuse heparin at 40 mL/hr
   Supply: heparin 25,000 units in 500 mL D5W
   How many units are infusing per hour?

5. Order: Infuse aminophylline at 60 mL/hr
   Supply: aminophylline 500 mg/250 mL D5W
   How many mg are infusing per hour?

6. Order: Infuse Bretylol (bretylium) 2 mg/min via infusion pump
   Supply: Bretylol (bretylium) 1 g/500 mL D5W
   How many mL/hr?

7. Order: lidocaine 3 mg/min via infusion pump
   Supply: lidocaine 2 g/500 mL D5W
   How many mL/hr?

8. Order: nitroglycerine 20 mcg/min via infusion pump
   Supply: nitroglycerin 50 mg/250 mL D5W
   How many mL/hr?

9. Order: Isuprel (isoproterenol) 5 mcg/min via infusion pump
   Supply: Isuprel (isoproterenol) 2 mg/250 mL D5W
   How many mL/hr?

10. Order: Intropin (dopamine) 5 mcg/kg/min via infusion pump
    Supply: Intropin (dopamine) 200 mg/250 mL D5W; weight, 70 kg
    How many mL/hr?

11. Order: Pitocin (oxytocin) 5 milliunits/min via infusion pump
    Supply: Pitocin (oxytocin) 15 units/250 mL NS
    Solve using the same equation used for questions 8 and 9. Use the equivalency
    1 unit = 1000 milliunits.
    How many mL/hr?

12. Order: Nipride (nitroprusside) 2 mcg/kg/min via infusion pump
    Supply: Nipride (nitroprusside) 50 mg/250 mL D5W; weight, 110 lb
    How many mL/hr?

PROFICIENCY TEST 1   Dimensional Analysis

Solve these problems using the dimensional analysis method. Set up the equation first, then cancel out any like measurement systems, reduce the fraction, and solve. Answers are given in Appendix A.

1. Order: Augmentin (amoxicillin) 500 mg q8h
   Supply: 125 mg/5 mL

2. Order: heparin 5000 units subcutaneous bid
   Supply: heparin 10,000 units/mL

3. Order: Lasix (furosemide) 20 mg IV bid
   Supply: Lasix (furosemide) 40 mg/4 mL

4. Order: Halcion (triazolam) 0.25 mg po at bedtime
   Supply: Halcion (triazolam) 0.125 mg/tablet

5. Order: Tylenol (acetaminophen) elixir 650 mg po q4h
   Supply: Tylenol (acetaminophen) elixir 325 mg/5 mL

6. Order: calcium gluconate 0.5 g IV × 1
   Supply: calcium gluconate 10%

7. Order: Lanoxin (digoxin) 125 mcg IV every day
   Supply: Lanoxin (digoxin) 0.25 mg/mL

8. Order: Amoxil (amoxicillin) 375 mg q6h
   Supply: Amoxil (amoxicillin) 125 mg/5 mL
   How many tsp?

9. Order: nitroglycerine 1/150 gr SL × 3
   Supply: 0.4-mg tablets

10. Order: Tylenol (acetaminophen) 5 gr q3–4h prn
    Supply: Tylenol (acetaminophen) elixir 325 mg/5 mL

11. Order: Deltasone (prednisone) 40 mg/m² × 1 dose; BSA, 0.44 m²
    What is the calculated dose?

12. Order: morphine 0.1 to 0.2 mg/kg IM; weight, 32 lb
    Supply: 10 mg/mL

13. Order: Ancef (cefazolin) 0.44 g IM q12h
    Supply: Ancef (cefazolin) vial
    Follow reconstitution directions to yield solution 330 mg/1 mL

14. Order: penicillin 1 million units
    Supply: penicillin vial
    Follow reconstitution directions to yield solution 500,000 units/1 mL.

15. Order: D5W 500 mL over 6 hr
    How many mL/hr?

16. Order: NS 1000 mL over 16 hr
    How many mL/hr?

17. Order: D5W 1000 mL over 10 hr
    Drop factor is 60 gtt/mL. How many gtts/minute?

18. Order: D5W 250 mL over 2 hr
    Drop factor is 15 gtts/mL. How many gtts/minute?

(continued)

19. Order: regular insulin 5 units/hr via infusion pump
Supply: regular insulin 125 units/125 mL NS
How many mL/hr?

20. Order: heparin 1500 units/hr via infusion pump
Supply: heparin 25,000 units/500 mL D5W
How many mL/hr?

21. Order: heparin 30 mL/hr via infusion pump
Supply: heparin 25,000 units/250 mL D5W
How many units infusing per hour?

22. Order: nitroglycerine 15 mcg/min per infusion pump
Supply: nitroglycerine 50 mg/250 mL D5W
How many mL/hr?

23. Order: Pronestyl (procainamide) 2 mg/min per infusion pump
Supply: Pronestyl (procainamide) 2 g/500 mL D5W
How many mL/hr?

24. Order: Dobutrex (dobutamine) 10 mcg/kg/min per infusion pump
Supply: Dobutrex (dobutamine) 500 mg/500 mL D5W; weight, 100 kg
How many mL/hr?

25. Order: Nipride (nitroprusside) 5 mcg/kg/min per infusion pump
Supply: Nipride (nitroprusside) 50 mg/250 mL D5W; weight, 220 lb
How many mL/hr?

26. Order: Blood glucose 300. Use formula $BG - 60 \times 0.02 =$ units insulin/hr
Supply: 100 units regular insulin in 100 mL NS
How many mL/hr?

27. Order: Blood glucose 400. Use same formula as number 26.
Supply: 100 units regular insulin in 100 mL NS
How many mL/hr?

28. Order: Starting dose Heparin 16 units/kg/hr
Supply: Heparin 25000 units in 500 mL
Patients weight 50 kg.
How many mL/hr?

29. Order: Heparin bolus dose 60 units/kg
Patients weight 110 lbs.
What is the bolus dose?

30. Order: Increase Heparin drip by 2 units/kg/hr
Supply: Heparin 25000 units/500 mL NS
Current rate: 21.5 mL/hr
Patients weight: 120 lb.
How many mL/hr?

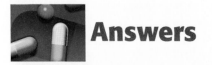

Answers

Self-Test 1 Calculation of Medications

1. $\dfrac{0.5\ \text{mg}\ \big|\ 1\ \text{tablet}}{\big|\ 0.25\ \text{mg}}$

$\dfrac{\overset{2}{\cancel{0.5}}\ \text{mg}\ \big|\ 1\ \cancel{\text{tablet}}}{\big|\ \underset{1}{\cancel{0.25}}\ \text{mg}}\ \bigg|\ \dfrac{2\times 1}{} = 2\ \text{tablets}$

2. $\dfrac{800{,}000\ \text{units}\ \big|\ 1\ \text{tablet}}{\big|\ 400{,}000\ \text{units}}$

$\dfrac{\overset{2}{\cancel{800{,}000}}\ \cancel{\text{units}}\ \big|\ 1\ \cancel{\text{tablet}}}{\big|\ \underset{1}{\cancel{400{,}000}}\ \cancel{\text{units}}}\ \bigg|\ \dfrac{2\times 1}{} = 2\ \text{tablets}$

3. $\dfrac{400\ \text{mg}\ \big|\ 5\ \text{mL}}{\big|\ 200\ \text{mg}}$

$\dfrac{\overset{2}{\cancel{400}}\ \text{mg}\ \big|\ 5\ \cancel{\text{mL}}}{\big|\ \underset{1}{\cancel{200}}\ \text{mg}}\ \bigg|\ \dfrac{2\times 5}{} = 10\ \text{mL}$

4. $\dfrac{10\ \text{mg}\ \big|\ 1\ \text{tablet}}{\big|\ 2.5\ \text{mg}}$

$\dfrac{\overset{4}{\cancel{10}}\ \text{mg}\ \big|\ 1\ \cancel{\text{tablet}}}{\big|\ \underset{1}{\cancel{2.5}}\ \text{mg}}\ \bigg|\ \dfrac{4\times 1}{} = 4\ \text{tablets}$

5. $\dfrac{60\ \text{mg}\ \big|\ 1\ \text{tablet}}{\big|\ 40\ \text{mg}}$

$\dfrac{\overset{3}{\cancel{60}}\ \text{mg}\ \big|\ 1\ \cancel{\text{tablet}}}{\big|\ \underset{2}{\cancel{40}}\ \text{mg}}\ \bigg|\ \dfrac{3\times 1}{2} = \dfrac{3}{2} = 1.5\ \text{or}\ 1\tfrac{1}{2}\ \text{tablets}$

6. $\dfrac{75\ \text{mg}\ \big|\ 1\ \text{mL}}{\big|\ 50\ \text{mg}}$

$\dfrac{\overset{3}{\cancel{75}}\ \text{mg}\ \big|\ 1\ \cancel{\text{mL}}}{\big|\ \underset{2}{\cancel{50}}\ \text{mg}}\ \bigg|\ \dfrac{3\times 1}{2} = \dfrac{3}{2} = 1.5\ \text{mL}$

7. $\dfrac{0.5 \text{ mg}}{} \Big| \dfrac{1 \text{ mL}}{0.25 \text{ mg}}$

$\dfrac{\overset{2}{\cancel{0.5}} \text{ mg}}{} \Big| \dfrac{1 \,\text{\textcircled{mL}}}{\underset{1}{\cancel{0.25}} \text{ mg}} \Big| \dfrac{2 \times 1}{1} = 2 \text{ mL}$

8. $\dfrac{1500 \text{ units}}{} \Big| \dfrac{1 \text{ mL}}{5000 \text{ units}}$

$\dfrac{\overset{3}{\cancel{1500}} \text{ units}}{} \Big| \dfrac{1 \,\text{\textcircled{mL}}}{\underset{10}{\cancel{5000}} \text{ units}} \Big| \dfrac{3 \times 1}{10} = \dfrac{3}{10} \text{ or } 0.3 \text{ mL}$

9. $\dfrac{15 \text{ mg}}{} \Big| \dfrac{1 \text{ mL}}{10 \text{ mg}}$

$\dfrac{\overset{3}{\cancel{15}} \text{ mg}}{} \Big| \dfrac{1 \,\text{\textcircled{mL}}}{\underset{2}{\cancel{10}} \text{ mg}} \Big| \dfrac{3 \times 1}{2} = \dfrac{3}{2} = 1.5 \text{ mL}$

10. $\dfrac{80 \text{ mg}}{} \Big| \dfrac{2 \text{ mL}}{125 \text{ mg}}$

$\dfrac{\overset{16}{\cancel{80}} \text{ mg}}{} \Big| \dfrac{2 \,\text{\textcircled{mL}}}{\underset{25}{\cancel{125}} \text{ mg}} \Big| \dfrac{16 \times 2}{25} = \dfrac{32}{25} = 1.28 \text{ or } 1.3 \text{ mL}$

Self-Test 2 Calculation of Medications Involving Equivalencies

1. $\dfrac{0.8 \text{ g}}{} \Big| \dfrac{1 \text{ tablet}}{400 \text{ mg}} \Big| \dfrac{1000 \text{ mg}}{1 \text{ g}}$

$\dfrac{0.8 \,\cancel{\text{g}}}{} \Big| \dfrac{1 \,\text{\textcircled{tablet}}}{\cancel{400} \text{ mg}} \Big| \dfrac{\cancel{1000} \text{ mg}}{1 \,\cancel{\text{g}}} \Big| \dfrac{0.8 \times 1 \times 10}{4 \times 1} = \dfrac{8}{4} = 2 \text{ tablets}$

2. $\dfrac{0.3 \text{ mg}}{} \Big| \dfrac{1 \text{ tablet}}{300 \text{ mcg}} \Big| \dfrac{1000 \text{ mcg}}{1 \text{ mg}}$

$\dfrac{0.3 \,\cancel{\text{mg}}}{} \Big| \dfrac{1 \,\text{\textcircled{tablet}}}{\cancel{300} \text{ mcg}} \Big| \dfrac{\cancel{1000} \text{ mcg}}{1 \,\cancel{\text{mg}}} \Big| \dfrac{0.3 \times 1 \times 10}{3 \times 1} = \dfrac{3}{3} = 1 \text{ tablet}$

3. $\dfrac{\frac{1}{2} \text{ gr}}{} \Big| \dfrac{1 \text{ tablet}}{30 \text{ mg}} \Big| \dfrac{60 \text{ mg}}{1 \text{ gr}}$

$\dfrac{\frac{1}{2} \,\cancel{\text{gr}}}{} \Big| \dfrac{1 \,\text{\textcircled{tablet}}}{\underset{1}{\cancel{30}} \text{ mg}} \Big| \dfrac{\overset{2}{\cancel{60}} \text{ mg}}{1 \,\cancel{\text{gr}}} \Big| \dfrac{\frac{1}{2} \times 1 \times 2}{1} = \dfrac{2}{2} = 1 \text{ tablet}$

4. $\dfrac{500\ \text{mg}}{}\ \Big|\ \dfrac{5\ \text{mL}}{250\ \text{mg}}\ \Big|\ \dfrac{1\ \text{tsp}}{5\ \text{mL}}$

$$\dfrac{\overset{2}{\cancel{500}}\ \text{mg}}{}\ \Bigg|\ \dfrac{\overset{1}{\cancel{5}}\ \text{mL}}{\underset{1}{\cancel{250}}\ \text{mg}}\ \Bigg|\ \dfrac{1\ \boxed{\text{tsp}}}{\underset{1}{\cancel{5}}\ \text{mL}}\ \Bigg|\ \dfrac{2 \times 1}{} = 2\ \text{tsp}$$

5. $\dfrac{100\ \text{mg}}{}\ \Big|\ \dfrac{5\ \text{mL}}{100\ \text{mg}}\ \Big|\ \dfrac{1\ \text{tsp}}{5\ \text{mL}}$

$$\dfrac{\overset{1}{\cancel{100}}\ \text{mg}}{}\ \Bigg|\ \dfrac{\overset{1}{\cancel{5}}\ \text{mL}}{\underset{1}{\cancel{100}}\ \text{mg}}\ \Bigg|\ \dfrac{1\ \boxed{\text{tsp}}}{\underset{1}{\cancel{5}}\ \text{mL}} = 1\ \text{tsp}$$

6. $\dfrac{1\ \text{mg}}{}\ \Big|\ \dfrac{1\ \text{mL}}{1000\ \text{mcg}}\ \Big|\ \dfrac{1000\ \text{mcg}}{1\ \text{mg}}$

$$\dfrac{1\ \text{mg}}{}\ \Bigg|\ \dfrac{1\ \boxed{\text{mL}}}{\underset{1}{\cancel{1000}}\ \text{mcg}}\ \Bigg|\ \dfrac{\overset{1}{\cancel{1000}}\ \text{mcg}}{\cancel{1}\ \text{mg}} = 1\ \text{mL}$$

7. $\dfrac{500\ \text{mg}}{}\ \Big|\ \dfrac{1\ \text{mL}}{1\ \text{g}}\ \Big|\ \dfrac{1\ \text{g}}{1000\ \text{mg}}$

$$\dfrac{\overset{1}{\cancel{500}}\ \text{mg}}{}\ \Bigg|\ \dfrac{1\ \boxed{\text{mL}}}{\cancel{1}\ \text{g}}\ \Bigg|\ \dfrac{\cancel{1}\ \text{g}}{\underset{2}{\cancel{1000}}\ \text{mg}} = \dfrac{1}{2}\ \text{or}\ 0.5\ \text{mL}$$

8. $1 : 1000 = 1\ \text{g in } 1000\ \text{mL}$

$\dfrac{0.4\ \text{mg}}{}\ \Big|\ \dfrac{1000\ \text{mL}}{1\ \text{g}}\ \Big|\ \dfrac{1\ \text{g}}{1000\ \text{mg}}$

$$\dfrac{0.4\ \text{mg}}{}\ \Bigg|\ \dfrac{\overset{1}{\cancel{1000}}\ \boxed{\text{mL}}}{\cancel{1}\ \text{g}}\ \Bigg|\ \dfrac{\cancel{1}\ \text{g}}{\underset{1}{\cancel{1000}}\ \text{mg}} = 0.4\ \text{mL}$$

9. $2\% = 2\ \text{g in } 100\ \text{mL}$

$\dfrac{30\ \text{mg}}{}\ \Big|\ \dfrac{100\ \text{mL}}{2\ \text{g}}\ \Big|\ \dfrac{1\ \text{g}}{1000\ \text{mg}}$

$$\dfrac{30\ \text{mg}}{}\ \Bigg|\ \dfrac{\overset{1}{\cancel{100}}\ \boxed{\text{mL}}}{\underset{2}{\cancel{2}}\ \text{g}}\ \Bigg|\ \dfrac{\cancel{1}\ \text{g}}{\underset{10}{\cancel{1000}}\ \text{mg}} = \dfrac{30}{10 \times 2} = \dfrac{30}{20} = 1.5\ \text{mL}$$

10. $\dfrac{\frac{1}{150}\ \text{gr}}{}\ \Big|\ \dfrac{1\ \text{mL}}{0.4\ \text{mg}}\ \Big|\ \dfrac{60\ \text{mg}}{1\ \text{gr}}$

$$\dfrac{\cancel{\frac{1}{150}}\ \text{gr}}{}\ \Bigg|\ \dfrac{1\ \boxed{\text{mL}}}{0.4\ \text{mg}}\ \Bigg|\ \dfrac{\cancel{60}\ \text{mg}}{\cancel{1}\ \text{gr}} = \dfrac{\frac{1}{150} \times 60}{0.4} = \dfrac{0.4}{0.4} = 1\ \text{mL}$$

Self-Test 3 Calculation of Medications Using Weight or BSA

1. $\dfrac{1 \text{ mg}}{\text{kg}} \;\bigg|\; \dfrac{1 \text{ mL}}{10 \text{ mg}} \;\bigg|\; 70 \text{ kg}$

$$\frac{1 \text{ mg}}{\text{kg}} \;\bigg|\; \frac{1\,\text{(mL)}}{10\ \text{mg}} \;\bigg|\; \overset{7}{70}\ \text{kg} = 7 \text{ mL}$$

2. $\dfrac{10 \text{ mg}}{\text{kg}} \;\bigg|\; \dfrac{5 \text{ mL}}{125 \text{ mg}} \;\bigg|\; 30 \text{ kg}$

$$\frac{10 \text{ mg}}{\text{kg}} \;\bigg|\; \frac{\overset{1}{5}\,\text{(mL)}}{\underset{25}{125}\ \text{mg}} \;\bigg|\; 30 \text{ kg} \;\bigg|\; \frac{10 \times 30}{25} = 12 \text{ mL}$$

3. $\dfrac{25 \text{ mg}}{\text{kg/day}} \;\bigg|\; \dfrac{5 \text{ mL}}{250 \text{ mg}} \;\bigg|\; 50 \text{ lb} \;\bigg|\; \dfrac{1 \text{ kg}}{2.2 \text{ lb}} \;\bigg|\; \dfrac{\text{day}}{4 \text{ doses}}$

$$\frac{25 \text{ mg}}{\text{kg / day}} \;\bigg|\; \frac{\overset{1}{5}\,\text{(mL)}}{\underset{5}{250}\ \text{mg}} \;\bigg|\; 50 \text{ lb} \;\bigg|\; \frac{1 \text{ kg}}{2.2 \text{ lb}} \;\bigg|\; \frac{\text{day}}{4 \text{ doses}} \;\bigg|\; \frac{25 \times 5 \times 1 \times 1}{5 \times 2.2 \times 4} = \frac{125}{44} = 2.84 \text{ mL per dose}$$

4. $\dfrac{0.4 \text{ mg}}{\text{kg/day}} \;\bigg|\; \dfrac{1 \text{ mL}}{4 \text{ mg}} \;\bigg|\; 25 \text{ lb} \;\bigg|\; \dfrac{1 \text{ kg}}{2.2 \text{ lb}} \;\bigg|\; \dfrac{\text{day}}{4 \text{ doses}}$

$$\frac{\overset{0.1}{0.4} \text{ mg}}{\text{kg / day}} \;\bigg|\; \frac{1\,\text{(mL)}}{\underset{1}{4}\ \text{mg}} \;\bigg|\; 25 \text{ lb} \;\bigg|\; \frac{1 \text{ kg}}{2.2 \text{ lb}} \;\bigg|\; \frac{\text{day}}{4 \text{ doses}} \;\bigg|\; \frac{0.1 \times 25}{2.2 \times 4} = \frac{2.5}{8.8} = 0.28 \text{ mL per dose}$$

5. $\dfrac{10 \text{ mg}}{\text{m}^2} \;\bigg|\; \dfrac{1 \text{ tablet}}{2.5 \text{ mg}} \;\bigg|\; 1.29 \text{ m}^2$

$$\frac{\overset{4}{10}\ \text{mg}}{\text{m}^2} \;\bigg|\; \frac{1\,\text{(tablet)}}{\underset{1}{2.5}\ \text{mg}} \;\bigg|\; 1.29 \text{ m}^2 \;\bigg|\; \frac{4 \times 1 \times 1.29}{} = 5.16 \text{ or } 5 \text{ tablets}$$

Self-Test 4 Reconstitution

1. $\dfrac{0.5 \text{ g}}{} \;\bigg|\; \dfrac{1 \text{ mL}}{250 \text{ mg}} \;\bigg|\; \dfrac{1000 \text{ mg}}{1 \text{ g}}$

$$\frac{0.5 \text{ g}}{} \;\bigg|\; \frac{1\,\text{(mL)}}{\underset{1}{250}\ \text{mg}} \;\bigg|\; \frac{\overset{4}{1000}\ \text{mg}}{1 \text{ g}} \;\bigg|\; \frac{0.5 \times 4}{1 \times 1} = 2 \text{ mL}$$

2. $\dfrac{1{,}000{,}000 \text{ units}}{} \;\bigg|\; \dfrac{1 \text{ mL}}{1{,}000{,}000 \text{ units}}$

$$\frac{1{,}000{,}000 \text{ units}}{} \;\bigg|\; \frac{1\,\text{(mL)}}{5{,}000{,}000 \text{ units}} = 1 \text{ mL}$$

3. $\dfrac{0.3 \text{ g}}{} \Bigg| \dfrac{1 \text{ mL}}{225 \text{ mg}} \Bigg| \dfrac{1000 \text{ mg}}{1 \text{ g}}$

$\dfrac{0.3 \cancel{\text{ g}}}{} \Bigg| \dfrac{1 \text{ \textcircled{mL}}}{\underset{45}{\cancel{225}} \text{ mg}} \Bigg| \dfrac{\overset{200}{\cancel{1000}} \text{ mg}}{1 \cancel{\text{ g}}} \Bigg| \dfrac{0.3 \times 1 \times 200}{45 \times 1} = \dfrac{60}{45} = 1.33 \text{ mL}$

4. $\dfrac{1500 \text{ mg}}{} \Bigg| \dfrac{5 \text{ mL}}{1.5 \text{ g}} \Bigg| \dfrac{1 \text{ g}}{1000 \text{ mg}}$

$\dfrac{\cancel{1500} \text{ mg}}{} \Bigg| \dfrac{\overset{1}{\cancel{5}} \text{ \textcircled{mL}}}{1.5 \cancel{\text{ g}}} \Bigg| \dfrac{1 \cancel{\text{ g}}}{\underset{2}{\cancel{1000}} \text{ mg}} \Bigg| \dfrac{15 \times 1 \times 1}{1.5 \times 2} \Bigg| \dfrac{15}{3} = 5 \text{ mL}$

5. $\dfrac{0.25 \text{ g}}{} \Bigg| \dfrac{1 \text{ mL}}{500 \text{ mg}} \Bigg| \dfrac{1000 \text{ mg}}{1 \text{ g}}$

$\dfrac{0.25 \cancel{\text{ g}}}{} \Bigg| \dfrac{1 \text{ \textcircled{mL}}}{\underset{1}{\cancel{500}} \text{ mg}} \Bigg| \dfrac{\overset{2}{\cancel{1000}} \text{ mg}}{1 \cancel{\text{ g}}} \Bigg| \dfrac{0.25 \times 2}{} = 0.5 \text{ mL}$

Self-Test 5 Basic IV Calculations and Drop Factors

1. $\dfrac{1000 \text{ mL}}{8 \text{ hr}} \Bigg|$

$\dfrac{\overset{250}{\cancel{1000}} \text{ \textcircled{mL}}}{\underset{2}{\cancel{8}} \text{ \textcircled{hr}}} \Bigg| \dfrac{250}{2} = 125 \text{ mL/hr}$

2. $\dfrac{500 \text{ mL}}{5 \text{ hr}} \Bigg|$

$\dfrac{\overset{100}{\cancel{500}} \text{ \textcircled{mL}}}{\underset{1}{\cancel{5}} \text{ \textcircled{hr}}} \Bigg| \dfrac{100}{} = 100 \text{ mL/hr}$

3. $\dfrac{250 \text{ mL}}{5 \text{ hr}} \Bigg|$

$\dfrac{\overset{50}{\cancel{250}} \text{ \textcircled{mL}}}{\underset{1}{\cancel{5}} \text{ \textcircled{hr}}} \Bigg| \dfrac{50}{} = 50 \text{ mL/hr}$

4. $\dfrac{500 \text{ mL}}{4 \text{ hr}} \Bigg|$

$\dfrac{\overset{125}{\cancel{500}} \text{ \textcircled{mL}}}{\underset{1}{\cancel{4}} \text{ \textcircled{hr}}} \Bigg| \dfrac{125}{} = 125 \text{ mL/hr}$

5.
$$\frac{250 \text{ mL}}{2 \text{ hr}} \left| \frac{20 \text{ gtts}}{\text{mL}} \right| \frac{1 \text{ hr}}{60 \text{ min}}$$

$$\frac{\overset{125}{\cancel{250}} \text{ mL}}{\underset{1}{\cancel{2}} \text{ hr}} \left| \frac{\overset{1}{\cancel{20}} \text{ \textcircled{gtts}}}{\text{mL}} \right| \frac{1 \text{ hr}}{\underset{3}{\cancel{60}} \text{ \textcircled{min}}} \left| \frac{125 \times 1 \times 1}{1 \times 3} = \frac{125}{3} = 41.6 \text{ or } 42 \text{ gtts/min}$$

6.
$$\frac{100 \text{ mL}}{30 \text{ min}} \left| \frac{15 \text{ gtts}}{\text{mL}} \right.$$

$$\frac{100 \text{ mL}}{\underset{2}{\cancel{30}} \text{ \textcircled{min}}} \left| \frac{\overset{1}{\cancel{15}} \text{ \textcircled{gtts}}}{\text{mL}} \right| \frac{100}{2} = 50 \text{ gtts/min}$$

7.
$$\frac{500 \text{ mL}}{4 \text{ hr}} \left| \frac{60 \text{ \textcircled{gtts}}}{\text{mL}} \right| \frac{1 \text{ hr}}{60 \text{ min}}$$

$$\frac{500 \text{ mL}}{4 \text{ hr}} \left| \frac{\overset{1}{\cancel{60}} \text{ gtts}}{\text{mL}} \right| \frac{1 \text{ hr}}{\underset{1}{\cancel{60}} \text{ \textcircled{min}}} \left| \frac{500 \times 1 \times 1}{4 \times 1} = \frac{500}{4} = 125 \text{ gtts/min}$$

8.
$$\frac{300 \text{ mL}}{90 \text{ min}} \left| \frac{60 \text{ gtts}}{\text{mL}} \right.$$

$$\frac{300 \text{ mL}}{\underset{3}{\cancel{90}} \text{ \textcircled{min}}} \left| \frac{\overset{2}{\cancel{60}} \text{ \textcircled{gtts}}}{\text{mL}} \right| \frac{600}{3} = 200 \text{ gtts/min}$$

9.
$$\frac{1000 \text{ mL}}{8 \text{ hr}} \left| \frac{20 \text{ gtts}}{\text{mL}} \right| \frac{1 \text{ hr}}{60 \text{ min}}$$

$$\frac{1000 \text{ mL}}{8 \text{ hr}} \left| \frac{\overset{1}{\cancel{20}} \text{ \textcircled{gtts}}}{\text{mL}} \right| \frac{1 \text{ hr}}{\underset{3}{\cancel{60}} \text{ \textcircled{min}}} \left| \frac{1000 \times 1 \times 1}{8 \times 3} = \frac{1000}{24} = 41.6 \text{ or } 42 \text{ gtts/min}$$

10.
$$\frac{500 \text{ mL}}{4 \text{ hr}} \left| \frac{10 \text{ gtts}}{\text{mL}} \right| \frac{1 \text{ hr}}{60 \text{ min}}$$

$$\frac{500 \text{ mL}}{4 \text{ hr}} \left| \frac{\overset{1}{\cancel{10}} \text{ \textcircled{gtts}}}{\text{mL}} \right| \frac{1 \text{ hr}}{\underset{6}{\cancel{60}} \text{ \textcircled{min}}} \left| \frac{500 \times 1 \times 1}{4 \times 6} = \frac{500}{24} = 20.8 \text{ or } 21 \text{ gtts/min}$$

Self-Test 6 Advanced IV Calculations

1.
$$\frac{1000 \text{ units}}{\text{hr}} \left| \frac{250 \text{ mL}}{25,000 \text{ units}} \right.$$

$$\frac{1000 \text{ units}}{\text{\textcircled{hr}}} \left| \frac{\overset{1}{\cancel{250}} \text{ \textcircled{mL}}}{\underset{100}{\cancel{25,000}} \text{ units}} \right| \frac{1000}{100} = 10 \text{ mL/hr}$$

2. $\dfrac{20 \text{ units}}{\text{hr}} \;\bigg|\; \dfrac{250 \text{ mL}}{125 \text{ units}}$

$\dfrac{20 \text{ units}}{\text{hr}} \;\bigg|\; \dfrac{250 \; \overset{2}{\text{mL}}}{\underset{1}{125} \text{ units}} \;\bigg|\; 2 \times 20 = 40 \text{ units/hr}$

3. $\dfrac{50 \text{ mg}}{\text{hr}} \;\bigg|\; \dfrac{250 \text{ mL}}{250 \text{ mg}}$

$\dfrac{50 \text{ mg}}{\text{hr}} \;\bigg|\; \dfrac{\overset{1}{250} \text{ mL}}{\underset{1}{250} \text{ mg}} = 50 \text{ mL/hr}$

4. $\dfrac{40 \text{ mL}}{\text{hr}} \;\bigg|\; \dfrac{25{,}000 \text{ units}}{500 \text{ mL}}$

$\dfrac{40 \text{ mL}}{\text{hr}} \;\bigg|\; \dfrac{\overset{50}{25{,}000} \text{ units}}{\underset{1}{500} \text{ mL}} \;\bigg|\; 40 \times 50 = 2000 \text{ units/hr}$

5. $\dfrac{60 \text{ mL}}{\text{hr}} \;\bigg|\; \dfrac{500 \text{ mg}}{250 \text{ mL}}$

$\dfrac{60 \text{ mL}}{\text{hr}} \;\bigg|\; \dfrac{\overset{2}{500} \text{ mg}}{\underset{1}{250} \text{ mL}} \;\bigg|\; 60 \times 2 = 120 \text{ mg/hr}$

6. $\dfrac{2 \text{ mg}}{\text{min}} \;\bigg|\; \dfrac{500 \text{ mL}}{1 \text{ g}} \;\bigg|\; \dfrac{1 \text{ g}}{1000 \text{ mg}} \;\bigg|\; \dfrac{60 \text{ min}}{1 \text{ hr}}$

$\dfrac{2 \text{ mg}}{\text{min}} \;\bigg|\; \dfrac{\overset{1}{500} \text{ mL}}{1 \text{ g}} \;\bigg|\; \dfrac{1 \text{ g}}{\underset{2}{1000} \text{ mg}} \;\bigg|\; \dfrac{60 \text{ min}}{1 \text{ hr}} \;\bigg|\; \dfrac{2 \times 60}{2} = \dfrac{120}{2} = 60 \text{ mL/hr}$

7. $\dfrac{3 \text{ mg}}{\text{min}} \;\bigg|\; \dfrac{500 \text{ mL}}{2 \text{ g}} \;\bigg|\; \dfrac{1 \text{ g}}{1000 \text{ mg}} \;\bigg|\; \dfrac{60 \text{ min}}{1 \text{ hr}}$

$\dfrac{3 \text{ mg}}{\text{min}} \;\bigg|\; \dfrac{\overset{1}{500} \text{ mL}}{2 \text{ g}} \;\bigg|\; \dfrac{1 \text{ g}}{\underset{2}{1000} \text{ mg}} \;\bigg|\; \dfrac{60 \text{ min}}{1 \text{ hr}} \;\bigg|\; \dfrac{3 \times 1 \times 1 \times 60}{2 \times 2 \times 1} = \dfrac{180}{4} = 45 \text{ mL/hr}$

8. $\dfrac{20 \text{ mcg}}{\text{min}} \;\bigg|\; \dfrac{250 \text{ mL}}{50 \text{ mg}} \;\bigg|\; \dfrac{1 \text{ mg}}{1000 \text{ mcg}} \;\bigg|\; \dfrac{60 \text{ min}}{1 \text{ hr}}$

$\dfrac{20 \text{ mcg}}{\text{min}} \;\bigg|\; \dfrac{\overset{5}{250} \text{ mL}}{\underset{1}{50} \text{ mg}} \;\bigg|\; \dfrac{1 \text{ mg}}{1000 \text{ mcg}} \;\bigg|\; \dfrac{60 \text{ min}}{1 \text{ hr}} \;\bigg|\; \dfrac{20 \times 5 \times 60}{1000} = \dfrac{6000}{1000} = 6 \text{ mL/hr}$

9. $\dfrac{5 \text{ mcg}}{\text{min}} \Bigg| \dfrac{250 \text{ mL}}{2 \text{ mg}} \Bigg| \dfrac{1 \text{ mg}}{1000 \text{ mcg}} \Bigg| \dfrac{60 \text{ min}}{1 \text{ hr}}$

$\dfrac{5 \text{ mcg}}{\text{min}} \Bigg| \dfrac{250 \text{ mL}}{2 \text{ mg}} \Bigg| \dfrac{1 \text{ mg}}{1000 \text{ mcg}} \Bigg| \dfrac{60 \text{ min}}{1 \text{ hr}} \Bigg| \dfrac{5 \times 60}{2 \times 4} = \dfrac{300}{8} = 37.5 \text{ or } 38 \text{ mL/hr}$

10. $\dfrac{5 \text{ mcg}}{\text{kg/min}} \Bigg| \dfrac{250 \text{ mL}}{200 \text{ mg}} \Bigg| \dfrac{1 \text{ mg}}{1000 \text{ mcg}} \Bigg| \dfrac{70 \text{ kg}}{} \Bigg| \dfrac{60 \text{ min}}{1 \text{ hr}}$

$\dfrac{5 \text{ mcg}}{\text{kg/min}} \Bigg| \dfrac{250 \text{ mL}}{200 \text{ mg}} \Bigg| \dfrac{1 \text{ mg}}{1000 \text{ mcg}} \Bigg| \dfrac{70 \text{ kg}}{} \Bigg| \dfrac{60 \text{ min}}{1 \text{ hr}} \Bigg| \dfrac{1 \times 1 \times 1 \times 70 \times 60}{40 \times 4 \times 1} = \dfrac{4200}{160} = 26.2 \text{ or } 26 \text{ mL/hr}$

11. $\dfrac{5 \text{ milliunits}}{\text{min}} \Bigg| \dfrac{250 \text{ mL}}{15 \text{ units}} \Bigg| \dfrac{1 \text{ unit}}{1000 \text{ milliunits}} \Bigg| \dfrac{60 \text{ min}}{1 \text{ hr}}$

$\dfrac{5 \text{ milliunits}}{\text{min}} \Bigg| \dfrac{250 \text{ mL}}{15 \text{ units}} \Bigg| \dfrac{1 \text{ unit}}{1000 \text{ milliunits}} \Bigg| \dfrac{60 \text{ min}}{1 \text{ hr}} \Bigg| \dfrac{1 \times 1 \times 1 \times 60}{3 \times 4 \times 1} = \dfrac{60}{12} = 5 \text{ mL/hr}$

12. $\dfrac{2 \text{ mcg}}{\text{kg/min}} \Bigg| \dfrac{250 \text{ mL}}{50 \text{ mg}} \Bigg| \dfrac{1 \text{ mg}}{1000 \text{ mcg}} \Bigg| \dfrac{110 \text{ lb}}{} \Bigg| \dfrac{1 \text{ kg}}{2.2 \text{ lb}} \Bigg| \dfrac{60 \text{ min}}{1 \text{ hr}}$

$\dfrac{2 \text{ mcg}}{\text{kg/min}} \Bigg| \dfrac{250 \text{ mL}}{50 \text{ mg}} \Bigg| \dfrac{1 \text{ mg}}{1000 \text{ mcg}} \Bigg| \dfrac{110 \text{ lb}}{} \Bigg| \dfrac{1 \text{ kg}}{2.2 \text{ lb}} \Bigg| \dfrac{60 \text{ min}}{1 \text{ hr}} \Bigg| \dfrac{1 \times 1 \times 1 \times 110 \times 1 \times 60}{25 \times 4 \times 2.2 \times 1} = \dfrac{6600}{220} = 30 \text{ mL/hr}$

Information Basic to Administering Drugs

LEARNING OBJECTIVES

1. Generic names and trade names

2. Drug classification and drug categories

3. Side effects and adverse effects

4. Basic knowledge essential for safe drug administration

5. Pharmacokinetics

6. Legal considerations: criminal and civil

7. Ethical principles in drug administration

8. Information on preparation and administration of medications

In previous chapters you learned drug forms and preparations, how to read prescriptions, and how to calculate dosages. This chapter provides the opportunity to focus on some of the nurse's responsibilities for drug therapy—drug knowledge, legal and ethical considerations, and, finally, specific points that may prove helpful in giving medications.

Drug Knowledge

Nursing drug handbooks are the best references for the nurse who needs a variety of information specifically designed to help assess, manage, evaluate, and teach the patient. The following headings represent the kind of information found in a nursing handbook.

- Generic and trade names
- Classification and category
- Side and adverse effects
- Pregnancy category
- Dosage and route
- Action

- Indications
- Contraindications and precautions
- Interactions and incompatibilities
- Nursing implications
- Signs of effectiveness
- Patient teaching

Two long-standing web sites that include drug information are the U.S. Food and Drug Administration (www.fda.gov) and Rx Med (www.rxmed.com). Nursing publishing companies include drug information on their web sites. Lippincott's is www.nursingcenter.com.

Generic and Trade Names

The generic name, which is not capitalized, is the official name given to a drug. In the United States a drug can only have one generic name. The letters USP (United States Pharmacopeia) following a generic name indicate that the drug meets government standards for purity and assay.

A trade name is the brand name under which a company manufactures a generic drug. While a drug has only one generic name, it may have several trade names. The trade name is capitalized and is sometimes followed by the symbol ®.

Example The generic name of Nubain® is nalbuphine.

Consumer groups have advocated that drugs be prescribed by generic name only so that the pharmacist may dispense the least expensive drug available on the market. The nurse should understand that generic drugs, because they are manufactured by different companies, are not exactly the same. Although the active ingredient in the drug meets standards of uniformity and purity, manufacturers use different fillers and dyes. These substances can cause adverse effects (e.g., severe nausea caused by the dye used in coloring).

Also, when a pharmacist dispenses the same drug with a different trade name, the patient may become confused and distressed about medication that appears unlike previous doses. While the active ingredient is the same, the medication size, shape, or color may vary according to trade name and manufacturer.

Drug Classification and Drug Category

Drug classification is a way to categorize drugs by the way they act against diseases or disorders, especially by their effect on a particular area of the body or on a particular condition. A diuretic, for instance, acts on the kidneys; an anticonvulsant prevents seizures. Because drug classifications are a quick reference to a drug's therapeutic actions, uses, and adverse effects, they provide the administering nurse with a drug's general indications, precautions, and nursing implications.

Category (in this text) refers to the way a drug works at the molecular, tissue, or body system level (e.g., beta blocker, SSRI).

Example The classification of **nalbuphine (Nubain)** is an opioid analgesic, and the category is narcotic antagonist/agonist. This drug's main action and use is to relieve pain; its adverse effects are sedation and respiratory depression. Sometimes it will decrease the effect of other opioids.

Side Effects and Adverse Effects

Side effects are non-therapeutic reactions to a drug. Because these reactions are transient, they may not require any nursing intervention. Side effects occur as a consequence of drug administration; often they are unrelated to the desired action of the drug.

Adverse effects are non-therapeutic effects that may be harmful to the patient and thus require lowering the dosage or discontinuing the drug. Because these effects can be life-threatening, they may require medical intervention.

Drowsiness is a **side effect** that occurs with some antihistamines. A serious decrease in white blood cells (WBCs) is an **adverse effect,** resulting in lowered resistance to infection. The nurse must watch for these effects, know how to manage them, and, if necessary, teach the patient about them.

Example **Nalbuphine (Nubain)** can cause these side effects: sedation headache, dizziness, nausea, vomiting, dry mouth, and sweating. **Nalbuphine,** in high doses, can cause these adverse effects: hypotension and drug addiction.

Pregnancy Category

The U.S. Food and Drug Administration (FDA) has established the following categories for pregnant women:

A: No risk to the fetus in any trimester

B: No adverse effect demonstrated in animals; no human studies available

C: Studies with animals have shown adverse reactions; no human studies are available; given only after risks to the fetus have been considered

D: Definite fetal risk exists; may be given despite risk to the fetus if needed for a life-threatening condition

X: Absolute fetal abnormality; not to be used anytime during pregnancy

A nurse administering a drug to any woman of child-bearing age should know the pregnancy categories. If the drug has a category of D or X, the nurse should inform the woman of that category's significance and determine whether there is any possibility of the woman being pregnant. If a woman has a confirmed pregnancy, the nurse should find out the pregnancy's current gestational week. The nurse also should use this circumstance as an opportunity to educate the client about the risks of *any* current medication (whether prescribed, over-the-counter, herbal, or nutritional supplement) and its known or potential effects on a fetus.

> **Example** **Nalbuphine (Nubain)** is pregnancy category C, which indicates possible fetal risk.

Dosage and Route

Information about the dosage and route of administration is crucial to protect against medication error. Most handbooks include, for each drug, appropriate dosage ranges for adults, the elderly, and children.

> **Example** **Nalbuphine (Nubain)** IM, subcutaneous, IV (adults)
>
> Usual dose: 10 mg q3–6h. Single dose not to exceed 20 mg. Total daily dose not to exceed 160 mg. Dose in children not determined.

Action

Action explains how the drug works—that is, what medical experts know or believe about how the drug acts to produce a therapeutic effect. This knowledge helps the nurse understand whether a drug should be taken with food or between meals, with other drugs or alone, orally, or parenterally.

The nurse who knows drug action can better assess, manage, and evaluate drug therapy. For example, if a particular drug is metabolized in the liver and kidney, then the nurse can apply this knowledge. Because patients with liver or kidney disease may not be able to metabolize or excrete certain drugs, this particular drug could accumulate in the body and possibly cause adverse effects.

> **Example** **Nalbuphine (Nubain)** binds to opiate receptors in the central nervous system (CNS) and alters the perception of and response to painful stimuli.

Indications

Indications give the reasons for using the drug. This information helps the nurse watch not only for expected effects and therapeutic response, but also for any side effects and adverse effects. One of the most common questions patients ask nurses is "Why am I getting this drug?" With a good understanding of indications, the nurse can answer the patient's question, describing the drug's expected effects.

Often a drug can be used for an indication "off label"—that is, for an indication other than the one(s) "labeled," or approved, by the FDA. The drug may be widely known to be effective in "off-label" conditions because of its side effects (e.g., Benadryl—generic diphenhydramine—causes sleep); or research studies may have proven the drug effective for that particular indication, but the drug hasn't yet been licensed as a treatment for it (e.g., Wellbutrin—generic bupropion—helps a patient stop smoking).

The nurse should become familiar with the typical off-label uses of particular drugs. If a medication order requests a drug for an indication other than the one for which it is labeled and approved, or other than off-label uses with which the nurse is familiar, the nurse should question the medication order.

> **Example** **Nalbuphine (Nubain)** is also used to alleviate moderate to severe pain.

Contraindications and Precautions

These terms refer to conditions in which a drug should be either given with caution or not given at all. For instance, patients who have exhibited a previous reaction to penicillin should be cautioned against taking that drug again; if a patient has poor kidney function, certain antibiotics must be administered with caution. Because the nurse has a responsibility to safeguard the patient and carry out effective nursing care, a knowledge of contraindications and precautions is important—especially in relation to patients with glaucoma, renal disease, or liver disease, and patients who are very young or very old.

Example | **Nalbuphine (Nubain)** is contraindicated if hypersensitivity to the drug exists or if the patient has a dependency on other opioids. Use this drug cautiously in head trauma, increased intracranial pressure (ICP), severe respiratory disease, undiagnosed abdominal pain, and pregnancy (depressed respirations in newborn). The drug's safety is not established in children.

Interactions and Incompatibilities

When more than one drug is administered at a time, unexpected or non-therapeutic responses may occur. Some interactions are desirable: for example, naloxone (Narcan) is a narcotic antagonist that reverses the effects of a morphine overdose. Other interactions, however, are undesirable: aspirin, for instance, should not be taken with an oral anticoagulant because that combination increases the possibility of an adverse effect (e.g., increased bleeding). The nurse must carefully consider some drug-herbal interactions as well.

Some drugs are incompatible and thus should not be mixed. Knowledge of incompatibilities is especially important when medications are combined for injection in IV administration. *Chemical incompatibility* usually produces a visible sign such as precipitation or color change. *Physical incompatibility,* however, may not give a visible sign, so the nurse should never combine drugs without checking a suitable reference.

A good rule of thumb: *When in doubt, do not mix.*

COMMON DRUGS AND DRUG CLASSIFICATIONS THAT CAUSE UNEXPECTED OR NON-THERAPEUTIC RESPONSES

Refer to a drug handbook for specific interactions:

- MAO inhibitors–anticonvulsants–lithium
- Tricyclic antidepressants–antifungals–methotrexate
- Alcohol–barbiturates–NSAIDs
- Aluminum–beta blockers–oral contraceptives
- Aminoglycosides–cimetidine–phenothiazines
- Antacids–clonidine–phenytoin
- Anticoagulants–cyclosporine–probenecid
- Heparin–digoxin–rifampin
- Coumadin–erythromycin–theophylline
- ASA–isoniazid

Interactions also may occur between drugs and certain foods. Here are some common examples. The calcium present in dairy products interferes with the absorption of tetracycline. Foods high in vitamin B6 can decrease the effect of an antiparkinsonian drug. Foods high in tyramine, such as wine and cheese, can precipitate a hypertensive crisis in patients taking monoamine oxidase (MAO) inhibitors. Grapefruit juice interferes with the absorption of multiple drugs.

Additionally, cigarette smoke—which can increase the liver's metabolism of drugs—may decrease drug effectiveness. People exposed even to secondhand cigarette smoke may require higher doses of medication.

Example **Nalbuphine (Nubain)** produces additive CNS depression with alcohol, antihistamines, and sedative/hypnotics. It can produce withdrawal in patients dependent on opioids and can diminish the analgesic effect. Exercise care when giving to patients receiving MAO inhibitors, because severe reactions are possible.

Nursing Implications

To administer a drug safely and to assess, manage, and teach the patient, the nurse needs a knowledge of implications: whether the drug should be taken with or without food; what specific vital signs to monitor; and what lab values may be affected by the drug or may need to be ordered to check the drug's effectiveness or toxicity.

Example Some nursing implications related to **nalbuphine (Nubain)** include the following: assess pain both before the dose and one hour after the dose; assess BP, pulse, and respiration both before the dose and periodically after the dose; assess for dependency and for tolerance.

Signs of Effectiveness

Few drug references actually list this heading, yet the nurse is expected to evaluate the drug regimen and to record and report observations. Knowledge of the drug's class, its action, and its use helps the nurse understand the expected therapeutic outcomes.

Ampicillin sodium, for instance, is a broad-spectrum antibiotic that is used for urinary, respiratory, and other infections. Signs of effectiveness might include these: normal temperature; the laboratory report of the WBC count, indicating a normal result; clear urine, no pain on urination, and no WBC in urine; decreased pus in an infected wound; wound healing; a patient showing alertness, interest in surroundings, and improved appetite.

Example For **nalbuphine (Nubain),** signs of effectiveness are relief of pain and sedation.

Teaching the Patient

The patient has a right to know the drug's name and dose, why the drug is ordered, and what effects to expect or watch for. A patient who will be taking a drug at home also needs specific information. Making sure that patients are knowledgeable about their drugs is a professional responsibility shared by three people: the physician or healthcare provider, the nurse, and the pharmacist.

Pharmacokinetics

When a drug is taken *orally,* the villi of the small intestine absorb it, and the bloodstream distributes it to the cells. The body metabolizes the drug to a greater or lesser extent and then excretes it. When a drug is given *parenterally,* it bypasses the gastrointestinal system, entering the circulation more quickly—or, in the case of the intravenous route, immediately. The general term **pharmacokinetics** includes these drug activities: absorption, distribution, biotransformation, and excretion.

Absorption

Effective absorption of an oral drug depends on several conditions: the degree of stomach acidity, the time required for the stomach to empty, whether food is present, the amount of contact with villi in the small intestine, and the flow of blood to the villi.

Other circumstances, too, may affect a drug's absorption. Enteric-coated (EC) tablets, for instance, are not meant to dissolve in the acidic stomach; they ordinarily pass through the stomach to the duodenum. When a patient receives an antacid along with an EC tablet, the pH of the stomach rises, perhaps causing the tablet to dissolve prematurely—which either can make the drug less potent or can irritate the gastric lining. Timed-release EC capsules that dissolve prematurely can deliver a huge dose of the drug, producing adverse effects.

Here's another example: laxatives increase gastrointestinal movement and decrease the time a drug is in contact with the villi of the small intestine, where most absorption occurs. The presence of food in the stomach, however, can impair absorption. In particular, foods that contain calcium, such as milk and cheese, form a complex with some drugs and inhibit absorption. Penicillin is a good example of a drug that should be taken on an empty stomach.

Distribution

Distribution describes the drug's movement through body fluids—chiefly the bloodstream—to the cells. Drugs do not travel freely in the blood; instead, most travel attached to plasma proteins, especially albumin. If a drug is not attached to a plasma protein, it can attach to cells and can effect them in various ways.

When the bloodstream contains more than one drug, the drugs may compete for binding with protein sites. One drug may displace another, leaving the displaced drug free to interact with the cells, and its effect on the cells will be more pronounced. Aspirin is a common drug that displaces others; it should not be given with oral anticoagulants, which are 99% bound to albumin. Because aspirin displaces the anticoagulant, it leaves the anticoagulant free to act at the cellular level, sometimes causing the toxic effect of bleeding.

Biotransformation

Biotransformation refers to the chemical change of a drug into a form that can be excreted. Most biotransformation occurs in the liver, because that's where oral drugs go first. The process, called the first-pass effect, begins when the drug is absorbed. Here, too, one drug can interfere with the effects of another. Barbiturates increase the liver's enzyme activity. Since this activity makes the body metabolize the drugs more rapidly, it reduces their effect. Conversely, acetaminophen (Tylenol) blocks the breakdown of penicillin in the liver, thereby increasing the effect of the drug.

Excretion

The major organ of excretion—the process by which the body removes a drug—is the kidney. Drug interactions may also occur at this point. The drug probenecid, for example, inhibits the excretion of penicillin and increases its length of action. Furosemide (Lasix), a diuretic, blocks the excretion of aspirin and can cause aspirin to produce adverse effects.

Drug interactions at the excretion stage are not necessarily harmful. For instance, narcotic antagonists are used intentionally to reverse the adverse effects of general anesthetics. This reversal action is termed *antagonism.* The term *synergism,* on the other hand, describes what happens when a second drug increases the intensity or prolongs the effect of a first drug. A narcotic and a minor tranquilizer together, for example, produce more pain relief than the narcotic alone. The nurse administering medications needs to be aware of possible interactions and must carefully evaluate the patient's response.

To minimize adverse interactions, the nurse should closely review the patient's drug profile, administer as low a dose as possible, know the actions, the side and adverse effects of the drugs administered, and monitor the patient. Continued monitoring is important, because some drug interactions may take several weeks to develop.

Tolerance

When a medication for pain or sleeping is administered frequently, the liver enzymes become skilled at rapid biotransforming. Thus less of the drug is available, and the drug is less effective in relieving pain or aiding sleep. This reaction may be labeled "addiction" because the patient complains that the drug is not working and asks for more; but in fact, it is a physiologic response rather than an addictive one. The patient requires more of the drug, or a drug with a different molecular structure.

> ## Cultural Considerations
>
> - Drug metabolism and side effects can vary among different cultures, races, and ethnic groups.
> - *Pharmacoanthropology* deals with differences in drug responses among racial and ethnic groups. *Ethnocultural perception* deals with various cultural perceptions and beliefs related to illness, disease, and drug therapy.
> - Assessing the personal beliefs of the patient and the family is an essential step in drug administration.
> - The nurse's communication about drugs must meet the cultural needs of the patient and family and must respect their culture and cultural practices.
>
> **CLINICAL ALERT!**

Cumulation

When a condition—such as liver or kidney disease—inhibits biotransformation or excretion, the drug accumulates in the body. The same thing can happen when a patient receives too much of a drug or takes a drug too frequently. This activity, called cumulation, can produce an adverse effect.

Other factors that affect drug action include these:

- Weight: Larger individuals need a higher dose.
- Age: People at either extreme of life respond more strongly. The liver and kidneys of infants are not well developed; in the elderly, systems are less efficient.
- Pathologic conditions, especially of liver and kidneys.
- Hypersensitivity to a drug, which causes an allergic reaction.
- Psychological and emotional state: Depression or anxiety can decrease or increase body metabolism and thus affect drug action.

Side effects and adverse reactions can occur in any system or organ. Drug knowledge will enhance the nurse's skill in observation and will lead to responsible and appropriate intervention.

Half-Life

The half-life of a drug, which correlates roughly with its duration of action, indicates how often the drug may be given to continue therapeutic effect. Literally, the half-life is the time required for half of the drug to be excreted and therefore no longer available for therapeutic use. For example, penicillin's half-life is 30 minutes: after 30 minutes, only half of the dose is still therapeutic. After 30 more minutes, only half of *that* dose is therapeutic, and so on, until most of the drug is eliminated. Then the patient needs another dose. In this case, the patient receives oral Penicillin every 6 to 8 hours. Another example is piroxicam (Feldene), which has a half-life of 48 to 72 hours and is given by mouth as a single dose once a day. Carisoprodol (Soma) has a half-life of 4 to 6 hours and is administered three to four times daily.

Therapeutic Range

To evaluate the effects of drug therapy, the nurse can monitor the drug concentration in the patient's blood or serum through the use of lab tests that measure the therapeutic level. The International System of Units (Système International d'Unités—SI) is a standard measurement system adopted by most countries. One of the units in SI is used to quantify the amount of drug in the blood or serum. (More details on SI can be found at http://www.bipm.org/en/si/.) Some drugs, such as Theo-Dur (theophylline), Dilantin (phenytoin), Lanoxin (digoxin), and others, require periodic measurements of the drug in order to ensure that the patient is receiving the right amount, or not receiving too much of the drug. Antibiotics often are measured with peak and trough therapeutic levels; the trough level is drawn from the blood before the next dose of antibiotic is due, to see if there is too much drug left in the body. The peak level is drawn from the blood after a dose of antibiotic, to see if there is enough drug in the body to have a therapeutic effect.

Herbs, Herbs, Herbs

CLINICAL ALERT!

- Herbal therapy is one of the oldest forms of medication. Today its use is worldwide, with more and more people taking herbal remedies.

- Herbal therapies and other alternative medications, however, *are not subject to FDA regulations.*

- Clients should consult with their healthcare provider before beginning herbal therapy, while taking herbal therapy, whenever they experience any side effects from the products, and before discontinuing herbal medications.

- The Office of Alternative Medicine, under the auspices of the National Institutes of Health, studies alternative medicine and therapies (see www.nccam.nih.gov).

- The Dietary Supplement Health and Education Act of 1994 clarified regulations for herbal remedies (see http://vm.cfsan.fda.gov/~dms/dietsupp.html).

- Healthcare providers need to be aware of potential drug interactions between herbal therapy and conventional drugs (both prescription and over-the-counter).

Legal Considerations

Nurses must know the scope of nursing practice in the state in which they function. They should be familiar not only with government regulations—federal, state, and local—that affect nursing, but also with the policies and procedures of the agency where they practice, which also have legal status. Failure to follow guidelines, or even just a lack of knowledge, can lead to liability. The web site for the National Council of State Boards of Nursing (www.ncsbn.org) gives information on nurse regulation and licensure in each state; up-to-date information on legal issues is available from the web site of the American Nurses Association (www.ana.org).

In Canada, the Health Protection Branch of the Department of National Health and Welfare (http://www.hc-sc.gc.ca/ahc-asc/index_e.html) maintains the quality and safety of drug development. (Details regarding the Canadian Food and Drugs Act appear on the same site.) For information about narcotics control, see the web page for the Canadian Narcotics Control Act: http://laws.justice.gc.ca/en/C-38.8/index.html.

Nursing practice is also affected by two other types of law: criminal and civil.

Criminal Law

Criminal law relates to offenses against the general public that are detrimental to society as a whole. Actions considered criminal are prosecuted by governmental authorities. If the defendant is judged guilty, the penalty may be a fine, imprisonment, or both.

Criminal charges include unlawful use, possession, or administration of a controlled substance. The Comprehensive Drug Abuse, Prevention and Control Act of 1970 classified drugs that are subject to abuse into one of five schedules, according to their medical usefulness and abuse potential.

Schedule I drugs have no valid use and are not available for prescription use (e.g., LSD).

Schedule II drugs, such as narcotics, have a valid medical use and are available for prescriptions, but they exhibit a high potential for abuse, and their misuse can lead to physical and psychological dependence. Labels for these drugs are marked with the symbol VII. In a hospital setting, an order for a narcotic might be valid for three days; once the three days have elapsed, however, a new order is required. A nurse who administers a controlled drug after its order has expired commits a medication error.

Schedule III, IV, and V drugs are classified as having less abuse potential than schedule II drugs, but they can cause some physical and psychological dependence. The labels VIII, VIV, and VV identify these drugs. Examples include Percodan (oxycodone), Fiorinal, diazepam (Valium), and Tylenol #3 (acetaminophen with codeine).

Schedule II, III, IV, and V drugs are stored in a locked cabinet or cart on nursing units, and a record is kept for each narcotic administered. Many hospitals use the Pyxis system, a computerized locked cabinet that dispenses controlled substances (Fig. 12-1). Controlled drugs are counted for each shift, and discrepancies are reported. Government and institutional policies specify how these drugs are stored and protected.

Nurses who become impaired (unable to function) because of alcohol or drug abuse leave themselves open to criminal action, as well as to disciplinary action by the state board of nursing. Many states have laws requiring mandatory reporting of impaired nurses.

Civil Law

Civil law is concerned with the legal rights and duties of private persons. When an individual believes that a wrong was committed against him or her personally, he or she can sue for damages in the form of money.

The legal wrong is called a tort. *Malpractice,* or negligence on the part of the nurse, involves four elements:

1. A claim that the nurse owed the patient a special duty of care—i.e., that a nurse–patient relationship existed.

2. A claim that the nurse failed to meet the required standard. To prove or disprove this element, both sides bring in expert witnesses to testify.

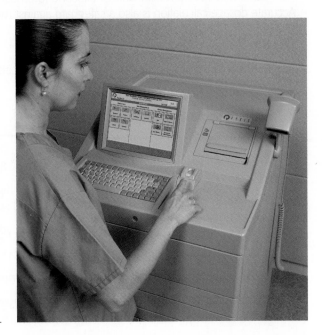

FIGURE 12-1

Pyxis Controlled Medication System. (With permission from Roach, S. [2004]. Introductory clinical pharmacology [7th ed.]. Philadelphia: Lippincott Williams & Wilkins, p. 18.)

3. A claim that harm or injury resulted because the nurse did not meet the required standard.

4. A claim of damages for which compensation is sought.

The nurse–patient relationship is a legal status that begins the moment a nurse actually provides nursing care to another person.

For administration of medications, a nurse is required by law to exercise the degree of skill and care that a reasonably prudent nurse with similar training and experience, practicing in the same community, would exercise under the same or similar circumstances. When a nursing student performs duties that are customarily performed by a registered nurse, the courts have held the nursing student to the higher standard of care, that of the registered nurse.

Mistakes in administering medications are among the most common causes of malpractice. Liability may result from administering the wrong dose, giving a medication to the wrong patient, giving a drug at the wrong time, or failing to administer a drug at the right time or in the proper manner.

A frequent cause of medication errors is either misreading the order of the physician or healthcare provider, or failing to check with the physician or healthcare provider when the order is questionable. Faulty technique in administering medications, especially injections that result in injury to the patient, is another common medication error.

Not all malpractice is a result of negligence. Malpractice claims are also founded on the daily interaction between the nurse and the patient; consequently, the nurse's personality plays a major role in fostering or preventing malpractice claims. All nurses should be familiar with the principles of psychology. The surest way to prevent claims is to recognize the patient as a human being who has emotional as well as physical needs, and to respond to these needs in a humane and competent manner.

If an error does occur, primary consideration must be given to the patient. Assessment of the patient is done first. The nurse notifies the physician and the immediate nursing supervisor; students notify the instructor. Error-in-medication forms are filled out, and appropriate action is taken under the direction of the physician or healthcare provider.

To prevent malpractice claims, the nurse must render, as consistently as possible, the best possible care to patients. Every nurse involved in direct care should regard prevention of malpractice claims as an integral part of daily nursing responsibilities, for two fundamental reasons:

1. Such measures result in higher-quality care.

2. All affirmative measures taken to minimize malpractice will minimize the nurse's exposure to personal liability.

How can a nurse avoid liability claims? First and foremost are the three checks and six rights (see p. 362). Accurate dosage calculation is also a safeguard against medication errors and potential liability claims.

OTHER SAFEGUARDS INCLUDE

- Know and follow institutional policies and procedures.

- Look up what you do not know.

- Do not leave medicines at the bedside.

- Chart carefully.

- Listen to the patient: "I never took that before," and the like.

- Check and double-check when a dose seems high. Most oral tablet doses range from 1/2 to 2 tablets. Most intramuscular, intradermal, and subcutaneous injections are less than 3 mL.

- Label any powder you dilute. Label any IV bag you use.

- When necessary, seek advice from competent professionals.

- Do not administer drugs prepared by another nurse.

- Keep drug knowledge up to date. Attend continuing education programs and update your nursing skills.

It is possible to render high-quality nursing care and never commit a medication error. Safe effective drug therapy is a combination of knowledge, skill, carefulness, and caring.

Medication Errors

- Prevent them.
- Don't make them.
- Don't be in a hurry.
- If you do make them, learn from your mistakes and don't make them again.

Reporting

- The nurse has a legal and ethical responsibility to report medication errors.
- Follow institutional policy in reporting and documenting medication errors.
- The FDA maintains a confidential database for medication errors: 1-800-23-ERROR. The FDA Medication Error web site is www.fda.gov/cder/drug/MedErrors.
- The National Coordinating Council for Medication Error Reporting and Prevention (NCCMERP) provides assistance on medication errors and promoting medication safety: 1-800-822-8772; the web site is www.nccmerp.org.

CLINICAL ALERT!

Ethical Principles in Drug Administration

Both moral and legal dimensions are involved in the administration of medications. Nurses are responsible for their actions. Here are two helpful web sites that relate to ethics: Nursing Ethics Resources (www.nursingethics.ca) and Nursing Ethics Network (www.nursingethicsnetwork.org).

The American Nurses Association Code of Ethics contains several statements that apply to drug therapy. Briefly stated, they are as follows:

1. The nurse provides services with respect for the patient's human dignity and uniqueness.

2. The nurse safeguards the patient's right to privacy.

3. The nurse acts to safeguard the patient from incompetent, unethical, or illegal practice.

4. The nurse assumes responsibility and accountability for nursing judgments and actions.

5. The nurse maintains competence in nursing.

When a nurse faces an ethical decision, several principles can serve as guides: autonomy, truthfulness, beneficence, nonmaleficence, confidentiality, justice, and fidelity.

Autonomy

Autonomy, or self-determination, is a form of personal liberty in which a person has the freedom to decide, knows the facts and understands them, and acts without outside force, deceit, or constraints. For the patient, this implies a right to be informed about drug therapy and a right to refuse medication. For the nurse, autonomy brings a responsibility to discuss drug information with the patient and to accept the patient's right to refuse. Autonomy also gives the nurse the right to refuse to participate in any drug therapy deemed to be unethical or unsafe for the patient.

Truthfulness

The nurse has an obligation not to lie. Telling the truth, however, is not the same as telling the whole truth. Ethically it is sometimes difficult to decide what may be concealed and what must be revealed.

In drug research the patient has a right to informed consent—to be told the truth before signing as a participant. In double-blind studies, used to determine effectiveness, patients are randomly assigned to an experimental group that receives the drug or to a control group that receives a placebo (a preparation devoid of pharmacologic effect). Neither the patient nor the nurse knows to which group he or she is assigned. To participate freely, the patient must receive full disclosure of risks and benefits and must understand the research design.

Beneficence

The principle of beneficence holds that the nurse should act in the patient's best interests. In fact, the respect due to the patient's freedom and to the patient's right to self-determination can sometimes limit the nurse's actions. If the nurse overrides a patient's wishes, deciding him- or herself what is best for the patient, the nurse is violating the patient's rights. Conflict can arise.

Nonmaleficence

The related but distinct principle of nonmaleficence holds that the nurse must not inflict harm on the patient and must prevent harm whenever possible. In drug therapy, every medication administered risks inducing some undesirable side effect and/or adverse effect. Chemotherapy, for example, may reduce the size of a tumor but may cause nausea, vomiting, decreased white cell count, and so forth. The nurse anticipates the untoward effects of drugs that may occur and acts to minimize them.

Confidentiality

Confidentiality is respect for the information that a nurse learns from professional involvement with patients. A patient's drug therapy and responses should be discussed only with people who have a right to know—that is, other professionals caring for the patient. The extent to which the family or significant others have a right to know depends on the specific situation and on the patient's wishes. These varying interests can cause conflict.

Justice

Justice refers to the patient's right to receive the right drug, the right dose, by the right route, at the right time. In addition, the patient has a right to the nurse's careful assessment, management, and evaluation of drug therapy, and to the nursing actions that promote the patient's safety and well-being. The nurse's obligation is to maintain a high standard of care.

Fidelity

A nurse should keep promises made to the patient. Statements such as "I'll be right back" and "I'll check the chart and let you know" create a covenant that should be respected.

Specific Points That May Be Helpful in Giving Medications

Three Checks and Six Rights

The nurse observes the three checks and six rights of medication administration.

Three Checks When Preparing Medications:

Read the label:

Check the drug label with medication administration record (MAR) when removing the container or unit dose package.

Check the drug label again immediately before pouring or opening the medication, or preparing the unit dose.

Check the drug label once more when replacing the container or before giving the unit dose to the patient.

Six Rights Before Administering Medications

1. Right medication
2. Right patient
3. Right dosage
4. Right route
5. Right time
6. Right documentation

Other rights that are important: the right to receive drug education, the right to refuse a drug, right drug preparation, right assessment, and right evaluation.

Medication Orders

A correct medication order bears the patient's name and room number, the date, the name of the drug (generic or trade), the dose of the drug, the route of administration, and the times to administer the drug.

It ends with the signature of the physician or healthcare provider.

Types of orders:

1. Standing order with termination

| **Example** | Keflex (cephalexin) 500 mg PO every 6 hours × 7 days |

2. Standing order without termination

| **Example** | Digoxin (Lanoxin) 0.5 mg PO every day |

3. A prn order

| **Example** | Demerol (meperidine) 50 mg IM q4h prn pain |

4. Single-dose order

| **Example** | atropine 0.3 mg subcutaneous 7:30 am on call to OR |

5. Stat order

| **Example** | morphine sulfate 4 mg IV stat |

Hospital guidelines provide for an automatic stop time on some classes of drugs; narcotic orders may be valid for only 3 days, antibiotics for 10 days. When first reading the order and transferring the order, the nurse must take care to note the expiration time, thus alerting all staff who pour medications. State laws and hospital policies vary.

Following are general guidelines in regards to several areas of medication administration:

Medication Orders for Physicians and Healthcare Providers

- Medical students may write orders on charts, but orders must be countersigned by a house physician before they are legal. Medical students are not licensed.

- In states that allow nurses or paramedical personnel to prescribe drugs, these care givers must follow hospital guidelines when carrying out orders.

- Do not carry out an order that is not clear or that is illegible. Check with the physician or healthcare provider who wrote the order. Do not assume anything.

- Do not carry out an order if a conflict exists with nursing knowledge. For example, Demerol (meperidine) 500 mg IM is above the average dose. Check with the physician or healthcare provider who wrote the order.

- Nursing students should not accept oral or telephone orders. The student should refer the physician to the instructor or staff nurse.

- Professional nurses may take oral or telephone orders in accord with institutional policy. The nurse must write these orders on the chart, and the physician or healthcare provider must sign them within 24 hours. Two nurses should listen to the order and verify it.

Knowledge Base

- Nurses should know the generic and trade names of drugs to be administered, as well as their class, average dose, routes of administration, use, side effects and adverse effects, contraindications, and nursing implications in administration. Nurses should also know what signs of effectiveness to look for and what drug interactions are possible. New or unfamiliar drugs require research.

- The nurse should be aware of the patient's diagnosis and medical history, especially relative to drugs taken. Be especially alert to OTC drugs, which patients often do not consider important. Check for allergies.

- Assess the patient's need for drug information. Be prepared to implement and evaluate a nursing care plan in drug therapy.

Medication Safety

- The patient has a right to considerate and respectful care, and the right to refuse a medication. The patient also has a right to know the name of the medication, what it is supposed to do, any side effects that may occur, and what to do should they occur.

- It is a fallacy that the nurse is no longer required to calculate or prepare drugs dispensed as unit dose. In some instances, the pharmacy may not have the exact dose on hand; or the nurse may need to administer a partial dose. The label must still be read three times.

- Labels must be clear. If not, return them to the pharmacy.

- In the ticket system, the Kardex is the main check against the medication ticket. If the medication ticket does not match the Kardex, further checking is necessary. First go to the chart and find the original order; then check through every order up until the current date to verify when the order changed. (The ticket system is rarely used.)

- In the unit dose mobile cart system, the nurse has the medication sheets of each patient together in a folder or on a computer printout. If unsure of an order, take the sheet to the patient's chart and check from the date ordered to the current date.

- If any doubt about a drug exists, do not administer it. Check further with the physician, the healthcare provider, the pharmacist, or a supervising nurse.

- Keys to a locked system or a Pyxis system are needed to obtain controlled drugs (e.g., narcotics) and to prevent others' access to medications.

- Pour oral medications first, then injections. For oral administration, use medical asepsis (clean technique). Injections require aseptic technique.

- Orders issued as "stat" take precedence and must be carried out immediately.

- Perform indicated nursing actions before administering certain medications. Example: Digitalis preparations require an apical heart rate, whereas antihypertensives require a blood pressure reading.

- Administer medications within 30 minutes of the time scheduled.

- Keep medications within sight at all times. Never leave medications unattended.

- Do not administer a medication if assessment shows that the drug is contraindicated or that an adverse effect may have occurred as a result of a previous dose. If you withhold a drug, notify the physician or healthcare provider who wrote the order.

Oral Medications—Tablets and Capsules

- Administer irritating oral drugs along with meals or a snack (unless contraindicated), to decrease gastric irritation.

- If the patient is nauseated or vomiting, withhold oral medications and notify the physician or the healthcare provider. Be sure to chart this action.

- Break a tablet only if it is scored.

- Never open capsules or break EC tablets. If the patient cannot swallow capsules or tablets, either ask the physician or healthcare provider to order a liquid, or check with the pharmacist.

- Check the tablets in a stock container. Are they the same size? Same color? If not, return them to the pharmacy.

- Hydrophilic capsules are not medications. They are labeled DO NOT EAT and are placed in stock containers of tablets and capsules to absorb dampness and to maintain the drug in a solid state.

Liquid Medications

- Read labels three times: (1) when removing the drug from storage, (2) when calculating the dose, and (3) after pouring the drug.

- Quiet and concentration are needed to pour drugs. Follow a routine in pouring. Methodology is the best safeguard in preventing error.

- Never return any poured drug to a stock bottle once the drug has been taken from the preparation room.

- Never combine medications from two stock bottles. Return both bottles to the pharmacy. It is the responsibility of the pharmacists to combine drugs.

- Some liquid medications require dilution. Check references for directions.

- Some liquids may have to be administered through a straw. Liquid iron preparations, for example, cause discoloring and should not come in contact with teeth.

- Pour liquids at eye level, using a medicine cup. Measure at the center of the meniscus. To keep from spilling the medication onto the label (which could make it unreadable), pour with the label up.

- After the patient has taken a liquid antacid, add 5 to 10 mL water to the cup, mix, and have the patient drink it as well. Because antacids are thick, some medication often remains in the cup.

- The nurse who pours medications is responsible for administering and charting.

- Do not give drugs that another nurse has poured.

- Aqueous or water-based solutions do not need to be shaken before pouring.

Giving Medications

- Follow the universal safeguards in administration of medication (see Chapter 13).

- **Always check the patient's ID band before administering medications (Fig. 12-2). If the patient does not have an ID band, have a responsible person identify the patient for you and obtain an ID band for the patient.**

- Listen to the patient's comments and act on them. If a patient says something like "That's not mine" or "I never took this before," check carefully, then return to the patient with the result of your investigation. Failure to do this will cause you to lose the patient's trust and confidence, and may result in a medication error.

- If a patient refuses a drug, find out why. First check the chart, to see if the drug was in fact ordered; then talk to the patient to understand his or her reasons. After charting the reason for refusal, notify the physician or healthcare provider who wrote the order.

- Watch to make sure the patient takes the drugs. Stay until oral drugs are swallowed.

- Keep drugs within view at all times.

- Never leave any drug at the bedside stand unless hospital policy permits this. If a medication is left with the patient, inform the patient why the drug is ordered, how to take it, and what to expect. Later, check to determine whether the drug was taken, and record the findings.

Charting

Documentation is the "sixth right" of medication administration. The always-quoted axiom is still true: "If it's not charted, it's not done."

- Chart all medications after administration.

- Chart single doses, stat doses, and prn medications immediately, and note the exact time when they were administered.

- Chart any nursing actions done before administering drugs (e.g., apical heart rate [with digoxin], or blood pressure [with antihypertensives]). The safest place to chart these actions is on the medication administration record where the drug is documented.

- If the drug was refused or was withheld (not given), write the reason on the nurse's notes and/or on the medication administration record, and notify the healthcare provider who ordered the medication. Also note the time you notified the healthcare provider, and any response.

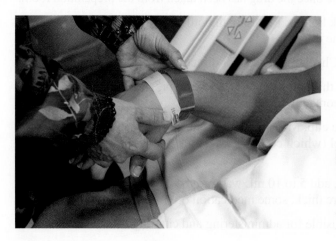

FIGURE 12-2

Checking the patient's armband. (With permission from Evans-Smith, P. [2005] Lippincott's atlas of medication administration [2nd ed.] Philadelphia: Lippincott Williams and Wilkins, p. 8.)

Evaluation

- Check for the expected effect of the drug. Did side effects or adverse effects occur? Perform indicated nursing actions. Record your observations.

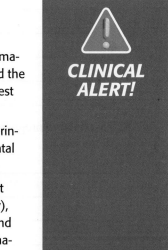

CLINICAL ALERT!

Age-Specific Considerations

- Neonatal clients—The nurse needs to consider the immaturity of organ function, the importance of weight, and the precision of dosage calculation (rounding to the nearest one hundredth).

- Pediatric clients—The nurse needs to remember the principles of atraumatic care and to consider developmental stages.

- Geriatric clients—The nurse needs to take into account decreasing organ function (especially liver and kidney), circulatory changes leading to decreased perfusion, and physical limitations (poor eyesight, decreased coordination, decreased ability to chew and/or swallow).

Error in Medication

- Report any error immediately to the charge nurse and the physician or healthcare provider.

- Always give primary concern to the patient.

- Fill out an error-in-medication form. Follow the physician's or healthcare provider's directions in caring for the patient.

CRITICAL THINKING: TEST YOUR CLINICAL SAVVY

Mr. T is a patient receiving a drug that is in a drug study.

A. As a nurse administering this drug, what is your ethical responsibility?

B. If the patient asks "Is it safe to take this drug?" what is an appropriate response? If the patient refuses to take the drug, what should you do?

C. You agree with the patient that he should not take the experimental drug. What are your ethical responsibilities? What are your legal responsibilities?

Mr. T discovers from the Internet that the drug he is taking is an experimental drug and that another drug with similar actions has been released by the FDA and is available by prescription.

D. How do you respond to the information that he has acquired? What are some questions that the patient should ask regarding information acquired over the Internet?

E. If the patient asks you whether he should continue to take the experimental drug, or whether he should discontinue his participation in the drug study and obtain a prescription for the similar drug, what is an appropriate response?

F. What reasons can you give Mr. T regarding the benefits of participating in a drug study?

SELF-TEST 1   **Basic Information**

Give the information requested. (Answers appear at the end of the chapter.)

1. List at least 10 kinds of information the nurse needs to know in order to administer drugs safely.

   _____   _____

   _____   _____

   _____   _____

   _____   _____

   _____   _____

2. List the five pregnancy categories used to identify the safety of drugs for the fetus and briefly define each.

   _____

   _____

   _____

   _____

   _____

3. Name the major organ for the following drug activities.

   a. Absorption _____   **c.** Biotransformation _____

   b. Distribution _____   **d.** Excretion _____

4. Define these terms:

   a. Tolerance _____

   _____

   _____

   b. Cumulation _____

   _____

   _____

5. List the four elements of negligence.

   _____,

   _____,

   _____, and

   _____

6. What is the standard by which a tort is judged?

   _____

   _____

   _____

(continued)

7. List at least five positive actions to avoid liability.

_____

_____

_____

_____

_____

8. List and briefly describe five ethical principles in drug therapy.

_____

_____

_____

_____

_____

9. What are the seven elements of a correct medication order?

_____

_____

_____

_____

_____

_____

10. When an order is not clear, what action should a nurse take?

_____

_____

Name: _____

Choose the correct answer. Answers are given in Appendix A.

1. Two drugs are given for different reasons, but drug Y interferes with the excretion of drug X. The effect of drug X would be

   a. increased
   b. decreased
   c. unchanged
   d. stopped

2. Major biotransformation of drugs occurs in the

   a. lungs
   b. kidney
   c. liver
   d. urine

3. Toxicity to a drug is more likely to occur when

   a. elimination of the drug is rapid
   b. the drug is bound to the plasma protein albumin
   c. the drug will not dissolve in the lipid layer of the cell
   d. the drug is free in the blood circulation

4. The term USP after a drug name indicates that the drug

   a. is made only in the United States
   b. meets official standards in the United States
   c. cannot be made by any other pharmaceutical company
   d. is registered by the US Public Health Service

5. When an order is written to be administered "as needed" it is called a

   a. standing order
   b. prn order
   c. single order
   d. stat order

6. Signs of effectiveness of a drug are based on what information?

   a. action and use
   b. untoward effects
   c. generic and trade names
   d. drug interaction

7. Drug classification is an aid in understanding

   a. use of the drug
   b. drug idiosyncrasy
   c. the trade name
   d. the generic name

(continued)

8. Names of many drugs include

   a. several generic, several trade names
   b. several generic, one trade name
   c. one generic, one trade name
   d. one generic, several trade names

9. Which pregnancy category is considered safe for the fetus?

   a. A
   b. B
   c. C
   d. D

10. What is the primary purpose of EC medications?

    a. improve taste
    b. delay absorption
    c. code the drug for identification
    d. make the drug easier to swallow

11. Which of the following drug preparations does *not* have to be shaken before pouring?

    a. magma
    b. gel
    c. suspension
    d. aqueous solution

12. Most oral drugs are absorbed in the

    a. mouth
    b. stomach
    c. small intestine
    d. large intestine

13. Nursing legal responsibilities associated with controlled substances include

    a. storage in a locked place
    b. assessing vital signs
    c. evaluating psychological response
    d. establishing automatic 24-hour stop orders

14. Characteristics of a schedule II drug include

    a. accepted medical use with a high abuse potential
    b. medically accepted drug with low-dependence possibility
    c. no accepted use in patient care
    d. unlimited renewals

15. The responsibilities of the nurse regarding medication in the hospital include all except

    a. prescribing drugs
    b. teaching patients
    c. regulating automatic expiration times of drugs
    d. preparing solutions

(continued)

16. Under what condition does a nurse have a right to refuse to administer a drug?

    a. The pharmacist ordered the drug.
    b. The drug is manufactured by two different companies.
    c. The drug is prescribed by a licensed physician.
    d. The dose is within the range given in the physicians desk reference.

17. When administering medication in the hospital, the nurse should

    a. chart medications before administering them
    b. chart only those drugs that she or he personally gave the patient
    c. chart all medications given for the day at one time
    d. determine the best method for giving the drugs

18. Which of the following illustrates a medication error?

    a. administering a 10 AM dose at 10:20 AM
    b. giving 2 tablets of gantrisin (sufisoxazole) 500 mg when 1 g is ordered
    c. pouring 5 mL of cough syrup when 1 tsp is ordered
    d. giving digoxin (Lanoxin) IM when digoxin po 0.25 mg is ordered

19. A nurse reads a medication order that is not clear. What action is indicated?

    a. Ask the charge nurse to explain the order.
    b. Ask a doctor at the nurses' station for help.
    c. Check the drug reference on the unit.
    d. Check with the doctor who wrote the order.

20. Which nursing action is illegal?

    a. Pouring medication from one stock bottle into another.
    b. Counting control drugs in the narcotic cabinet or Pyxis each shift.
    c. Labeling a vial of powder after dissolving it.
    d. Refusing to carry out an order that is confusing.

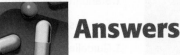

Answers

Self-Test I Basic Information

1. Generic/trade name, drug class and drug classification, pregnancy category, dose and route, action, use, side/adverse effects, contraindications/precautions, interactions/ incompatibilities, nursing implications, evaluation of effectiveness, patient teaching

2. **A.** No risk to fetus
   B. No adverse effects in animals, but no human studies
   C. Animals show adverse effects; calculated risk to fetus
   D. Fetal risk exists
   X. Absolute fetal abnormality

3. **a.** Small intestines
   b. Blood
   c. Liver
   d. Kidney

4. **a.** Repeated administration of a drug increases microsomal enzyme activity in the liver. The drug is broken down more quickly and its effectiveness is decreased.
   b. Biotransformation is inhibited and the drug level remains high. Adverse effects are more likely to occur.

5. A claim that a nurse–patient relationship existed

   The nurse was required to meet a standard of care

   A claim that harm or injury occurred because the standard was not met

   A claim of damages for which compensation is sought

6. Whether the nurse exercised the degree of skill and care that a reasonably prudent nurse with similar training and experience, practicing in the same community, would exercise under the same or similar circumstances

7. Know policies and practices of the institution.
   Research unfamiliar drugs.
   Do not leave medicines at the bedside.
   Chart carefully.
   Listen to the patient's complaints.
   Check yourself (eg, read labels three times).
   Label anything you dilute.
   Keep up to date.

8. Autonomy: freedom to decide based on knowledge with no constraint
   Truthfulness: truth telling that can create a dilemma. Is it absolute or is there a beneficent deceit?
   Beneficence: obligation to help others
   Nonmaleficence: do no harm
   Confidentiality: keep secrets
   Justice: rights of an individual
   Fidelity: keep promises

9. Patient's name and room, date, name of drug, dose, route, times of administration, doctor's or health care provider's signature

10. The nurse does not administer the drug and checks with the physician or health care provider who wrote the order.

1. Standard precautions

2. Systems of administration

3. Guidelines for administrati
drugs
Oral
Parenteral—IM, subcuta
IV, IVPB, intradermal

4. Administering Injections
Topical—skin, mucous
membrane

5. Special Considerations
Neonatal and Pediatric
Geriatric

CHAPTER

13

Administration Procedures

Throughout this text we have calculated dosages and studied information related to drug therapy. This chapter is the "how to" chapter—describing the actual methods of administering drugs orally, parenterally, and topically. The adages "practice makes perfect" and "one picture is worth a thousand words" apply. Administering medications is a skilled activity that requires practice—with supervision—to ensure correct technique. As this chapter covers only the basics, you will want to work with a medication administration skill book and a pharmacology textbook as well.

Every institution has a standard procedure for administering medications, which depends on the way its drugs are dispensed: by unit-dose, in multidose containers, or a combination of the two. Institutional procedure may call for the use of a mobile cart with medication administration records, or a locked medication dispensing system, or the use of a computer printout or a bar code device.

Whatever the procedure's specifications, follow them carefully. Step-by-step attention to detail is the best safeguard to ensure the patient's six rights.

Standard Precautions Applied to Administration of Medications

When you are administering drugs, there's a chance that the patient's blood, body fluids, or tissues can come into contact with your skin or mucous membranes. So you always risk potential exposure to a long list of viruses, including these: hepatitis A (HAV), hepatitis B (HBV), hepatitis C (HCV), hepatitis D (HDV), hepatitis E (HEV), and the human immunodeficiency virus (HIV).

The Centers for Disease Control and Prevention (CDC) in Atlanta recommends standard precautions in caring for all patients and when handling equipment that's contaminated with blood or blood-streaked body fluids. In 1996, the term *standard precautions* replaced "universal precautions." *Transmission-based precautions* are those used with patients who have a suspected infection. For more information on these procedures, see the CDC web site: http://www.cdc.gov/ncidod/dhqp/index.html

The following points, based on CDC guidelines, can help you determine appropriate safeguards in giving medications. The safeguards you need to follow depend on the type of contact you have with patients.

General Safeguards in Administering Medications

1. Oral medications: Handwashing is adequate. If there's a possibility of exposure to blood or body secretions, wear gloves.

2. Injections: Both handwashing and gloves are required. Do not recap needles. Carefully dispose of used sharps, either by holding the sharp away from you in a puncture-proof container or by using a needle-guard device.

3. Heparin locks, IV catheters, and IV needles: Wash your hands and wear gloves when inserting or removing IV needles and catheters. Dispose of used sharps in a puncture-proof container, or use a needleguard device.

4. Secondary administration sets or IVPB sets: Before removing this equipment from the main IV tubing, wash your hands and put on gloves. Either use a needleless device or place used needles in a puncture-proof container.

5. Application of medication to mucous membranes: Wash your hands and wear gloves (see the following guidelines for using gowns, masks, and protective eyewear).

6. Applications to skin: Before applying such drug forms as transdermal patches or applying lotions, ointments or creams, wash your hands and wear gloves.

Hands

1. With each patient, always wash your hands twice: before preparing medications and after administering medications.

2. Wash your hands after removing your gloves, gown, mask, and protective eyewear, and wash them again before leaving any patient's room where you have used them.

3. If your hands have come into contact with a patient's blood or body fluids, wash them *immediately.*

4. Wash your hands after handling any equipment soiled with blood or body fluids.

Gloves

1. While administering medications, wear gloves for any direct ("hands-on") contact with a patient's blood, bodily fluids, or secretions.

2. Wear gloves when handling materials or equipment contaminated with blood or body fluids.

3. Whenever you use gloves, you must change them after completing procedures for each patient, and between patients.

Gowns

When administering medications, you need to wear a gown if there's a risk that your clothing may become contaminated with a patient's blood or body fluids.

Masks, Protective Eyewear, and Face Shields

1. A mask is required when you are caring for a patient on strict or respiratory isolation procedures.

2. Masks and protective eyewear or face shields are required when a medication procedure may cause blood or body fluids to splash directly onto your face, eyes, or mucous membranes.

3. You must wear masks and protective eyewear during any medication procedure known to cause aerosolization of fluids that contain chemicals or body fluids.

Management of Used Needles and Sharps

1. All used needles, syringes, sharps, stylets, butterfly needles, and IV catheters must be discarded in appropriate, labeled, puncture-proof containers.

2. Do not break, bend, or recap needles after using them. Immediately place needles in a puncture-proof container.

3. Wear gloves and exercise caution when removing heparin locks, IV catheters, and IV needles. Place them in a puncture-proof container. Never remove the IV needle from the IV tubing by hand. Instead,

use either a clamp or the needle unlocking device on the sharps container. It's best to use needleless systems or needleguard devices.

4. As you dispose of a sharp, keep your eyes on the sharps (puncture-proof) container.

Needleless Systems and Needleguard Devices

Needleless systems, used to reduce the risk of needlesticks and blood-borne pathogens, work in several ways. Some syringes have a needleguard device that retracts the needle into the syringe or a cap after it is used. Needleless adapters for syringes withdraw medication from vials (Fig. 13-1). Needleless systems are also available for IV tubing (Fig. 13-2) and for use at the patient's IV site. All needleless equipment must be discarded into sharp containers.

Management of Materials Other Than Needles and Sharps

Paper cups, plastic cups, and other equipment not contaminated with blood or body fluids may be discarded according to routine hospital procedures. In situations that require strict or respiratory isolation precautions, follow the institution's established protocol.

Management of Nurse Exposed to Blood or Body Fluids

If a personal needlestick, an injury, or a skin laceration causes contact with the blood or blood-streaked body fluids of any patient, *act immediately:* Squeeze the area of contact if appropriate, wash the area

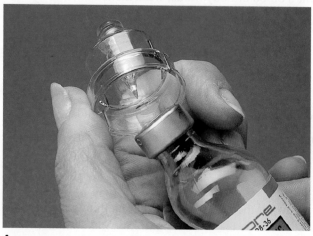

A

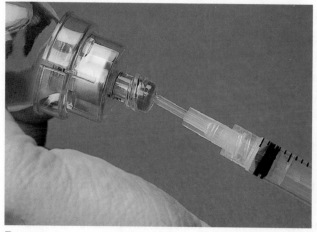

B

FIGURE 13-1

(A) Needleless system adapter for vial. (B) Use syringe (without needle) to withdraw medication.

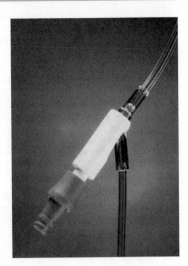

FIGURE 13-2
Needleless system for IV tubing

with soap and copious amounts of water, and apply an acceptable antiseptic. If mucous membrane exposure occurs, flush the exposed areas with copious amounts of warm water. Follow the protocol established by the healthcare institution for management of needlestick injury or accidental exposure to blood or body fluids.

Systems of Administration

Institutions establish their own systems for administering medication. You might need to use tickets, the mobile cart, a locked medication cabinet near the patient's bedside, and/or computer printouts.

Unit-dose packaging is the most widely used system. Drugs are dispensed by the pharmacy and placed in individual patient drawers, either on a mobile cart, or in a locked cabinet at the patient's bedside. The mobile cart can be wheeled into the patient's room so that you can prepare medications at the bedside for administration.

A newer system uses a scanner device, scanning the patient's ID band, the nurse's ID, the medication administration record, and the medication in unit dose packaging. If the scan reveals any discrepancy, the device alerts the nurse.

The ticket system, rarely used, works with drugs that are dispensed in multidose containers. The nurse prepares the drugs in a medication room and then carries them on a tray to the patient.

Medication Administration Record

The Medication Administration Record (MAR), a daily (24 hours) record of what medications are ordered for the patient, also documents the medications given by the nurse. Most MARs consist of a computerized printout (Fig. 13-3), with key identifying information—the patient's name, ID number, room, date of admission, age, diagnosis, gender, and attending physician—printed at the top. Orders written during the shift have to be added to the printout by hand, a procedure that can lead to medication errors. Therefore hospitals require that every shift, the nurse must check the MAR against the original orders in the chart, to make sure that the orders are correct.

Each healthcare setting will have different guidelines on charting medications. Generally, routine medications are assigned a scheduled time on the MAR. After the nurse gives the medication, a line is drawn through the time and initialed. If the medication is refused or held, the time is circled and initialed and then a reason given why the medication was not given. Prn meds are not assigned a scheduled time on the MAR, rather, after the medication is given, the time is then written on the MAR, a line crossed through that time and then initialed. Different medications may be given at different scheduled times throughout the day, for example Coumadin is given at 1700 or 1800 in the evening, so that the therapeutic effect is maximized. Follow institutional guidelines for medication administration times.

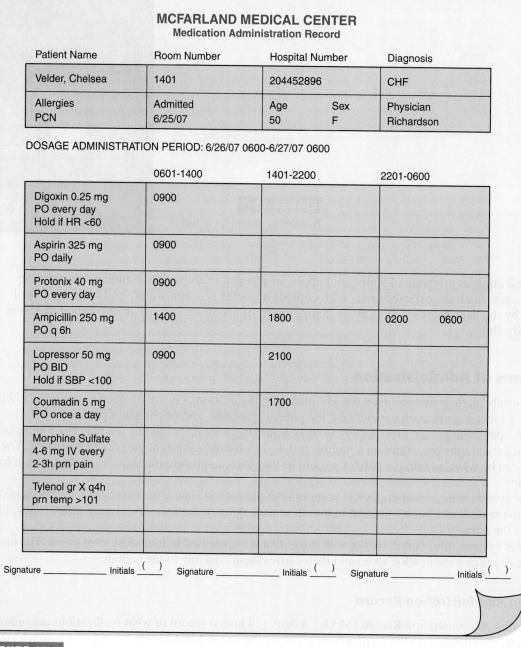

MCFARLAND MEDICAL CENTER
Medication Administration Record

Patient Name	Room Number	Hospital Number		Diagnosis
Velder, Chelsea	1401	204452896		CHF
Allergies PCN	Admitted 6/25/07	Age 50	Sex F	Physician Richardson

DOSAGE ADMINISTRATION PERIOD: 6/26/07 0600-6/27/07 0600

	0601-1400	1401-2200	2201-0600	
Digoxin 0.25 mg PO every day Hold if HR <60	0900			
Aspirin 325 mg PO daily	0900			
Protonix 40 mg PO every day	0900			
Ampicillin 250 mg PO q 6h	1400	1800	0200	0600
Lopressor 50 mg PO BID Hold if SBP <100	0900	2100		
Coumadin 5 mg PO once a day		1700		
Morphine Sulfate 4-6 mg IV every 2-3h prn pain				
Tylenol gr X q4h prn temp >101				

Signature _____ Initials __( )__   Signature _____ Initials __( )__   Signature _____ Initials __( )__

FIGURE 13-3

A sample 24-hour computerized medication record. Scheduled drugs are listed at the top of the sheet and PRN orders at the bottom. Military time is used. The nurse draws a line through the time administered, and initialed to indicate that the drug was administered, then signs at the bottom of the sheet.

Ticket System

This system transfers a medication order to three places: a medication ticket, the patient's medication sheet, and the patient's Kardex file, which contains the nursing care plan. Tickets for all patients are kept in a central location. The nurse sorts them according to time of administration and compares them with the Kardex entry. If there is a discrepancy, the nurse checks the original order on the patient's chart, using three-check system:

Check 1: Separate the first patient's tickets and place them together in a pile; read each ticket, locate the medication in the medication cart or medication room, and verify that the label matches the ticket.

Check 2: Compare the dose on the ticket with the label, then calculate and pour the amount of the drug.
Check 3: Before discarding the unit-dose packet or returning the container to the shelf, read the order and the label again, verifying the poured dose.

Having finished these checks, place each medication on a tray with the ticket in front to identify it. Then dispense the medication to the patient, identifying the patient by ID band and keeping the medications in sight. Complete any required nursing assessment (e.g., obtain a blood pressure or heart rate). Administer the drugs, then take the medication tray to the next patient and follow the same procedure. After giving all the medications, chart them on each patient's chart. If you give a stat medication, chart it and destroy the ticket.

This system has a number of disadvantages: Since every order must be transcribed to three different places, that opens three opportunities for error. Also, tickets can be lost or misplaced; an error may occur while the nurse is choosing the stock medication; and if the tickets become mixed, a medication may go to the wrong patient. Medications requiring assessment need some kind of tag, for identification, and locating the chart of each patient takes a lot of time.

Mobile Cart System

In this system, pharmacy dispenses unit-dose medications directly to the patient's drawer in the mobile cart, which is labeled with the patient's name. The cart contains all the equipment the nurse might require to administer medications.

When a drug is ordered, the nurse transcribes the order to only one place: the patient's medication administration record, either in a medication book on the cart or in the patient's chart.

Here's the appropriate procedure: When it's time to administer medications, wash your hands and roll the cart to the bedside of the first patient. Identify the patient verbally by name, unlock the cart, and open the medication book to that patient's medication sheet.

Before giving the medication, check the sheet for special nursing actions required, such as obtaining a blood pressure or heart rate. Carry out the orders, record the results, and decide whether to withhold the medication or to administer it.

First check: Place the patient's drawer on the top of the cart. Read each medication order, starting with the first medication listed. If you're giving a dose, choose the unit-dose from the drawer and compare the label with the order (Fig. 13-4). Check the label.

Second check: After comparing the order with the unit measure, compute the dose. Then open or prepare the unit-dose, and pour the amount.

Third check: Label the unit dose, read the order again, and verify the dose. After preparing all the patient's medications, read the name on the medicine sheet, check the patient's ID band, and administer the drugs. Remain with the patient until he or she has taken the medications; then provide any comfort measures, wash your hands, and return to the cart to chart the drugs administered. Replace the patient's drawer and roll the cart to the next patient. When all the medications have been administered, return the mobile cart to its designated area.

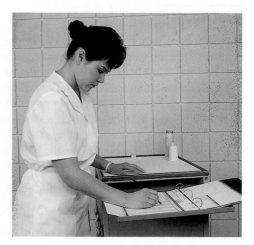

FIGURE 13-4

The nurse compares the medication with the order. (With permission from Roach, S. [2004]. *Introductory clinical pharmacology* [7th ed.]. Philadelphia: Lippincott Williams & Wilkins, p. 16.)

This system has several advantages. Two professionals—the pharmacist and the nurse—check the medication in the drawer. All the medication administration records are together on the cart, which saves time. The nurse can carry out assessment and can chart the results before pouring any medication. Immediately after administering the drugs, the nurse can sign for them.

Note that with the ticket system and the mobile cart system, you must *check the label three times:* when choosing the drug, when pouring the dose or opening the medication, and before replacing the container or giving the unit-dose to the patient.

In a variation of the mobile cart system, the medications are locked in a cabinet at or near the patient's bedside. As with the original mobile cart system, the pharmacy fills the cabinet with the unit-dose medications. Medication administration records are in the patient chart, which is in the cabinet; and the nurse prepares the medications in the same manner, using the three checks and the six rights. Having the medications and the patient's chart closer to the patient's bedside saves time for both the patient and the nurse.

Many hospitals are using the computerized narcotic cart or cabinet (Pyxis system) to dispense all medications (controlled substances and non-controlled medications). The computer in the cart or cabinet stores a record of each medication, when it is due, and lists this information for each patient. The nurse simply goes to the Pyxis with the medication administration record (MAR) and removes the unit-doses for each patient by accessing the computer. This system provides yet another check to make sure that the right patient receives the right medication, the right dose, at the right time.

Computer Scanning

Like the mobile cart system, this system uses a portable computer scanning device, which stores information about the patient and the medication. The unit-dose packaging used with this system shows bar codes. The nurse's process is simple: Prepare the medications and check each one against the medication administration record. Use the scanning device to scan the patient's ID band, your own ID, the medication package, and the medication administration record. If the computer detects no discrepancy, you can continue to administer the medications as described in the previous paragraph.

Computer Order Entry

Some institutions have computerized medication procedures, which enable doctors or prescribing healthcare providers to input medication orders directly onto the computer. The pharmacy receives the order and adds it to the patient's drug profile; subsequently the nursing unit receives a computer printout that lists the medications and times of administration (the frequency of updates varies according to the hospital). This system presents several advantages: Neither the nurse nor the pharmacist has to interpret the handwriting of the doctor or healthcare provider. The nurse does not have to transfer the written orders to an MAR—lessening the chance for error while also saving time. Moreover, a computer check identifies possible interactions among the patient's medications and alerts the nurse and the pharmacist.

Routes of Administration

Oral Route

Regardless of which system you use to prepare the medications, the procedure for administering drugs requires specific steps. The oral route is the least expensive, the safest, and also the easiest to administer.

For oral administration, you first identify the patient verbally by name, check the ID band, and make sure the patient is alert and able to swallow. If so, assist him/her to a sitting position. Give oral solids first, along with a full glass of water whenever possible (unless contraindicated). Then give oral liquid medications. Watch to be sure that the patient has swallowed all the drugs. Discard the paper and/or plastic cups according to routine hospital procedure, unless the patient is on strict or respiratory isolation. For this condition, use special isolation bags. Finally, make the patient comfortable, wash your hands, and chart the medications given.

Special considerations for oral administration include the following:

- Check expiration dates on all labels. Never administer expired drugs.
- Check patients for allergies to drugs. This should be a routine procedure.
- Some drugs are best taken on an empty stomach; others may be taken with food.

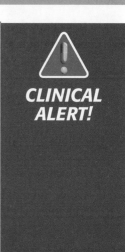

Medication Errors

CLINICAL ALERT!

- Medication errors can cause unnecessary side effects, adverse effects, illnesses, and sometimes death.
- Medication errors are among the most common medical errors, harming at least 1.5 million people every year, according to the Institute of Medicine of the National Academies.
- The three most common errors are administering an improper dose, administering the wrong drug, and using the wrong route of administration.
- Medication errors are preventable. As a nurse, you can prevent medication errors by following the six rights of medication administration and the three checks of medication identification. For information on medication errors, visit the FDA web site (www.fda.gov/cder/drug/MedErrors/reports.htm).

- Be aware of foods or fluids that are safe for ingesting with the drug, and those that are contraindicated.
- Even if the patient is NPO (nothing by mouth), the patient may need to receive certain drugs (e.g., an anticonvulsant for a patient with epilepsy). Check with the doctor or healthcare provider to determine whether you can administer oral medication with a small amount of water.
- When administering solid stock medications, pour them first into the container lid and then into a paper cup, using medical asepsis. Do not touch the medication. You can combine several solids in the cup, but you should first pour each medication into a separate cup. Check all unit-dose medications three times before you discard the package container.
- To break a scored tablet, use medical asepsis: clean (not sterile) technique. One method is to place the tablet in a paper towel, fold the towel over and, with your thumbs and index fingers in apposition, break the tablet along the score line. You can also use commercial pill splitters. Don't break any tablets that are not scored.
- If the patient has difficulty swallowing solids, first determine whether the medication is available in a liquid form. Don't crush enteric-coated and film-coated tablets, and don't open capsules; instead, check with the pharmacist for alternative forms. If opening a capsule won't compromise the medication inside it, you can open the capsule and mix the drug with a small amount of applesauce, custard, or other soft food that will make the medication more palatable and easy to swallow.
- If crushing a pill won't compromise its medication, you can crush it, preferably using a commercial "pill crusher." You can also crush a pill using a mortar and pestle; just make sure to clean both implements before and after crushing, so no residue remains. To help a patient swallow the medication, you can mix a crushed drug with water or semisolids, such as applesauce or custard.
- Be knowledgeable about food–drug, drug–drug, and herb-drug interactions, and always act to safeguard the patient.

Special Considerations for Liquid Medications

- Shake liquid medications (magmas, gels, suspensions) thoroughly before pouring; otherwise the drug in the liquid may settle to the bottom.

- Pour liquids at eye level, then place them on a flat surface to accurately measure the dose. When pouring liquids, keep the label face up so it will not become stained. Before recapping, wipe the lip of the bottle with a paper towel.

- Note any unusual color change or precipitate in a liquid. If such a change occurs, do not use the medication. Send the container to the pharmacy with a note describing what you've observed.

- Check references to determine how to disguise liquids that are distasteful or irritating. Two possibilities are to mix them with juice or to administer them through a straw after diluting well. Because liquid iron preparations stain the teeth, have the patient take them through a straw placed in the back of the mouth. Always dilute tinctures.

- Don't dilute liquid cough mixtures. Besides their antitussive action, they have a secondary soothing (demulcent) effect on the mucous membranes.

Parenteral Route

You can give medications by IM, subcutaneous, IVPB, or IV routes, or intradermally. Use the parenteral route when a patient cannot take the drug orally, or when you want to obtain a rapid systemic effect, or when the oral route would destroy a drug or render it ineffective. With parenteral routes, use aseptic technique.

Choosing the Site for Intradermal, Intramuscular, or Subcutaneous Injections

Avoid the following areas: bony prominences, large blood vessels, nerves, sensitive areas, bruises, hardened areas, abrasions, and inflamed areas; also areas contraindicated from previous medical procedures, such as mastectomies, renal shunts, and grafts. The site for intramuscular injections should be able to accept 3 mL; if you're giving repeated injections, rotate sites.

Preparation of the Skin

Clean the site with an alcohol pad, using a circular motion from the center out. Grasping the area firmly between your thumb and forefinger, insert the needle with a dartlike motion (Fig. 13-5). If the area is obese, you can spread the skin rather than pinching it together.

Syringes for Injection

The most common syringe used for injections is a standard 3-mL size, marked in minims and in milliliters to the nearest tenth. The precision (tuberculin) syringe is marked in half minims and milliliters to the near-

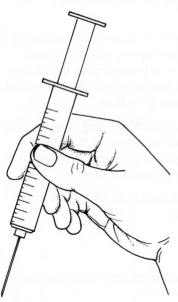

FIGURE 13-5

An injection is administered with a quick, dart-like motion into taut skin that has been spread or bunched together.

est hundredth. There are two insulin syringes: a regular 1-mL size marked to 100 units, and a 0.5-mL size (low-dose) insulin syringe marked to 50 units.

Needles for Injections

Needles are chosen both for their length and for their gauge (the diameter of the needle opening). The *length* of needles varies from 5/16 to 2 inches, as appropriate to the route. Here's the *gauge* principle: The higher the gauge number, the finer the needle.

The finest needle currently available for routine injections is the 28-gauge needle on the insulin syringe. Gauge numbers 25, 26, and 28 are used in subcutaneous injections for adults, and in IM injections for children and emaciated patients. Numbers 23 and 22 are used for IM injections; 20 and 21 are for IV therapy; and 16 and 18 are for blood transfusions.

Angle of Insertion

INTRAMUSCULAR. For an intramuscular injection, hold the syringe at a right angle to the skin. Give the injection at a 90-degree angle (Fig. 13-6). Intramuscular sites have a good blood supply, and absorption is rapid.

SUBCUTANEOUS. For subcutaneous injections, hold the syringe at a 45-degree angle when you insert the needle. You can administer some subcutaneous injections at a 90-degree angle if the subcutaneous layer of fat is thick and the needle is short. Be careful to reach the correct site. When in doubt, use the 45-degree angle. Subcutaneous sites have a poor blood supply, and absorption is prolonged (Fig. 13-6).

INTRADERMAL. If you're doing skin testing for allergies and tuberculosis, use a 26-gauge or other fine needle. Hold the syringe at a 15-degree angle (Fig. 13-6).

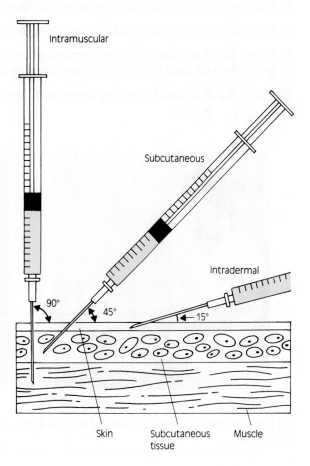

FIGURE 13-6

Comparison of angles of intersection for intramuscular, subcutaneous, and intradermal injections.

Preparing the Dose

To prevent incompatibility of drugs, ordinarily you draw up only one medication in a syringe. If you're giving two drugs in one syringe, first determine that the drugs are compatible and then follow the procedure for mixing.

DRUGS THAT ARE LIQUIDS IN VIALS

1. Clean the top of the vial with an alcohol pad.

2. Draw up into the syringe an amount of air equivalent to the desired amount of solution (Fig. 13-7A).

3. Inject the needle (or needleless device) through the rubber diaphragm into the vial.

4. Expel air from the syringe into the vial. This increases the pressure in the vial and makes it easier to withdraw medication.

5. Invert the vial, hold it at eye level, and draw up the desired amount into the syringe (Fig. 13-7B).

6. Withdraw the needle or needleless device quickly from the vial.

DRUGS THAT ARE POWDERS IN VIALS

1. Clean the top of the vial with an alcohol pad.

2. Draw up the amount of calculated diluent from a vial of distilled water or normal saline for injection. If a different diluent is indicated, follow pharmaceutical directions.

3. Add the diluent to the powder, and roll the vial between your hands to make the powder dissolve.

4. Label the vial with the solution made, your initials, and the date and time.

5. Clean the top of the vial again.

6. Draw up into the syringe an amount of air equivalent to the amount of solution desired.

7. Inject the needle or needleless device through the rubber diaphragm into the vial.

8. Expel the air into the vial. This increases pressure in the vial and makes it easier to remove medication. Invert the vial, hold it at eye level, and draw up the desired amount of medication into the syringe.

9. Check the directions for storing any remaining drug.

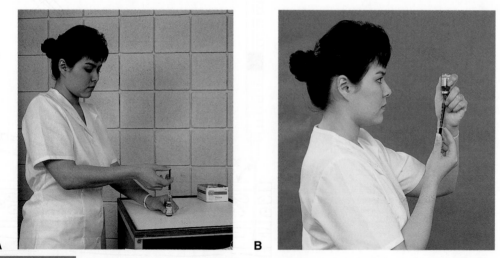

A   **B**

FIGURE 13-7

(A) Injecting air into the vial. **(B)** Invert the vial and draw up the desired amount of medication into the syringe.

Note: When the whole amount of powder contained in a vial is needed for an IVPB medication, you can use a reconstitution device as a way of diluting the powder without a syringe.

DRUGS IN GLASS AMPULES

1. Tap the top of the ampule with your finger to clear out any drug.

2. Place an opened alcohol pad around the neck of the ampule.

3. Hold the ampule sideways.

4. Place your thumbs above the ampule neck, and your index fingers below it.

5. Press down with your thumbs to break the ampule.

6. Invert the ampule, hold it at eye level, insert the syringe needle or needleless device, and withdraw the dose (Fig. 13-8). Important: Do not add air before removing the dose, because if you do, medication will spray from the ampule.

UNIT-DOSE CARTRIDGE AND HOLDER

Insert the cartridge into the metal or plastic holder, and screw it into place. Move the plunger forward until it engages the shaft of the cartridge. Then twist the plunger until it is locked into the cartridge. The holder is reusable, but the cartridge is not. Place the cartridge in a sharps container after use.

UNIT-DOSE PREFILLED SYRINGES

The medication is already in the syringe. Some prefilled syringes are simple and require no action other than removing the needle cover; others are packaged for compactness, and include directions for preparing the syringe for use. These prefilled syringes are disposable.

MIXING TWO MEDICATIONS IN ONE SYRINGE

General Principles

1. Consult a standard reference to determine that the drugs are compatible.

2. When in doubt about compatibility, prepare medications separately and administer them into different injection sites.

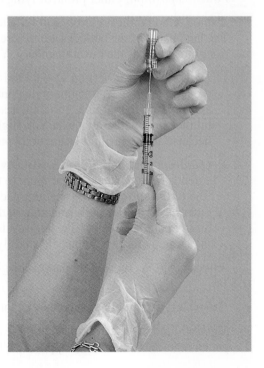

FIGURE 13-8

Invert the ampule for withdrawal. (© B. Proud.)

3. When medications are in both a vial and an ampule, draw up the medication from the vial first; then add the medication from the ampule. Discard the ampule in a sharps container.

4. When you're preparing two types of insulin in one syringe, first draw into the syringe the vial containing regular insulin. (Regular insulin has not been adulterated with protein as have other insulins such as protamine zinc insulin.)

Method

1. Clean both vials with an alcohol pad.

2. Choose one vial as the primary. Example: With vials of a narcotic and a nonnarcotic, the narcotic is the primary. With two insulins, regular insulin is the primary.

3. Inject air into the second vial, in an amount equaling the medication to be withdrawn. Do not let the needle touch the medication.

4. Inject air into the primary vial, in an amount equaling the medication to be withdrawn, and then withdraw the medication in the usual way. Make sure there are no air bubbles.

5. Insert the needle or needleless device into the second vial. Don't touch the plunger, because if you do, you might push the primary medication into the second vial.

6. Slowly withdraw the needed amount of drug from the second vial. The two medications are now combined.

7. Remove the needle or needleless device from the second vial and carefully recap it. Note: Some authorities suggest changing the needle after withdrawing medication from the primary vial. Such a change may result in air bubbles; so to obtain an accurate dose, be careful when you withdraw the second medication.

Identifying the Injection Site—Adults

INTRAMUSCULAR

Common sites are the dorsogluteal, the ventrogluteal, the vastus lateralis, and the deltoid muscles.

Dorsogluteal Site: the thick gluteal muscles of the buttocks.

Patient's position: either prone or lying on the side, with both buttocks fully exposed.

Method: Choose the area very carefully to avoid striking the sciatic nerve, major blood vessels, or bone. The landmarks of the buttocks are the crest of the posterior ilium as the superior boundary, and the inferior gluteal fold as the lower boundary. You can identify the exact site in either of these two ways:

1. *Diagonal landmark* (Fig. 13-9): Find the posterior superior iliac spine and the greater trochanter of the femur. Draw an imaginary diagonal line between these two points, and give the injection lateral and superior to that line, 1 to 2 inches below the iliac crest (to avoid hitting the iliac bone). If you hit the bone, withdraw the needle slightly and continue the procedure. This is the preferred method, because all the landmarks are bony prominences.

2. *Quadrant landmark* (Fig. 13-10): Divide the buttocks into imaginary quadrants. Your vertical line extends from the crest of the ilium to the gluteal fold. Your horizontal line extends from the medial fold of the buttock to the lateral aspect of the buttock. Next, locate the upper aspect of the upper outer quadrant. Give the injection in this area, 1 to 2 inches below the crest of the ilium (to avoid hitting bone). To select the precise site, palpate the crest of the ilium. If you hit the bone when injecting, withdraw the needle slightly and continue the procedure.

Ventrogluteal Site: the ventral part of the gluteal muscle, which has no large nerves or blood vessels and less fat.

Patient's position: either supine, lying on the side, sitting, or standing.

Method: Find the greater trochanter, the anterior superior iliac spine, and the iliac crest. Stand by the patient's knee. Use the hand opposite to the patient's leg (i.e., left leg, right hand). First, open an

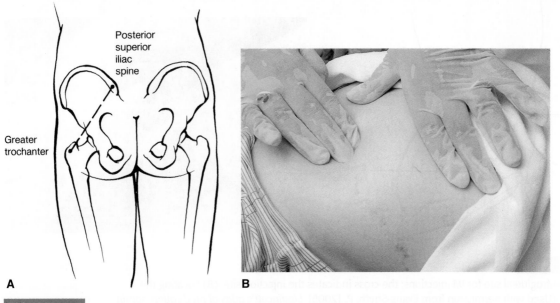

FIGURE 13-9

(**A**) Identification of the dorsogluteal site using a diagonal between the bony prominences. (**B**) Locating the exact site.

alcohol pad. Then place the palm of your hand on the greater trochanter. Point your index finger toward the anterior superior iliac spine, and point your middle finger toward the iliac crest. The injection site lies in the center of the triangle, between your middle finger and index finger (Fig. 13-11). Before giving the injection, place the alcohol pad over the site. Use the alcohol pad to prep the area from the center out. Then remove your hand and proceed with the injection in the usual manner.

Vastus Lateralis Site: the lateral thigh.

Patient's position: either supine, lying on the side, or standing.

Method: Measure one hand's width below the greater trochanter and one hand's width above the knee (Fig. 13-12). Ask the patient to point the big toe to the center of his body, an action that relaxes the vastus muscle. Give the injection in the lateral thigh.

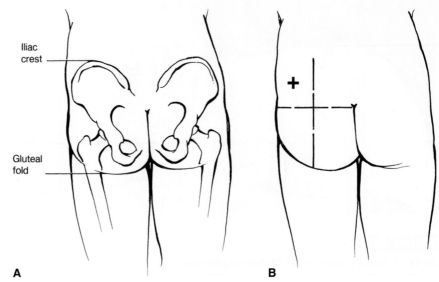

FIGURE 13-10

(**A**) Identification of the dorsogluteal injection site using quadrants. Draw an imaginary line from the iliac crest to the gluteal fold and from the medial to the lateral buttock. (**B**) The cross indicates the injection area.

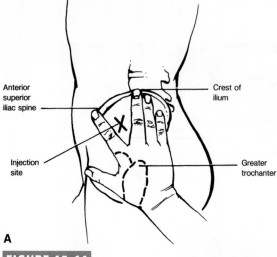

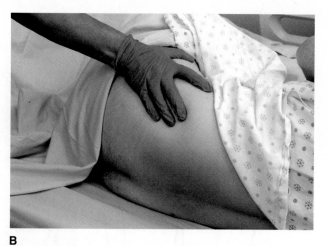

A

B

(**A**) The ventrogluteal site for IM injections; the cross indicates the injection site. (**B**) Locating the exact site. (Used with permission from Evans-Smith, P. [2005]. *Lippincott's atlas of medication administration* [2nd ed.]. Philadelphia: Lippincott Williams & Wilkins, p. 31.)

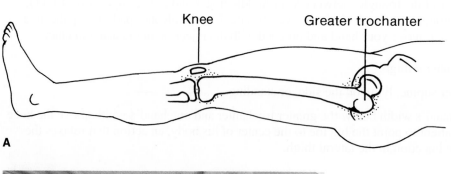

A

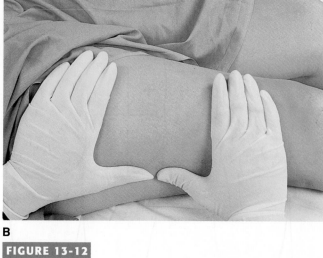

B

(**A**) Vastus lateralis injection site. (**B**) Locating the site.

Deltoid Site: the lateral aspect of the upper arm, at the deltoid, a small muscle close to the radial and brachial arteries. Use this site for IM injections only if specifically ordered, and inject no more than 2 mL of medication.

Patient's position: either sitting or lying down.

Method: The boundaries are the lower edge of the acromion process (shoulder bone) and the axilla (armpit) (Fig. 13-13). Give the injection into the lateral arm between these two points, about 2 inches below the acromion process.

Subcutaneous Sites: commonly, the upper arms, anterior thighs, lower abdomen, and upper back (Fig. 13-14). Insulin subcutaneous is administered in the arm, lower abdomen, and thigh. Heparin subcutaneous is given in the lower abdomen.

Method: To avoid reaching muscle, give the injection at a 45-degree angle. You can give subcutaneous injections at a 90-degree angle if the subcutaneous layer of fat is thick. Inject no more than 1 mL of medication.

Intradermal (Intracutaneous) Site: the inner aspect of the forearm. The intradermal site is used for skin testing for allergies and diseases such as tuberculosis. Intradermal skin testing requires follow-up evaluations to determine if the skin test is positive. Injecting an antigen causes an antigen–antibody sensitivity reaction if the individual is susceptible. If the test is positive, the area will become raised, warm, and reddened.

Method: Clean the skin with an alcohol pad and allow the skin to dry. Place your nondominant hand around the arm from below and pull the skin tightly to make the forearm tissue taut. Hold the syringe in your four fingers and thumb, with the bevel (opening) of the needle up. Then insert the needle about 1/8 inch, almost parallel to the skin (Fig. 13-15A). You will be able to see the needle under the skin. Inject the solution so that it raises a small wheal (a raised bump or a blister) (Fig. 13-15B). Afterward, remove the needle and allow the injection site to dry. Do not massage the skin. Place both the needle and the syringe in a sharps container. Finally, make the patient comfortable, wash your hands, and chart the procedure.

Identifying the Injection Site—Children

The site for the IM injection in a child depends on the child's age, the child's size, and the volume and density of medication being administered. Infants cannot tolerate volumes greater than 0.5 mL in a single site. Older infants or small children can tolerate 1 mL in a single site. Needle gauges range from 21 to 25 gauge.

The preferred site for infants is the vastus lateralis muscle (Fig. 13-16). After the child has been walking for more than a year, you can use the dorsogluteal site; usually, however, that site is not recommended for children less than 5 years old. For the older child and adolescent, you can use the same injection sites as for adults.

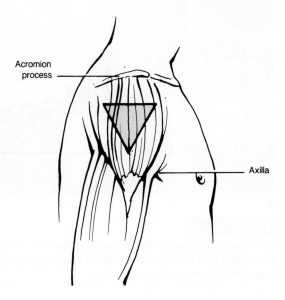

FIGURE 13-13

The deltoid muscle site for IM injections. The triangle indicates the injection site.

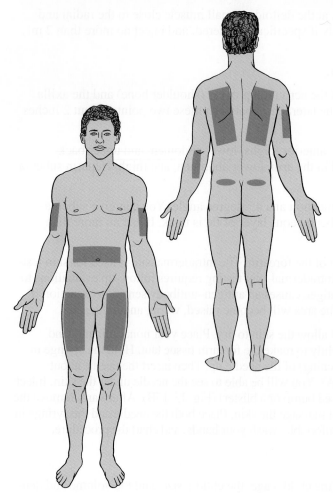

FIGURE 13-14

Sites for subcutaneous injection. The deltoid muscle may be used for subcutaneous injections or, when ordered, for small intramuscular injections.

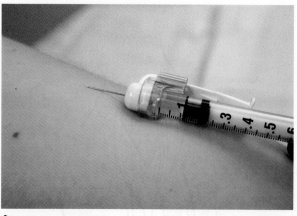
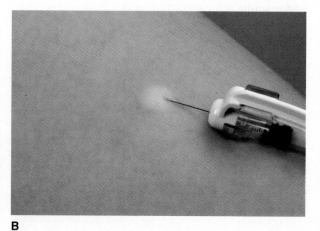

A   **B**

FIGURE 13-15

(**A**) Inserting the needle almost level with the skin. (**B**) Observing for wheal while injecting medication. (Used with permission from Evans-Smith, P. [2005]. *Taylor's clinical nursing Skills.* Philadelphia: Lippincott Williams & Wilkins, p. 132.)

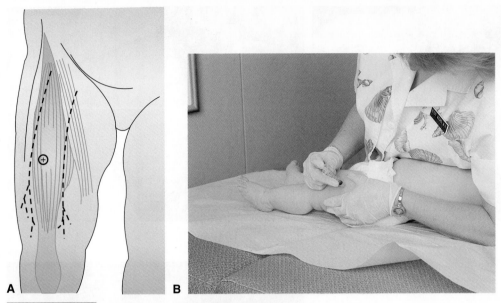

(A) For infants under walking age, use the vastus lateralis muscle for intramuscular injections. **(B)** Technique for administering an intramuscular injection to an infant. Note the way the nurse uses her body to restrain and stabilize the infant. (With permission from Pillitteri, A. [2002]. *Maternal and child health nursing* [4th ed.]. Philadelphia: Lippincott Williams & Wilkins, p. 1102.)

Administering Injections

Handwashing and gloves are required.

1. Identify the patient verbally by name.

2. Check the patient's ID band.

3. Before administering the injection, perform any necessary assessment (e.g., checking vital signs, apical rate, or site integrity).

4. Explain the procedure to the patient.

5. Ask the patient where the last injection was given. Choose a different site, because the sites should be rotated.

6. Clean the area with an alcohol pad, using a circular motion from the center out.

7. Place the alcohol pad between your fingers or lay it on the patient's skin above the site.

8. Remove the needle cover.

9. Make the skin taut by mounding the tissue between your thumb and index finger or by spreading the tissue firmly.

10. Dart the needle in quickly (Fig. 13-17A).

11. Hold the barrel with your nondominant hand, and with your dominant hand pull the plunger back. This action, called aspiration, makes sure the needle is not in a blood vessel (Fig. 13-17B).

12. If blood enters the syringe, withdraw the needle, discard both the needle and the syringe into a sharps container, and prepare another injection.

13. If no blood is aspirated, inject the medication slowly (Fig. 13-17C).

14. Remove the needle quickly.

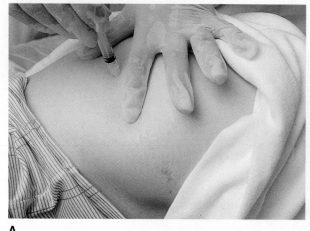

A

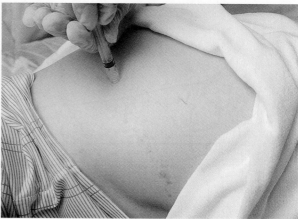

B

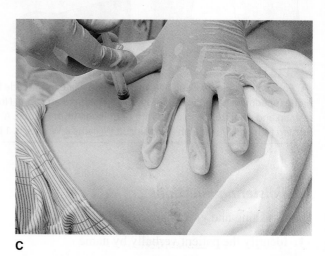

C

FIGURE 13-17

(**A**) Dart the needle into the skin; (**B**) aspirate slowly; (**C**) inject medication slowly.

15. To inhibit bleeding, press down on the area with the alcohol pad or a dry gauze pad.

16. Do not recap the needle. Dispose of the needle and syringe in a sharps container. Make the patient comfortable, wash your hands, and chart the medication, documenting the site of injection.

Special Injection Techniques

SUBCUTANEOUS HEPARIN (OR LOW MOLECULAR WEIGHT HEPARIN SUCH AS LOVENOX)
A heparin injection indicates several changes in routine injection technique. Because heparin is an anticoagulant, you must take care to minimize tissue trauma; slow bleeding at the site of the injection can cause bruising. Wear gloves. Give the injection with a fine (25-gauge) 1/2-inch needle into the lower abdominal fold, at least 2 inches from the umbilicus.

1. After drawing up the dose, change the needle to prevent leakage along the tract. (For Lovenox injections, the dose comes pre-mixed with an air bubble in the prefilled syringe. Do not expel the air bubble before administration.)

2. After prepping the skin with an alcohol pad, allow the skin to dry.

3. With your nondominant hand, bunch the tissue to a depth of at least 1/2 inch.

4. Inject the needle at a 90-degree angle.

5. To minimize tissue damage, do not aspirate.

6. Inject the medication slowly.

7. Hold the needle in place for 10 seconds.

8. Remove the needle quickly.

9. Do not massage the area. If the site bleeds, apply pressure with a dry gauze pad or alcohol pad for 1 to 2 minutes.

SUBCUTANEOUS INSULIN

Insulin is administered with a special insulin syringe, measured in 100 units or 50 units (low dose insulin syringe). Figure 13-14 shows the sites for insulin injection.

1. Draw up the ordered dose in the correct insulin syringe. If you're mixing two insulins, follow the correct procedure (see p. 159).

2. With another nurse, double check the dose in the insulin syringe.

3. Clean the skin with an alcohol pad and allow the skin to dry.

4. Bunch the tissue with your nondominant hand, to a depth of at least 1/2 inch.

5. Inject the needle at a 45-degree or 90-degree angle.

6. To minimize tissue damage, do not aspirate.

7. Inject the medication slowly.

8. Remove the needle quickly.

9. Do not massage the area. If the site bleeds, apply pressure with a dry gauze pad or alcohol pad for 1 to 2 minutes.

You can also administer insulin with a prefilled insulin pen or insulin device. The pen or insulin device has a needle attached for each injection, and a dial on the pen or insulin device measures the correct insulin dose. The technique matches the one described above, but you must hold the device for 6–10 seconds before removing it from the skin. Dispose of the needle in a sharps container.

To administer insulin continuously by the subcutaneous route, use an insulin pump, typically near the abdominal area of the patient. The pump's preset rate delivers the insulin via tubing through a needle inserted in the subcutaneous tissue. You can adjust the settings according to the patient's insulin needs. Change the sites every 2–3 days or as needed.

Z-TRACK TECHNIQUE FOR INTRAMUSCULAR INJECTIONS

Some medications, such as iron dextran (Imferon) and hydroxyzine (Vistazine), are irritating to the tissues and can stain the skin. The Z-track method, used at the dorsogluteal site, can prevent medication from seeping into the needle tract and onto the skin.

1. After preparing the medication, change the needle to prevent leakage along the tract.

2. Add 0.2 mL of air to the syringe. As the medication is injected, the air will rise to the top of the syringe and will be administered last—thus sealing off the medication and preventing it from leaking onto the skin.

3. Prepare the patient and the site in the usual manner.

4. Use the fingers on your nondominant hand to retract the tissue to the side. Hold this position during the injection (Fig. 13-18).

5. Inject at a 90-degree angle, as usual. Before giving this injection, be sure to aspirate (Fig. 13-19).

6. After giving the injection, count 10 seconds.

7. Then remove the needle quickly.

8. Remove the hand that has been retracting the tissue.

9. Do not massage the site.

10. Using an alcohol pad or dry gauze pad, press down on the site to inhibit bleeding.

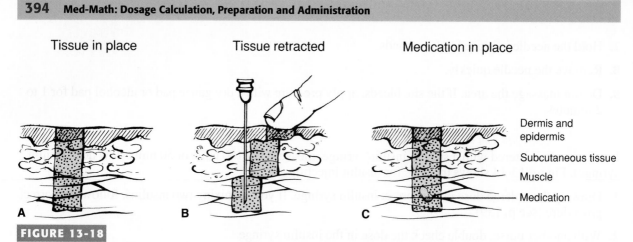

FIGURE 13-18

Z-track technique—dorsogluteal site. The tissue is retracted to one side and held there until the injection is given. When the hand is removed, the tissue closes over the injection tract, preventing medication from rising to the surface.

IV Administration

Intravenous drugs may be given in a number of ways: continuous IV infusion; secondary or piggyback IV infusion; IV push (slow or fast); and flushing of an IV heparin lock or INT (intermittent needle therapy). Because intravenous medications introduce the drug directly into the bloodstream—thus having an immediate effect—you must follow strict asepsis technique.

Several types of IV needles are appropriate for inserting into a vein. The most common is the cathlon or "over the needle," in which a plastic catheter covers the needle. After inserting the needle in the vein, you withdraw the needle, and the plastic catheter stays in place for a specified amount of time.

Usually, IV needles are inserted in the hand or forearm (Fig. 13-20). For longterm intravenous therapy, however, you can insert a central venous catheter (Fig. 13-21) or use a peripherally inserted central catheter (PICC) (Fig. 13-22). Information on IV calculations is found in Chapters 8 and 9.

Basic guidelines regarding peripheral IV therapy:

1. Use aseptic technique for insertion of IV needle.

2. Use an occlusive dressing to secure IV needle. Most healthcare settings use a clear plastic dressing over the IV needle site so that constant monitoring of the site can occur.

3. Verify IV fluids and IV medications orders before administration. Calculate the correct dose. Check an approved compatibility guide to determine the compatibility of IV fluids and IV medications. Flush IV tubing between administration of incompatible solutions.

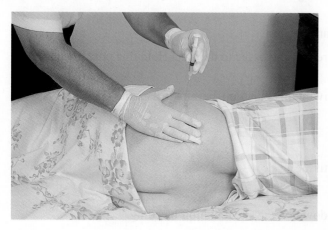

FIGURE 13-19

Displacing tissue in a Z-track manner and darting needle into tissue.

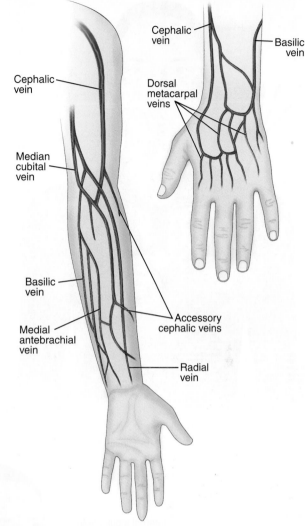

FIGURE 13-20

Infusion sites available in the hand or forearm. (Used with permission from Taylor, C. [2008]. *Fundamentals of nursing* [6th ed.]. Philadelphia: Lippincott Williams & Wilkins, p. 1709.)

4. Infuse IV fluids and IV medications according to policy and procedures of the institution. Use an infusion pump if available.

5. Monitor and assess the IV site frequently and according to institutional guidelines. Monitor the IV site for: swelling, color, temperature and pain.

6. Follow institutional guidelines for changing the IV site, changing the IV fluids and changing the IV tubing. Generally, a peripheral IV site is changed every 72 hours; IV fluids every 24 hours and IV tubing every 72–96 hours.

   For further information about IV insertion and IV medication administration, consult a nursing pharmacology or a nursing fundamentals textbook.

Application to Skin and Mucous Membranes

Topical drug preparations have two purposes: to cause a local effect or to act systematically. To create a systemic effect, the drug must be absorbed into the circulation.

Buccal Tablet (standard precautions: handwashing and gloves)

Identify the patient verbally by name. Check the ID band, explain the procedure, and then give the tablet to the patient. The patient should place the tablet between the gum and cheek. Withhold food and liquids until

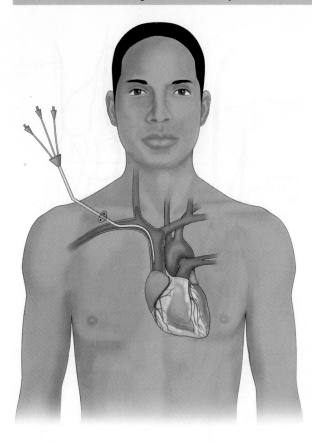

FIGURE 13-21

Triple lumen central venous catheter (TLC or CVC). (Used with permission from Taylor, C. [2008]. *Fundamentals of nursing* [6th ed.]. Philadelphia: Lippincott Williams & Wilkins, p. 1708.)

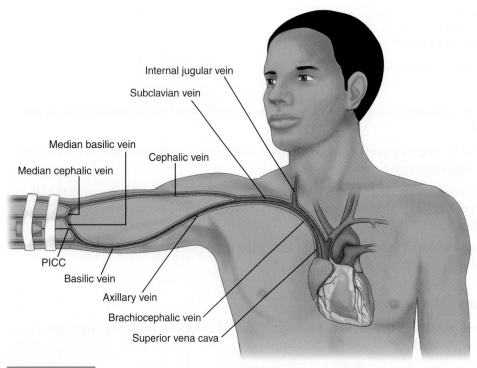

Internal jugular vein

Subclavian vein

Median basilic vein

Cephalic vein

Median cephalic vein

PICC

Basilic vein

Axillary vein

Brachiocephalic vein

Superior vena cava

FIGURE 13-22

Peripherally inserted central catheter (PICC). (Used with permission from Taylor, C. [2008]. *Fundamentals of nursing* [6th ed.]. Philadelphia: Lippincott Williams & Wilkins, p. 1706.)

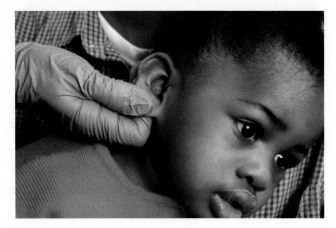

FIGURE 13-23

Technique for administering eardrops in children under 3 years old. (Used with permission from Evans-Smith, P. [2005]. *Taylor's clinical nursing skills.* Philadelphia: Lippincott Williams & Wilkins, p. 173.)

the tablet is dissolved, and warn the patient not to disturb the tablet. Medication applied across mucous membranes causes rapid systemic absorption. To minimize irritation, alternate doses between cheeks.

Ear Drops (standard precautions: handwashing and gloves)

The ear drops, labeled either "otic" or "auric," should be warmed to body temperature. Identify the patient verbally by name, check the patient's ID band, and explain the procedure. Help the patient into a comfortable position: either sitting upright, head tilted toward the unaffected side or lying on side with the affected ear up. With a dropper, draw the medication into the dropper. Straighten the ear canal by pulling the pinna up and back (for an adult) or down and back (for a child 3 years or younger; Fig. 13-23).

Placing the tip of the dropper at the opening of the canal, instill the medication into the canal (Fig. 13-24). The patient should then rest on the unaffected side for 10 to 15 minutes. If the patient wishes, place a cotton ball in the canal. Make sure the patient is comfortable, and then wash your hands and chart the medication.

Eye Drops or Ointment (standard precautions: handwashing and gloves)

Identify the patient verbally by name, check the patient's ID band, and explain the procedure. Hand the patient a tissue. The patient may sit or lie down. If exudate is present, you may need to cleanse the eyelid with cotton or gauze and either normal saline or distilled water for the eye. Eye medications—which must be labeled "ophthalmic" or "for the eye"—come in either a monodrop container (a container with a drop-like lid); in a bottle with a dropper; or as an ophthalmic ointment. Gently draw the patient's lower eyelid down to create a sac (Fig. 13-25). Instruct the patient to look up. Then instill the liquid medication into the

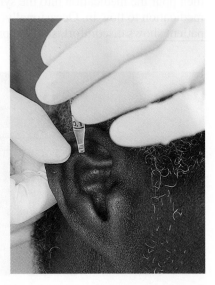

FIGURE 13-24

Straighten the ear canal and instill the medication.

Ear Drop Administration

- Should the ear pinna be pulled up or down with adults?
- Should the ear pinna be pulled up or down with children?
- Adults are usually taller than children, so the ear pinna is pulled "up" and back for ear drops.
- Children younger than 3 years old are smaller than adults, so the ear pinna is pulled "down" and back for ear drops.

CLINICAL ALERT!

lower conjunctival sac, taking care not to touch the membrane. If you're administering ophthalmic ointment, spread a small amount from the inner to the outer canthus of the eye.

After either of these procedures, instruct the patient to close their eyelids gently and rotate their eyes. The patient may use a tissue to wipe away excess medication. Also, after instilling eye drops, have the patient apply gentle pressure with the index finger to the inner canthus for a minute. This action keeps the medication from entering the tear duct.

To prevent cross-contamination, each patient should have individual medication containers. If the medication impairs the patient's vision, provide a safe environment. Make the patient comfortable. Then dispose of the gloves according to institutional procedure, wash your hands, and chart the medication.

Nasogastric Route (standard precautions: handwashing and gloves)

When possible, obtain the medication in liquid form. Before opening capsules or crushing tablets, check with the pharmacist for alternatives. Use either a bulb syringe or a 60-mL syringe.

First, dilute the medication with water. The fluid mixture should be at room temperature. After identifying the patient verbally by name, check the patient's ID band and explain the procedure. Elevate the head of the bed to 30 degrees. Put on your gloves and insert the syringe into the tube; then remove the clamp on the tube. To check the position of the tube in the stomach, place a stethoscope on the stomach and insert about 15 mL of air. If you hear a swishing sound, the stethoscope is in the proper place. Then aspirate the stomach's contents. You can also test the stomach contents for acidity by using pH paper, if it's available.

Close off the tube by bending it back on itself (Fig. 13-26). Holding the syringe and bent tube in your nondominant hand, remove the bulb or plunger and leave the syringe in place.

Flush the tube with at least 30 mL of warm water to ensure patency (Fig. 13-27). Clamp the tube, and then pour the medication into the syringe (Fig. 13-28). Release the tubing, so that gravity will cause the medication to flow in. Occasionally, you may apply slight pressure with the plunger of the syringe. If the patient shows discomfort, stop the procedure and wait until he or she appears relaxed.

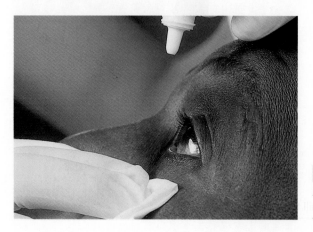

FIGURE 13-25

Applying eye drops: Gently draw the lower eyelid down to create a pocket. Insert the medication into this pocket.

Eye and Ear Abbreviations

CLINICAL ALERT!

- The Joint Commission has identified abbreviations—including those for eye and ear medications—that can cause confusion. Although The Joint Commission does not prohibit the following abbreviations, *it's best to avoid using them:*

- AS (left ear), AD (right ear), AU (both ears). These are often confused with the terms for eyes: OS (left eye), OD (right eye), OU (both eyes).

- Recommendations: Write out the phrases "left ear," "right ear," or "both ears," as appropriate. It's okay to use the eye abbreviations, but if you want to be particularly safe, write them out: "left eye," "right eye," "both eyes." Be sure to write out "every day" or "daily" rather than using the abbreviation "qd," which is easily confused with "OD."

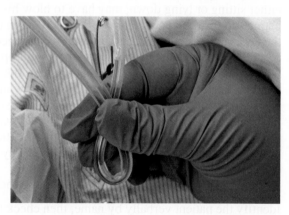

FIGURE 13-26

Bend the tube back on itself to close the tube. (Used with permission from Taylor, C. [2008]. *Fundamentals of nursing* [6th ed.]. Philadelphia: Lippincott Williams & Wilkins, p. 1473.)

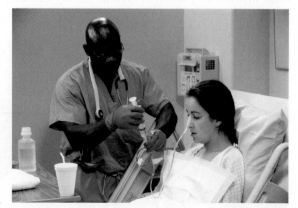

FIGURE 13-27

Flush the tube with at least 30 mL water. (Used with permission from Taylor, C. [2008]. *Fundamentals of nursing* [6th ed.]. Philadelphia: Lippincott Williams & Wilkins, p. 1473.)

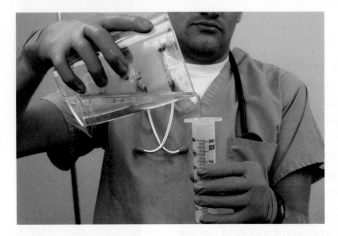

FIGURE 13-28

Pour the medications into the syringe. (Used with permission from Taylor, C. [2008]. *Fundamentals of nursing* [6th ed.]. Philadelphia: Lippincott Williams & Wilkins, p. 1470.)

Before all the medication flows in, flush the tube by adding at least 30 mL of water to the syringe. Shut the tube by bending it back on itself before the syringe completely empties. Then clamp the tube and remove the syringe. Make the patient comfortable. If possible, leave the head of the bed elevated. Dispose of your gloves according to institutional procedures, and finish by washing your hands and charting the medication.

Nose Drops (standard precautions: handwashing and gloves)

Identify the patient verbally by name, check the patient's ID band, and explain the procedure. The patient, either sitting or lying down, may have to blow his nose gently to clear the nasal passageway. Have the patient tilt his head back. If the patient is lying in bed, place a pillow under his shoulders to hyperextend the neck (unless contraindicated). Insert the dropper about one-third of the way into first one nostril, then the other. Do not touch the nostril. Instill the nose drops (Fig. 13-29), and then instruct the patient to maintain the position for 1 to 2 minutes. If the patient feels the medication flowing down his throat, he may sit up and bend his head down so the medication will flow into the sinuses instead.

To prevent cross-contamination, the patient should have his own medication container. After making the patient comfortable, wash your hands and chart the medication.

If a nasal spray is ordered, push the tip of patient's nose up and then place the nozzle tip just inside the nares, so when you give the medication, the spray is aiming toward the back of the nose.

Rectal Suppository (standard precautions: handwashing and gloves)

Identify the patient verbally by name, then check the patient's ID band and explain the procedure. Encourage the patient to defecate (unless the suppository is ordered for this purpose). Position the patient in the left lateral recumbent position (Fig. 13-30). After moistening the suppository with a water-soluble lubricant, instruct the patient to breathe slowly and deeply through the mouth. To open the anal sphincter, ask

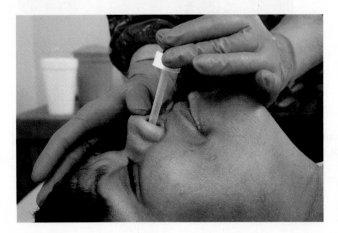

FIGURE 13-29

Administering nose drops. (Used with permission from Evans-Smith, P. [2005]. *Taylor's clinical nursing skills.* Philadelphia: Lippincott Williams & Wilkins, p. 178.)

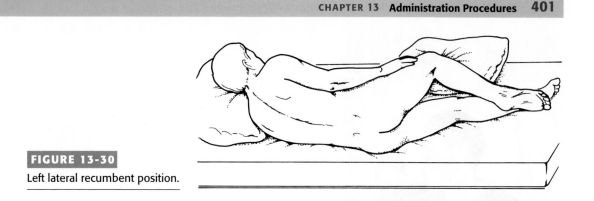

FIGURE 13-30

Left lateral recumbent position.

the patient to "bear down" as if having a bowel movement. Using a gloved finger, insert the suppository past the sphincter. You will feel the suppository move into the canal. Wipe away excess lubricant, and encourage the patient to retain the suppository as long as possible. Make the patient comfortable. Then dispose of gloves according to institutional procedure, wash your hands, and chart the medication.

The patient may insert her own suppository if she is able and wishes to do so. Provide a glove, lubricant, and suppository. After insertion, check to make sure that the suppository is in place and is not in the bed.

Respiratory Inhaler (standard precautions: handwashing and gloves)

An inhaler is a small, pressurized metal container that holds medication. Inhalers come in these forms: a metered dose (MDI) inhaler, accompanied by a mouthpiece; a metered dose inhaler with an extender; or a dry powder inhaler (DPI) (Fig. 13-31).

First, identify the patient verbally by name, check the patient's ID band, and explain the procedure. Then teach the patient to follow these general directions (Fig. 13-32).

1. Shake the inhaler well immediately before you use it.

2. Remove the cap from the mouthpiece.

3. Breathe out fully, expel as much air as you can, and hold your breath.

4. Place the mouthpiece in your mouth and close your lips around it. Keep the metal inhaler upright.

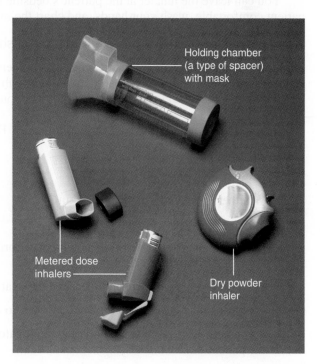

Holding chamber (a type of spacer) with mask

Metered dose inhalers

Dry powder inhaler

FIGURE 13-31

Examples of metered dose inhalers and spacers. (Used with permission from Taylor, C. [2008]. *Fundamentals of nursing* [6th ed.]. Philadelphia: Lippincott Williams & Wilkins, p. 810.)

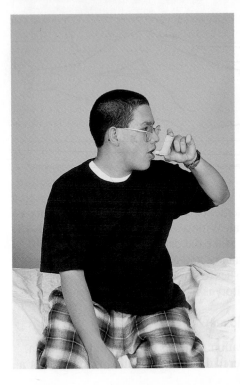

FIGURE 13-32

Many children with asthma use a metered dose inhaler to administer a bronchodilator. (With permission from Pillitteri, A. [2002]. *Maternal and child health nursing* [4th ed.]. Philadelphia: Lippincott Williams & Wilkins, p. 1210.)

5. While breathing in deeply and slowly, use your index finger to fully depress the metal inhaler.

6. Remove the inhaler from your mouth and release your finger. Hold your breath for several seconds.

7. Wait 1 minute. Then shake the inhaler again and repeat the steps for each prescribed inhalation. (An order might read "Proventil inhaler 2 puffs qid.")

8. At least once a day, clean the mouthpiece and cap by rinsing them in warm running water. After they have dried, replace the mouthpiece and cap on the inhaler.

   You can leave the inhaler at the patient's bedside stand if the institution's policy permits. Make the patient comfortable, wash your hands, and chart the medication.

Skin Applications (standard precautions: handwashing and gloves)

Identify the patient verbally by name, check the patient's ID band, and explain the procedure. Avoid personal contact with the medication so that you don't absorb any of the drug. Apply the medication with either a tongue blade, a glove, a gauze pad, or a cotton-tipped applicator. Cleanse the area as appropriate before beginning a new application.

Many kinds of medications are applied topically. Before you proceed, obtain the following information:

- How to prepare the skin
- How to apply the medication
- Whether to cover or uncover the skin

These are some typical drug preparations:

- Powders: The patient's skin should be dry. Sprinkle the medication on your gloved hands, then apply it. Use sparingly to avoid caking.
- Lotions: Using a gloved hand or gauze pad, pat the medication on lightly.
- Creams: Using gloves, rub the medication into the patient's skin.
- Ointments: Using a gloved hand or an applicator, apply an even coat and then place a dressing on the patient's skin.

After any of these procedures, make the patient comfortable and dispose of gloves according to institutional policy. Then wash your hands and chart the medication.

Nitroglycerin Ointment (standard precautions: handwashing and gloves)

Identify the patient verbally by name, check the patient's ID band, and explain the procedure. Take a baseline blood pressure and record it. (Note that because nitroglycerin is a potent vasodilator, it may cause a drop in the blood pressure after application.) To protect yourself from contact with the drug, put on gloves. Then remove the previous dose and cleanse the skin.

Measure the prescribed dose in inches on the ruled paper that comes with the ointment. Select a non-hairy site on the patient's trunk—chest, upper arm, abdomen, or upper back. If necessary, shave the area. (*Note:* Seek advice before shaving.) Spread the measured ointment on the ruled paper and apply the ointment in a thin layer about 6 × 6 inches. Do not rub it in. Place the ruled paper with the ointment on the skin and then apply tape; some sources recommend covering the area with plastic wrap and taping the plastic in place. Within 30 minutes, check the patient's blood pressure.

If the patient gets a headache (a common side effect of Nitroglycerin) or if his blood pressure lowers, have him stay in bed until the blood pressure returns to normal. Treat the headaches with an ordered pain medication. After making the patient comfortable, dispose of the gloves according to institutional procedure, wash your hands, and chart the medication.

Transdermal Disks, Patches, and Pads (standard precautions: handwashing and gloves)

All of these products are unit-dose adhesive bandages, consisting of a semipermeable membrane that allows medication to be released continuously over time. Some patches are effective for 24 hours, some for 72 hours, and some last as long as one week.

The skin at the site should be free of hair and not subject to excessive movement; therefore, avoid distal extremities. At each administration, change the site. If the patch loosens with bathing, apply a new pad.

Medications appropriate for this route include hormones, nitroglycerin, antihypertensive drugs such as clonidine (Catapres), and antimotion sickness drugs such as scopolamine.

Identify the patient verbally by name, check the patient's ID band, and explain the procedure. Select a site where the skin is clear and dry, with no signs of irritation. Open the packet and remove the cover from the adhesive transdermal drug. Don't touch the inside of the pad. Apply the pad to the skin, pressing firmly to be certain all edges adhere. Chart on the pad the date, time, and your initials. Then make the patient comfortable, wash your hands, and chart the medication.

Sublingual Tablets (standard precautions: handwashing and gloves)

The most common sublingual medication is nitroglycerin, which is prescribed to alleviate symptoms of angina pectoris. If a patient does not feel relief within 5 minutes, you can administer a second and then a third tablet at 5-minute intervals. If the pain continues after 15 minutes, notify the physician.

To administer a sublingual tablet, first identify the patient verbally by name, check the patient's ID band, and explain the procedure. Instruct the patient to sit down and to place the tablet under her tongue. If the patient is unable to place the tablet under the tongue, the nurse should do it, and should wear a glove. The patient should not swallow or chew the tablet, but allow it to dissolve. Make sure the patient does not eat or drink anything with the tablet, because that will interfere with the effectiveness of the medication. Stay with the patient until the pain has stopped. For more information, consult an appropriate text. To conclude, wash your hands and chart the medication.

Vaginal Suppository or Tablet (standard precautions: handwashing and gloves)

Identify the patient verbally by name, check the patient's ID band, and explain the procedure. Ask her to void in a bed pan. (If the perineal area has excessive secretions, you may need to perform perineal care after the patient voids.) Insert the suppository or tablet into the applicator. Then assist the patient into a lithotomy position (lying on her back, with knees flexed and legs apart) and drape her, leaving the perineal area exposed. Put on gloves.

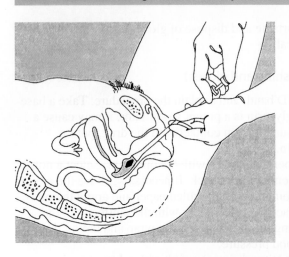

Separate the labia majora and identify the vaginal opening. Then insert the applicator down and back (Fig. 13-33), and eject the suppository or tablet into the vagina. (If the patient wishes, she can do this procedure herself.) You may also insert the suppository—using gloved fingers—into the vagina. Place a pad at the vaginal opening to collect secretions, and make the patient comfortable before you leave.

Wash the applicator with soap and water, wrap it in a paper towel, and leave it at the bedside. Dispose of gloves and equipment according to institutional procedure, and chart the medication.

Vaginal Cream or Vaginal Tablet (standard precautions: handwashing and gloves)

Vaginal cream is packaged either in a prefilled disposable syringe or in a tube with its own applicator. To fill the applicator, remove the cap from the tube and screw the top of the tube into the applicator's barrel. Squeeze the tube and fill the barrel to the prescribed dose. Then unscrew the tube from the applicator and cap it.

Prepare the patient as described in the previous section. Insert the applicator down and back, and press the plunger to empty the barrel of medication (Fig. 13-33). The patient may do this herself if she wishes. After removing the applicator, place a pad at the vaginal opening to collect secretions. Before you leave, make sure the patient is comfortable. She should remain in bed for a minimum of 20 minutes.

If the applicator is a prefilled unit dose, dispose of it according to institutional policy. If it is reusable, wash it with soap and water, and place it in a clean paper towel on the bedside stand. Dispose of your gloves, and chart the medication.

Special Considerations

The basics of medication administration apply to all age groups. However, administering drugs to pediatric and geriatric patients requires special considerations.

Neonatal and Pediatric Considerations

Dosages of medications for neonatal and pediatric administration are briefly covered in Chapter 10.

Differences in medication administration are mainly developmental; consult a nursing pediatric textbook for specifics and for special skills needed.

Here are some suggestions for administering oral medication to children:

- Before you administer an oral medication, offer the child a popsicle, which will numb her taste buds.

- Mix the drug with a teaspoon of puréed fruit, ice cream, or syrup. Using essential foodstuffs is not a good idea, because the child may refuse those foods later.

- Have older children pinch their nostrils closed and drink the medication through a straw. Because this technique interferes with their ability to smell, it keeps them from tasting the medication.

- For infants, use a specially manufactured medication nipple or pacifier.

IM administration in children:

- Explain the procedure to the child, using terms he can easily understand.
- Predetermine the injection site to make sure the muscle is large enough to accommodate the amount and type of medication.
- To reduce the pain of deep needle administration, you can subcutaneously inject a local anesthetic such as lidocaine. A topical anesthetic can help reduce the pain of a needlestick.
- A child's behavior and movements are unpredictable, so have someone help you hold the child.
- Distract the child with conversation or a toy.
- Insert the needle quickly and inject the medication slowly.
- Use a decorative adhesive bandage to cover the injection site.

Geriatric Considerations

Before administering medications to geriatric clients, consider these factors: decreasing organ function (especially of liver and kidney); circulatory changes leading to decreased perfusion; and physical limitations (poor eyesight, decreased coordination, decreased ability to chew and/or swallow).

Here are some suggestions for administering oral tablets and liquids to geriatric patients:

- Before administering a liquid medication, offer the patient a popsicle, which will numb the taste buds.
- If crushing a tablet won't compromise its medication, you can crush it and mix the fragments with a teaspoon of puréed fruit, ice cream, or syrup.
- Patients who are post-CVA often have problems with tongue mobility and/or a decreased gag reflex. To promote swallowing, you may have to place the tablet or capsule in the patient's mouth, toward the pharynx and on the unaffected side. Afterward, thoroughly check the patient's mouth to determine whether she has swallowed the tablet or capsule. CVA patients with a feeding tube (Nasogastric, oralgastric or PEG tube) can receive their medications through the tube.

Subcutaneous and/or IM administration in geriatric clients:

- Explain the procedure to the client.
- Predetermine the injection site, to make sure there is sufficient subcuticular tissue or the muscle is large enough to accommodate the amount and type of medication.
- Distract the client with conversation.
- Insert the needle quickly and inject the medication slowly.

CRITICAL THINKING: TEST YOUR CLINICAL SAVVY

A client in your outpatient clinic is to receive an IM injection. The drug literature states that the preferred site is the gluteus maximus or vastus lateralis.

A. When would the deltoid muscle be preferable over either of these sites? What are the contraindications for using the deltoid muscle?

B. The client requests the injection in the deltoid. What is your response in light of the recommended site in the drug literature?

C. If a patient is bedridden, which site would you choose for an IM injection, and why?

D. Even though you are not actually touching the injection site, why are gloves necessary when giving IM injections?

SELF TEST 1   Standard Precautions

Complete the statements about standard precautions in medication administration. Answers appear at the end of the chapter.

1. Standard precautions should be applied when administering medications

    a. to all patients

    b. only to patients with HIV or hepatitis B virus

2. The type of precaution to be used by the nurse depends on _____

    _____.

3. Administering medications, the nurse must wear gloves when _____

    _____

    and_____.

4. After the nurse administers an injection, the syringe should be placed

    _____

    _____.

5. Five precautions stressed by the CDC are _____, _____,

    _____, _____,

    and_____.

6. If you're administering medications, you should wash your hands when

    a. _____

    b. _____

    c. _____

    d. _____

7. Standard precautions while administering ear drops or eye drops medications are

    _____

    _____

8. A nurse should wear a gown to protect his or her uniform whenever

    _____

    _____

9. The nurse should wear protective eyewear whenever _____

    _____

    _____.

10. Wear a mask when _____

    _____or_____

    _____.

SELF TEST 2	Medication Administration

Complete the statements about medication administration. Answers appear at the end of the chapter.

1. The primary reason patients should have individual eye medication is to _____
   _____.

2. Two methods of checking the positioning of a nasogastric tube are
   _____

   and _____.

3. For administration of a rectal suppository, the patient should lie
   _____

   _____.

4. How should each of the following be applied to a patient's skin?
   a. powders _____
   b. lotions _____
   c. creams _____
   d. ointments _____

5. How many sublingual nitroglycerin tablets may a patient take to relieve pain?

   _____

   At what time interval? _____

6. Identify these administration procedures as parenteral or non-parenteral.
   a. subcutaneous injection _____   **f.** nitroglycerin ointment _____
   b. sublingual tablet _____   **g.** respiratory inhaler _____
   c. vaginal suppository _____   **h.** nasogastric route _____
   d. nose drops _____   **i.** intradermal _____
   e. IM injection _____   **j.** rectal suppository _____

7. How should the nurse insert a vaginal applicator? _____
   _____

   _____

8. How should the nurse prepare the patient's skin for an injection?
   _____

   _____

9. List three reasons for administering medication by injection. _____
   _____

   _____

   _____

10. What is the difference in administering ear drops to an adult and to a 2-year-old child?
    _____

    _____

Date: June 26, 2007
Time: 0900
Vital Signs: Temperature 101.5 oral. Respiratory Rate: 32 breaths/minute. Apical heart rate: 75/minute. Blood Pressure: 98/50. Drug Allergies: Penicillin. No complaints of pain.

You will administer the medications appropriately based on this data. Document on the MAR. Use the guidelines on page 377. Answers appear at the end of the chapter.

SELF TEST 3   **Medication Administration Record**

MCFARLAND MEDICAL CENTER
Medication Administration Record

Patient Name	Room Number	Hospital Number		Diagnosis
Velder, Chelsea	1401	204452896		CHF

Allergies	Admitted	Age	Sex	Physician
PCN	6/25/07	50	F	Richardson

DOSAGE ADMINISTRATION PERIOD: 6/26/07 0600-6/27/07 0600

	0601-1400	1401-2200	2201-0600	
Digoxin 0.25 mg PO every day Hold if HR <60	0900			
Aspirin 325 mg PO daily	0900			
Protonix 40 mg PO every day	0900			
Ampicillin 250 mg PO q 6h	1400	1800	0200	0600
Lopressor 50 mg PO BID Hold if SBP <100	0900	2100		
Coumadin 5 mg PO once a day		1700		
Morphine Sulfate 4-6 mg IV every 2-3h prn pain				
Tylenol gr X q4h prn temp >101				

Signature _____ Initials _( )_   Signature _____ Initials _( )_   Signature _____ Initials _( )_

PROFICIENCY TEST 1 – PART A   **Administration Procedures**

Name: _____

Choose the correct answer for each of these questions. Answers appear in Appendix A.

1. A nurse's first check when preparing medication is:

   a. checking the patient's armband before administration

   b. checking the order while pouring the liquid medication

   c. checking the unit dose label with the order

   d. checking the unit dose packaging after it is disposed

2. Which actions of the medication computer scanning device help prevent medication errors?

   a. verifying patient's identity by scanning the patient's armband

   b. verifying the correct medication by scanning the bar code on the unit dose packaging

   c. verifying the correct time by scanning the medication administration record (MAR)

   d. all of the above

3. Checking the medication administration record (MAR) before administering medication enables the nurse to determine

   a. the name of the pharmacist who ordered the medication

   b. the correct administration time of the medication

   c. any previous medication errors

   d. orders for intake and output

4. When pouring an oral liquid medication, the nurse should

   a. place the cup on the tabletop and bend over to get the right level

   b. hold the cup in the hand and pour to the top of the meniscus

   c. hold the cup at eye level and pour to the center of the meniscus

   d. rest the cup on a flat surface and pour to the meniscus line

5. Which of these statements regarding injections from powders is *false?*

   a. Read the label twice before drawing up, and once after.

   b. Draw up one medication at a time.

   c. Always use sterile water as a diluent.

   d. Pull back on the plunger before injecting the medication.

6. Injecting a specific amount of air into the vial beforehand helps in withdrawing medication from a vial. Which of these statements explains this action?

   a. It creates a partial vacuum in the vial.

   b. It makes the pressure in the vial greater than atmospheric pressure.

   c. It makes the pressure in the vial the same as atmospheric pressure.

   d. It makes the pressure in the vial less than atmospheric pressure.

(continued)

7. If a patient has difficulty swallowing medications, which oral form of drug may be crushed?

    a. sugar-coated tablet

    b. enteric-coated tablet

    c. buccal tablet

    d. capsule

8. A major advantage in the unit-dose system of drug administration is that

    a. the drug supply is always available

    b. no error is possible

    c. the drugs are less expensive than stock distribution

    d. the pharmacist provides a second professional check

9. When a drug is to be administered sublingually, the patient should be instructed to

    a. drink a full glass of water when swallowing

    b. rinse the mouth with water after taking the drug

    c. chew the tablet and allow saliva to collect under the tongue

    d. hold the medication under the tongue until it dissolves

10. Ampules differ from vials in that ampules

    a. are always glass containers

    b. contain only one dose

    c. contain solids as well as liquids

    d. are not used for injections

11. The Z-track technique for injections can be used to

    a. administer more than one drug at a single site

    b. inhibit hematoma formation by promoting drug absorption

    c. prevent skin discoloration by inhibiting drug seepage

    d. reduce allergic reactions at the injection site

12. Which action is correct when giving a Z-track injection?

    a. Retract the skin and hold it to one side while giving the medication.

    b. Massage the skin after giving the injection.

    c. After the needle has been inserted, do not pull back the plunger.

    d. Inject the medication quickly.

13. Which angle of injection is correctly matched with the route of administration?

    a. intradermal—45-degree angle

    b. IM—90-degree angle

    c. subcutaneous—30-degree angle

    d. Z track—45-degree angle

(continued)

14. A patient asks how to put in eye drops. The nurse instructs the patient to place the drops

   a. into the lower conjunctival sac

   b. under the upper lid

   c. directly on the cornea

   d. in the inner canthus

15. When administering a vaginal suppository, which statement is false?

   a. Use standard precautions.

   b. The patient may insert the medication.

   c. The patient should be lying on her back.

   d. The applicator must be kept sterile.

16. When applying the next dose of a transdermal medication, the nurse should

   a. shave the new area and prepare with povidone–iodine

   b. cleanse the previous area and use a different site

   c. rotate the use of arms and legs as sites

   d. allow the previous patch to remain on the skin

17. When an injection is irritating to the tissues, which muscle is the preferred site?

   a. deltoid—subcutaneous

   b. dorsogluteal—Z track

   c. ventrogluteal—intradermal

   d. vastus lateralis—IM

18. Discomfort of an injection is reduced when the needle is inserted

   a. slowly into loose tissue

   b. slowly into firm tissue

   c. rapidly into loose tissue

   d. rapidly into firm tissue

19. After administering an injection, the nurse should

   a. immediately recap the needle

   b. break the needle off the syringe for safety

   c. place the used syringe in a nearby sharps container

   d. put on gloves to carry the syringe to the utility room

20. Which statement is incorrect for administering drugs to mucous membranes?

   a. Eye medications must be labeled ophthalmic.

   b. Patients may insert their own rectal suppositories.

   c. Apply sublingual medications to the space between the teeth and cheek.

   d. The nurse may leave eye medications on the patient's bedside stand.

(continued)

PROFICIENCY TEST 1 – PART B   **Administration Procedures**

Decide whether the following actions are correct or incorrect, according to the precautions to follow when administering medications. Explain your choice. Answers appear in Appendix A.

1. A nurse wears gloves to remove an IV heparin lock from a patient's arm. This action is

   _____

   _____

2. A nurse who has just removed a gown and gloves puts them into the disposal container in the patient's room and leaves the room. This action is

   _____

   _____

3. In the medication room, a nurse puts on gloves to prepare an IV for administration. This action is

   _____

   _____

4. A nurse puts on a mask to administer an oral medication to a patient on respiratory isolation precautions. This action is

   _____

   _____

5. A nurse applies standard precautions in caring for all patients on the unit. This action is

   _____

   _____

6. A nurse wears gloves to place a transdermal pad behind a patient's ear. This action is

   _____

   _____

7. A nurse puts on gloves and gown to administer 500 mL of a vaginal douche to a lethargic patient. This action is

   _____

   _____

8. A nurse whose finger has been stuck with a contaminated IV needle carefully washes his/her hands with soap and water, and applies a band-aid to the site. Because the patient's diagnosis is a brain tumor, the nurse decides no further action is necessary. This action is

9. A nurse giving an injection to a patient decides not to wear gloves. This action is

   _____

   _____

(continued)

PROFICIENCY TEST 1—PART B   **Administration Procedures (Continued)**

10. A nurse puts on gloves to administer an oral tablet to an alert patient with a positive HIV blood count. This action is

_____

_____

11. After administering an injection, the nurse carefully caps the needle. This action is

_____

_____

_____

12. A nurse wears gloves to apply nitroglycerin ointment to a patient's chest, even though there is no break in the skin. This action is

_____

_____

_____

13. A nurse decides not to wear gloves when administering eye drops, because they are too bulky. This action is

_____

_____

_____

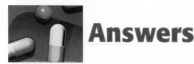

Answers

Self-Test 1 Standard Precautions

1. To all patients. There is a risk of potential exposure to hepatitis virus and HIV that may not have been detected by standard laboratory methods.

2. The type of contact the nurse has with the patient.

3. When there is any direct "hands-on" contact with patient's blood, bodily fluids, or secretions; when handling materials or equipment contaminated with blood or body fluids.

4. In a labeled, puncture-proof container.

5. Handwashing, gloves, gowns, masks, and protective eyewear.

6. a. Before preparing medications and after administering medicines to each patient.

   b. After removing gloves, gowns, masks, and protective eyewear, and before leaving each patient.

   c. Immediately when soiled with the patient's blood or body fluids.

   d. After handling equipment soiled with blood or body fluids.

7. Handwashing and gloves.

8. The nurse's clothing may become contaminated with a patient's blood or body fluids.

9. A nurse is in extremely close contact with the patient and there is the possibility of the patient's blood or blood-tinged fluids being splashed or sprayed into the nurse's eyes or mucous membranes.

10. The patient is placed on strict or respiratory isolation precautions. Carrying out a medication procedure may cause blood or body fluids to splash directly onto the nurse's face.

Self-Test 2 Medication Administration

1. Prevent cross-contamination.

2. Aspirate stomach contents and check for pH or place a stethoscope on the stomach and insert 15 mL of air. A swishing sound indicates proper placement.

3. On the left side, left lateral recumbent position.

4. a. Sprinkle on gloved hands and apply, use sparingly to prevent caking.

   b. Pat on lightly with gloved hand or gauze pad.

   c. Rub into skin while wearing gloves.

   d. Use a gloved hand to apply an even coat, and cover with a dressing

5. Three tablets, 5 minutes apart.

6. a. parenteral

   b. non-parenteral

   c. non-parenteral

   d. non-parenteral

   e. parenteral

   f. non-parenteral

   g. non-parenteral

   h. non-parenteral

   i. parenteral

   j. non-parenteral

7. down and back

8. Rub the skin with an alcohol pad in a circular motion from the center of the site out.

9. The drug would be destroyed orally, a rapid effect is desired, the patient is unable to take the drug orally.

10. In the adult, pull the ear back and up. In a 2-year-old child, pull the ear back and down.

Self-Test 3 Medication Administration Record

MCFARLAND MEDICAL CENTER
Medication Administration Record

Patient Name	Room Number	Hospital Number		Diagnosis
Velder, Chelsea	1401	204452896		CHF

Allergies	Admitted	Age	Sex	Physician
PCN	6/25/07	50	F	Richardson

DOSAGE ADMINISTRATION PERIOD: 6/26/07 0600-6/27/07 0600

	0601-1400	1401-2200	2201-0600
Digoxin 0.25 mg PO every day Hold if HR <60	0900 AH HR: 75		
Aspirin 325 mg PO daily	0900 AH		
Protonix 40 mg PO every day	0900 AH		
Ampicillin 250 mg PO q 6h	(1400) DISCONTINUE	(1800) DUE to PATIENT	(0200) (0600) ALLERGY
Lopressor 50 mg PO BID Hold if SBP <100	B/P 98/50 AH (0900)	2100	
Coumadin 5 mg PO once a day		1700	
Morphine Sulfate 4-6 mg IV every 2-3h prn pain			
Tylenol gr X q4h prn temp >101	900 AH Temp 101.5		

Signature _Andrew Hughes_ Initials _(AH)_ Signature _____ Initials _____ Signature _____ Initials _____

Proficiency Test Answers

Chapter 1

Test 1: Arithmetic

A. a)
$$\begin{array}{r} 647 \\ \times\ \ 38 \\ \hline 5176 \\ 1941\ \ \\ \hline 24586 \end{array}$$

b)
$$\frac{\overset{1}{\cancel{8}}}{\underset{3}{\cancel{9}}} \times \frac{\overset{\overset{1}{\cancel{4}}}{\cancel{12}}}{\underset{1}{\cancel{32}}} = \frac{1}{3}$$

c)
$$\begin{array}{r} 0.56 \\ \times\ 0.17 \\ \hline 392 \\ 56\ \ \\ \hline 0.0952 \end{array}$$

B. a)
$$\begin{array}{r} 9.670 = 9.67 \\ 82\overline{)793.000} \\ \underline{738}\ \ \ \ \ \ \\ 55\,0\ \ \ \ \\ \underline{49\,2}\ \ \ \ \\ 5\,80\ \\ \underline{5\,74}\ \\ 60 \end{array}$$

b)
$$5\frac{1}{4} \div \frac{7}{4} = \frac{\overset{3}{\cancel{21}}}{\underset{1}{\cancel{4}}} \times \frac{\overset{1}{\cancel{4}}}{\underset{1}{\cancel{7}}} = 3$$

c)
$$\begin{array}{r} 20. \\ 0.015\overline{)0.300} \end{array}$$

C. a) $\dfrac{7}{15} + \dfrac{8}{15} = \dfrac{15}{15} = 1$

b) $\dfrac{3}{8} + \dfrac{2}{5} =$
$$\frac{15}{40} + \frac{16}{40} = \frac{31}{40}$$

c) $0.825 + 0.1 = 0.925$

D. a) $\dfrac{11}{15} - \dfrac{7}{10} =$
$$\frac{44}{60} - \frac{42}{60} = \frac{2}{60} = \frac{1}{30}$$

b) $\dfrac{8}{15} - \dfrac{4}{15} = \dfrac{4}{15}$

c) $1.56 - 0.2 =$
$$\begin{array}{r} 1.56 \\ \underline{-0.2}\ = 1.36 \\ 1.36 \end{array}$$

E. a) $\dfrac{1}{18}$
$$\begin{array}{r} 0.055 = 0.06 \\ 18\overline{)1.000} \\ \underline{90}\ \ \ \ \\ 100\ \\ \underline{90}\ \\ 100 \end{array}$$

b) $\dfrac{3}{8}$
$$\begin{array}{r} 0.375 = 0.38 \\ 8\overline{)3.000} \\ \underline{2\,4}\ \ \ \ \\ 60\ \ \\ \underline{56}\ \ \\ 40\ \\ \underline{40}\ \end{array}$$

F. a)

$$0.35 = \frac{\overset{7}{\overset{35}{\cancel{100}}}}{\underset{20}{\cancel{100}}} = \frac{7}{20}$$

b)

$$0.08 = \frac{\overset{2}{\overset{8}{\cancel{100}}}}{\underset{25}{\cancel{100}}} = \frac{2}{25}$$

G. a) 0.4

  b) 0.8

  c) 0.83

  d) 0.3

H. a)

$$\frac{\frac{5}{20}}{\frac{12}{3}} = \frac{5}{3} \begin{array}{l} 1.666 = 1.67 \\ \overline{)5.00} \\ \quad \underline{3} \\ \quad 20 \\ \quad \underline{18} \\ \quad\;\; 20 \\ \quad\;\; \underline{18} \\ \quad\quad 20 \\ \quad\quad \underline{18} \end{array}$$

b)

$$\frac{\frac{1}{7}}{\frac{84}{12}} = \frac{1}{12} \begin{array}{l} 0.083 = 0.08 \\ \overline{)1.00} \\ \;\; \underline{96} \\ \;\; 40 \\ \;\; \underline{36} \\ \quad 4 \end{array}$$

c)

$$\frac{6}{13} \begin{array}{l} 0.461 = 0.46 \\ \overline{)6.00} \\ \;\; \underline{5\,2} \\ \;\; 80 \\ \;\; \underline{78} \\ \quad 20 \\ \quad \underline{13} \end{array}$$

I. a) 5.3   **b)** 0.63   **c)** 0.924

J. a) ratio: $\frac{1}{3}\% = 1:300$

decimal: $\dfrac{\frac{1}{3}}{100} = \frac{1}{3} \div 100 = 0.0033$

fraction: $\frac{1}{3} \times \frac{1}{100} = \frac{1}{300}$

$1:300$

0.0033

b) ratio:

$0.8\% = \underset{\smile}{00.8} = 0.008 = 1:125$

$\dfrac{\frac{1}{8}}{\underset{125}{\cancel{1000}}} = \frac{1}{125} = 1:125$

decimal:

$0.8\% = \dfrac{0.8}{100} \begin{array}{l} .008 \\ \overline{)0.800} \end{array} = 0.008 = 0.008$

fraction: $0.8\% = \dfrac{\frac{8}{10}}{100} = \frac{8}{10} \div 100 = \frac{8}{10} \times \frac{1}{100} = \dfrac{\frac{1}{8}}{\underset{125}{\cancel{1000}}} = \frac{1}{125}$

K. a) $\dfrac{7}{100} = \underset{\smile}{00.7} = 7\%$

b) $1:10 = \dfrac{1}{10} = \underset{\smile}{0.10} = 10\%$

c) $0.008 = \underset{\smile}{0.008} \qquad 0.8\%$

L. a) $\dfrac{32}{128} = \dfrac{4}{x}$

$\dfrac{\overset{1}{\cancel{32}}x}{\underset{1}{\cancel{32}}} = \dfrac{\overset{4}{\cancel{128}} \times 4}{\underset{1}{\cancel{32}}}$

$x = 16$

b) $8:72::5:x$

$\dfrac{\overset{1}{\cancel{8}}}{\underset{1}{\cancel{8}}} x = \dfrac{\overset{9}{\cancel{72}} \times 5}{\underset{1}{\cancel{8}}}$

$x = 45$

c) $\dfrac{0.4}{0.12} = \dfrac{x}{8}$

$0.12x = 0.4 \times 8$

$\dfrac{\cancel{0.12}}{\cancel{0.12}} x = \dfrac{0.4 \times 8}{0.12}$

$x = \dfrac{3.2}{0.\underset{\smile}{12}} \begin{array}{l} 26.66 = 27 \\ \overline{)3.2000} \\ \;\; \underline{2\,4} \\ \;\; 80 \\ \;\; \underline{72} \\ \quad 80 \\ \quad \underline{72} \\ \quad\;\; 8 \end{array}$

$x = 27$

Chapter 2

Test 1: Abbreviations

1. Twice a day
2. Do not use hs. Use "at bedtime."
3. When necessary
4. Write out "both eyes"
5. By mouth
6. By rectum
7. Sublingually
8. Swish and swallow
9. Do not use tiw. Use "three times weekly."
10. Milliliter
11. Every 4 hours
12. Do not use cc. Use "milliliter."
13. Do not use sc. Use "subcutaneous."
14. Do not use AU. Use "both ears."
15. Gram
16. After meals
17. Do not use qd. Use "every day."
18. Immediately
19. Every 12 hours
20. Three times a day
21. Do not use OS. Write out "left eye"
22. Kilogram
23. Every night
24. Every hour
25. Do not use OD. Write out "right eye"
26. Milliequivalent
27. Before meals
28. Four times a day
29. Milligram
30. Intramuscularly
31. Do not use qod. Use "every other day."
32. Twice a week
33. Nasogastric tube
34. Every 8 hours
35. Liter
36. Microgram
37. Every 6 hours
38. Do not use µg. Use "microgram" or "mcg."
39. Do not use U. Use "unit."
40. Teaspoon
41. Do not use AD. Use "right ear."
42. Grain
43. Intravenously
44. Suspension
45. Tablespoon
46. Intravenous piggyback
47. Minim
48. Gram
49. Every 2 hours
50. Every 3 hours

Test 2: Reading Prescriptions

1. Nembutal one hundred milligrams at the hour of sleep, as needed, by mouth (eg, 10 PM or 2200)
2. Propranolol hydrochloride forty milligrams by mouth twice a day (eg, 10 AM, 6 PM)
3. Ampicillin one gram intravenous piggyback every 6 hours (eg, 6 AM, 12 noon, 6 PM, 12 midnight)
4. Demerol fifty milligrams intramuscularly every 4 hours as needed for pain
5. Tylenol three hundred twenty-five milligrams, two tablets by mouth immediately. (Give two tablets of Tylenol. Each tablet is 325 mg.)
6. Pilocarpine drops two in both eyes every 3 hours (eg, 3 AM, 6 AM, 9 AM, 12 noon, 3 PM, 6 PM, 9 PM, 12 midnight). Do not use OU; write "both eyes."
7. Scopolamine eight-tenths of a milligram subcutaneously immediately
8. Elixir of digoxin twenty-five hundredths of a milligram by mouth every day (eg, 10 AM). Do not use qd; write "every day."
9. Kaochlor thirty milliequivalents by mouth twice a day (eg, 10 AM and 6 PM)
10. Liquaemin sodium six thousand units subcutaneously every 4 hours (eg, 2 AM, 6 AM, 10 AM, 2 PM, 6 PM, 10 PM)
11. Tobramycin seventy milligrams intramuscularly every 8 hours (eg, 6 AM, 2 PM, 10 PM or 2200)
12. Prednisone ten milligrams by mouth every other day (eg, even days of the month at 10 AM). You might substitute "odd days of the month."
13. Milk of magnesia one tablespoon by mouth at the hour of sleep every night (eg, 10 PM)
14. Septra one double-strength tablet every day by mouth (eg, 10 AM)
15. Morphine sulfate fifteen milligrams subcutaneously immediately and ten milligrams every 4 hours as needed. The stat time given determines when the next dose can be administered. (Next dose must be *at least 4 hours later.*)

Test 3: Interpreting Written Prescription Orders

1. Colace one hundred milligrams by mouth three times a day (eg, 10 AM, 2 PM, 6 PM)

2. Ativan one milligram intravenous push times one dose now.

3. Ten milliequivalents potassium chloride in one hundred cubic centimeters of normal saline over one hour, times one dose. Should be one hundred "milliliters".

4. Tylenol number three two tablets by mouth every four hours as needed for pain

5. Heparin twenty-five thousand international units in two hundred fifty cubic centimeters dextrose five percent in water at five hundred units per hour. Should write out "international unit." Should write out "500 units." Should write out "mL."

6. Ticlid two hundred fifty milligrams one tablet by mouth twice a day (eg, 10 AM, 6 PM)

7. Lopressor 25 milligrams by mouth twice a day (eg, 10 AM, 6 PM)

8. Benadryl 25 milligrams by mouth every hour of sleep (eg, every night at 10 PM or 2200); should write "at bedtime"

Chapter 3

Test 1: Exercises in Equivalents and Mixed Conversions

1. 0.1	**11.** 30	**21.** 100	**31.** 10
2. 30	**12.** 1/5	**22.** 1	**32.** 1
3. 1000	**13.** 15	**23.** 0.6	**33.** 1000
4. 5	**14.** 2.2	**24.** 0.01	**34.** 0.6 mg
5. 15	**15.** 1000	**25.** 1000	**35.** gr 1/2
6. 0.01	**16.** 0.06	**26.** 0.0005 mg	**36.** 120 mg
7. 1	**17.** 1	**27.** 0.0006 g	**37.** gr 4
8. 200	**18.** 16	**28.** 0.25 mg	**38.** 0.48 mg
9. 0.03	**19.** 45	**29.** 0.001	**39.** gr 15
10. 0.5	**20.** 40°	**30.** 125	**40.** 98.6°

Chapter 4

Test 1: Labels and Packaging

1. **a. 1.** Individually wrapped and labeled drugs

    2. Large stock containers of drugs

  b. 1. Glass container holding a single dose. Container must be broken to reach the drug. Any portion not used must be discarded.

    2. Glass or plastic container with a sealed top that allows medication to be kept sterile

  c. 1. Drug applied to skin or mucous membranes to achieve a local effect. May be absorbed into the circulation and causes a systemic effect.

    2. Drugs given by injection include subcutaneous, IM, IV, and IVPB

  d. 1. Brand or proprietary name of manufacturer. Identified by symbol ®.

    2. Official name of a drug as listed in the USP

  e. 1. Liquid sterile medication ready to administer

    2. Powder or crystals diluted according to specific directions. Date and time of preparation must be written on the label, and the expiration date noted.

2. **a.** 4   **c.** 2   **e.** 1

  b. 2   **d.** 1

3. 1. g   **4.** i   **7.** j   **9.** c
   2. e   **5.** d   **8.** a   **10.** b
   3. h   **6.** f

Test 2: Interpreting a Label

1. Fortaz
2. Ceftazidime
3. Intravenous, intramuscular
4. Varies: 1.8 mL, 3.6 mL, 5.3 mL, 10.6 mL
5. 500 mg, 1 g
6. Reconstitute with sterile water for injection, bacteriostatic water for injection, or 0.5% or 1% lidocaine hydrochloride injection. Dilute with 1.5 mL, approximate available volume 1.8 mL to equal 500 mg (intramuscular route); add 3.0 mL, approximate available volume 3.6 mL to equal 1 g (intramuscular route); add 5.0 mL, approximate available volume 5.3 mL to equal 500 mg (intravenous route); add 10.0 mL, approximate available volume 10.6 mL to equal 1 g (intravenous infusion). Shake well.
7. Powder
8. Protect from light. Maintains satisfactory potency for 24 hours at room temperature or for 7 days under refrigeration. Solutions in sterile water for injection that are frozen immediately after constitution in the original container are stable for 3 months when stored at −20°C. Once thawed, solutions should not be refrozen. Thawed solutions may be stored for up to 8 hours at room temperature or for 4 days in a refrigerator.
9. Not shown
10. 500 mg or 1 g (adults)
11. Federal law prohibits dispensing without prescription. This vial is under reduced pressure. Addition of diluent generates a positive pressure. Color changes do not affect potency.

Chapter 5

Test 1: Drug Preparations and Equipment

1. Diabetes mellitus, alcoholism
2. Two teaspoons or less
3. Subcutaneous, IM, IVPB, and IV
4. **a.** The date
   b. The nurse's initials
   c. The dilution made
   d. The time
5. Aseptic technique is required in preparing and administering drugs parenterally (IM, subcutaneous, IV, IVPB).
6. Milk of magnesia
7. Before an oral suspension is poured, the liquid must always be shaken.
8. Aerosol powders, creams, ointments, pastes, suppositories, transdermal medications
9. Ease in administering; prolonged action
10. An ointment is a semisolid preparation in a petroleum or lanolin base for topical use.

11. **1.** Pour to a line. Never estimate a dose.
    2. Pour liquids at eye level.
12. **a.** The natural curve of the surface of a liquid in a container
    b. Diameter or width of a needle. The higher the gauge number, the finer the needle.
13. Route of administration, size and condition of the patient, amount of adipose tissue present at the site
14. **1.** When the last number is 5 or more, add 1 to the previous number.
    2. When the last number is 4 or less, drop the number.
15. The equipment used
    3-mL syringe—nearest 10th in milliliters
    precision syringe—nearest 100th in milliliters
    medicine cup—metric, apothecary, or household lines

Chapter 6

Test 1: Calculation of Oral Doses

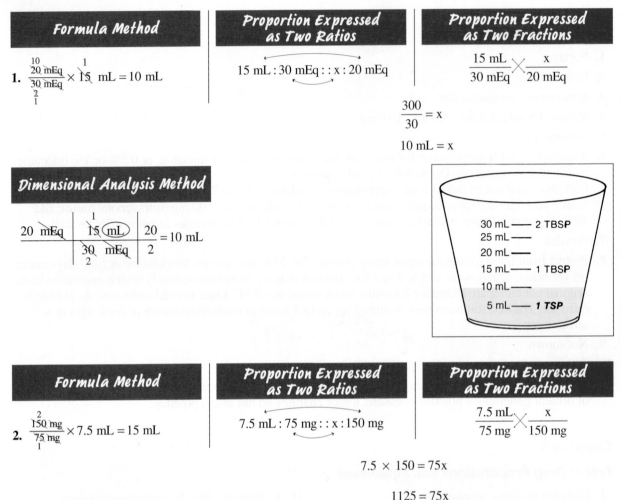

Formula Method

$$1. \quad \frac{\overset{10}{\cancel{20 \text{ mEq}}}}{\underset{2}{\underset{1}{\cancel{30 \text{ mEq}}}}} \times \overset{1}{\cancel{15}} \text{ mL} = 10 \text{ mL}$$

Proportion Expressed as Two Ratios

$$15 \text{ mL} : 30 \text{ mEq} : : \text{x} : 20 \text{ mEq}$$

Proportion Expressed as Two Fractions

$$\frac{15 \text{ mL}}{30 \text{ mEq}} \times \frac{\text{x}}{20 \text{ mEq}}$$

$$\frac{300}{30} = \text{x}$$

$$10 \text{ mL} = \text{x}$$

Dimensional Analysis Method

$$\frac{20 \text{ mEq}}{} \left| \frac{\overset{1}{\cancel{15}} \; \cancel{\text{mL}}}{\underset{2}{\cancel{30}} \; \cancel{\text{mEq}}} \right| \frac{20}{2} = 10 \text{ mL}$$

Formula Method

$$2. \quad \frac{\overset{2}{\cancel{150 \text{ mg}}}}{\underset{1}{\cancel{75 \text{ mg}}}} \times 7.5 \text{ mL} = 15 \text{ mL}$$

Proportion Expressed as Two Ratios

$$7.5 \text{ mL} : 75 \text{ mg} : : \text{x} : 150 \text{ mg}$$

Proportion Expressed as Two Fractions

$$\frac{7.5 \text{ mL}}{75 \text{ mg}} \times \frac{\text{x}}{150 \text{ mg}}$$

$$7.5 \times 150 = 75\text{x}$$

$$1125 = 75\text{x}$$

$$15 \text{ mL} = \text{x}$$

Dimensional Analysis Method

$$\frac{\overset{2}{\cancel{150}} \; \cancel{\text{mg}}}{} \left| \frac{7.5 \; \cancel{\text{mL}}}{\underset{1}{\cancel{75}} \; \cancel{\text{mg}}} \right| \frac{2 \times 7.5}{1} = 15 \text{ mL}$$

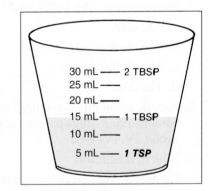

Formula Method

3. $\dfrac{\overset{1}{\cancel{0.125 \text{ mg}}}}{\underset{\underset{1}{2}}{\cancel{0.250 \text{ mg}}}} \times \overset{5}{\cancel{10}} = 5 \text{ mL}$

Proportion Expressed as Two Ratios

$10 \text{ mL} : 0.25 \text{ mg} :: x : 0.125 \text{ mg}$

Proportion Expressed as Two Fractions

$\dfrac{10 \text{ mL}}{0.25 \text{ mg}} \times \dfrac{x}{0.125 \text{ mg}}$

$$10 \times 0.125 = 0.25x$$

$$\frac{1.25}{0.25} = x$$

$$5 \text{ mL} = x$$

Dimensional Analysis Method

$\dfrac{\overset{1}{\cancel{0.125}} \ \cancel{\text{mg}}}{} \ \bigg| \ \dfrac{10 \ \text{(mL)}}{\underset{2}{\cancel{0.25}} \ \cancel{\text{mg}}} \ \bigg| \ \dfrac{10}{2} = 5 \text{ mL}$

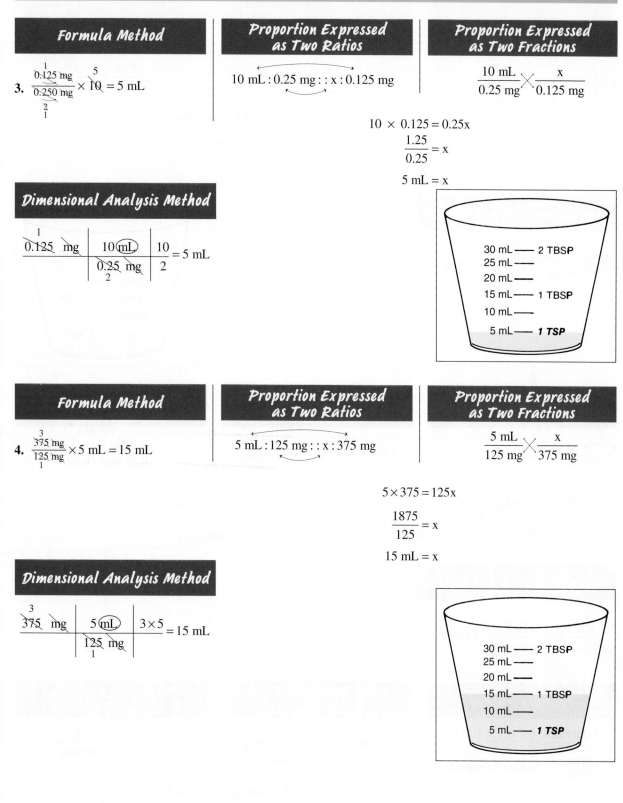

Formula Method

4. $\dfrac{\overset{3}{\cancel{375 \text{ mg}}}}{\underset{1}{\cancel{125 \text{ mg}}}} \times 5 \text{ mL} = 15 \text{ mL}$

Proportion Expressed as Two Ratios

$5 \text{ mL} : 125 \text{ mg} :: x : 375 \text{ mg}$

Proportion Expressed as Two Fractions

$\dfrac{5 \text{ mL}}{125 \text{ mg}} \times \dfrac{x}{375 \text{ mg}}$

$$5 \times 375 = 125x$$

$$\frac{1875}{125} = x$$

$$15 \text{ mL} = x$$

Dimensional Analysis Method

$\dfrac{\overset{3}{\cancel{375}} \ \cancel{\text{mg}}}{} \ \bigg| \ \dfrac{5 \ \text{(mL)}}{\underset{1}{\cancel{125}} \ \cancel{\text{mg}}} \ \bigg| \ 3 \times 5 = 15 \text{ mL}$

Formula Method	Proportion Expressed as Two Ratios	Proportion Expressed as Two Fractions

5. $\dfrac{\overset{2}{40} \text{ mg}}{\underset{1}{20} \text{ mg}} \times 2.5 \text{ mL} = 5 \text{ mL}$

2.5 mL : 20 mg : : x : 40 mg

$\dfrac{2.5 \text{ mL}}{20 \text{ mg}} \times \dfrac{\text{x}}{40 \text{ mg}}$

$$2.5 \times 40 = 20\text{x}$$

$$\frac{100}{20} = \text{x}$$

$$5 \text{ mL} = \text{x}$$

Dimensional Analysis Method

$\dfrac{\overset{2}{40} \text{ mg}}{} \Bigg| \dfrac{2.5 \text{ mL}}{\underset{1}{20} \text{ mg}} \Bigg| \dfrac{2 \times 2.5}{} = 5 \text{ mL} = \text{x}$

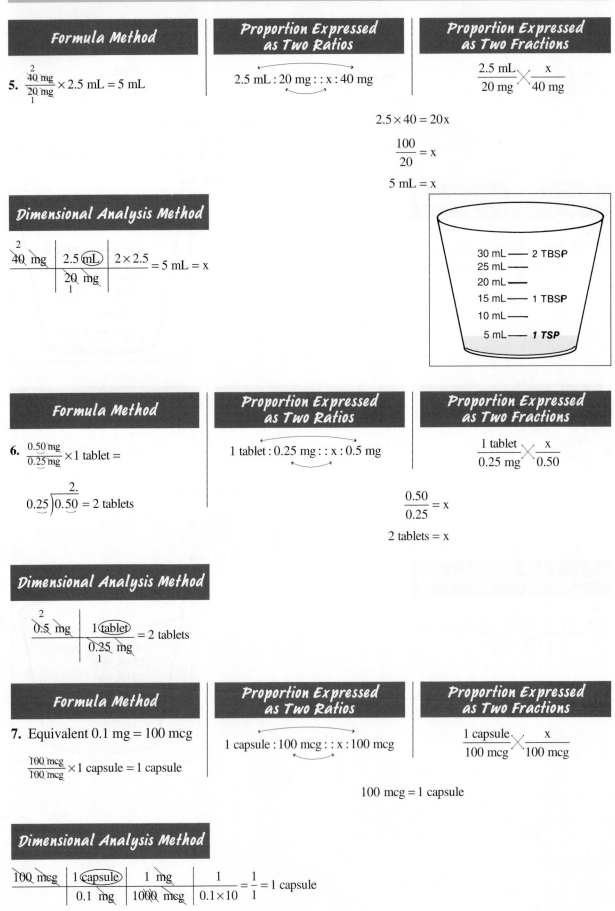

30 mL —— 2 TBSP	
25 mL ——	
20 mL ——	
15 mL —— 1 TBSP	
10 mL ——	
5 mL —— *1 TSP*	

Formula Method	Proportion Expressed as Two Ratios	Proportion Expressed as Two Fractions

6. $\dfrac{0.50 \text{ mg}}{0.25 \text{ mg}} \times 1 \text{ tablet} =$

1 tablet : 0.25 mg : : x : 0.5 mg

$\dfrac{1 \text{ tablet}}{0.25 \text{ mg}} \times \dfrac{\text{x}}{0.50}$

$0.25 \overset{2.}{\overline{)0.50}} = 2 \text{ tablets}$

$$\frac{0.50}{0.25} = \text{x}$$

$$2 \text{ tablets} = \text{x}$$

Dimensional Analysis Method

$\dfrac{\overset{2}{0.5} \text{ mg}}{} \Bigg| \dfrac{1 \text{ tablet}}{\underset{1}{0.25} \text{ mg}} = 2 \text{ tablets}$

Formula Method	Proportion Expressed as Two Ratios	Proportion Expressed as Two Fractions

7. Equivalent 0.1 mg = 100 mcg

1 capsule : 100 mcg : : x : 100 mcg

$\dfrac{1 \text{ capsule}}{100 \text{ mcg}} \times \dfrac{\text{x}}{100 \text{ mcg}}$

$\dfrac{100 \text{ mcg}}{100 \text{ mcg}} \times 1 \text{ capsule} = 1 \text{ capsule}$

$$100 \text{ mcg} = 1 \text{ capsule}$$

Dimensional Analysis Method

$\dfrac{100 \text{ mcg}}{} \Bigg| \dfrac{1 \text{ capsule}}{0.1 \text{ mg}} \Bigg| \dfrac{1 \text{ mg}}{1000 \text{ mcg}} \Bigg| \dfrac{1}{0.1 \times 10} = \dfrac{1}{1} = 1 \text{ capsule}$

Formula Method	Proportion Expressed as Two Ratios	Proportion Expressed as Two Fractions

8. $\dfrac{\overset{5}{\cancel{250}\ \text{mg}}}{\underset{2}{\cancel{100}\ \text{mg}}} \times 1\ \text{tablet} = \dfrac{5}{2} = 2\dfrac{1}{2}$ tablets

1 tablet : 100 mg : : x : 250 mg

$\dfrac{1\ \text{tablet}}{100\ \text{mg}} \diagup\diagdown \dfrac{\text{x}}{250\ \text{mg}}$

$$\dfrac{250}{100} = \text{x}$$

$$2.5\ \text{tablet} = \text{x}$$

$$\text{or } 2\dfrac{1}{2}\ \text{tablets}$$

Dimensional Analysis Method

$\dfrac{\overset{2.5}{\cancel{250}\ \text{mg}}}{} \ \Big|\ \dfrac{1\ \text{tablet}}{\underset{1}{\cancel{100}\ \text{mg}}} \ \Big|\ 2.5 \times 1 = 2.5$ tablets or $2\dfrac{1}{2}$ tablets

Formula Method	Proportion Expressed as Two Ratios	Proportion Expressed as Two Fractions

9. Equivalent 0.5 g = 500 mg

$\dfrac{\overset{2}{\cancel{500}\ \text{mg}}}{\underset{1}{\cancel{250}\ \text{mg}}} \times 1\ \text{capsule} = 2$ capsule

1 capsule : 250 mg : : x : 500 mg

$\dfrac{1\ \text{capsule}}{250\ \text{mg}} \diagup\diagdown \dfrac{\text{x}}{500\ \text{mg}}$

$$\dfrac{500}{250} = \text{x}$$

$$2\ \text{capsules} = \text{x}$$

Dimensional Analysis Method

$0.5\ \cancel{\text{g}} \ \Big|\ \dfrac{1\ \text{capsule}}{\underset{1}{\cancel{250}\ \text{mg}}} \ \Big|\ \dfrac{\overset{4}{\cancel{1000}\ \text{mg}}}{1\ \cancel{\text{g}}} \ \Big|\ 0.5 \times 4 = 2$ capsules

Formula Method	Proportion Expressed as Two Ratios	Proportion Expressed as Two Fractions

10. Equivalent 0.3 mg = 300 mcg

$\dfrac{\overset{1}{\cancel{300}\ \text{mcg}}}{\underset{1}{\cancel{300}\ \text{mcg}}} \times 1\ \text{tablet} = 1$ tablet

1 tablet : 300 mcg : : x : 300 mcg

$\dfrac{1\ \text{tablet}}{300\ \text{mcg}} \diagup\diagdown \dfrac{\text{x}}{300\ \text{mcg}}$

$$\dfrac{300}{300} = \text{x}$$

$$1\ \text{tablet} = \text{x}$$

Dimensional Analysis Method

$0.3\ \cancel{\text{mg}} \ \Big|\ \dfrac{1\ \text{tablet}}{300\ \cancel{\text{mcg}}} \ \Big|\ \dfrac{1000\ \cancel{\text{mcg}}}{1\ \cancel{\text{mg}}} \ \Big|\ \dfrac{0.3 \times 10}{3} = 1$ tablet

Test 2: Calculation of Oral Doses (Test 2)

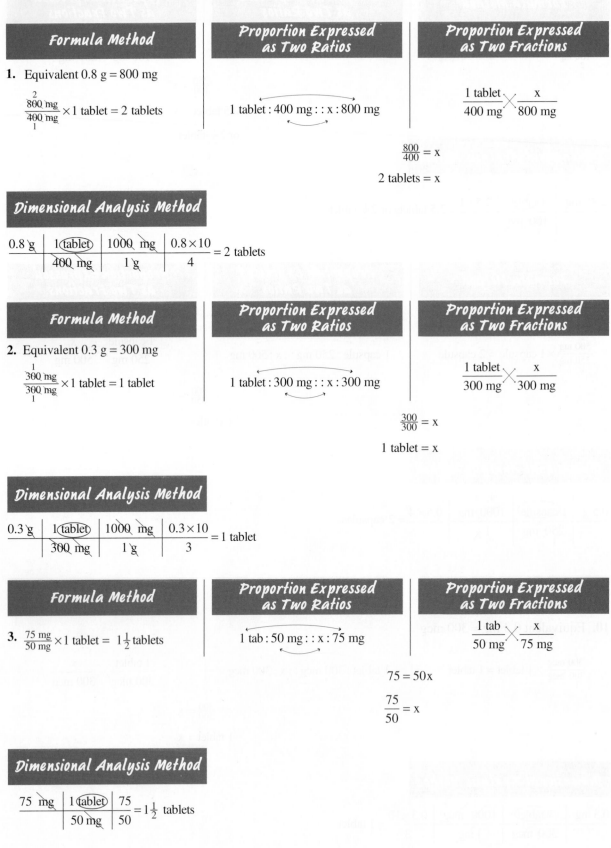

Formula Method	Proportion Expressed as Two Ratios	Proportion Expressed as Two Fractions

1. Equivalent 0.8 g = 800 mg

$$\frac{\overset{2}{\cancel{800}} \text{ mg}}{\underset{1}{\cancel{400}} \text{ mg}} \times 1 \text{ tablet} = 2 \text{ tablets}$$

1 tablet : 400 mg : : x : 800 mg

$$\frac{1 \text{ tablet}}{400 \text{ mg}} \times \frac{x}{800 \text{ mg}}$$

$$\frac{800}{400} = x$$

2 tablets = x

Dimensional Analysis Method

$$\frac{0.8 \cancel{g}}{} \left| \frac{1 \text{ tablet}}{400 \cancel{mg}} \right| \frac{1000 \cancel{mg}}{1 \cancel{g}} \left| \frac{0.8 \times 10}{4} = 2 \text{ tablets} \right.$$

Formula Method	Proportion Expressed as Two Ratios	Proportion Expressed as Two Fractions

2. Equivalent 0.3 g = 300 mg

$$\frac{\overset{1}{\cancel{300}} \text{ mg}}{\underset{1}{\cancel{300}} \text{ mg}} \times 1 \text{ tablet} = 1 \text{ tablet}$$

1 tablet : 300 mg : : x : 300 mg

$$\frac{1 \text{ tablet}}{300 \text{ mg}} \times \frac{x}{300 \text{ mg}}$$

$$\frac{300}{300} = x$$

1 tablet = x

Dimensional Analysis Method

$$\frac{0.3 \cancel{g}}{} \left| \frac{1 \text{ tablet}}{300 \cancel{mg}} \right| \frac{1000 \cancel{mg}}{1 \cancel{g}} \left| \frac{0.3 \times 10}{3} = 1 \text{ tablet} \right.$$

Formula Method	Proportion Expressed as Two Ratios	Proportion Expressed as Two Fractions

3. $\frac{75 \text{ mg}}{50 \text{ mg}} \times 1 \text{ tablet} = 1\frac{1}{2} \text{ tablets}$

1 tab : 50 mg : : x : 75 mg

$$\frac{1 \text{ tab}}{50 \text{ mg}} \times \frac{x}{75 \text{ mg}}$$

$$75 = 50x$$

$$\frac{75}{50} = x$$

Dimensional Analysis Method

$$\frac{75 \text{ mg}}{} \left| \frac{1 \text{ tablet}}{50 \text{ mg}} \right| \frac{75}{50} = 1\frac{1}{2} \text{ tablets}$$

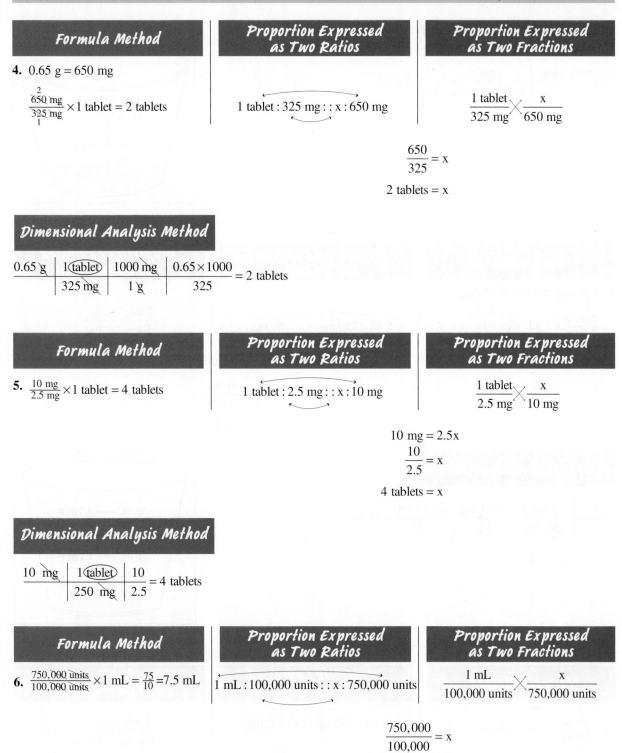

Formula Method	Proportion Expressed as Two Ratios	Proportion Expressed as Two Fractions
4. 0.65 g = 650 mg		

$$\frac{\overset{2}{\cancel{650\ mg}}}{\underset{1}{\cancel{325\ mg}}} \times 1\ tablet = 2\ tablets$$

1 tablet : 325 mg : : x : 650 mg

$$\frac{1\ tablet}{325\ mg} \diagup \frac{x}{650\ mg}$$

$$\frac{650}{325} = x$$

$$2\ tablets = x$$

Dimensional Analysis Method

$$\frac{0.65\ \cancel{g}}{} \ \left|\ \frac{1\ \text{(tablet)}}{325\ \cancel{mg}}\ \right|\ \frac{1000\ \cancel{mg}}{1\ \cancel{g}}\ \right|\ \frac{0.65 \times 1000}{325} = 2\ tablets$$

Formula Method	Proportion Expressed as Two Ratios	Proportion Expressed as Two Fractions
5. $\frac{10\ mg}{2.5\ mg} \times 1\ tablet = 4\ tablets$	1 tablet : 2.5 mg : : x : 10 mg	$\frac{1\ tablet}{2.5\ mg} \diagup \frac{x}{10\ mg}$

$$10\ mg = 2.5x$$

$$\frac{10}{2.5} = x$$

$$4\ tablets = x$$

Dimensional Analysis Method

$$\frac{10\ \cancel{mg}}{} \ \left|\ \frac{1\ \text{(tablet)}}{250\ \cancel{mg}}\ \right|\ \frac{10}{2.5} = 4\ tablets$$

Formula Method	Proportion Expressed as Two Ratios	Proportion Expressed as Two Fractions
6. $\frac{750,000\ \cancel{units}}{100,000\ \cancel{units}} \times 1\ mL = \frac{75}{10} = 7.5\ mL$	1 mL : 100,000 units : : x : 750,000 units	$\frac{1\ mL}{100,000\ units} \diagup \frac{x}{750,000\ units}$

$$\frac{750,000}{100,000} = x$$

$$7.5\ mL = x$$

Dimensional Analysis Method

$$\frac{750,000 \text{ units}}{1} \left| \frac{1 \text{ mL}}{100,000 \text{ units}} \right| \frac{75}{10} = 7.5 \text{ mL}$$

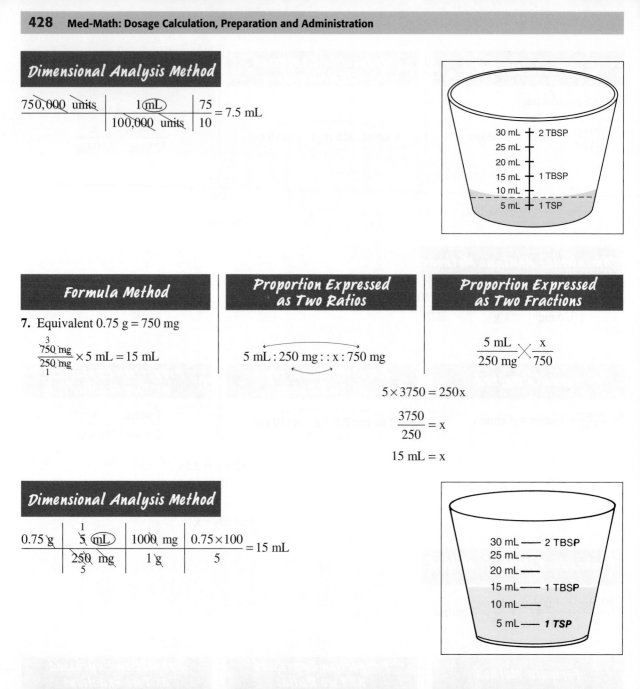

Formula Method

7. Equivalent 0.75 g = 750 mg

$$\frac{\overset{3}{750 \text{ mg}}}{\underset{1}{250 \text{ mg}}} \times 5 \text{ mL} = 15 \text{ mL}$$

Proportion Expressed as Two Ratios

5 mL : 250 mg : : x : 750 mg

Proportion Expressed as Two Fractions

$$\frac{5 \text{ mL}}{250 \text{ mg}} \times \frac{x}{750}$$

$$5 \times 3750 = 250x$$

$$\frac{3750}{250} = x$$

$$15 \text{ mL} = x$$

Dimensional Analysis Method

$$\frac{0.75 \text{ g}}{1} \left| \frac{\overset{1}{5} \text{ mL}}{\underset{5}{250} \text{ mg}} \right| \frac{1000 \text{ mg}}{1 \text{ g}} \left| \frac{0.75 \times 100}{5} = 15 \text{ mL} \right.$$

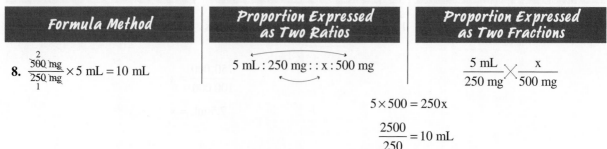

Formula Method

8. $\dfrac{\overset{2}{500 \text{ mg}}}{\underset{1}{250 \text{ mg}}} \times 5 \text{ mL} = 10 \text{ mL}$

Proportion Expressed as Two Ratios

5 mL : 250 mg : : x : 500 mg

Proportion Expressed as Two Fractions

$$\frac{5 \text{ mL}}{250 \text{ mg}} \times \frac{x}{500 \text{ mg}}$$

$$5 \times 500 = 250x$$

$$\frac{2500}{250} = 10 \text{ mL}$$

Dimensional Analysis Method

$$\frac{\overset{2}{\cancel{500}}\ \cancel{mg}}{}\ \bigg|\ \frac{5\ \cancel{mL}}{\underset{1}{\cancel{250}}\ \cancel{mg}}\ \bigg|\ \frac{2\times 5}{}=10\ mL$$

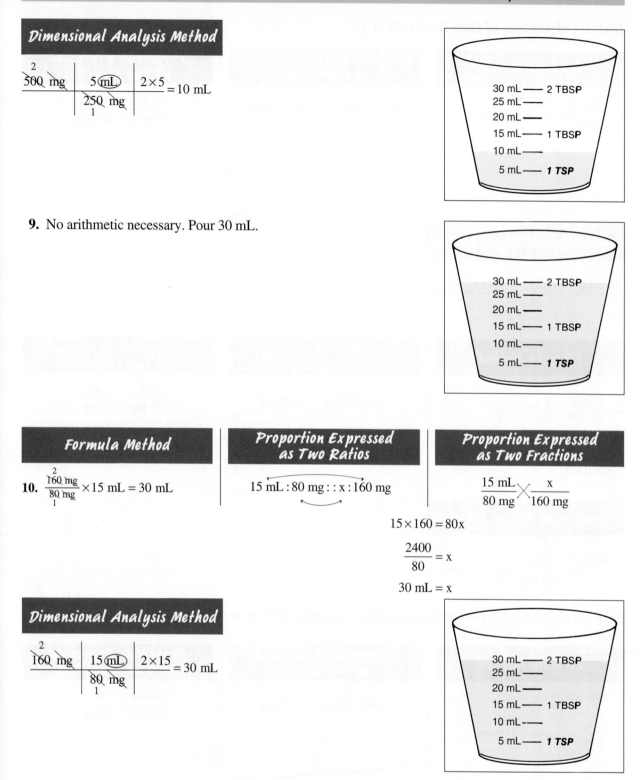

9. No arithmetic necessary. Pour 30 mL.

Formula Method	Proportion Expressed as Two Ratios	Proportion Expressed as Two Fractions
10. $\dfrac{\overset{2}{\cancel{160}\ \cancel{mg}}}{\underset{1}{\cancel{80}\ \cancel{mg}}}\times 15\ mL = 30\ mL$	$15\ mL : 80\ mg :: x : 160\ mg$	$\dfrac{15\ mL}{80\ mg}\times\dfrac{x}{160\ mg}$

$$15\times 160 = 80x$$

$$\frac{2400}{80}=x$$

$$30\ mL = x$$

Dimensional Analysis Method

$$\frac{\overset{2}{\cancel{160}}\ \cancel{mg}}{}\ \bigg|\ \frac{15\ \cancel{mL}}{\underset{1}{\cancel{80}}\ \cancel{mg}}\ \bigg|\ \frac{2\times 15}{}=30\ mL$$

Test 3: Calculation of Oral Doses (Test 3)

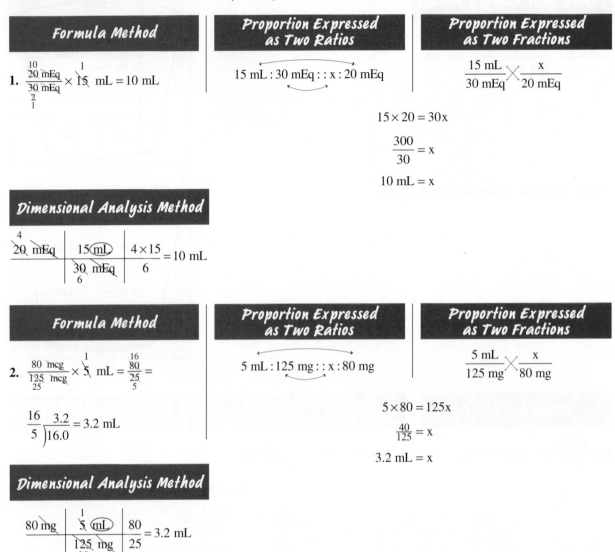

| Formula Method | Proportion Expressed as Two Ratios | Proportion Expressed as Two Fractions |

1. $\dfrac{\overset{10}{\cancel{20}} \text{ mEq}}{\underset{2}{\cancel{30}} \text{ mEq}} \times \overset{1}{\cancel{15}} \text{ mL} = 10 \text{ mL}$

$15 \text{ mL} : 30 \text{ mEq} :: x : 20 \text{ mEq}$

$\dfrac{15 \text{ mL}}{30 \text{ mEq}} \times \dfrac{x}{20 \text{ mEq}}$

$15 \times 20 = 30x$

$\dfrac{300}{30} = x$

$10 \text{ mL} = x$

Dimensional Analysis Method

$\dfrac{\overset{4}{\cancel{20}} \text{ mEq}}{1} \left| \dfrac{15 \text{ mL}}{\underset{6}{\cancel{30}} \text{ mEq}} \right| \dfrac{4 \times 15}{6} = 10 \text{ mL}$

| Formula Method | Proportion Expressed as Two Ratios | Proportion Expressed as Two Fractions |

2. $\dfrac{\overset{16}{\cancel{80}} \text{ mcg}}{\underset{25}{\cancel{125}} \text{ mcg}} \times \overset{1}{\cancel{5}} \text{ mL} = \dfrac{\overset{16}{\cancel{80}}}{\underset{5}{\cancel{25}}} =$

$5 \text{ mL} : 125 \text{ mg} :: x : 80 \text{ mg}$

$\dfrac{5 \text{ mL}}{125 \text{ mg}} \times \dfrac{x}{80 \text{ mg}}$

$5 \times 80 = 125x$

$\dfrac{40}{125} = x$

$3.2 \text{ mL} = x$

$\dfrac{16}{5} \, \overset{3.2}{\overline{)16.0}} = 3.2 \text{ mL}$

Dimensional Analysis Method

$\dfrac{80 \text{ mg}}{1} \left| \dfrac{\overset{1}{\cancel{5}} \text{ mL}}{\underset{25}{\cancel{125}} \text{ mg}} \right| \dfrac{80}{25} = 3.2 \text{ mL}$

If you do not have a dropper bottle, you could use a syringe without the needle to obtain the dose.

| Formula Method | Proportion Expressed as Two Ratios | Proportion Expressed as Two Fractions |

3. $0.02 \text{ g} = 20 \text{ mg}$

$1 \text{ tablet} : 10 \text{ mg} :: x : 20 \text{ mg}$

$\dfrac{1 \text{ tablet}}{10 \text{ mg}} \times \dfrac{x}{20 \text{ mg}}$

$\dfrac{\overset{2}{\cancel{20}} \text{ mg}}{\underset{1}{\cancel{10}} \text{ mg}} \times 1 \text{ tablet} = 2 \text{ tablets}$

$\dfrac{20}{10} = x$

$2 \text{ tablets} = x$

Dimensional Analysis Method

$\dfrac{0.02 \text{ g}}{} \left| \dfrac{1 \text{ tablet}}{\underset{1}{\cancel{10}} \text{ mg}} \right| \dfrac{\overset{100}{\cancel{1000}} \text{ mg}}{1 \text{ g}} \left| \dfrac{0.02 \times 100}{} = 2 \text{ tablets} \right.$

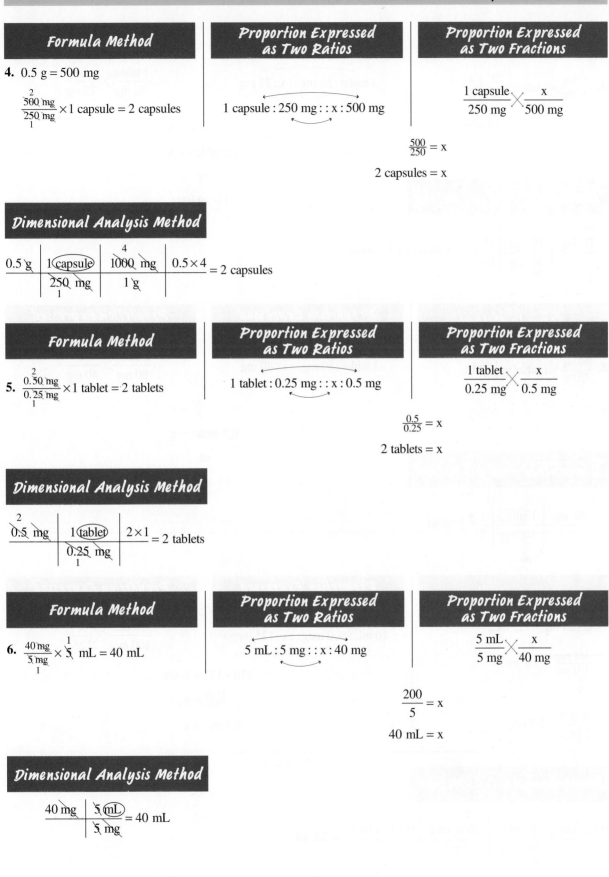

Formula Method	Proportion Expressed as Two Ratios	Proportion Expressed as Two Fractions
4. $0.5 \text{ g} = 500 \text{ mg}$ $\dfrac{\overset{2}{\cancel{500 \text{ mg}}}}{\underset{1}{\cancel{250 \text{ mg}}}} \times 1 \text{ capsule} = 2 \text{ capsules}$	$1 \text{ capsule} : 250 \text{ mg} :: \text{x} : 500 \text{ mg}$	$\dfrac{1 \text{ capsule}}{250 \text{ mg}} \diagdown \dfrac{\text{x}}{500 \text{ mg}}$

$$\frac{500}{250} = \text{x}$$

$$2 \text{ capsules} = \text{x}$$

Dimensional Analysis Method

$$\frac{0.5 \cancel{\text{ g}}}{} \left| \frac{1 \, \text{capsule}}{\underset{1}{250 \cancel{\text{ mg}}}} \right| \frac{\overset{4}{1000} \cancel{\text{ mg}}}{1 \cancel{\text{ g}}} \right| \frac{0.5 \times 4}{} = 2 \text{ capsules}$$

Formula Method	Proportion Expressed as Two Ratios	Proportion Expressed as Two Fractions
5. $\dfrac{\overset{2}{0.50 \text{ mg}}}{\underset{1}{0.25 \text{ mg}}} \times 1 \text{ tablet} = 2 \text{ tablets}$	$1 \text{ tablet} : 0.25 \text{ mg} :: \text{x} : 0.5 \text{ mg}$	$\dfrac{1 \text{ tablet}}{0.25 \text{ mg}} \diagdown \dfrac{\text{x}}{0.5 \text{ mg}}$

$$\frac{0.5}{0.25} = \text{x}$$

$$2 \text{ tablets} = \text{x}$$

Dimensional Analysis Method

$$\frac{\overset{2}{0.5} \cancel{\text{ mg}}}{} \left| \frac{1 \, \text{tablet}}{\underset{1}{0.25 \cancel{\text{ mg}}}} \right| \frac{2 \times 1}{} = 2 \text{ tablets}$$

Formula Method	Proportion Expressed as Two Ratios	Proportion Expressed as Two Fractions
6. $\dfrac{40 \text{ mg}}{\underset{1}{5 \text{ mg}}} \times \overset{1}{5} \text{ mL} = 40 \text{ mL}$	$5 \text{ mL} : 5 \text{ mg} :: \text{x} : 40 \text{ mg}$	$\dfrac{5 \text{ mL}}{5 \text{ mg}} \diagdown \dfrac{\text{x}}{40 \text{ mg}}$

$$\frac{200}{5} = \text{x}$$

$$40 \text{ mL} = \text{x}$$

Dimensional Analysis Method

$$\frac{40 \cancel{\text{ mg}}}{} \left| \frac{5 \, \cancel{\text{mL}}}{5 \cancel{\text{ mg}}} \right| = 40 \text{ mL}$$

Formula Method	Proportion Expressed as Two Ratios	Proportion Expressed as Two Fractions

7. $\dfrac{\overset{3}{\cancel{75}\text{ mg}}}{\underset{2}{\cancel{50}\text{ mg}}} \times 1 \text{ tablet} = \dfrac{3}{2}\,\overline{)3.0}^{\,1.5}$

$= 1\frac{1}{2}$ tablets

1 tablet : 50 mg : : x : 75 mg

$\dfrac{1 \text{ tablet}}{50 \text{ mg}} \times \dfrac{\text{x}}{75 \text{ mg}}$

$\dfrac{75}{50} = \text{x}$

1.5 tablets = x

or

$1\frac{1}{2}$ tablets

Dimensional Analysis Method

$\dfrac{\overset{15}{\cancel{75}}\text{ mg}}{} \left| \dfrac{1\,\text{(tablet)}}{\underset{10}{\cancel{50}}\text{ mg}} \right| \dfrac{15}{10} = 1.5 \text{ tablets or } 1\frac{1}{2} \text{ tablets}$

Formula Method	Proportion Expressed as Two Ratios	Proportion Expressed as Two Fractions

8. $\dfrac{\overset{1}{\cancel{40}}\text{ mg}}{\underset{2}{\cancel{80}}\text{ mg}} \times 1 \text{ tablet} = \frac{1}{2} \text{ tablet}$

1 tablet : 80 mg : : x : 40 mg

$\dfrac{1 \text{ tablet}}{80 \text{ mg}} \times \dfrac{\text{x}}{40 \text{ mg}}$

$\dfrac{40}{80} = \text{x}$

0.5 tablet = x

or

$1\frac{1}{2}$ tablets

Dimensional Analysis Method

$\dfrac{\overset{1}{\cancel{40}}\text{ mg}}{} \left| \dfrac{1\,\text{(tablet)}}{\underset{2}{\cancel{80}}\text{ mg}} \right| \dfrac{1}{2} = \frac{1}{2} \text{ tablet}$

Formula Method	Proportion Expressed as Two Ratios	Proportion Expressed as Two Fractions

9. 0.125 mg = 125 mcg

$\dfrac{\overset{1}{\cancel{125}\text{ mcg}}}{\underset{4\ 2}{\cancel{500}\text{ mcg}}} \times \overset{5}{\cancel{10}}\ \text{mL} =$

$\dfrac{5}{2}\,\overline{)5.0}^{\,2.5} = 2.5 \text{ mL}$

10 mL : 500 mcg : : x : 125 mcg

$\dfrac{10 \text{ mL}}{500 \text{ mcg}} \times \dfrac{\text{x}}{125}$

$10 \times 125 = 500\text{x}$

$\dfrac{1250}{500} = \text{x}$

2.5 mL = x

Dimensional Analysis Method

$\dfrac{0.125\ \cancel{\text{mg}}}{} \left| \dfrac{10\,\cancel{\text{(mL)}}}{\underset{1}{\cancel{500}}\ \cancel{\text{mcg}}} \right| \dfrac{\overset{2}{\cancel{1000}}\ \cancel{\text{mcg}}}{1\ \cancel{\text{mg}}} \right| \dfrac{0.125 \times 10 \times 2}{} = 2.5 \text{ mL}$

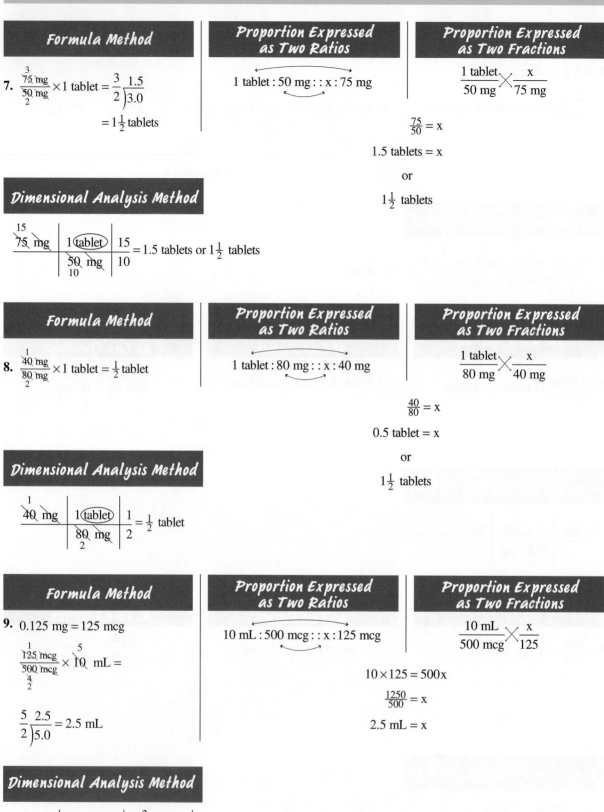

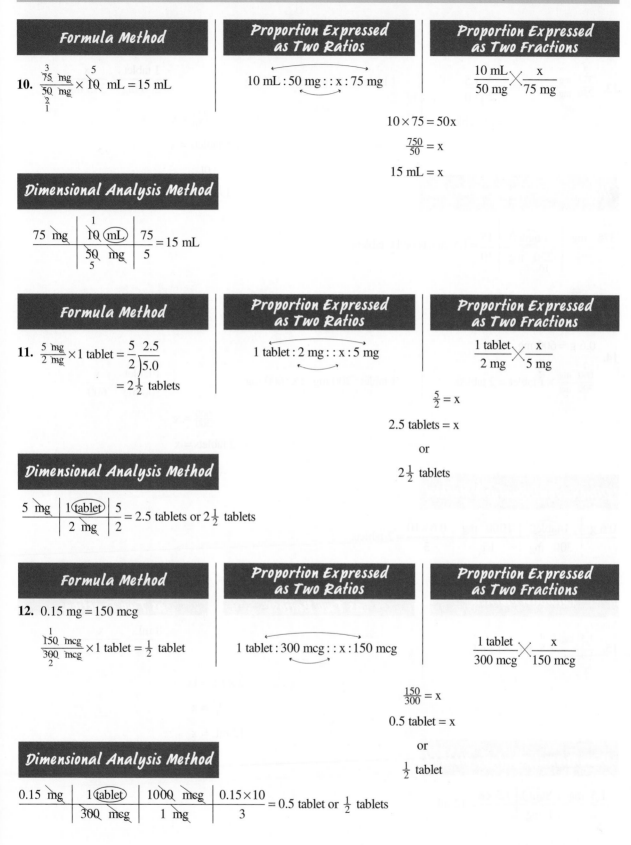

Formula Method	Proportion Expressed as Two Ratios	Proportion Expressed as Two Fractions
10. $\dfrac{\overset{3}{\cancel{75}}\ \cancel{mg}}{\underset{2}{\cancel{50}}\ \cancel{mg}} \times \overset{5}{\cancel{10}}\ mL = 15\ mL$	$10\ mL : 50\ mg : : x : 75\ mg$	$\dfrac{10\ mL}{50\ mg} \underset{\diagdown}{\diagup} \dfrac{x}{75\ mg}$

$$10 \times 75 = 50x$$
$$\frac{750}{50} = x$$
$$15\ mL = x$$

Dimensional Analysis Method

$$\frac{\cancel{75}\ \cancel{mg} \quad \left| \quad \overset{1}{\cancel{10}}\ \text{(mL)} \quad \right| \quad 75}{\qquad \left| \quad \underset{5}{\cancel{50}}\ \cancel{mg} \quad \right| \quad 5} = 15\ mL$$

Formula Method	Proportion Expressed as Two Ratios	Proportion Expressed as Two Fractions
11. $\dfrac{5\ \cancel{mg}}{2\ \cancel{mg}} \times 1\ tablet = \dfrac{5}{2}\ \begin{array}{r} 2.5 \\ \hline 5.0 \end{array}$ $= 2\frac{1}{2}\ tablets$	$1\ tablet : 2\ mg : : x : 5\ mg$	$\dfrac{1\ tablet}{2\ mg} \underset{\diagdown}{\diagup} \dfrac{x}{5\ mg}$

$$\frac{5}{2} = x$$
$$2.5\ tablets = x$$
or
$$2\frac{1}{2}\ tablets$$

Dimensional Analysis Method

$$\frac{5\ \cancel{mg} \quad \left| \quad 1\ \text{(tablet)} \quad \right| \quad 5}{\qquad \left| \quad 2\ \cancel{mg} \quad \right| \quad 2} = 2.5\ tablets\ or\ 2\frac{1}{2}\ tablets$$

Formula Method	Proportion Expressed as Two Ratios	Proportion Expressed as Two Fractions
12. $0.15\ mg = 150\ mcg$ $\dfrac{\overset{1}{\cancel{150}}\ \cancel{mcg}}{\underset{2}{\cancel{300}}\ \cancel{mcg}} \times 1\ tablet = \dfrac{1}{2}\ tablet$	$1\ tablet : 300\ mcg : : x : 150\ mcg$	$\dfrac{1\ tablet}{300\ mcg} \underset{\diagdown}{\diagup} \dfrac{x}{150\ mcg}$

$$\frac{150}{300} = x$$
$$0.5\ tablet = x$$
or
$$\frac{1}{2}\ tablet$$

Dimensional Analysis Method

$$\frac{0.15\ \cancel{mg} \quad \left| \quad 1\ \text{(tablet)} \quad \right| \quad 1000\ \cancel{mcg} \quad \left| \quad 0.15 \times 10 \right.}{\qquad \left| \quad 300\ \cancel{mcg} \quad \right| \quad 1\ \cancel{mg} \quad \left| \quad 3 \right.} = 0.5\ tablet\ or\ \frac{1}{2}\ tablets$$

Formula Method	**Proportion Expressed as Two Ratios**	**Proportion Expressed as Two Fractions**

13. $\dfrac{\overset{3}{\cancel{375}} \text{ mg}}{\underset{2}{\cancel{250}} \text{ mg}} \times 1 \text{ tablet} = \dfrac{3}{2}\overline{\smash{\big)}3.0}^{\,1.5}$

$= 1\frac{1}{2}$ tablets

1 tablet : 250 mg : : x : 375 mg

$\dfrac{1 \text{ tablet}}{250 \text{ mg}} \diagup \dfrac{\text{x}}{375 \text{ mg}}$

$\dfrac{375}{250} = \text{x}$

1.5 tablets = x

or

$1\frac{1}{2}$ tablets

Dimensional Analysis Method

$\dfrac{\overset{15}{\cancel{375}} \text{ mg}}{} \bigg| \dfrac{1 \text{ tablet}}{\underset{10}{\cancel{250}} \text{ mg}} \bigg| \dfrac{15}{10} = 1.5 \text{ tablets or } 1\frac{1}{2} \text{ tablets}$

Formula Method	**Proportion Expressed as Two Ratios**	**Proportion Expressed as Two Fractions**

14. 0.6 g = 600 mg

$\dfrac{\overset{2}{\cancel{600}} \text{ mg}}{\underset{1}{\cancel{300}} \text{ mg}} \times 1 \text{ tablet} = 2 \text{ tablets}$

1 tablet : 300 mg : : x : 600 mg

$\dfrac{1 \text{ tablet}}{300 \text{ mg}} \diagup \dfrac{\text{x}}{600}$

$\dfrac{600}{300} = \text{x}$

2 tablets = x

Dimensional Analysis Method

$\dfrac{0.6 \text{ g}}{} \bigg| \dfrac{1 \text{ tablet}}{300 \text{ mg}} \bigg| \dfrac{1000 \text{ mg}}{1 \text{ g}} \bigg| \dfrac{0.6 \times 10}{3} = 2 \text{ tablets}$

Formula Method	**Proportion Expressed as Two Ratios**	**Proportion Expressed as Two Fractions**

15. $\dfrac{\overset{3}{\cancel{1.5}} \text{ mg}}{\underset{\underset{1}{2}}{\cancel{1.0}} \text{ mg}} \times \overset{4}{\cancel{8}} \text{ mL} = 12 \text{ mL}$

8 mL : 1 mg : : x : 1.5 mg

$\dfrac{8 \text{ mL}}{1 \text{ mg}} \diagup \dfrac{\text{x}}{1.5 \text{ mg}}$

$8 \times 1.5 = 1\text{x}$

$\dfrac{12}{1} = \text{x}$

12 mL = x

Dimensional Analysis Method

$\dfrac{1.5 \text{ mg}}{} \bigg| \dfrac{8 \text{ mL}}{1 \text{ mg}} \bigg| \dfrac{1.5 \times 8}{1} = 12 \text{ mL}$

Use a syringe without the needle to measure the dose.

Formula Method	Proportion Expressed as Two Ratios	Proportion Expressed as Two Fractions

16. $\dfrac{\overset{2}{\cancel{25.0}}\ \text{mg}}{\underset{1}{\cancel{12.5}}\ \text{mg}} \times 5\ \text{mL} = 10\ \text{mL}$

5 mL : 12.5 mg : : x : 25 mg

$\dfrac{5\ \text{mL}}{12.5\ \text{mg}} \times \dfrac{\text{x}}{25\ \text{mg}}$

$$5 \times 25 = 12.5\text{x}$$
$$\frac{125}{12.5} = \text{x}$$
$$10\ \text{mL} = \text{x}$$

Dimensional Analysis Method

$\dfrac{\overset{2}{\cancel{25}}\ \text{mg}}{\underset{1}{\cancel{12.5}}\ \text{mg}} \left|\ 5\ \widehat{\text{mL}}\ \right|\ \dfrac{2 \times 5}{} = 10\ \text{mL}$

Formula Method	Proportion Expressed as Two Ratios	Proportion Expressed as Two Fractions

17. $\dfrac{\overset{3}{\cancel{60}}\ \text{mg}}{\underset{2}{\cancel{40}}\ \text{mg}} \times 0.6\ \text{mL} = \dfrac{1.8}{2} = 0.9\ \text{mL}$

0.6 mL : 40 mg : : x : 60 mg

$\dfrac{0.6\ \text{mL}}{40\ \text{mg}} \times \dfrac{\text{x}}{60\ \text{mg}}$

$$0.6 \times 60 = 40\text{x}$$
$$\frac{36}{40} = \text{x}$$
$$0.9\ \text{mL} = \text{x}$$

Dimensional Analysis Method

$\dfrac{\overset{3}{\cancel{60}}\ \text{mg}}{\underset{2}{\cancel{40}}\ \text{mg}} \left|\ 0.6\ \widehat{\text{mL}}\ \right|\ \dfrac{3 \times 0.6}{2} = 0.9\ \text{mL}$

Formula Method	Proportion Expressed as Two Ratios	Proportion Expressed as Two Fractions

18. 0.5 g = 500 mg

$\dfrac{\overset{2}{\cancel{500}}\ \text{mg}}{\underset{1}{\cancel{250}}\ \text{mg}} \times 5\ \text{mL} = 10\ \text{mL}$

5 mL : 250 mg : : x : 500 mg

$\dfrac{5\ \text{mL}}{250\ \text{mg}} \times \dfrac{\text{x}}{500\ \text{mg}}$

$$500 \times 5 = 250\text{x}$$
$$\frac{2500}{250} = \text{x}$$
$$10\ \text{mL} = \text{x}$$

Dimensional Analysis Method

$0.5\ \cancel{\text{g}} \left|\ 5\ \widehat{\text{mL}}\ \right|\ \dfrac{\overset{4}{\cancel{1000}}\ \text{mg}}{1\ \cancel{\text{g}}} \left|\ \dfrac{0.5 \times 5 \times 4}{} = 10\ \text{mL}\right.$

with denominator $\underset{1}{\cancel{250}}\ \text{mg}$

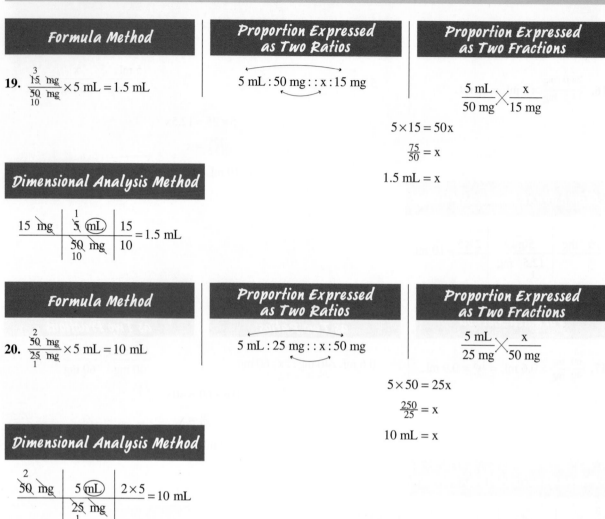

Formula Method	Proportion Expressed as Two Ratios	Proportion Expressed as Two Fractions

19. $\dfrac{\overset{3}{\cancel{15}}\ mg}{\underset{10}{\cancel{50}}\ mg}\times 5\ mL = 1.5\ mL$ 5 mL : 50 mg : : x : 15 mg

$\dfrac{5\ mL}{50\ mg}\times\dfrac{x}{15\ mg}$

$5\times 15 = 50x$

$\dfrac{75}{50} = x$

$1.5\ mL = x$

Dimensional Analysis Method

$\dfrac{15\ \cancel{mg}}{\underset{10}{\cancel{50}}\ \cancel{mg}}\ \Big|\ \dfrac{\overset{1}{\cancel{5}}\ \boxed{mL}}{}\ \Big|\ \dfrac{15}{10} = 1.5\ mL$

Formula Method	Proportion Expressed as Two Ratios	Proportion Expressed as Two Fractions

20. $\dfrac{\overset{2}{\cancel{50}}\ mg}{\underset{1}{\cancel{25}}\ mg}\times 5\ mL = 10\ mL$ 5 mL : 25 mg : : x : 50 mg

$\dfrac{5\ mL}{25\ mg}\times\dfrac{x}{50\ mg}$

$5\times 50 = 25x$

$\dfrac{250}{25} = x$

$10\ mL = x$

Dimensional Analysis Method

$\dfrac{\overset{2}{\cancel{50}}\ \cancel{mg}}{\underset{1}{\cancel{25}}\ \cancel{mg}}\ \Big|\ \dfrac{5\ \boxed{mL}}{}\ \Big|\ 2\times 5 = 10\ mL$

Chapter 7

Test 1: Calculations of Liquid Injections

Formula Method	Proportion Expressed as Two Ratios	Proportion Expressed as Two Fractions

1. Equivalent 0.1 g = 100 mg

$\dfrac{\overset{1}{\cancel{100}}\ mg}{\underset{2}{\cancel{200}}\ mg}\times 3\ mL = \dfrac{3}{2}\overline{)\overset{1.5}{3.0}}$ 3 mL : 200 mg : : x : 100 mg

$\dfrac{3\ mL}{200\ mg}\times\dfrac{x}{100\ mg}$

$3\times 100 = 200x$

$\dfrac{300}{200} = x$

$1.5\ mL = x$

Give 1.5 mL IM.

Dimensional Analysis Method

$\dfrac{0.1\ \cancel{g}}{}\ \Big|\ \dfrac{3\ \boxed{mL}}{200\ \cancel{mg}}\ \Big|\ \dfrac{\overset{5}{\cancel{1000}}\ \cancel{mg}}{1\ \cancel{g}}\ \Big|\ 0.1\times 3\times 5 = 1.5\ mL$

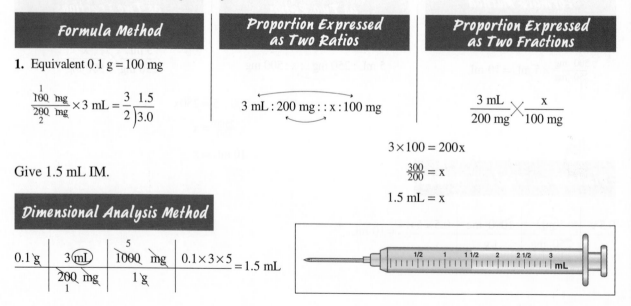

Formula Method	Proportion Expressed as Two Ratios	Proportion Expressed as Two Fractions

2. $\dfrac{\overset{1}{\cancel{5}}\ \text{mg}}{\underset{3}{\cancel{15}}\ \text{mg}} \times 1\ \text{mL} = \dfrac{1}{3}$ $3\overline{)1.000}^{.333}$

$1\ \text{mL} : 15\ \text{mg} :: x : 5\ \text{mg}$

$\dfrac{1\ \text{mL}}{15\ \text{mg}} \times \dfrac{x}{5\ \text{mg}}$

$\dfrac{5}{15} = x$

$0.33\ \text{mL} = x$

Give 0.33 mL IV.

Dimensional Analysis Method

$\dfrac{\overset{1}{\cancel{5}}\ \text{mg}}{} \ \Big|\ \dfrac{1\ \cancel{\text{mL}}}{\underset{3}{\cancel{15}}\ \text{mg}}\ \Big|\ \dfrac{1}{3} = 0.33\ \text{mL}$

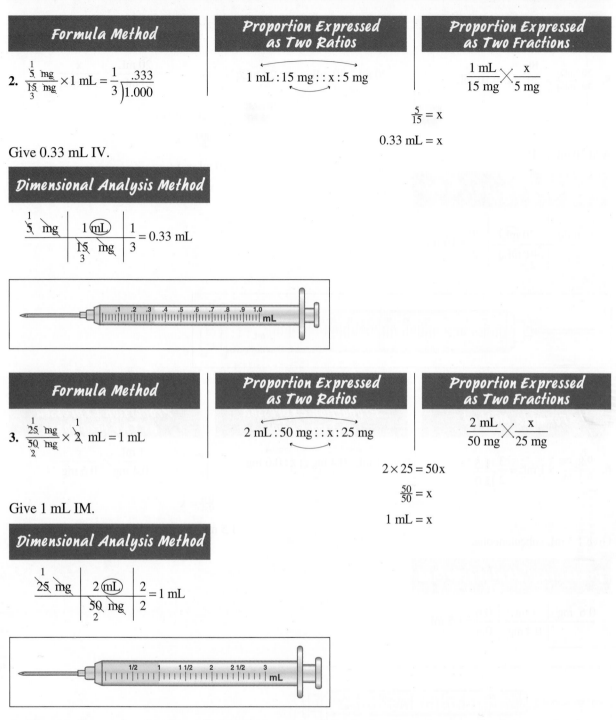

Formula Method	Proportion Expressed as Two Ratios	Proportion Expressed as Two Fractions

3. $\dfrac{\overset{1}{\cancel{25}}\ \text{mg}}{\underset{2}{\cancel{50}}\ \text{mg}} \times \overset{1}{\cancel{2}}\ \text{mL} = 1\ \text{mL}$

$2\ \text{mL} : 50\ \text{mg} :: x : 25\ \text{mg}$

$\dfrac{2\ \text{mL}}{50\ \text{mg}} \times \dfrac{x}{25\ \text{mg}}$

$2 \times 25 = 50x$

$\dfrac{50}{50} = x$

$1\ \text{mL} = x$

Give 1 mL IM.

Dimensional Analysis Method

$\dfrac{\overset{1}{\cancel{25}}\ \text{mg}}{} \ \Big|\ \dfrac{2\ \cancel{\text{mL}}}{\underset{2}{\cancel{50}}\ \text{mg}}\ \Big|\ \dfrac{2}{2} = 1\ \text{mL}$

4. 20 units. Remember that Humulin insulin is a type of regular insulin and so must be drawn up first into the syringe.

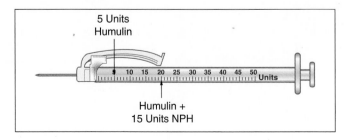

5 Units
Humulin

Humulin +
15 Units NPH

Formula Method	Proportion Expressed as Two Ratios	Proportion Expressed as Two Fractions

5. $\dfrac{\overset{1}{\cancel{20}}\ \text{mEq}}{\underset{2}{\cancel{40}}\ \text{mEq}} \times \overset{10}{\cancel{20}}\ \text{mL} = 10\ \text{mL}$ $\underset{1}{}$

20 mL : 40 mEq :: x : 20 mEq

$\dfrac{20\ \text{mL}}{40\ \text{mEq}} \times \dfrac{\text{x}}{20\ \text{mEq}}$

$20 \times 20 = 40\text{x}$

$\dfrac{400}{40} = \text{x}$

$10\ \text{mL} = \text{x}$

Add 10 mL to IV.

Dimensional Analysis Method

$\dfrac{\overset{1}{\cancel{20}}\ \text{mEq}}{\ }\ \bigg|\ \dfrac{20\ \cancel{\text{mL}}}{\underset{2}{\cancel{40}}\ \text{mEq}}\ \bigg|\ \dfrac{20}{2} = 10\ \text{mL}$

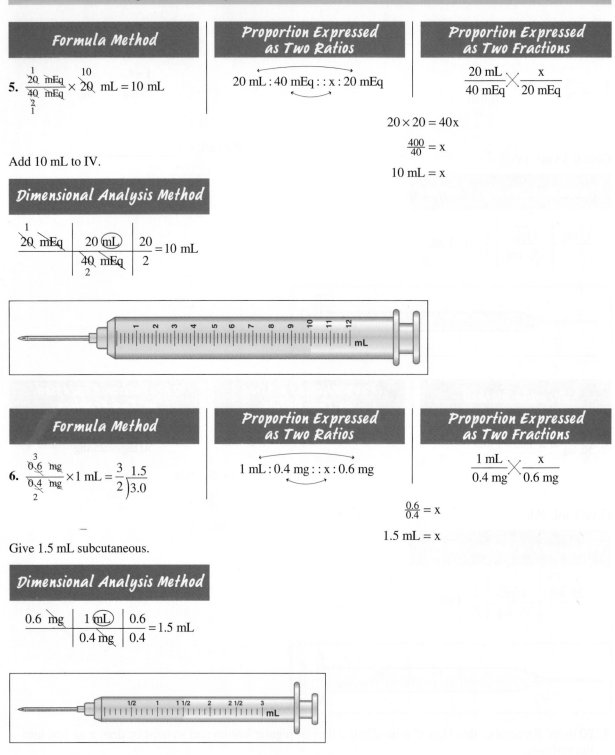

Formula Method	Proportion Expressed as Two Ratios	Proportion Expressed as Two Fractions

6. $\dfrac{\overset{3}{\cancel{0.6}}\ \text{mg}}{\underset{2}{\cancel{0.4}}\ \text{mg}} \times 1\ \text{mL} = \dfrac{3}{2}\overline{\smash{\big)}\,\dfrac{1.5}{3.0}}$

1 mL : 0.4 mg :: x : 0.6 mg

$\dfrac{1\ \text{mL}}{0.4\ \text{mg}} \times \dfrac{\text{x}}{0.6\ \text{mg}}$

$\dfrac{0.6}{0.4} = \text{x}$

$1.5\ \text{mL} = \text{x}$

Give 1.5 mL subcutaneous.

Dimensional Analysis Method

$\dfrac{0.6\ \text{mg}}{\ }\ \bigg|\ \dfrac{1\ \cancel{\text{mL}}}{0.4\ \text{mg}}\ \bigg|\ \dfrac{0.6}{0.4} = 1.5\ \text{mL}$

Formula Method	Proportion Expressed as Two Ratios	Proportion Expressed as Two Fractions
7. $\dfrac{\overset{2}{\cancel{0.8}}\ \text{mg}}{\underset{1}{\cancel{0.4}}\ \text{mg}} \times 1\ \text{mL} = 2\ \text{mL}$	$1\ \text{mL} : 0.4\ \text{mg} :: x : 0.8\ \text{mg}$	$\dfrac{1\ \text{mL}}{0.4\ \text{mg}} \times \dfrac{x}{0.8\ \text{mg}}$ $\dfrac{0.8}{0.4} = x$ $2\ \text{mL} = x$

Give 2 mL IV.

Dimensional Analysis Method

$$\frac{0.8\ \cancel{\text{mg}}}{} \left| \frac{1\ \cancel{\text{mL}}}{0.4\ \cancel{\text{mg}}} \right| \frac{0.8}{0.4} = 2\ \text{mL}$$

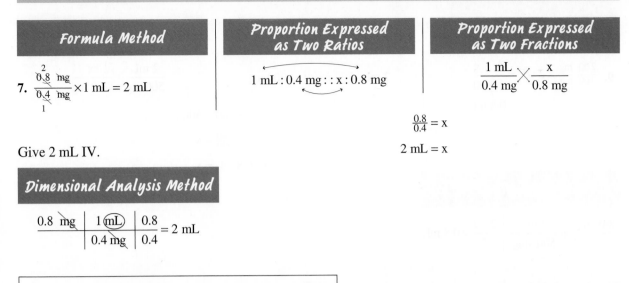

8. Equivalent 0.5 g = 500 mg

Formula Method	Proportion Expressed as Two Ratios	Proportion Expressed as Two Fractions
$\dfrac{\overset{2}{\cancel{500}}\ \text{mg}}{\underset{1}{\cancel{250}}\ \text{mg}} \times 1\ \text{mL} = 2\ \text{mL}$	$1\ \text{mL} : 250\ \text{mg} :: x : 500\ \text{mg}$	$\dfrac{1\ \text{mL}}{250\ \text{mg}} \times \dfrac{x}{500\ \text{mg}}$ $\dfrac{500}{250} = x$ $2\ \text{mL} = x$

Dimensional Analysis Method

$$\frac{0.5\ \cancel{\text{g}}}{} \left| \frac{1\ \cancel{\text{mL}}}{250\ \cancel{\text{mg}}} \right| \frac{\overset{4}{\cancel{1000}}\ \cancel{\text{mg}}}{1\ \cancel{\text{g}}} \right| \frac{0.5 \times 4}{} = 2\ \text{mL}$$

Add 2 mL to IV.

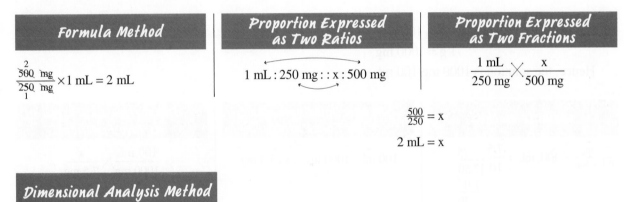

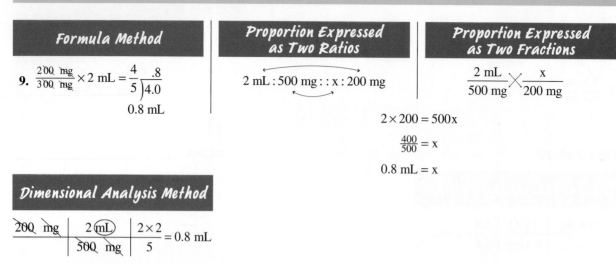

Formula Method	Proportion Expressed as Two Ratios	Proportion Expressed as Two Fractions
9. $\frac{200 \text{ mg}}{300 \text{ mg}} \times 2 \text{ mL} = \frac{4}{5} \frac{.8}{)4.0}$ 0.8 mL	2 mL : 500 mg : : x : 200 mg	$\frac{2 \text{ mL}}{500 \text{ mg}} \times \frac{x}{200 \text{ mg}}$

$$2 \times 200 = 500x$$
$$\frac{400}{500} = x$$
$$0.8 \text{ mL} = x$$

Dimensional Analysis Method

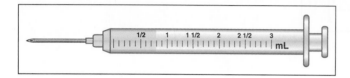

$$\frac{200 \text{ mg}}{} \left| \frac{2 \text{ mL}}{500 \text{ mg}} \right| \frac{2 \times 2}{5} = 0.8 \text{ mL}$$

Give 0.8 mL IM.

10. Equivalent 1:100 means 1 g in 100 mL

$$1 \text{ g} = 1000 \text{ mg}$$

Hence, the solution is 1000 mg/100 mL.

Formula Method	Proportion Expressed as Two Ratios	Proportion Expressed as Two Fractions
$\frac{7.5 \text{ mg}}{1000 \text{ mg}} \times 100 \text{ mL} = \frac{7.5}{10} \frac{.75}{)7.50}$ $\frac{7\ 0}{50}$ $\frac{50}{}$ 0.75 or 0.8 mL	100 mL : 1000 mg : : x : 7.5 mg	$\frac{100 \text{ mL}}{1000 \text{ mg}} \times \frac{x}{7.5 \text{ mg}}$

$$100 \times 7.5 = 1000x$$
$$\frac{7500}{1000} = x$$
$$0.75 \text{ or } 0.8 \text{ mL} = x$$

Dimensional Analysis Method

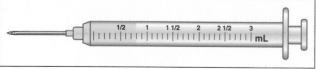

$$7.5 \text{ mg} \left| \frac{\overset{1}{100} \text{ mL}}{1 \text{ g}} \right| \frac{1 \text{ g}}{\underset{10}{1000} \text{ mg}} \left| \frac{7.5}{10} \right. = 0.75 \text{ or } 0.8 \text{ mL}$$

Give 0.8 mL subcutaneous.

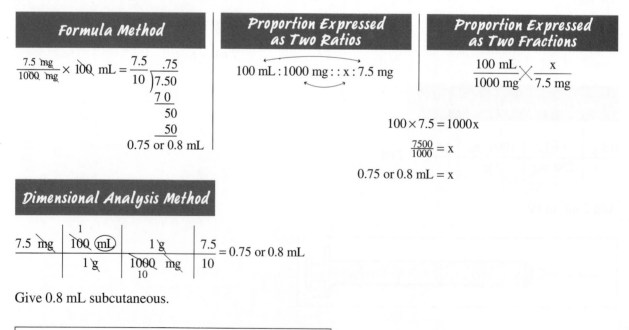

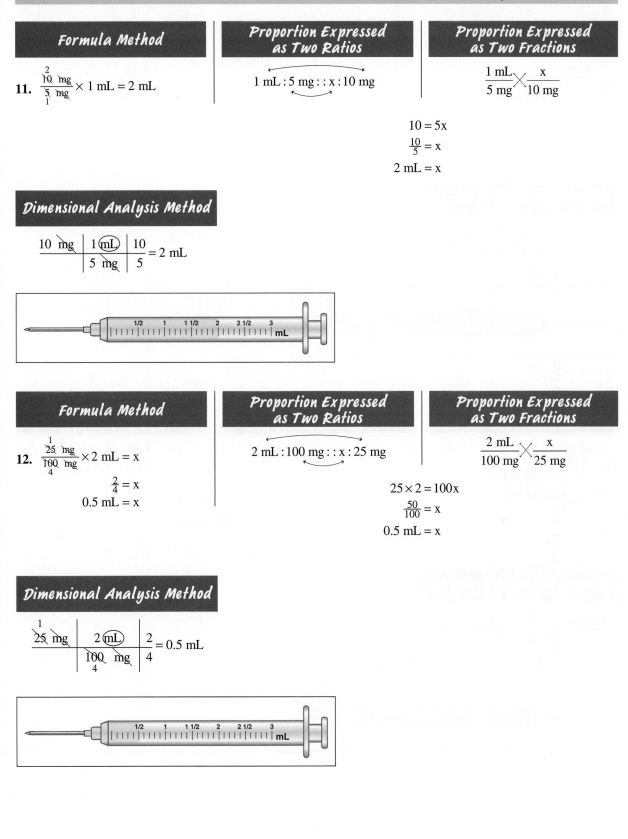

Formula Method	Proportion Expressed as Two Ratios	Proportion Expressed as Two Fractions

11. $\dfrac{\overset{2}{\cancel{10}} \text{ mg}}{\underset{1}{\cancel{5}} \text{ mg}} \times 1 \text{ mL} = 2 \text{ mL}$

1 mL : 5 mg : : x : 10 mg

$\dfrac{1 \text{ mL}}{5 \text{ mg}} \diagtimes \dfrac{x}{10 \text{ mg}}$

$$10 = 5x$$
$$\frac{10}{5} = x$$
$$2 \text{ mL} = x$$

Dimensional Analysis Method

$\dfrac{10 \text{ mg}}{} \ \left|\ \dfrac{1 \text{ mL}}{5 \text{ mg}}\ \right|\ \dfrac{10}{5} = 2 \text{ mL}$

Formula Method	Proportion Expressed as Two Ratios	Proportion Expressed as Two Fractions

12. $\dfrac{\overset{1}{\cancel{25}} \text{ mg}}{\underset{4}{\cancel{100}} \text{ mg}} \times 2 \text{ mL} = x$

$$\frac{2}{4} = x$$
$$0.5 \text{ mL} = x$$

2 mL : 100 mg : : x : 25 mg

$\dfrac{2 \text{ mL}}{100 \text{ mg}} \diagtimes \dfrac{x}{25 \text{ mg}}$

$$25 \times 2 = 100x$$
$$\frac{50}{100} = x$$
$$0.5 \text{ mL} = x$$

Dimensional Analysis Method

$\dfrac{\overset{1}{\cancel{25}} \text{ mg}}{} \ \left|\ \dfrac{2 \text{ mL}}{\underset{4}{\cancel{100}} \text{ mg}}\ \right|\ \dfrac{2}{4} = 0.5 \text{ mL}$

Formula Method	Proportion Expressed as Two Ratios	Proportion Expressed as Two Fractions
13. $\dfrac{50 \text{ mg}}{25 \text{ mg}} \times 1 \text{ mL} = x$ $2 \text{ mL} = x$	$1 \text{ mL} : 25 \text{ mg} :: x : 50 \text{ mg}$	$\dfrac{1 \text{ mL}}{25 \text{ mg}} \times \dfrac{x}{50 \text{ mg}}$

$$\frac{50}{25} = x$$
$$2 \text{ mL} = x$$

Dimensional Analysis Method

$$\frac{50 \text{ mg}}{\,} \left|\, \frac{1 \text{ mL}}{25 \text{ mg}} \,\right| \frac{50}{25} = 2 \text{ mL}$$

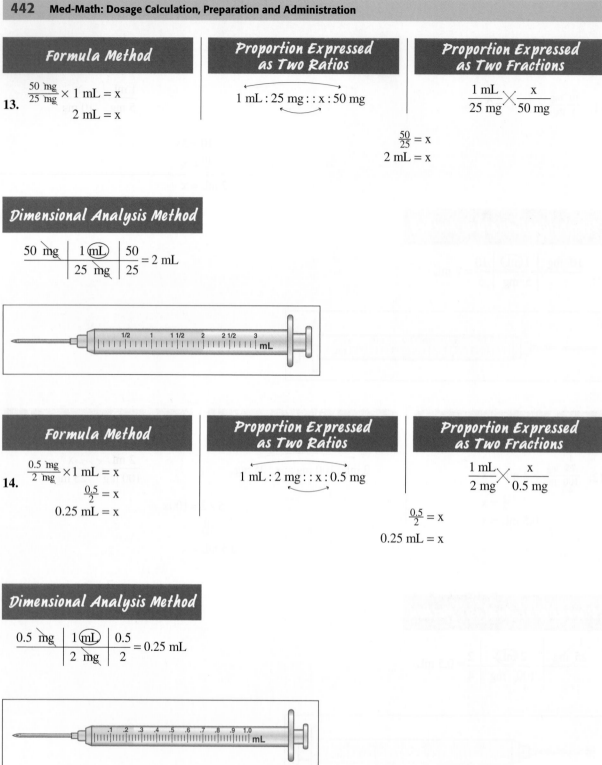

Formula Method	Proportion Expressed as Two Ratios	Proportion Expressed as Two Fractions
14. $\dfrac{0.5 \text{ mg}}{2 \text{ mg}} \times 1 \text{ mL} = x$ $\dfrac{0.5}{2} = x$ $0.25 \text{ mL} = x$	$1 \text{ mL} : 2 \text{ mg} :: x : 0.5 \text{ mg}$	$\dfrac{1 \text{ mL}}{2 \text{ mg}} \times \dfrac{x}{0.5 \text{ mg}}$

$$\frac{0.5}{2} = x$$
$$0.25 \text{ mL} = x$$

Dimensional Analysis Method

$$\frac{0.5 \text{ mg}}{\,} \left|\, \frac{1 \text{ mL}}{2 \text{ mg}} \,\right| \frac{0.5}{2} = 0.25 \text{ mL}$$

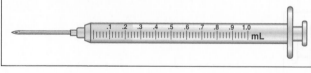

15. Equivalent 0:2 Gm = 200 mg

Formula Method	Proportion Expressed as Two Ratios	Proportion Expressed as Two Fractions

$$\frac{\overset{1}{\cancel{200}}\ \cancel{mg}}{\underset{1}{\cancel{200}}\ \cancel{mg}} \times 2\ mL = x$$

$$2\ mL = x$$

2 mL : 200 mg : : x : 200 mg

$$\frac{2\ mL}{200\ mg} \times \frac{x}{200\ mg}$$

$$2 \times 200 = 200x$$
$$400 = 200x$$
$$\frac{400}{200} = x$$
$$2\ mL = x$$

Dimensional Analysis Method

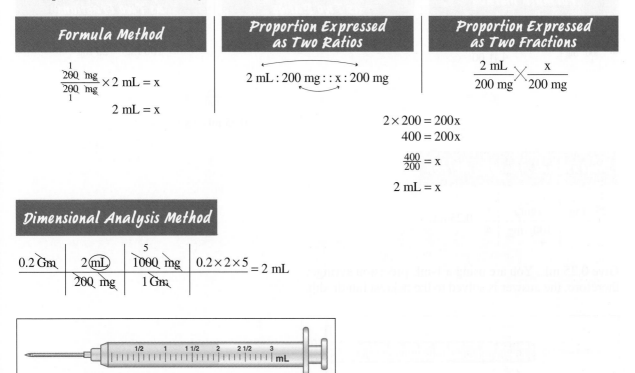

$$\frac{0.2\ \cancel{Gm}}{} \left|\ \frac{2\ \textcircled{mL}}{200\ \cancel{mg}}\ \right|\ \frac{\overset{5}{\cancel{1000}}\ \cancel{mg}}{1\ \cancel{Gm}}\ \right|\ 0.2 \times 2 \times 5 = 2\ mL$$

Test 2: Calculations of Liquid Injections

Formula Method	Proportion Expressed as Two Ratios	Proportion Expressed as Two Fractions

1. $\dfrac{\overset{2}{\cancel{10}}\ \cancel{mg}}{\underset{3}{\cancel{15}}\ \cancel{mg}} \times 1\ mL = \dfrac{2}{3}\ \overset{0.66}{\overline{)2.00}}$

0.66 mL 0.7 mL

1 mL : 15 mg : : x : 10 mg

$$\frac{1\ mL}{15\ mg} \times \frac{x}{10\ mg}$$

$$\frac{10}{15} = x$$

0.66 or 0.7 mL = x

Dimensional Analysis Method

$$\frac{10\ \cancel{mg}}{}\ \left|\ \frac{1\ \textcircled{mL}}{15\ \cancel{mg}}\ \right|\ \frac{10}{15} = 0.66\ or\ 0.7\ mL$$

Give 0.7 mL IV.

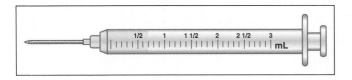

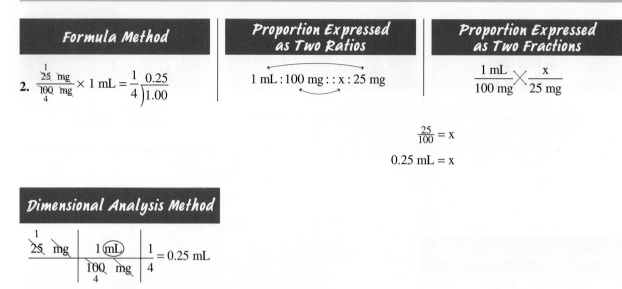

$$\frac{\overset{1}{\cancel{25}} \text{ mg}}{\underset{4}{\cancel{100}} \text{ mg}} \times 1 \text{ mL} = \frac{1}{4} \overline{)\, \frac{0.25}{1.00}}$$

$$1 \text{ mL} : 100 \text{ mg} :: x : 25 \text{ mg}$$

$$\frac{1 \text{ mL}}{100 \text{ mg}} \times \frac{x}{25 \text{ mg}}$$

$$\frac{25}{100} = x$$

$$0.25 \text{ mL} = x$$

Dimensional Analysis Method

$$\frac{\overset{1}{\cancel{25}} \text{ mg}}{\underset{4}{\cancel{100}} \text{ mg}} \,\bigg|\, \frac{1 \,\text{(mL)}}{} \,\bigg|\, \frac{1}{4} = 0.25 \text{ mL}$$

Give 0.25 mL. You are using a 1-mL precision syringe; therefore, the answer is solved to the nearest hundredth.

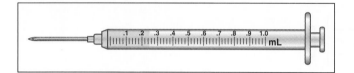

3. Equivalent 0.1 g = 100 mg

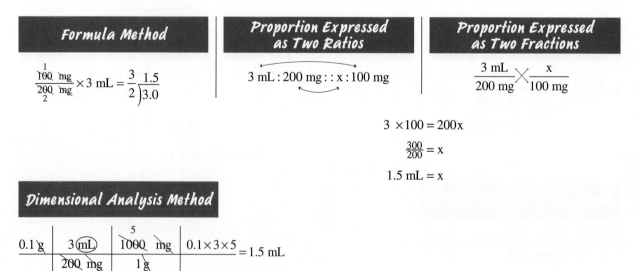

$$\frac{\overset{1}{\cancel{100}} \text{ mg}}{\underset{2}{\cancel{200}} \text{ mg}} \times 3 \text{ mL} = \frac{3}{2} \overline{)\, \frac{1.5}{3.0}}$$

$$3 \text{ mL} : 200 \text{ mg} :: x : 100 \text{ mg}$$

$$\frac{3 \text{ mL}}{200 \text{ mg}} \times \frac{x}{100 \text{ mg}}$$

$$3 \times 100 = 200x$$

$$\frac{300}{200} = x$$

$$1.5 \text{ mL} = x$$

Dimensional Analysis Method

$$0.1 \,\cancel{g} \,\bigg|\, 3 \,\text{(mL)} \,\bigg|\, \frac{\overset{5}{\cancel{1000}} \text{ mg}}{1 \,\cancel{g}} \,\bigg|\, \frac{0.1 \times 3 \times 5}{} = 1.5 \text{ mL}$$

Give 1.5 mL IM.

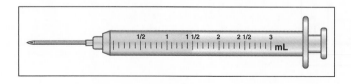

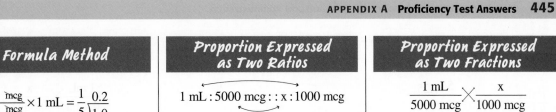

4. $\dfrac{\overset{1}{\cancel{1000}}\ \cancel{mcg}}{\underset{5}{\cancel{5000}}\ \cancel{mcg}} \times 1\ mL = \dfrac{1}{5} \overset{0.2}{\overline{\smash{)}1.0}}$

1 mL : 5000 mcg :: x : 1000 mcg

$$\dfrac{1\ mL}{5000\ mcg} \times \dfrac{x}{1000\ mcg}$$

$$\dfrac{1000}{5000} = x$$

$$0.2\ mL = x$$

Dimensional Analysis Method

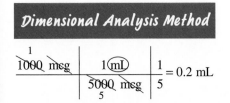

$\dfrac{\overset{1}{\cancel{1000}}\ \cancel{mcg}}{} \left|\ \dfrac{1\ \boxed{mL}}{\underset{5}{\cancel{5000}}\ \cancel{mcg}}\ \right|\ \dfrac{1}{5} = 0.2\ mL$

Give 0.2 mL IM.

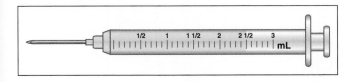

5. Equivalent 1% means 1 g in 100 mL

$$1\ g = 1000\ mg$$

Hence, the solution is 1000 mg in 100 mL.

Formula Method

$\dfrac{\overset{5}{\cancel{25}}\ \cancel{mg}}{\underset{\underset{2}{10}}{\cancel{1000}}\ \cancel{mg}} \times \overset{1}{\cancel{100}}\ mL = \dfrac{5}{2} \overset{2.5}{\overline{\smash{)}5.0}}$

Proportion Expressed as Two Ratios

100 mL : 1000 mg :: x : 25 mg

Proportion Expressed as Two Fractions

$$\dfrac{100\ mL}{1000\ mg} \times \dfrac{x}{25\ mg}$$

$$100 \times 25 = 1000x$$

$$\dfrac{2500}{1000} = x$$

$$2.5\ mL = x$$

Dimensional Analysis Method

$\dfrac{25\ \cancel{mg}}{}\ \left|\ \dfrac{\overset{1}{\cancel{100}}\ \boxed{mL}}{\cancel{1}\ \cancel{g}}\ \right|\ \dfrac{\cancel{1}\ \cancel{g}}{\underset{10}{\cancel{1000}}\ \cancel{mg}}\ \right|\ \dfrac{25}{10} = 2.5\ mL$

Prepare 2.5 mL.

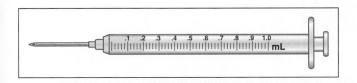

Formula Method	Proportion Expressed as Two Ratios	Proportion Expressed as Two Fractions
6. $\frac{0.5\,mg}{0.4\,mg} \times 1\,mL = \frac{1.25}{4\overline{)5.00}}$ $\quad\quad 1.25$ or 1.3 mL	$1\,mL : 0.4\,mg :: x : 0.5\,mg$	$\frac{1\,mL}{0.4\,mg} \times \frac{x}{0.5\,mg}$

$$\frac{0.5\,mg}{0.4\,mg} = x$$

$$1.25 \text{ or } 1.3 \text{ mL} = x$$

Dimensional Analysis Method

$$\frac{0.5\ \cancel{mg}}{} \left| \frac{1\ \cancel{mL}}{0.4\ \cancel{mg}} \right| \frac{0.5}{0.4} = 1.25 \text{ or } 1.3 \text{ mL}$$

Give 1.3 mL subcutaneous.

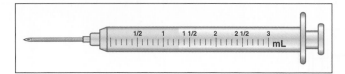

7. 13 units. Humulin insulin is a type of regular insulin and so must be drawn up first into the syringe.

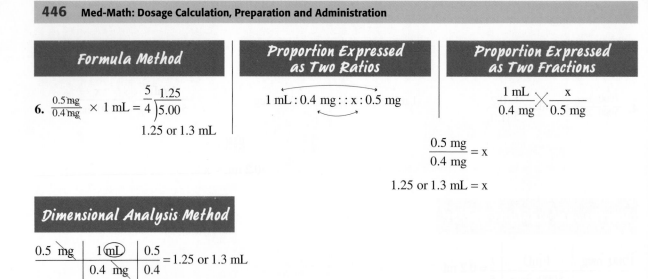

Formula Method	Proportion Expressed as Two Ratios	Proportion Expressed as Two Fractions
8. $\frac{1.2\,mEq}{0.5\,mEq} \times 1\,mL = \frac{2.4}{0.5\overline{)1.20}}$	$1\,mL : 0.5\,mEq :: x : 1.2\,mEq$	$\frac{1\,mL}{0.5\,mEq} \times \frac{x}{1.2\,mEq}$

$$\frac{1.2}{0.5} = x$$

$$2.4 \text{ mL} = x$$

Dimensional Analysis Method

$$\frac{1.2\ \cancel{mEq}}{} \left| \frac{1\ \cancel{mL}}{0.5\ \cancel{mEq}} \right| \frac{1.2}{0.5} = 2.4 \text{ mL}$$

Add 2.4 mL to the IV stat.

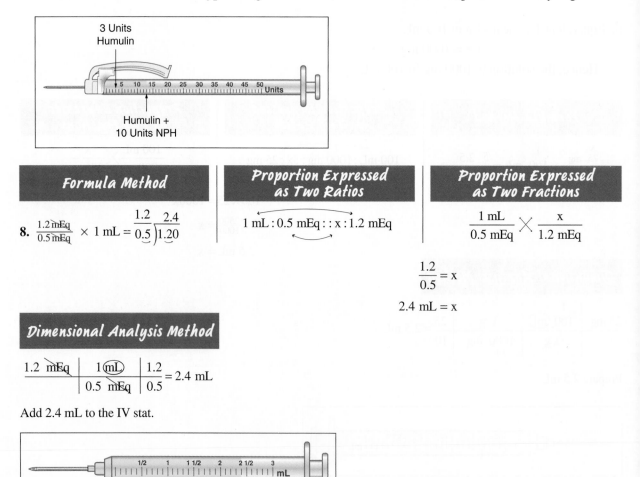

Formula Method	Proportion Expressed as Two Ratios	Proportion Expressed as Two Fractions

$$9.\quad \frac{\overset{3}{\cancel{75\ mg}}}{\underset{2}{\cancel{50\ mg}}} \times 1\ mL = \frac{3}{2} \overset{1.5}{\big)3.0}$$

1 mL : 50 mg : : x : 75 mg

$$\frac{1\ mL}{50\ mg} \times \frac{x}{75\ mg}$$

$$\frac{75}{50} = x$$

$$1.5\ mL = x$$

Dimensional Analysis Method

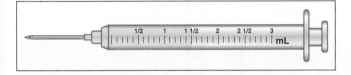

$$\frac{1}{\cancel{75}\ mg} \left| \frac{1\ \textcircled{mL}}{\underset{2}{\cancel{50}\ mg}} \right| \frac{3}{2} = 1.5\ mL$$

Give 1.5 mL IM.

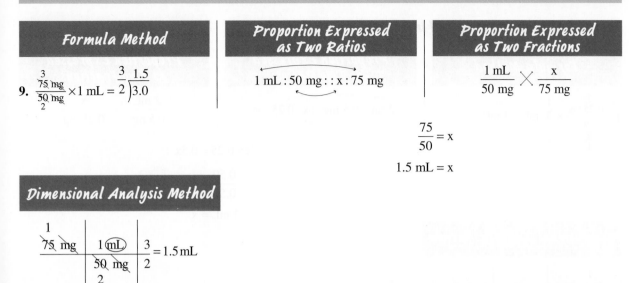

10. Equivalent 1:1000 means 1 g in 1000 mL

$$1\ g = 1000\ mg$$

Hence, the solution is 1000 mg in 1000 mL.

$$500\ mcg = 0.5\ mg$$

Formula Method	Proportion Expressed as Two Ratios	Proportion Expressed as Two Fractions

$$\frac{0.5\ mg}{\cancel{1000}\ mg} \times \overset{1}{\cancel{1000}}\ mL = 0.5\ mL$$

1000 mL : 1000 mg : : x : 0.5 mg

$$\frac{1000\ mL}{\underset{1}{\cancel{1000}\ mg}} \times \frac{x}{0.5\ mg}$$

$$1000 \times 0.5\ mg = 1000x$$

$$\frac{500}{1000} = x$$

$$0.5\ mL = x$$

Dimensional Analysis Method

$$\frac{1}{\cancel{500}\ mcg} \left| \frac{1000\ \textcircled{mL}}{1\ \cancel{g}} \right| \frac{1\ \cancel{g}}{\cancel{1000}\ mg} \left| \frac{1\ \cancel{mg}}{\underset{2}{\cancel{1000}\ \cancel{mcg}}} \right| \frac{1}{2} = 0.5\ mL$$

Give 0.5 mL subcutaneous stat.

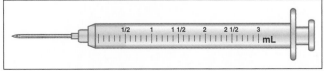

Test 3: Calculations of Liquid Injections

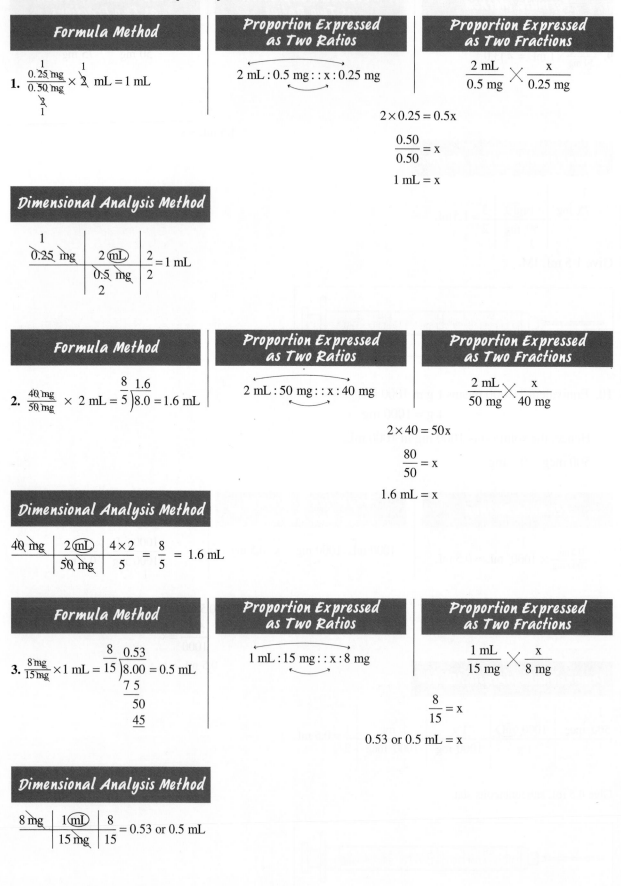

Formula Method

1. $\dfrac{\overset{1}{0.25\ mg}}{\underset{2}{0.50\ mg}} \times \overset{1}{\underset{1}{2}}\ mL = 1\ mL$

Proportion Expressed as Two Ratios

2 mL : 0.5 mg : : x : 0.25 mg

Proportion Expressed as Two Fractions

$\dfrac{2\ mL}{0.5\ mg} \times \dfrac{x}{0.25\ mg}$

$2 \times 0.25 = 0.5x$

$\dfrac{0.50}{0.50} = x$

$1\ mL = x$

Dimensional Analysis Method

$\dfrac{\overset{1}{0.25\ mg}}{} \Bigg| \dfrac{2\ mL}{0.5\ mg} \Bigg| \dfrac{2}{2} = 1\ mL$

Formula Method

2. $\dfrac{40\ mg}{50\ mg} \times 2\ mL = \overset{8}{5}\overset{1.6}{\overline{)8.0}} = 1.6\ mL$

Proportion Expressed as Two Ratios

2 mL : 50 mg : : x : 40 mg

Proportion Expressed as Two Fractions

$\dfrac{2\ mL}{50\ mg} \times \dfrac{x}{40\ mg}$

$2 \times 40 = 50x$

$\dfrac{80}{50} = x$

$1.6\ mL = x$

Dimensional Analysis Method

$\dfrac{40\ mg}{} \Bigg| \dfrac{2\ mL}{50\ mg} \Bigg| \dfrac{4 \times 2}{5} = \dfrac{8}{5} = 1.6\ mL$

Formula Method

3. $\dfrac{8\ mg}{15\ mg} \times 1\ mL = \overset{8}{15}\overset{0.53}{\overline{)8.00}} = 0.5\ mL$

$\underline{7\ 5}$

50

$\underline{45}$

Proportion Expressed as Two Ratios

1 mL : 15 mg : : x : 8 mg

Proportion Expressed as Two Fractions

$\dfrac{1\ mL}{15\ mg} \times \dfrac{x}{8\ mg}$

$\dfrac{8}{15} = x$

0.53 or 0.5 mL = x

Dimensional Analysis Method

$\dfrac{8\ mg}{} \Bigg| \dfrac{1\ mL}{15\ mg} \Bigg| \dfrac{8}{15} = 0.53\ or\ 0.5\ mL$

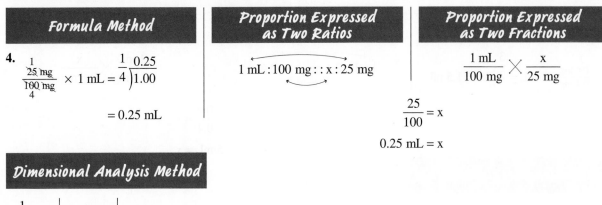

Formula Method	Proportion Expressed as Two Ratios	Proportion Expressed as Two Fractions

4.

$$\dfrac{\overset{1}{\cancel{25\text{ mg}}}}{\underset{4}{\cancel{100\text{ mg}}}} \times 1\text{ mL} = \dfrac{1}{4}\!\!\begin{array}{r}0.25\\ \overline{)1.00}\end{array}$$

$$= 0.25\text{ mL}$$

1 mL : 100 mg : : x : 25 mg

$$\dfrac{1\text{ mL}}{100\text{ mg}} \times \dfrac{x}{25\text{ mg}}$$

$$\dfrac{25}{100} = x$$

$$0.25\text{ mL} = x$$

Dimensional Analysis Method

$$\dfrac{\overset{1}{\cancel{25\text{ mg}}}}{} \;\bigg|\; \dfrac{1\;\textcircled{mL}}{\underset{4}{\cancel{100\text{ mg}}}} \;\bigg|\; \dfrac{1}{4} \;=\; 0.25\text{ mL}$$

Use the 1-mL precision syringe.

Formula Method	Proportion Expressed as Two Ratios	Proportion Expressed as Two Fractions

5.

$$\dfrac{200\text{ mg}}{500\text{ mg}} \times 2\text{ mL} \quad \dfrac{4}{5}\!\!\begin{array}{r}0.8\\ \overline{)4.0}\end{array} = 0.8\text{ mL}$$

2 mL : 500 mg : : x : 200 mg

$$\dfrac{2\text{ mL}}{500\text{ mg}} \times \dfrac{x}{200\text{ mg}}$$

$$2 \times 200 = 500x$$

$$\dfrac{400}{500} = x$$

$$0.8\text{ mL} = x$$

Dimensional Analysis Method

$$\dfrac{200\text{ mg}}{} \;\bigg|\; \dfrac{2\;\textcircled{mL}}{500\text{ mg}} \;\bigg|\; \dfrac{2 \times 2}{5} \;=\; \dfrac{4}{5} \;=\; 0.8\text{ mL}$$

Formula Method	Proportion Expressed as Two Ratios	Proportion Expressed as Two Fractions

6.

$$\dfrac{\overset{3}{\cancel{1500\text{ mcg}}}}{\underset{10}{\cancel{5000\text{ mcg}}}} \times 1\text{ mL} = \dfrac{3}{10}\!\!\begin{array}{r}0.3\\ \overline{)3.0}\end{array}$$

$$= 0.3\text{ mL}$$

1 mL : 5000 mcg : : x : 1500 mcg

$$\dfrac{1\text{ mL}}{5000\text{ mcg}} \times \dfrac{x}{1500\text{ mcg}}$$

$$\dfrac{1500}{5000} = x$$

$$0.3\text{ mL} = x$$

Dimensional Analysis Method

$$\dfrac{\overset{3}{\cancel{1500\text{ mcg}}}}{} \;\bigg|\; \dfrac{1\;\textcircled{mL}}{\underset{10}{\cancel{5000\text{ mcg}}}} \;\bigg|\; \dfrac{3}{10} = 0.3\text{ mL}$$

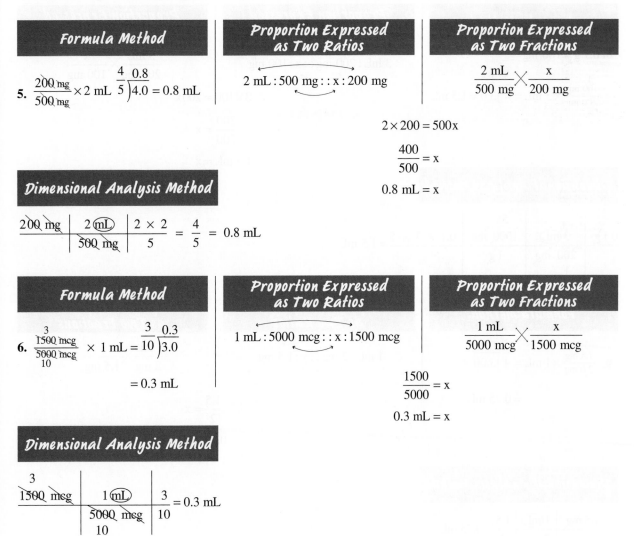

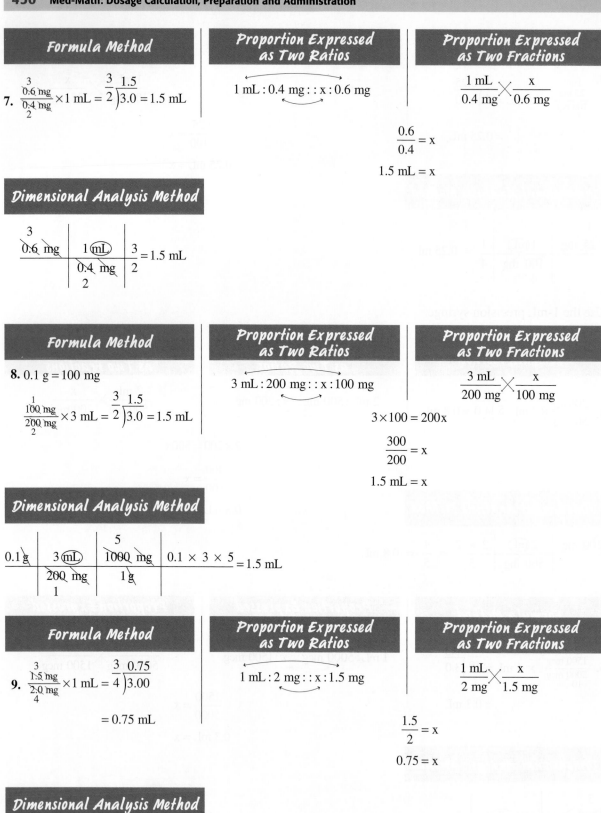

Formula Method	Proportion Expressed as Two Ratios	Proportion Expressed as Two Fractions

7. $\dfrac{\overset{3}{0.6\ \text{mg}}}{\underset{2}{0.4\ \text{mg}}} \times 1\ \text{mL} = \dfrac{3}{2} \overline{)3.0}^{\,1.5} = 1.5\ \text{mL}$

1 mL : 0.4 mg : : x : 0.6 mg

$\dfrac{1\ \text{mL}}{0.4\ \text{mg}} \times \dfrac{x}{0.6\ \text{mg}}$

$$\dfrac{0.6}{0.4} = x$$

$$1.5\ \text{mL} = x$$

Dimensional Analysis Method

$\dfrac{\overset{3}{0.6\ \text{mg}}}{} \left| \dfrac{1\ \text{mL}}{\underset{2}{0.4\ \text{mg}}} \right| \dfrac{3}{2} = 1.5\ \text{mL}$

Formula Method	Proportion Expressed as Two Ratios	Proportion Expressed as Two Fractions

8. 0.1 g = 100 mg

$\dfrac{\overset{1}{100\ \text{mg}}}{\underset{2}{200\ \text{mg}}} \times 3\ \text{mL} = \dfrac{3}{2} \overline{)3.0}^{\,1.5} = 1.5\ \text{mL}$

3 mL : 200 mg : : x : 100 mg

$\dfrac{3\ \text{mL}}{200\ \text{mg}} \times \dfrac{x}{100\ \text{mg}}$

$$3 \times 100 = 200x$$

$$\dfrac{300}{200} = x$$

$$1.5\ \text{mL} = x$$

Dimensional Analysis Method

$\dfrac{0.1\ \text{g}}{} \left| \dfrac{3\ \text{mL}}{\underset{1}{200\ \text{mg}}} \right| \dfrac{\overset{5}{1000\ \text{mg}}}{1\ \text{g}} \left| \dfrac{0.1 \times 3 \times 5}{} = 1.5\ \text{mL} \right.$

Formula Method	Proportion Expressed as Two Ratios	Proportion Expressed as Two Fractions

9. $\dfrac{\overset{3}{1.5\ \text{mg}}}{\underset{4}{2.0\ \text{mg}}} \times 1\ \text{mL} = \dfrac{3}{4} \overline{)3.00}^{\,0.75}$

$= 0.75\ \text{mL}$

1 mL : 2 mg : : x : 1.5 mg

$\dfrac{1\ \text{mL}}{2\ \text{mg}} \times \dfrac{x}{1.5\ \text{mg}}$

$$\dfrac{1.5}{2} = x$$

$$0.75 = x$$

Dimensional Analysis Method

$\dfrac{1.5\ \text{mg}}{} \left| \dfrac{1\ \text{mL}}{2\ \text{mg}} \right| \dfrac{1.5}{2} = 0.75\ \text{mL}$

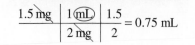

Use a 1-mL precision syringe.

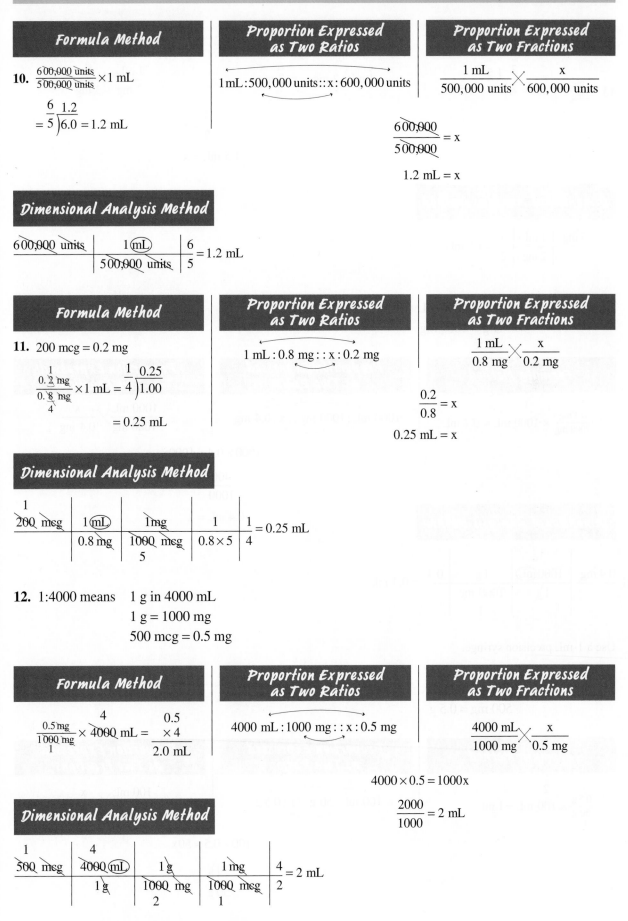

Formula Method

10. $\dfrac{600{,}000 \text{ units}}{500{,}000 \text{ units}} \times 1 \text{ mL}$

$= \dfrac{6}{5}\overset{1.2}{\overline{)6.0}} = 1.2 \text{ mL}$

Proportion Expressed as Two Ratios

$1 \text{ mL} : 500{,}000 \text{ units} :: x : 600{,}000 \text{ units}$

Proportion Expressed as Two Fractions

$\dfrac{1 \text{ mL}}{500{,}000 \text{ units}} \times \dfrac{x}{600{,}000 \text{ units}}$

$\dfrac{600{,}000}{500{,}000} = x$

$1.2 \text{ mL} = x$

Dimensional Analysis Method

$\dfrac{600{,}000 \text{ units}}{} \ \bigg|\ \dfrac{1 \text{ mL}}{500{,}000 \text{ units}} \ \bigg|\ \dfrac{6}{5} = 1.2 \text{ mL}$

Formula Method

11. $200 \text{ mcg} = 0.2 \text{ mg}$

$\dfrac{\overset{1}{0.2} \text{ mg}}{\underset{4}{0.8} \text{ mg}} \times 1 \text{ mL} = \dfrac{1}{4}\overset{0.25}{\overline{)1.00}}$

$= 0.25 \text{ mL}$

Proportion Expressed as Two Ratios

$1 \text{ mL} : 0.8 \text{ mg} :: x : 0.2 \text{ mg}$

Proportion Expressed as Two Fractions

$\dfrac{1 \text{ mL}}{0.8 \text{ mg}} \times \dfrac{x}{0.2 \text{ mg}}$

$\dfrac{0.2}{0.8} = x$

$0.25 \text{ mL} = x$

Dimensional Analysis Method

$\dfrac{\overset{1}{200} \text{ mcg}}{} \ \bigg|\ \dfrac{1 \text{ mL}}{0.8 \text{ mg}} \ \bigg|\ \dfrac{1 \text{ mg}}{1000 \text{ mcg}} \ \bigg|\ \dfrac{1}{0.8 \times 5} \ \bigg|\ \dfrac{1}{4} = 0.25 \text{ mL}$

12. 1:4000 means 1 g in 4000 mL

1 g = 1000 mg

500 mcg = 0.5 mg

Formula Method

$\dfrac{0.5 \text{ mg}}{\underset{1}{1000} \text{ mg}} \times \overset{4}{4000} \text{ mL} = \dfrac{\begin{array}{c} 0.5 \\ \times 4 \end{array}}{2.0 \text{ mL}}$

Proportion Expressed as Two Ratios

$4000 \text{ mL} : 1000 \text{ mg} :: x : 0.5 \text{ mg}$

Proportion Expressed as Two Fractions

$\dfrac{4000 \text{ mL}}{1000 \text{ mg}} \times \dfrac{x}{0.5 \text{ mg}}$

$4000 \times 0.5 = 1000x$

$\dfrac{2000}{1000} = 2 \text{ mL}$

Dimensional Analysis Method

$\dfrac{1}{500 \text{ mcg}} \ \bigg|\ \dfrac{\overset{4}{4000} \text{ mL}}{1 \text{ g}} \ \bigg|\ \dfrac{1 \text{ g}}{\underset{2}{1000} \text{ mg}} \ \bigg|\ \dfrac{1 \text{ mg}}{\underset{1}{1000} \text{ mcg}} \ \bigg|\ \dfrac{4}{2} = 2 \text{ mL}$

Formula Method	Proportion Expressed as Two Ratios	Proportion Expressed as Two Fractions
13. $\dfrac{3\,mg}{2\,mg} \times 1\ mL = \dfrac{\overset{3}{2\overline{)3.0}}^{1.5}}{} = 1.5\ mL$	$1\ mL : 2\ mg :: x : 3\ mg$	$\dfrac{1\ mL}{2\ mg} \times \dfrac{x}{3\ mg}$

$$\frac{3}{2} = x$$

$$1.5\ mL = x$$

Dimensional Analysis Method

$$\frac{3\ mg}{} \left| \frac{1\ \widehat{mL}}{2\ mg} \right| \frac{3}{2} = 1.5\ mL$$

14. 1:1000 means   1 g = 1000 mL

1 g = 1000 mg

Formula Method	Proportion Expressed as Two Ratios	Proportion Expressed as Two Fractions
$\dfrac{0.4\,mg}{1000\,mg} \times \overset{1}{1000}\ mL = 0.4\ mL$	$1000\ mL : 1000\ mg :: x : 0.4\ mg$	$\dfrac{1000\ mL}{1000\ mg} \times \dfrac{x}{0.4\ mg}$

$$1000 \times 0.4 = 1000x$$

$$\frac{400}{1000} = x$$

$$0.4\ mL = x$$

Dimensional Analysis Method

$$0.4\ mg \left| \frac{\overset{1}{1000}\ \widehat{mL}}{1\ g} \right| \frac{1\ g}{\underset{1}{1000}\ mg} \left| 0.4 \right. = 0.4\ mL$$

Use a 1-mL precision syringe.

15. 50% means   50 g in 100 mL

500 mg = 0.5 g

Formula Method	Proportion Expressed as Two Ratios	Proportion Expressed as Two Fractions
$\dfrac{0.5\,g}{\underset{1}{50\,g}} \times \overset{2}{100}\ mL = 1\ mL$	$100\ mL : 50\ g :: x : 0.5\ g$	$\dfrac{100\ mL}{50\ g} \times \dfrac{x}{0.5\ g}$

$$100 \times 0.5 = 50x$$

$$\frac{50\ g}{50\ g} = x$$

Dimensional Analysis Method

$$\dfrac{1}{\cancel{500}\ \cancel{mg}}\ \Bigg|\ \dfrac{\overset{2}{\cancel{100}}\ \cancel{\textcircled{mL}}}{\underset{1}{\cancel{50}}\ \cancel{g}}\ \Bigg|\ \dfrac{1\ \cancel{g}}{\underset{2}{\cancel{1000}}\ \cancel{mg}}\ \Bigg|\ \dfrac{2}{2}\ =1\ \text{mL}$$

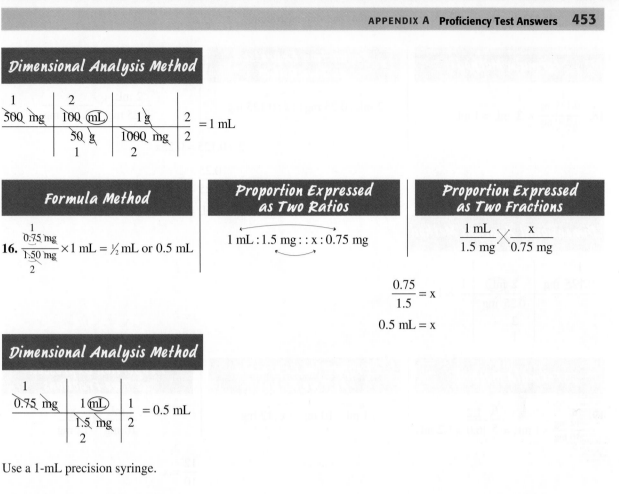

Formula Method

16. $\dfrac{\overset{1}{\cancel{0.75\ \text{mg}}}}{\underset{2}{\cancel{1.50\ \text{mg}}}}\times 1\ \text{mL}=\tfrac{1}{2}\ \text{mL or }0.5\ \text{mL}$

Proportion Expressed as Two Ratios

$$1\ \text{mL}:1.5\ \text{mg}::x:0.75\ \text{mg}$$

Proportion Expressed as Two Fractions

$$\dfrac{1\ \text{mL}}{1.5\ \text{mg}}\times\dfrac{x}{0.75\ \text{mg}}$$

$$\dfrac{0.75}{1.5}=x$$

$$0.5\ \text{mL}=x$$

Dimensional Analysis Method

$$\dfrac{1}{\cancel{0.75}\ \cancel{mg}}\ \Bigg|\ \dfrac{1\ \cancel{\textcircled{mL}}}{\underset{2}{\cancel{1.5}}\ \cancel{mg}}\ \Bigg|\ \dfrac{1}{2}\ =0.5\ \text{mL}$$

Use a 1-mL precision syringe.

17. 20% means   20 g in 100 mL

100 mg = 0.1 g

Formula Method

$\dfrac{0.1\,\text{g}}{\underset{1}{\cancel{20\,\text{g}}}}\times\overset{5}{\cancel{100}}\ \text{mL}=0.5\ \text{mL}$

Proportion Expressed as Two Ratios

$$100\ \text{mL}:20\ \text{g}::x:0.1\ \text{g}$$

Proportion Expressed as Two Fractions

$$\dfrac{100\ \text{mL}}{20\ \text{g}}\times\dfrac{x}{0.1\ \text{g}}$$

$$100\times0.1=20x$$

$$\dfrac{10}{20}=x$$

$$0.5\ \text{mL}=x$$

Dimensional Analysis Method

$$\dfrac{1}{\cancel{100}\ \cancel{mg}}\ \Bigg|\ \dfrac{\overset{5}{\cancel{100}}\ \cancel{\textcircled{mL}}}{\underset{1}{\cancel{20}}\ \cancel{g}}\ \Bigg|\ \dfrac{1\ \cancel{g}}{\underset{10}{\cancel{1000}}\ \cancel{mg}}\ \Bigg|\ \dfrac{5}{10}\ =0.5\ \text{mL}$$

Use a 1-mL precision syringe.

Formula Method	Proportion Expressed as Two Ratios	Proportion Expressed as Two Fractions

18. $\dfrac{\overset{1}{\cancel{0.125\text{ mg}}}}{\underset{2}{\cancel{0.250\text{ mg}}}} \times \overset{1}{\cancel{2}}$ mL = 1 mL

2 mL : 0.25 mg : : x : 0.125 mg

$\dfrac{2\text{ mL}}{0.25\text{ mg}} \times \dfrac{\text{x}}{0.125\text{ mg}}$

$$2 \times 0.125 = 0.25\text{x}$$

$$\dfrac{0.25}{0.25} = \text{x}$$

$$1\text{ mL} = \text{x}$$

Dimensional Analysis Method

$$\dfrac{\overset{1}{\cancel{0.125\text{ mg}}}}{} \;\bigg|\; \dfrac{\overset{1}{\cancel{2}}\ \cancel{(\text{mL})}}{\underset{\underset{1}{2}}{0.25\text{ mg}}} \;\bigg|\; \dfrac{1}{} = 1\text{ mL}$$

Formula Method	Proportion Expressed as Two Ratios	Proportion Expressed as Two Fractions

19. $\dfrac{\overset{6}{\cancel{12\text{ mg}}}}{\underset{5}{\cancel{10\text{ mg}}}} \times 1\text{ mL} = \dfrac{6}{5}\overset{1.2}{\overline{)6.0}} = 1.2\text{ mL}$

1 mL : 10 mg : : x : 12 mg

$\dfrac{1\text{ mL}}{10\text{ mg}} \times \dfrac{\text{x}}{12\text{ mg}}$

$$\dfrac{12}{10} = \text{x}$$

$$1.2\text{ mL} = \text{x}$$

Dimensional Analysis Method

$$\dfrac{\overset{6}{\cancel{12\text{ mg}}}}{} \;\bigg|\; \dfrac{1\ \cancel{(\text{mL})}}{\underset{5}{\cancel{10\text{ mg}}}} \;\bigg|\; \dfrac{6}{5} = 1.2\text{ mL}$$

Formula Method	Proportion Expressed as Two Ratios	Proportion Expressed as Two Fractions

20. $\dfrac{\overset{5}{\cancel{10\text{ mEq}}}}{\underset{\underset{1}{2}}{\cancel{40\text{ mEq}}}} \times \overset{1}{\cancel{20}}\ \text{mL} = 5\text{ mL}$

20 mL : 40 mEq : : x : 10 mEq

$\dfrac{20\text{ mL}}{40\text{ mEq}} \times \dfrac{\text{x}}{10\text{ mEq}}$

$$20 \times 10 = 40\text{x}$$

$$\dfrac{200}{40} = \text{x}$$

$$5\text{ mL} = \text{x}$$

Dimensional Analysis Method

$$\dfrac{\cancel{10\text{ mEq}}}{} \;\bigg|\; \dfrac{1\ \ \cancel{(\text{mL})}}{\underset{2}{\cancel{40\text{ mEq}}}} \;\bigg|\; \dfrac{10}{2} = 5\text{ mL}$$

Test 4: Mental Drill in Liquids-for-Injection Problems

1. 2 mL IM
2. 5 mL IV
3. 2 mL IM
4. 1 mL IM
5. 0.5 mL IM
6. 1 mL IM

7. 0.75 mL or 0.8 mL subcutaneous
8. 1 mL subcutaneous
9. 20 mL IV
10. 2.5 mL IM
11. 0.8 mL IM
12. 2 mL IM

13. 2 mL IV
14. 1.5 mL IM
15. 1.5 mL IM
16. 0.35 mL or 0.4 mL IM
17. 1.5 mL subcutaneous
18. 1.5 mL IM

Test 5: Injections from Powders

1. **a.** 1.5 mL, sterile water

   b. 280 mg/mL

   c.

Formula Method	Proportion Expressed as Two Ratios	Proportion Expressed as Two Fractions
$\frac{250 \text{ mg}}{280 \text{ mg}} \times 1 \text{ mL} = x$ $0.89 \times 1 \text{ mL} = x$ $0.89 \text{ or } 0.9 \text{ mL} = x$	$1 \text{ mL} : 280 \text{ mg} :: x : 250 \text{ mg}$	$\frac{1 \text{ mL}}{280 \text{ mg}} \times \frac{x}{250 \text{ mg}}$

$$\frac{250}{280} = x$$

$$0.89 \text{ mL} = x$$

or

$$0.9 \text{ mL} = x$$

Dimensional Analysis Method

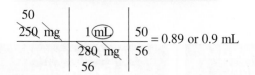

$$\frac{\overset{50}{\cancel{250}} \text{ mg}}{} \Bigg| \frac{1\, \textcircled{mL}}{\underset{56}{\cancel{280}} \text{ mg}} \Bigg| \frac{50}{56} = 0.89 \text{ or } 0.9 \text{ mL}$$

   d. 0.9 mL

   e. 280 mg/mL, date, time, expiration date (7 days after reconstitution), initials

   f. Refrigerate; stable for 7 days

2. **a.** 2 mL sterile water for injection

   b. 1 g/2.6 mL

   c.

Formula Method	Proportion Expressed as Two Ratios	Proportion Expressed as Two Fractions
$\frac{1 \text{ g}}{1 \text{ g}} \times 2.6 \text{ mL} = 2.6 \text{ mL}$	$2.6 \text{ mL} : 1 \text{ g} :: x : 1 \text{ g}$	$\frac{2.6 \text{ mL}}{1 \text{ g}} \times \frac{x}{1 \text{ g}}$

$$x = 2.6 \text{ mL}$$

Dimensional Analysis Method

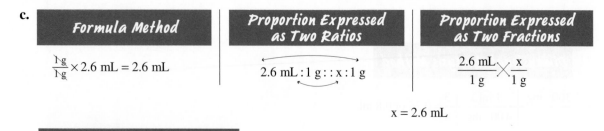

$$\frac{1\, \text{g}}{} \Bigg| \frac{2.6\, \textcircled{mL}}{1\, \text{g}} \Bigg| \frac{2.6}{} = 2.6 \text{ mL}$$

    d. 2.6 mL

    e. Nothing is left in the vial.

    f. Discard the vial in a proper receptacle.

3. a. 1.8 mL sterile water for injection

   b. 250 mg/mL

   c.

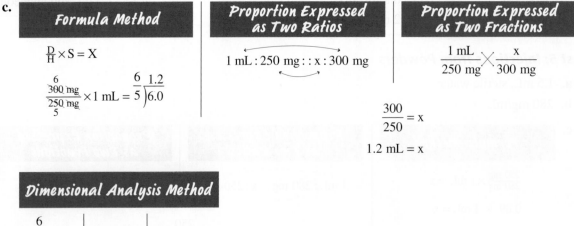

Formula Method	Proportion Expressed as Two Ratios	Proportion Expressed as Two Fractions
$\frac{D}{H} \times S = X$	$1\ mL : 250\ mg :: x : 300\ mg$	$\frac{1\ mL}{250\ mg} \times \frac{x}{300\ mg}$

$$\frac{\overset{6}{\cancel{300\ mg}}}{\underset{5}{\cancel{250\ mg}}} \times 1\ mL = \begin{array}{r} {}^{6}\ 1.2 \\ 5\overline{)6.0} \end{array}$$

$$\frac{300}{250} = x$$

$$1.2\ mL = x$$

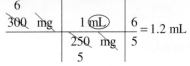

Dimensional Analysis Method

$$\frac{\overset{6}{\cancel{300}}\ mg}{} \ \Big|\ \frac{1\ \textcircled{mL}}{\underset{5}{\cancel{250}}\ mg} \ \Big|\ \frac{6}{5} = 1.2\ mL$$

   d. 1.2 mL

   e. Discard the vial. Directions say solution must be used within 1 hour.

   f. No. Discard the vial in an appropriate receptacle.

4. a. 2 mL sterile water for injection

   b. 400 mg/mL

   c.

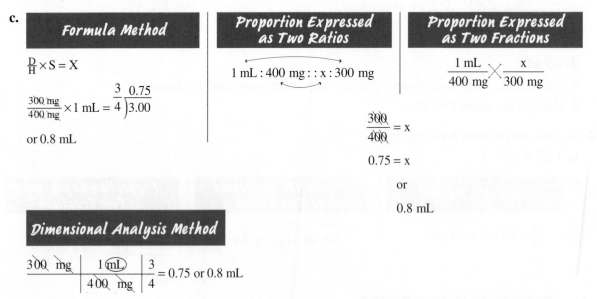

Formula Method	Proportion Expressed as Two Ratios	Proportion Expressed as Two Fractions
$\frac{D}{H} \times S = X$	$1\ mL : 400\ mg :: x : 300\ mg$	$\frac{1\ mL}{400\ mg} \times \frac{x}{300\ mg}$

$$\frac{\cancel{300\ mg}}{\cancel{400\ mg}} \times 1\ mL = \begin{array}{r} {}^{3}\ 0.75 \\ 4\overline{)3.00} \end{array}$$

or 0.8 mL

$$\frac{\cancel{300}}{\cancel{400}} = x$$

$$0.75 = x$$

or

$$0.8\ mL$$

Dimensional Analysis Method

$$\frac{\cancel{300}\ mg}{} \ \Big|\ \frac{1\ \textcircled{mL}}{\cancel{400}\ mg} \ \Big|\ \frac{3}{4} = 0.75\ or\ 0.8\ mL$$

   d. 0.8 mL

   e. 400 mg/mL, date, time, expiration date (1 week after reconstitution), initials

   f. Refrigerate; stable for 1 week

5. a. 2.5 mL sterile water for injection

b. 330 mg/mL

c.

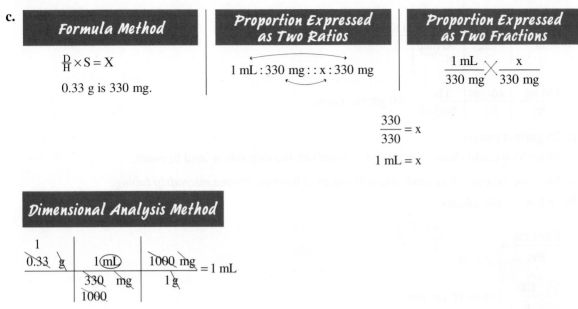

Formula Method	Proportion Expressed as Two Ratios	Proportion Expressed as Two Fractions
$\frac{D}{H} \times S = X$ 0.33 g is 330 mg.	1 mL : 330 mg : : x : 330 mg	$\frac{1\ mL}{330\ mg} \times \frac{x}{330\ mg}$

$$\frac{330}{330} = x$$

$$1\ mL = x$$

Dimensional Analysis Method

$$\frac{1}{0.33\ g} \Bigg| \frac{1\ mL}{330\ mg} \Bigg| \frac{1000\ mg}{1\ g} = 1\ mL$$

d. 1 mL IM

e. 330 mg/mL, date, time, expiration date (96 days after reconstitution), initials

f. Refrigerate; stable for 96 hours

Chapter 8

Test 1: Basic IV Problems

1. a. You have 1000 mL running at 150 mL/hr, therefore

$$\frac{\frac{20}{1000}}{\frac{150}{3}} = \frac{20}{3} \; 20.0 = \text{approximately 6.6 hours}$$

Dimensional Analysis Method

$$\frac{200}{1000\ mL} \Bigg| \frac{hr}{150\ mL} \Bigg| \frac{200}{30} = 6.6 \text{ hours}$$

b. 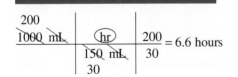 $\frac{\text{number mL} \times \text{TF}}{\text{number min}} = \text{gtt/min}$

$\frac{150 \times 10}{60} = 25\text{gtt/min macro}$

$\frac{150 \times 60}{60} = 150\text{gtt/min micro}$

Choose macrotubing.

Dimensional Analysis Method

$$\frac{150 \text{ mL}}{\text{hr}} \left| \frac{\overset{1}{10} \text{ gtt}}{\text{mL}} \right| \frac{1 \text{ hr}}{\underset{6}{60} \text{ min}} \right| \frac{150}{6} = 25 \text{ gtt/min macro}$$

$$\frac{150 \text{ mL}}{\text{hr}} \left| \frac{60 \text{ gtt}}{\text{mL}} \right| \frac{1 \text{ hr}}{60 \text{ min}} = 150 \text{ gtt/min micro}$$

c. 25 gtt/min macro

Note: You could choose microtubing; however, the drip rate is hard to count.

2. a. Because the amount is small and will run over 6 hours, choose *microdrip tubing*.

b.   6 hours = 360 minutes

$$\frac{100 \times \overset{1}{60}}{\underset{6}{360}} =$$

$$\frac{100}{6} = 16.6 \text{ or } 17 \text{ gtt/min}$$

Dimensional Analysis Method

$$\frac{100 \text{ mL}}{6 \text{ hr}} \left| \frac{\overset{1}{60} \text{ gtt}}{\text{mL}} \right| \frac{1 \text{ hr}}{\underset{1}{60} \text{ min}} \right| \frac{100}{6} = 16.6 \text{ or } 17 \text{ gtt/min}$$

3. a. Because the stock bag is 250 mL NS, you would aseptically allow 100 mL to run off. This will leave 150 mL NS. If using an infusion pump, you could set the volume to be infused at 150 mL.

b. *Microdrip* because

3 hours = 180 minutes

$$\text{Macro: } \frac{150 \times \overset{1}{15}}{\underset{12}{180}} =$$

$$\frac{150}{12} = 12.5 \text{ or } 13 \text{ gtt/min}$$

$$\text{Micro: } \frac{150 \times \overset{1}{60}}{\underset{3}{180}} =$$

$$\frac{150}{3} = 50 \text{ gtt/min}$$

c. 50 gtt/min (microdrip)

Note: It would not be incorrect to choose the macrodrip. However, 50 gtt/min provides a better flow.

Dimensional Analysis Method

$$\frac{\overset{50}{\cancel{150}\ \cancel{mL}}}{\underset{1}{\cancel{3}\ \cancel{hr}}}\ \left|\ \frac{1}{\overset{15\cancel{(gtt)}}{\cancel{mL}}}\ \right|\ \frac{1\ \cancel{hr}}{\underset{4}{\cancel{60}\ \cancel{(min)}}}\ \right|\ \frac{50}{4} = 12.5\ \text{or}\ 13\ \text{gtt/min}$$

$$\frac{\overset{50}{\cancel{150}\ \cancel{mL}}}{\underset{1}{\cancel{3}\ \cancel{hr}}}\ \left|\ \frac{1}{\overset{60\cancel{(gtt)}}{\cancel{mL}}}\ \right|\ \frac{1\ \cancel{hr}}{\underset{1}{\cancel{60}\ \cancel{(min)}}}\ \right|\ \frac{50}{} = 50\ \text{gtt/min}$$

4. 21 mL/hr

Step 1. $\frac{\text{number mL}}{\text{number hr}} = \text{mL/hr}$

$$\frac{500\ \text{mL}}{24\ \text{hr}} \quad \begin{array}{r} 20.8 \\ 24\,\overline{)500.0} \\ \underline{48} \\ 20\,0 \\ \underline{19\,2} \end{array} = 21\ \text{mL/hr}$$

Step 2 is not necessary because you have an infusion pump that delivers milliliters per hour.

Dimensional Analysis Method

$$\frac{500\ \cancel{(mL)}}{24\ \cancel{(hr)}}\ \left|\ \frac{500}{24}\right. = 20.8\ \text{or}\ 21\ \text{mL/hr}$$

5. Use a reconstitution device to add 100 mg powder to 250 mL D5W and give IVPB over 1 hour (60 min); TF = 10 gtts/mL.

$$\frac{\text{number mL} \times \text{TF}}{\text{number min}} = \text{gtt/min}$$

$$\frac{250 \times 10}{60} = \quad \begin{array}{r} 250 \\ 6 \end{array} \quad \begin{array}{r} 41.6 \\ \overline{)250.0} \end{array} = 42\ \text{gtt/min}$$

Label the IVPB.
Set the rate at 42 gtt/min.

Dimensional Analysis Method

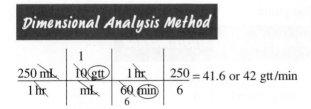

$$\frac{250\ \cancel{mL}}{1\ \cancel{hr}}\ \left|\ \frac{\overset{1}{10\cancel{(gtt)}}}{\cancel{mL}}\ \right|\ \frac{1\ \cancel{hr}}{\underset{6}{\cancel{60}\ \cancel{(min)}}}\ \right|\ \frac{250}{6} = 41.6\ \text{or}\ 42\ \text{gtt/min}$$

6 a. Order is 500 mg. Stock is 1 g in 10 mL.

1 g = 1000 mg

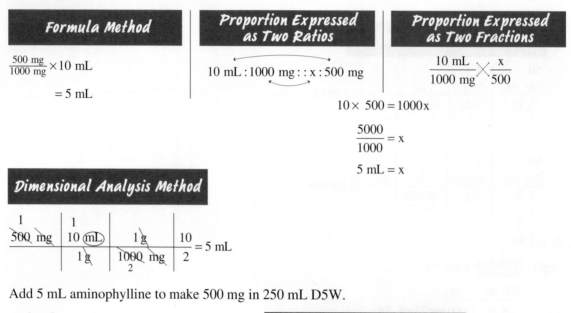

Formula Method	Proportion Expressed as Two Ratios	Proportion Expressed as Two Fractions
$\frac{500 \text{ mg}}{1000 \text{ mg}} \times 10 \text{ mL}$ $= 5 \text{ mL}$	10 mL : 1000 mg : : x : 500 mg	$\frac{10 \text{ mL}}{1000 \text{ mg}} \times \frac{x}{500}$ $10 \times 500 = 1000x$ $\frac{5000}{1000} = x$ $5 \text{ mL} = x$

Dimensional Analysis Method

$$\frac{1}{500 \text{ mg}} \left| \frac{1}{10 \text{ mL}} \right| \frac{1 \text{ g}}{1 \text{ g}} \left| \frac{10}{1000 \text{ mg}} \right| \frac{10}{2} = 5 \text{ mL}$$

Add 5 mL aminophylline to make 500 mg in 250 mL D5W.

b. $\frac{\text{number mL}}{\text{number hr}} = \text{mL/hr}$

$\frac{250 \text{ mL}}{8 \text{ hr}} = 31.2 = 31 \text{ mL/hr}$

mL/hr = microgtt/min

No math necessary.

Microdip: 31 mL/hr = 31 gtt/min

Label IV.

Set the rate at 31 gtt/min.

Dimensional Analysis Method

$$\frac{250 \text{ mL}}{8 \text{ hr}} \left| \frac{125}{4} \right. = 31 \text{ mL/hr}$$

7. 2800 mL

Logic: The patient gets 125 mL/hr and there are 24 hours in a day; four times a day the patient receives Cefoxitin. That leaves 20 hours (24 − 4) times 125 mL/hr:

$$\begin{array}{r} 125 \\ \times\ 20 \\ \hline 2500 \text{ mL} \end{array}$$

The patient gets 75 mL q6h and, therefore, is receiving 75 mL four times in 24 hours.

So $\begin{array}{r} 75 \\ \times\ 4 \\ \hline 300 \end{array}$ $\begin{array}{r} 2500 \text{ mL} \\ +\ 300 \text{ mL} \\ \hline 2800 \text{ mL} \end{array}$

8. a. 90 mL/hr—no math necessary—using an infusion pump

b.

$\frac{\text{total number mL}}{\text{mL/hr}} = \text{hr}$

$$\begin{array}{r} 11.1 \\ 90\ )\overline{1000.0} \\ \underline{90} \\ 100 \\ \underline{90} \\ 10\ 0 \end{array}$$

Dimensional Analysis Method

$$\frac{1000 \text{ mL}}{\text{hr}} \left| \frac{100}{90 \text{ mL}} \right| \frac{100}{9} = 11.1 \text{ hr}$$

Approximately 11 hours

9. 50 mg

   You have 0.5 g in 500 mL. 0.5 g = 500 mg. The solution is 500 mg in 500 mL. Reducing this amount equals 1 mg in 1 mL. Because the patient is receiving 50 mL/hour, the patient is receiving 50 mg aminophylline per hour.

10. **a.** You need 75 mL D5W. Take a 100-mL bag of D5W and aseptically remove 25 mL. Add 5 mL Bactrim to the 75 mL. Time is 60 minutes. The order is 75 mL/hour. No math is necessary. You have a pump in milliliters per hour.

    Label the IVPB.

    b. Set the pump:

    For 60 minutes:

    Secondary volume (mL): 75

    Secondary rate (mL/hr): 75

    For 90 minutes: $\dfrac{75 \times 60}{90} = 50$ mL/hr

    Secondary volume (mL): 75

    Secondary rate (mL/hr): 50

11. $\frac{3}{4} \times 150$ mL $= 112.5$ mL Isocal

    150 mL $- 112.5$ mL $= 37.5$ mL water

12. $\frac{1}{2} \times 500$ mL $= 250$ mL Vivonex

    500 mL $- 250$ mL $= 250$ mL water

13. $25\% = 0.25 = \frac{1}{4}$ (use any of these)

    $\frac{1}{4} \times 400$ mL $= 100$ mL Osmolite

    400 mL $- 100$ mL $= 300$ mL water

14. 500 mL Isocal

    0 mL water

Chapter 9

Test 1: Special IV Calculations

1.

Formula Method	Proportion Expressed as Two Ratios	Proportion Expressed as Two Fractions
$\dfrac{15 \text{ units/hr}}{125 \text{ units}} \times 250 \text{ mL} = X$ (reduced: $\frac{1}{1}$ and $\frac{2}{}$) $15 \times 2 = 30$ mL/hr on a pump	250 mL : 125 units : : x : 15 units	$\dfrac{x \text{ mL}}{15 \text{ units}} \times \dfrac{250 \text{ mL}}{125 \text{ units}}$ $15 \times 250 = 125x$ $\dfrac{3750}{125} = x$ 30 mL/hr

Set the pump.

Total number mL: 250

mL/hr: 30

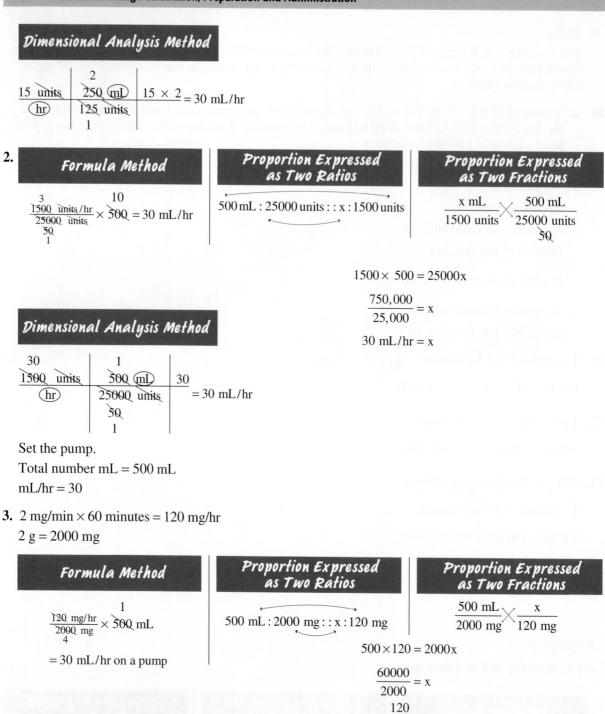

Dimensional Analysis Method

$$\frac{15 \ \text{units}}{\text{hr}} \ \bigg| \ \frac{\overset{2}{250} \ \text{mL}}{\underset{1}{125} \ \text{units}} \ \bigg| \ 15 \times 2 = 30 \ \text{mL/hr}$$

2.

Formula Method

$$\frac{\overset{3}{1500} \ \text{units/hr}}{\underset{\underset{1}{50}}{25000} \ \text{units}} \times \overset{10}{500} = 30 \ \text{mL/hr}$$

Proportion Expressed as Two Ratios

$$500 \ \text{mL} : 25000 \ \text{units} :: x : 1500 \ \text{units}$$

Proportion Expressed as Two Fractions

$$\frac{x \ \text{mL}}{1500 \ \text{units}} \times \frac{500 \ \text{mL}}{\underset{50}{25000} \ \text{units}}$$

$$1500 \times 500 = 25000x$$

$$\frac{750,000}{25,000} = x$$

$$30 \ \text{mL/hr} = x$$

Dimensional Analysis Method

$$\frac{\overset{30}{1500} \ \text{units}}{\text{hr}} \ \bigg| \ \frac{\overset{1}{500} \ \text{mL}}{\underset{\underset{1}{50}}{25000} \ \text{units}} \ \bigg| \ 30 = 30 \ \text{mL/hr}$$

Set the pump.

Total number mL = 500 mL

mL/hr = 30

3. $2 \ \text{mg/min} \times 60 \ \text{minutes} = 120 \ \text{mg/hr}$

$2 \ \text{g} = 2000 \ \text{mg}$

Formula Method

$$\frac{120 \ \text{mg/hr}}{\underset{4}{2000} \ \text{mg}} \times \overset{1}{500} \ \text{mL}$$

$$= 30 \ \text{mL/hr on a pump}$$

Proportion Expressed as Two Ratios

$$500 \ \text{mL} : 2000 \ \text{mg} :: x : 120 \ \text{mg}$$

Proportion Expressed as Two Fractions

$$\frac{500 \ \text{mL}}{2000 \ \text{mg}} \times \frac{x}{120 \ \text{mg}}$$

$$500 \times 120 = 2000x$$

$$\frac{60000}{2000} = x$$

$$\frac{120}{4} = x$$

$$30 \ \text{mL} = x$$

Dimensional Analysis Method

$$\frac{2 \ \text{mg}}{\text{min}} \ \bigg| \ \frac{500 \ \text{mL}}{2 \ \text{g}} \ \bigg| \ \frac{1 \ \text{g}}{\underset{\underset{1}{2}}{1000} \ \text{mg}} \ \bigg| \ \frac{\overset{30}{60} \ \text{min}}{1 \ \text{hr}} \ \bigg| \ 30 = 30 \ \text{mL/hr}$$

Set the pump.

Total number mL: 500

mL/hr: 30

4. a. Add diltiazem to the IV.

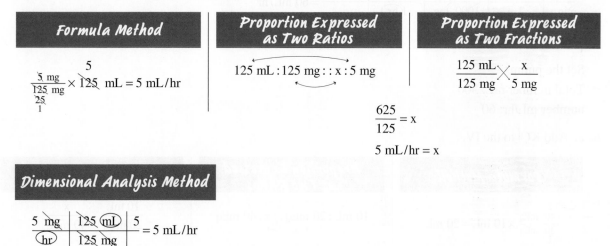

Formula Method	Proportion Expressed as Two Ratios	Proportion Expressed as Two Fractions

$$\dfrac{\overset{1}{\cancel{5} \text{ mg}}}{\underset{\underset{1}{\cancel{25}}}{\cancel{125} \text{ mg}}} \times \overset{4}{\cancel{100}} \text{ mL} = 4 \text{ mL/hr}$$

$$100 \text{ mL} : 125 \text{ mg} :: x : 5 \text{ mg}$$

$$\dfrac{100 \text{ mL}}{125 \text{ mg}} \times \dfrac{x}{5 \text{ mg}}$$

$$100 \times 5 = 125x$$

$$\dfrac{500}{125} = x$$

$$4 \text{ mL/hr}$$

Dimensional Analysis Method

$$\dfrac{\overset{1}{\cancel{5}} \text{ mg}}{\cancel{hr}} \bigg| \dfrac{100 \cancel{\text{mL}}}{\underset{25}{\cancel{125} \text{ mg}}} \bigg| \dfrac{100}{25} = 4 \text{ mL/hr}$$

Second way: If you add 25 mL of drug to the 100 mL D5W, you make 125 mL (a 1:1 solution). Because the order is 5 mg/hour, set the pump at 5 mL/hr.

Formula Method	Proportion Expressed as Two Ratios	Proportion Expressed as Two Fractions

$$\dfrac{\overset{1}{\cancel{5} \text{ mg}}}{\underset{\underset{1}{\cancel{25}}}{\cancel{125} \text{ mg}}} \times \overset{5}{\cancel{125}} \text{ mL} = 5 \text{ mL/hr}$$

$$125 \text{ mL} : 125 \text{ mg} :: x : 5 \text{ mg}$$

$$\dfrac{125 \text{ mL}}{125 \text{ mg}} \times \dfrac{x}{5 \text{ mg}}$$

$$\dfrac{625}{125} = x$$

$$5 \text{ mL/hr} = x$$

Dimensional Analysis Method

$$\dfrac{5 \text{ mg}}{\cancel{hr}} \bigg| \dfrac{125 \cancel{\text{mL}}}{125 \cancel{\text{mg}}} \bigg| 5 = 5 \text{ mL/hr}$$

It is considered better to remove fluid from the IV bag so the volume remains the same.

b.

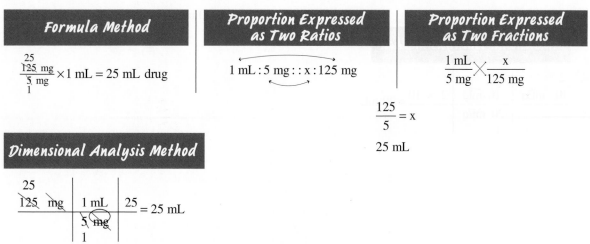

Formula Method	Proportion Expressed as Two Ratios	Proportion Expressed as Two Fractions

$$\dfrac{\overset{25}{\cancel{125} \text{ mg}}}{\underset{1}{\cancel{5} \text{ mg}}} \times 1 \text{ mL} = 25 \text{ mL drug}$$

$$1 \text{ mL} : 5 \text{ mg} :: x : 125 \text{ mg}$$

$$\dfrac{1 \text{ mL}}{5 \text{ mg}} \times \dfrac{x}{125 \text{ mg}}$$

$$\dfrac{125}{5} = x$$

$$25 \text{ mL}$$

Dimensional Analysis Method

$$\dfrac{\overset{25}{\cancel{125}} \text{ mg}}{} \bigg| \dfrac{1 \text{ mL}}{\underset{1}{\cancel{5} \text{ mg}}} \bigg| \dfrac{25}{} = 25 \text{ mL}$$

Remove 25 mL IV fluid from the IV bag and add 25 mL diltiazem = 100 mL total.

5. $2 \text{ g} = 2000 \text{ mg}$

Order calls for 4 mg/min. Pumps are set in mL/hr. Multiply $4 \text{ mg/min} \times 60 \text{ min} = 240 \text{ mg/hr}$.

Formula Method	**Proportion Expressed as Two Ratios**	**Proportion Expressed as Two Fractions**
$\dfrac{\overset{60}{\cancel{240}} \text{ mg/hr}}{\underset{\underset{1}{4}}{\cancel{2000}} \text{ mg}} \times \overset{1}{\cancel{500}} \text{ mL} = 60 \text{ mL/hr}$	$500 \text{ mL} : 2000 \text{ mg} :: x : 240 \text{ mg}$	$\dfrac{500 \text{ mL}}{2000 \text{ mg}} \times \dfrac{x}{240 \text{ mg}}$

$$500 \times 240 = 2000x$$
$$\frac{120,000}{2000} = x$$
$$\frac{240}{4} = x$$
$$60 \text{ mL} = x$$

Dimensional Analysis Method
$\dfrac{\overset{2}{\cancel{4}} \text{ mg}}{\text{min}} \left| \dfrac{\overset{1}{500} \text{ mL}}{\underset{1}{\cancel{2}} \text{ g}} \right. \left| \dfrac{1 \text{ g}}{\underset{\underset{1}{\cancel{2}}}{\cancel{1000}} \text{ mg}} \right| \dfrac{\overset{30}{\cancel{60}} \text{ min}}{1 \text{ hr}} \left| \dfrac{2 \times 30}{1} = 60 \text{ mL/hr} \right.$

Set the pump.

Total number mL: 500

number mL/hr: 60

6. a. Add KCl to the IV.

Formula Method	**Proportion Expressed as Two Ratios**	**Proportion Expressed as Two Fractions**
$\dfrac{\overset{2}{\cancel{40}} \text{ mEq}}{\underset{1}{\cancel{20}} \text{ mEq}} \times 10 \text{ mL} = 20 \text{ mL}$	$10 \text{ mL} : 20 \text{ mEq} :: x : 40 \text{ mEq}$	$\dfrac{10 \text{ mL}}{20 \text{ mEq}} \times \dfrac{x}{40 \text{ mEq}}$

$$10 \times 40 = 20x$$
$$\frac{400}{20} = x$$
$$20 \text{ mL} = x$$

Dimensional Analysis Method
$\dfrac{\overset{2}{\cancel{40}} \text{ mEq}}{} \left| \dfrac{10 \text{ mL}}{\underset{1}{\cancel{20}} \text{ mEq}} \right| \dfrac{2 \times 10}{1} = 20 \text{ mL}$

b. Remove 20 mL IV fluid and add the 20 mL of KCl to make 1000 mL.

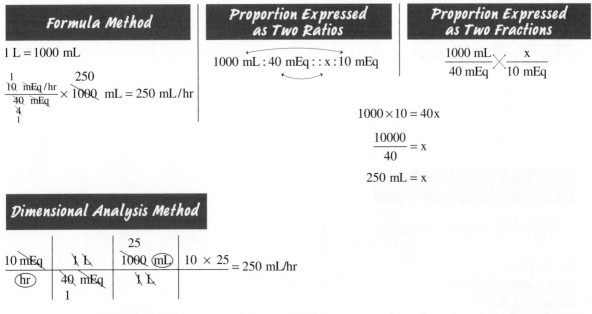

1 L = 1000 mL

$$\frac{\overset{1}{\cancel{10}}\text{ mEq/hr}}{\underset{4}{\cancel{40}}\text{ mEq}} \times \overset{250}{\cancel{1000}}\text{ mL} = 250 \text{ mL/hr}$$

Proportion Expressed as Two Ratios

1000 mL : 40 mEq : : x : 10 mEq

Proportion Expressed as Two Fractions

$$\frac{1000 \text{ mL}}{40 \text{ mEq}} \times \frac{x}{10 \text{ mEq}}$$

$$1000 \times 10 = 40x$$

$$\frac{10000}{40} = x$$

$$250 \text{ mL} = x$$

Dimensional Analysis Method

$$\frac{10 \text{ mEq}}{\text{hr}} \mid \frac{1 \text{ L}}{\cancel{40}\text{ mEq}} \mid \frac{\overset{25}{\cancel{1000}}\text{ mL}}{1 \text{ L}} \quad \frac{10 \times 25}{1} = 250 \text{ mL/hr}$$

Set pump at 250 mL/hr. This is a large volume and KCl is a potent electrolyte; therefore, the patient must be on a cardiac monitor for safety. Check the order with the doctor or healthcare provider.

Total number mL: 1000

number mL/hr: 250

7. 2 g = 2000 mL

Order calls for 1 mg/min. Pumps are set in mL/hr. Multiply 1 mg/min × 60 mg = 60 mg/hr.

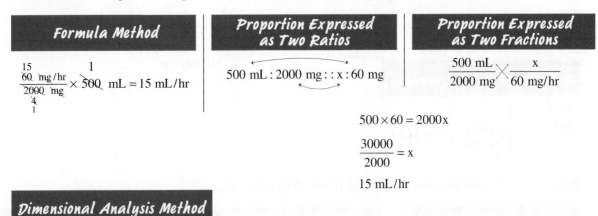

$$\frac{\overset{15}{\cancel{60}}\text{ mg/hr}}{\underset{4}{\cancel{2000}}\text{ mg}} \times \overset{1}{\cancel{500}}\text{ mL} = 15 \text{ mL/hr}$$

Proportion Expressed as Two Ratios

500 mL : 2000 mg : : x : 60 mg

Proportion Expressed as Two Fractions

$$\frac{500 \text{ mL}}{2000 \text{ mg}} \times \frac{x}{60 \text{ mg/hr}}$$

$$500 \times 60 = 2000x$$

$$\frac{30000}{2000} = x$$

$$15 \text{ mL/hr}$$

Dimensional Analysis Method

$$\frac{1 \text{ mg}}{\text{min}} \mid \frac{\overset{1}{\cancel{500}}\text{ mL}}{2 \text{ g}} \mid \frac{1 \text{ g}}{\underset{2}{\cancel{1000}}\text{ mg}} \mid \frac{\overset{30}{\cancel{60}}\text{ min}}{1 \text{ hr}} \quad \frac{30}{2} = 15 \text{ mL/hr}$$

Set the pump.

Total number mL: 500

number mL/hr: 15

8. Use a reconstitution device (see Chapter 8) to add 50 mg of drug to 500 mL D5W.

$$\frac{\text{number mL}}{\text{number hr}} = \text{mL/hr}$$

$$\frac{500 \text{ mL}}{6 \text{ hr}} \quad 6\overline{\smash{)}\begin{array}{r}83.0 \\ 500.0 \end{array}} = 83 \text{ mL/hr}$$
$$\begin{array}{r} 48 \\ \hline 20 \\ 18 \\ \hline 2\,0 \\ 1\,8 \\ \hline \end{array}$$

Dimensional Analysis Method

$$\frac{500 \, \cancel{\text{mL}}}{6 \, \cancel{\text{hr}}} \,\bigg|\, \frac{500}{6} = 83.33 \text{ or } 83 \text{ mL/hr}$$

Set the pump.

Total number mL: 500

number mL/hr: 83

9. Add vasopressin to the IV.

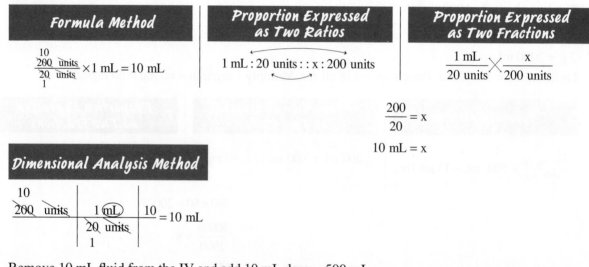

Formula Method	Proportion Expressed as Two Ratios	Proportion Expressed as Two Fractions
$\frac{\overset{10}{\cancel{200}} \text{ units}}{\underset{1}{\cancel{20}} \text{ units}} \times 1 \text{ mL} = 10 \text{ mL}$	$1 \text{ mL} : 20 \text{ units} :: \text{x} : 200 \text{ units}$	$\frac{1 \text{ mL}}{20 \text{ units}} \times \frac{\text{x}}{200 \text{ units}}$

$$\frac{200}{20} = \text{x}$$

$$10 \text{ mL} = \text{x}$$

Dimensional Analysis Method

$$\frac{\overset{10}{\cancel{200}} \text{ units}}{} \,\bigg|\, \frac{1 \, \cancel{\text{mL}}}{\underset{1}{\cancel{20}} \text{ units}} \,\bigg|\, \frac{10}{1} = 10 \text{ mL}$$

Remove 10 mL fluid from the IV and add 10 mL drug = 500 mL.

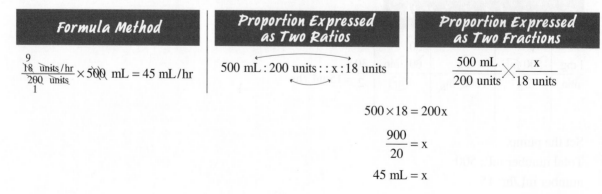

Formula Method	Proportion Expressed as Two Ratios	Proportion Expressed as Two Fractions
$\frac{\overset{9}{\cancel{18}} \text{ units/hr}}{\underset{1}{\cancel{200}} \text{ units}} \times \cancel{500} \text{ mL} = 45 \text{ mL/hr}$	$500 \text{ mL} : 200 \text{ units} :: \text{x} : 18 \text{ units}$	$\frac{500 \text{ mL}}{200 \text{ units}} \times \frac{\text{x}}{18 \text{ units}}$

$$500 \times 18 = 200 \text{x}$$

$$\frac{900}{20} = \text{x}$$

$$45 \text{ mL} = \text{x}$$

Dimensional Analysis Method

$$\frac{18 \text{ units}}{\text{hr}} \left| \frac{500 \text{ mL}}{200 \text{ units}} \right| \frac{18 \times 5}{2} = 45 \text{ mL/hr}$$

Set the pump.

Total number mL: 500

number mL/hr: 45

10. Order: 250 mcg/min

Solution: 500 mg in 500 mL D5W

Step 1. $\frac{500 \text{ mg}}{500 \text{ mL}} = 1 \text{ mg/mL}$

Step 2. 1 mg = 1000 mcg/mL

Step 3. Divide by 60 to get mcg/min. $\frac{1000}{60} = 16.67$ mcg/min.

Step 4.

Formula Method

$$\frac{250 \text{ mcg/min}}{16.67 \text{ mcg/min}} \times 1 \text{ mL} = x$$

14.99 or 15 mL

Proportion Expressed as Two Ratios

$$1 \text{ mL} : 16.67 \text{ mcg/min} :: x : 250 \text{ mcg/min}$$

Proportion Expressed as Two Fractions

$$\frac{1 \text{ mL}}{16.67 \text{ mcg/min}} \times \frac{x}{250 \text{ mcg/min}}$$

$$250 = 16.67x$$

$$\frac{250}{16.67} = x$$

$$14.99 \text{ or } 15 \text{ mL} = x$$

Dimensional Analysis Method

$$\frac{1}{250 \text{ mcg}} \left| \frac{500 \text{ mL}}{500 \text{ mg}} \right| \frac{1 \text{ mg}}{1000 \text{ mcg}} \left| \frac{60 \text{ min}}{1 \text{ hr}} \right| \frac{60}{4} = 15 \text{ mL/hr}$$

Set the pump.

Total mL: 500

mL/hr: 15

11. Order: 2.5 mcg/kg/min

Solution: 400 mg in 250 mL

Weight: 60 kg

Multiply 60 kg × 2.5 mcg = 150 mcg.

Step 1. $\dfrac{400 \text{ mg}}{250 \text{ mL}} = 1.6 \text{ mg/mL}$

Step 2. $1.6 \times 1000 = 1600 \text{ mcg/mL}$

Step 3.   Divide by 60 $\dfrac{1600}{60} = 26.67 \text{ mcg/min}$

Step 4.

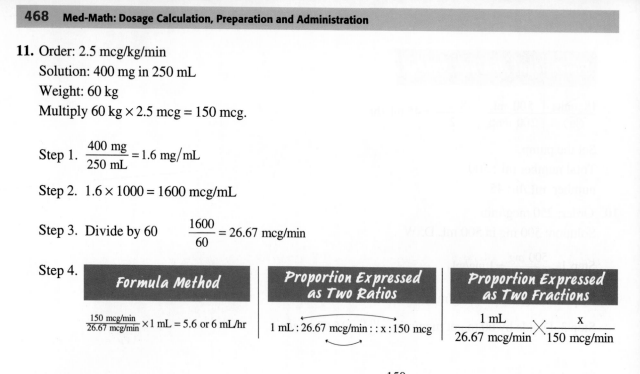

Formula Method	Proportion Expressed as Two Ratios	Proportion Expressed as Two Fractions
$\dfrac{150 \text{ mcg/min}}{26.67 \text{ mcg/min}} \times 1 \text{ mL} = 5.6 \text{ or } 6 \text{ mL/hr}$	$1 \text{ mL} : 26.67 \text{ mcg/min} :: x : 150 \text{ mcg}$	$\dfrac{1 \text{ mL}}{26.67 \text{ mcg/min}} \times \dfrac{x}{150 \text{ mcg/min}}$

$$\frac{150}{26.67} = 5.6 \text{ or } 6 \text{ mL/hr}$$

Dimensional Analysis Method

$$\frac{2.5 \text{ mcg}}{\text{kg / min}} \left| \frac{\overset{1}{250} \text{ mL}}{\underset{}{600} \text{ mg}} \right| \frac{1 \text{ mg}}{\underset{4}{1000} \text{ mcg}} \left| \frac{60 \text{ min}}{1 \text{ hr}} \right| 60 \text{ kg} \left| \frac{2.5 \times 6 \times 6}{4 \times 4} = 5.625 \text{ or } 6 \text{ mL/hr} \right.$$

Set the pump.

Total number mL: 250

number mL/hr: 6

12. Order: 2 milliunits/min

Solution: 9 units in 150 mL NS

Step 1. $\dfrac{9 \text{ units}}{150 \text{ mL}} = 0.06 \text{ units/mL}$

Step 2.   1 unit = 1000 milliunits $0.06 \times 1000 = 60 \text{ milliunits/mL}$

Step 3.   Divide by 60 $\dfrac{60}{60} = 1 \text{ milliunit/min}$

Step 4.

Formula Method	Proportion Expressed as Two Ratios	Proportion Expressed as Two Fractions

$$\frac{2 \text{ milliunits/min}}{1 \text{ milliunit/min}} \times 1 \text{ mL} = x$$

$$2 \text{ mL} = x$$

$1 \text{ mL} : 1 \text{ milliunit/min} :: x : 2 \text{ milliunits/min}$

$$\frac{1 \text{ mL}}{1 \text{ milliunit/min}} \diagdown \frac{x}{2 \text{ milliunits/min}}$$

$$2 = x$$

$$2 \text{ mL} = x$$

Dimensional Analysis Method

$$\frac{2 \text{ milliunits}}{\text{minute}} \left| \frac{15\cancel{0} \cancel{(mL)}}{9 \text{ units}} \right| \frac{1 \text{ unit}}{10\cancel{00} \text{ milliunits}} \left| \frac{6\cancel{0} \text{ minute}}{1 \cancel{(hr)}} \right| \frac{2 \times 15 \times 6}{9 \times 10} = 2 \text{ mL/hr}$$

Set the pump.

Total number mL: 150 mL

number mL/hr: 2

---

13. **a.** Correct; $100 \text{ mg/m}^2 \times 1.7 = 170 \text{ mg}$

b. $1 \text{ L} = 1000 \text{ mL}$

$$\frac{\text{number mL}}{\text{number hr}} = \text{mL/hr}$$

$$24 \overline{\smash{\big)}\, 1000.0} = 42 \text{ mL/hr}$$
$$\begin{array}{r} 41.6 \\ \underline{96} \\ 40 \\ \underline{24} \\ 160 \\ \underline{144} \end{array}$$

Dimensional Analysis Method

$$\frac{1 \cancel{L}}{24 \cancel{(hr)}} \left| \frac{1000 \cancel{(mL)}}{1 \cancel{L}} \right| \frac{1000}{24} = 41.66 \text{ or } 42 \text{ mL/hr}$$

Set the pump.

Total number mL: 1000

number mL/hr: 42

---

14. Order: 5 mcg/kg/min

Solution: 50 mg in 250 mL

Weight: 90 kg

Multiply: $5 \text{ mcg} \times 90 \text{ kg} = 450 \text{ mcg/min}$

Step 1. $\dfrac{50 \text{ mg}}{250 \text{ mL}} = 0.2 \text{ mg/mL}$

Step 2. $0.2 \times 1000 = 200 \text{ mcg/mL}$

Step 3. Divide by 60 $\quad \dfrac{200}{60} = 3.33 \text{ mcg/min}$

Step 4.

Formula Method	Proportion Expressed as Two Ratios	Proportion Expressed as Two Fractions
$\dfrac{450 \text{ mcg/min}}{3.33 \text{ mcg/min}} \times 1 \text{ mL} = 135 \text{ mL}$	1 mL : 3.33 mcg/min : : x : 450 mcg/min	$\dfrac{1 \text{ mL}}{3.33 \text{ mcg}} \times \dfrac{x}{450 \text{ mcg}}$

$$\frac{450}{3.33} = x$$

$$135 \text{ mL} = x$$

Dimensional Analysis Method

$$\frac{1}{\cancel{5} \text{ mcg}} \Bigg| \frac{1}{\cancel{250} \text{ mL}} \Bigg| \frac{1 \text{ mg}}{\cancel{1000} \text{ mcg}} \Bigg| \frac{\cancel{60} \text{ min}}{\cancel{1} \text{ hr}} \Bigg| 90 \text{ kg} \Bigg| \frac{60 \times 90}{10 \times 4} = 135 \text{ mL/hr}$$

(kg / min, 50 mg →10, 1000 mcg →4)

Set the pump.

Total number mL: 250 mL

number mL/hr: 135 mL/hr

15. Order: 2 mcg/min

Solution: 4 mg in 250 mL

Step 1. $\quad \dfrac{4 \text{ mg}}{250 \text{ mL}} = 0.016 \text{ mg/mL}$

Step 2. $\quad 0.016 \text{ mg} \times 1000 = 16 \text{ mcg}$

Step 3. Divide by 60 $\quad \dfrac{16}{60} = 0.267 \text{ mcg/min}$

Step 4.

Formula Method	Proportion Expressed as Two Ratios	Proportion Expressed as Two Fractions
$\dfrac{2 \text{ mcg/min}}{0.267 \text{ mcg/min}} \times 1 \text{ mL}$ $= 7.49 \text{ or } 8 \text{ mL}$	1 mL : 0.267 mcg/min : : x : 2 mcg/min	$\dfrac{1 \text{ mL}}{0.267 \text{ mcg/min}} \times \dfrac{x}{2 \text{ mcg/min}}$

$$\frac{2}{0.267} = x$$

$$7.49 \text{ or } 8 \text{ mL} = x$$

Dimensional Analysis Method

$$\frac{1}{\cancel{2} \text{ mcg}} \Bigg| \frac{1}{\cancel{250} \text{ mL}} \Bigg| \frac{1 \text{ mg}}{\cancel{1000} \text{ mcg}} \Bigg| \frac{\cancel{60} \text{ minute}}{\cancel{1} \text{ hr}} \Bigg| \frac{15}{2} = 7.5 \text{ or } 8 \text{ mL/hr}$$

(min, 4 mg →2, 4→1, 60 minute →15)

Set the pump.

Total number mL: 250 mL

number mL/hr: 8 mL/hr

16. a. Yes. 40 units × 90 kg = 3600 units

b. Yes. Increase rate by 2 units/kg/hr

2 units × 90 kg = 180 units

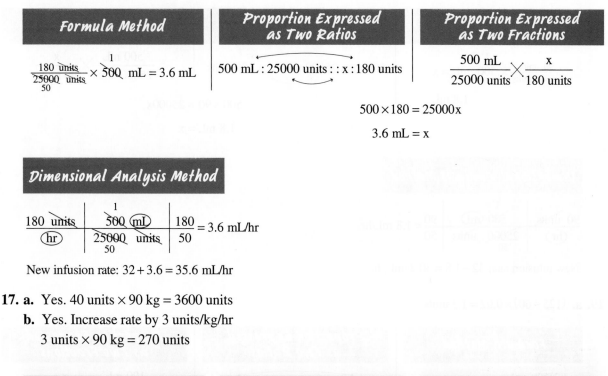

Formula Method	Proportion Expressed as Two Ratios	Proportion Expressed as Two Fractions

$$\frac{\overset{}{180 \text{ units}}}{\underset{50}{25000 \text{ units}}} \times \overset{1}{500} \text{ mL} = 3.6 \text{ mL}$$

500 mL : 25000 units : : x : 180 units

$$\frac{500 \text{ mL}}{25000 \text{ units}} \times \frac{x}{180 \text{ units}}$$

$$500 \times 180 = 25000x$$

$$3.6 \text{ mL} = x$$

Dimensional Analysis Method

$$\frac{180 \text{ units}}{\text{hr}} \left| \frac{\overset{1}{500} \text{ mL}}{\underset{50}{25000} \text{ units}} \right| \frac{180}{50} = 3.6 \text{ mL/hr}$$

New infusion rate: 32 + 3.6 = 35.6 mL/hr

17. a. Yes. 40 units × 90 kg = 3600 units

b. Yes. Increase rate by 3 units/kg/hr

3 units × 90 kg = 270 units

Formula Method	Proportion Expressed as Two Ratios	Proportion Expressed as Two Fractions

$$\frac{\overset{}{270 \text{ units}}}{\underset{50}{25000 \text{ units}}} \times \overset{1}{500} \text{ mL} =$$

$$\frac{270}{50} = x$$

$$5.4 \text{ mL}$$

500 mL : 25000 units : : x : 270 units

$$\frac{500 \text{ mL}}{2500 \text{ units}} \times \frac{x}{270 \text{ units}}$$

$$500 \times 270 = 25000x$$

$$5.4 \text{ mL} = x$$

Dimensional Analysis Method

$$\frac{270 \text{ units}}{} \left| \frac{\overset{1}{500} \text{ mL}}{\underset{50}{25000} \text{ units}} \right| \frac{270}{50} = 5.4 \text{ mL/hr}$$

New infusion rate: 32 + 5.4 = 37.4 mL/hr

18. a. No. Bolus

    b. Yes. Decrease by 1 unit/kg/hr

        1 unit × 90 kg = 90 units

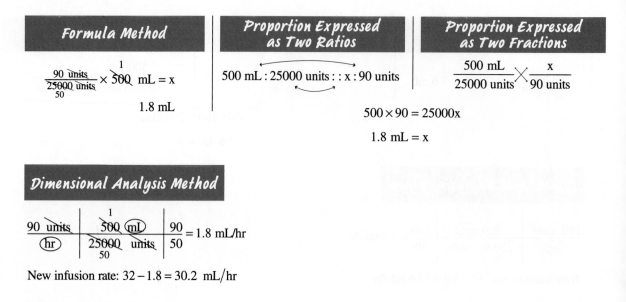

Formula Method	Proportion Expressed as Two Ratios	Proportion Expressed as Two Fractions
$\dfrac{90 \text{ units}}{25000 \text{ units}} \times 500 \text{ mL} = x$ 1.8 mL	500 mL : 25000 units : : x : 90 units $500 \times 90 = 25000x$ $1.8 \text{ mL} = x$	$\dfrac{500 \text{ mL}}{25000 \text{ units}} \times \dfrac{x}{90 \text{ units}}$

Dimensional Analysis Method

$$\frac{90 \text{ units}}{\text{hr}} \;\Big|\; \frac{500 \text{ mL}}{25000 \text{ units}} \;\Big|\; \frac{90}{50} = 1.8 \text{ mL/hr}$$

New infusion rate: $32 - 1.8 = 30.2$ mL/hr

19. a. $(125 - 60) \times 0.02 = 1.3$ units

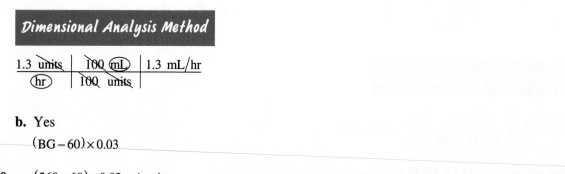

Formula Method	Proportion Expressed as Two Ratios	Proportion Expressed as Two Fractions
$\dfrac{1.3 \text{ units}}{100 \text{ units}} \times 100 \text{ mL} = 1.3 \text{ mL}$	100 mL : 100 units : : x : 1.3 units $100 \times 1.3 = 100x$ 1.3 mL	$\dfrac{100 \text{ mL}}{100 \text{ units}} \times \dfrac{x}{1.3 \text{ units}}$

Dimensional Analysis Method

$$\frac{1.3 \text{ units}}{\text{hr}} \;\Big|\; \frac{100 \text{ mL}}{100 \text{ units}} \;\Big|\; 1.3 \text{ mL/hr}$$

    b. Yes

       $(BG - 60) \times 0.03$

20. a. $(260 - 60) \times 0.02 = 4$ units

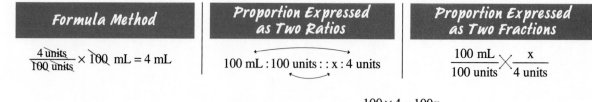

Formula Method	Proportion Expressed as Two Ratios	Proportion Expressed as Two Fractions
$\dfrac{4 \text{ units}}{100 \text{ units}} \times 100 \text{ mL} = 4 \text{ mL}$	100 mL : 100 units : : x : 4 units $100 \times 4 = 100x$ 4 mL	$\dfrac{100 \text{ mL}}{100 \text{ units}} \times \dfrac{x}{4 \text{ units}}$

Dimensional Analysis Method

$$\frac{4 \ \text{units}}{\text{hr}} \ \bigg| \ \frac{100 \ \text{mL}}{100 \ \text{units}} = 4 \ \text{mL/hr}$$

b. Yes. $(BG - 60) \times 0.03$

Chapter 10

Test 1: Infants and Children Dosage Problems

1. Safe dose 0.5 mg to 1 mg/dose IM. The order is safe.

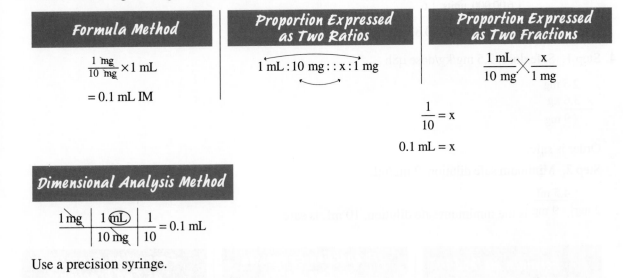

Formula Method	Proportion Expressed as Two Ratios	Proportion Expressed as Two Fractions
$\frac{1 \ \text{mg}}{10 \ \text{mg}} \times 1 \ \text{mL}$ $= 0.1 \ \text{mL IM}$	$1 \ \text{mL} : 10 \ \text{mg} :: \text{x} : 1 \ \text{mg}$	$\frac{1 \ \text{mL}}{10 \ \text{mg}} \times \frac{\text{x}}{1 \ \text{mg}}$

$$\frac{1}{10} = \text{x}$$

$$0.1 \ \text{mL} = \text{x}$$

Dimensional Analysis Method

$$\frac{1 \ \text{mg}}{} \ \bigg| \ \frac{1 \ \text{mL}}{10 \ \text{mg}} \ \bigg| \ \frac{1}{10} = 0.1 \ \text{mL}$$

Use a precision syringe.

2. Safe dose: 20 to 40 mg/kg/24 hours given q8h.

Low Dose	High Dose
20 mg	40 mg
× 10 kg	× 10 kg
200 mg/24 h	400 mg/24 h

Order is 125 mg q8h (3 doses).

125 mg × 3 doses = 375. Dose is safe.

No math necessary. Supply is 125 mg/5 mL.

Give 5 mL.

3. Safe dose: 50,000 units/kg × 1 dose

50,000 units
×   10 kg
500,000 units

The order is safe.

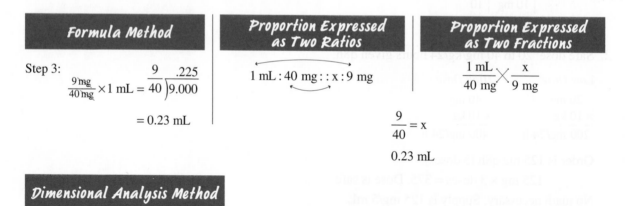

Formula Method	**Proportion Expressed as Two Ratios**	**Proportion Expressed as Two Fractions**
$\dfrac{500{,}000 \text{ units}}{600{,}000 \text{ units}} \times 1 \text{ mL} = \dfrac{5}{6} = 0.83 \text{ mL}$	1 mL : 600,000 units : : x : 500,000 units	$\dfrac{1 \text{ mL}}{600{,}000 \text{ units}} \times \dfrac{\text{x}}{500{,}000 \text{ units}}$

$$\frac{500{,}000}{600{,}000} = \text{x}$$

0.83 mL

Dimensional Analysis Method

$$\frac{500{,}000 \text{ units}}{} \left| \frac{1 \text{ mL}}{600{,}000 \text{ units}} \right| \frac{5}{6} = 0.83 \text{ mL}$$

Use a precision syringe. Give 0.83 mL IM.

4. Step 1. Safe dose: 2.5 mg/kg/dose q8h

$$\begin{array}{r} 2.5 \text{ mg} \\ \times\ 3.6 \text{ kg} \\ \hline 9 \text{ mg} \end{array}$$

Order is safe.

Step 2. Minimum safe dilution: 2 mg/mL

$$2 \text{ mg}\overline{)\ 9 \text{ mg}}^{\ 4.5 \text{ mL}}$$ is the minimum safe dilution. 10 mL is safe.

Formula Method	**Proportion Expressed as Two Ratios**	**Proportion Expressed as Two Fractions**
Step 3: $\dfrac{9 \text{ mg}}{40 \text{ mg}} \times 1 \text{ mL} = 40\overline{)9.000}^{\ .225}$ $= 0.23 \text{ mL}$	1 mL : 40 mg : : x : 9 mg	$\dfrac{1 \text{ mL}}{40 \text{ mg}} \times \dfrac{\text{x}}{9 \text{ mg}}$

$$\frac{9}{40} = \text{x}$$

0.23 mL

Dimensional Analysis Method

$$\frac{9 \text{ mg}}{} \left| \frac{1 \text{ mL}}{40 \text{ mg}} \right| \frac{9}{40} = 0.23 \text{ mL}$$

Use a precision syringe to draw up 0.23 mL.

Step 4. Add about 5 mL D5½NS to the Buretrol. Add the 0.23 mL drug. Add more D5½NS to make 10 mL.

Step 5. Set the pump at 20 because 20 mL in 1 hour will deliver the 10 mL in 30 min.

Step 6. When the IV is completed, add a flush of 20 mL D5½NS to the Buretrol to clear the tubing of medication.

5. Safe dose: infants and children younger than 3 years: 10 to 40 mg. The dose is safe.

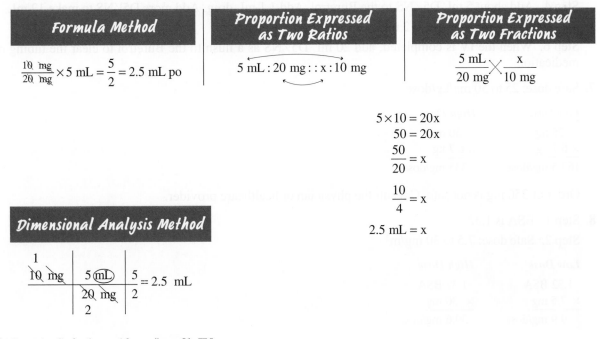

Formula Method	Proportion Expressed as Two Ratios	Proportion Expressed as Two Fractions
$\dfrac{10 \text{ mg}}{20 \text{ mg}} \times 5 \text{ mL} = \dfrac{5}{2} = 2.5 \text{ mL po}$	$5 \text{ mL} : 20 \text{ mg} :: x : 10 \text{ mg}$	$\dfrac{5 \text{ mL}}{20 \text{ mg}} \times \dfrac{x}{10 \text{ mg}}$

$$5 \times 10 = 20x$$
$$50 = 20x$$
$$\frac{50}{20} = x$$
$$\frac{10}{4} = x$$
$$2.5 \text{ mL} = x$$

Dimensional Analysis Method

$$\frac{1}{\cancel{10} \text{ mg}} \left| \frac{5 \text{ mL}}{\cancel{20} \text{ mg}} \right| \frac{5}{2} = 2.5 \text{ mL}$$

6. Step 1. Safe dose: 10 mg/kg q8h IV

$$\begin{array}{r} 10 \text{ mg} \\ \times\ 5.5 \text{ kg} \\ \hline 55 \text{ mg q8h} \end{array}$$

Dose is safe.

Step 2. Minimum safe dilution: 5 mg/mL; infuse over 1 hour.

$$5 \text{ mg}\overline{)54 \text{ mg}}^{\,10.8 \text{ mL}} = 11 \text{ mL}; \text{ infuse over 1 hour}$$

Step 3. To the 500-mg powder add 10 mL sterile water for injection to make 50 mg/mL.

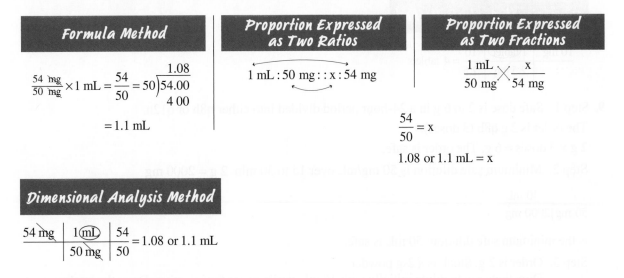

Formula Method	Proportion Expressed as Two Ratios	Proportion Expressed as Two Fractions
$\dfrac{54 \text{ mg}}{50 \text{ mg}} \times 1 \text{ mL} = \dfrac{54}{50} = 50\overline{)54.00}^{\,1.08}$ $\dfrac{4\ 00}{}$ $= 1.1 \text{ mL}$	$1 \text{ mL} : 50 \text{ mg} :: x : 54 \text{ mg}$	$\dfrac{1 \text{ mL}}{50 \text{ mg}} \times \dfrac{x}{54 \text{ mg}}$ $\dfrac{54}{50} = x$ $1.08 \text{ or } 1.1 \text{ mL} = x$

Dimensional Analysis Method

$$\frac{54 \text{ mg}}{} \left| \frac{1 \text{ mL}}{50 \text{ mg}} \right| \frac{54}{50} = 1.08 \text{ or } 1.1 \text{ mL}$$

Withdraw 1.1 mL of the drug, label the vial, refrigerate.

Step 4. Add about 5 mL D5½NS to the Buretrol. Add 1.1 mL drug. Add more D5½NS to make 12 mL.

Step 5. Set the pump for 12 (12 mL over 1 hour).

Step 6. When the IV is completed, add 20 mL D5½NS as a flush to the Buretrol to clear the tubing of medication.

7. Safe dose: 25 to 50 mg/kg/dose

Low Dose	*High Dose*
25 mg	50 mg
× 6.7 kg	× 6.7 kg
167.5 mg/dose	335 mg/dose

Order of 350 mg is not safe. Consult the physician or healthcare provider.

8. Step 1. BSA is 1.32

Step 2. Safe dose: 7.5 to 30 mg/m²

Low Dose	*High Dose*
1.32 BSA	1.32 BSA
× 7.5 mg	× 30 mg
9.9 mg/dose	39.6 mg/dose

Step 3. Order is 10 mg. Dose is safe.

Step 4.

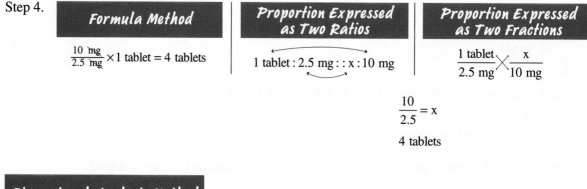

Formula Method	**Proportion Expressed as Two Ratios**	**Proportion Expressed as Two Fractions**
$\frac{10 \text{ mg}}{2.5 \text{ mg}} \times 1 \text{ tablet} = 4 \text{ tablets}$	$1 \text{ tablet} : 2.5 \text{ mg} : : x : 10 \text{ mg}$	$\frac{1 \text{ tablet}}{2.5 \text{ mg}} \times \frac{x}{10 \text{ mg}}$

$$\frac{10}{2.5} = x$$

4 tablets

Dimensional Analysis Method

$$\frac{10 \text{ mg}}{} \quad \frac{1 \text{ tablet}}{2.5 \text{ mg}} \quad \frac{10}{2.5} = 4 \text{ tablets}$$

9. Step 1: Safe dose is 2 to 6 g in a 24-hour period divided into either q8h or q12h.

The order is 2 g q8h (3 doses).

2 g × 3 doses = 6 g. The order is safe.

Step 2. Minimum safe dilution is 50 mg/mL over 15 to 30 min. 2 g = 2000 mg

$$50 \text{ mg} \overline{)2000 \text{ mg}}^{40 \text{ mL}}$$

is the minimum safe dilution: 50 mL is safe.

Step 3. Order is 2 g. Stock is a 2-g powder.
Directions say to dilute initially with 10 mL sterile water for injection. Draw the total amount into a syringe.

Step 4. Add about 20 mL D5⅓NS to the Buretrol. Add the medication from the syringe. Then add more D5½NS to make 50 mL.

Step 5. Set the pump for 100. It will deliver 50 mL in 30 min.

Step 6. When the IV is completed, add 20 mL D5½NS as a flush to the Buretrol to clear the tubing of medication.

10. Usual dose is 1 to 1.5 mg/kg/dose.

$$\frac{35 \text{ lb}}{2.2} = 15.91 \text{ kg}$$

Low Dose

$$\begin{array}{r} 1 \text{ mg} \\ \times 15.91 \text{ kg} \\ \hline 15.91 \text{ mg/dose} \end{array}$$

High Dose

$$\begin{array}{r} 1.5 \text{ mg} \\ \times 15.91 \text{ kg} \\ \hline 23.87 \text{ mg/dose} \end{array}$$

20 mg is a safe dose.

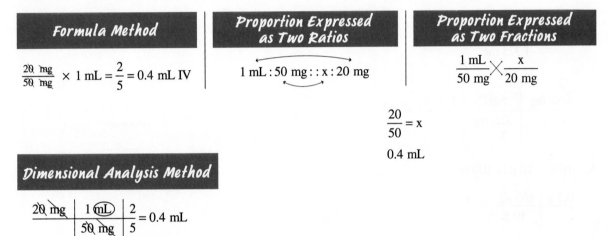

Formula Method

$$\frac{20 \text{ mg}}{50 \text{ mg}} \times 1 \text{ mL} = \frac{2}{5} = 0.4 \text{ mL IV}$$

Proportion Expressed as Two Ratios

$$1 \text{ mL} : 50 \text{ mg} :: x : 20 \text{ mg}$$

Proportion Expressed as Two Fractions

$$\frac{1 \text{ mL}}{50 \text{ mg}} \times \frac{x}{20 \text{ mg}}$$

$$\frac{20}{50} = x$$

0.4 mL

Dimensional Analysis Method

$$\frac{20 \text{ mg}}{} \left| \frac{1 \text{ mL}}{50 \text{ mg}} \right| \frac{2}{5} = 0.4 \text{ mL}$$

Use a precision syringe to draw up 0.4 mL. Follow hospital policy to give Demerol IVP.

Chapter 11

Test 1: Dimensional Analysis

1. $\dfrac{500 \text{ mg}}{} \left| \dfrac{5 \text{ mL}}{125 \text{ mg}} \right.$

$$\frac{\overset{4}{500 \text{ mg}}}{} \left| \frac{5 \text{ mL}}{\underset{1}{125 \text{ mg}}} \right| \frac{4 \times 5}{} = 20 \text{ mL}$$

2. $\dfrac{5000 \text{ units}}{} \left| \dfrac{1 \text{ mL}}{10000 \text{ units}} \right.$

$$\frac{\overset{1}{5000 \text{ units}}}{} \left| \frac{1 \text{ mL}}{\underset{2}{10000 \text{ units}}} \right| \frac{1}{2} = \frac{1}{2} \text{ or } 0.5 \text{ mL}$$

3. $\dfrac{20 \text{ mg}}{} \bigg| \dfrac{4 \text{ mL}}{40 \text{ mg}}$

$\dfrac{\overset{1}{\cancel{20} \text{ mg}}}{} \bigg| \dfrac{4 \text{ } \cancel{\text{mL}}}{\underset{2}{\cancel{40} \text{ mg}}} \bigg| \dfrac{4}{2} = 2 \text{ mL}$

4. $\dfrac{0.25 \text{ mg}}{} \bigg| \dfrac{1 \text{ tablet}}{0.125 \text{ mg}}$

$\dfrac{\overset{2}{\cancel{0.25} \text{ mg}}}{} \bigg| \dfrac{1 \text{ } \cancel{\text{tablet}}}{\underset{1}{\cancel{0.125} \text{ mg}}} \bigg| \dfrac{2 \times 1}{} = 2 \text{ tablets}$

5. $\dfrac{650 \text{ mg}}{} \bigg| \dfrac{5 \text{ mL}}{325 \text{ mg}}$

$\dfrac{\overset{2}{\cancel{650} \text{ mg}}}{} \bigg| \dfrac{5 \text{ } \cancel{\text{mL}}}{\underset{1}{\cancel{325} \text{ mg}}} \bigg| \dfrac{2 \times 5}{} = 10 \text{ mL}$

6. $10\% = 10 \text{ g in } 100 \text{ mL}$

$\dfrac{0.5 \text{ g}}{} \bigg| \dfrac{100 \text{ mL}}{10 \text{ g}}$

$\dfrac{\overset{1}{\cancel{0.5} \text{ g}}}{} \bigg| \dfrac{100 \text{ } \cancel{\text{mL}}}{\underset{20}{\cancel{10} \text{ g}}} \bigg| \dfrac{100}{20} = 5 \text{ mL}$

7. $\dfrac{125 \text{ mcg}}{} \bigg| \dfrac{1 \text{ mL}}{0.25 \text{ mg}} \bigg| \dfrac{1 \text{ mg}}{1000 \text{ mcg}}$

$\dfrac{\overset{1}{\cancel{125} \text{ mcg}}}{} \bigg| \dfrac{1 \text{ } \cancel{\text{mL}}}{0.25 \text{ mg}} \bigg| \dfrac{1 \text{ } \cancel{\text{mg}}}{\underset{8}{\cancel{1000} \text{ mcg}}} \bigg| \dfrac{1 \times 1 \times 1}{0.25 \times 8} = \dfrac{1}{2} \text{ or } 0.5 \text{ mL}$

8. $\dfrac{375 \text{ mg}}{} \bigg| \dfrac{5 \text{ mL}}{125 \text{ mg}} \bigg| \dfrac{1 \text{ tsp}}{5 \text{ mL}}$

$\dfrac{\overset{15}{\cancel{375} \text{ mg}}}{} \bigg| \dfrac{5 \text{ } \cancel{\text{mL}}}{\underset{5}{\cancel{125} \text{ mg}}} \bigg| \dfrac{1 \text{ } \cancel{\text{tsp}}}{5 \text{ } \cancel{\text{mL}}} \bigg| \dfrac{15 \times 5 \times 1}{5 \times 5} = \dfrac{75}{25} \text{ or } 3 \text{ tsp}$

9. $\dfrac{\frac{1}{150}\ \text{g}}{}$ | $\dfrac{1\ \text{tablet}}{0.4\ \text{mg}}$ | $\dfrac{60\ \text{mg}}{1\ \text{grain}}$

$\dfrac{\frac{1}{150}\ \cancel{\text{g}}}{}\ \Big|\ \dfrac{1\ \cancel{\text{tablet}}}{0.4\ \cancel{\text{mg}}}\ \Big|\ \dfrac{60\ \cancel{\text{mg}}}{1\ \cancel{\text{grain}}}\ \Big|\ \dfrac{\frac{1}{150}\times 60}{0.4}=\dfrac{\frac{60}{150}}{0.4}=\dfrac{0.4}{0.4}=1\ \text{tablet}$

10. Use 1 gr = 65 mg for Tylenol

$\dfrac{5\ \text{grain}}{}\ \Big|\ \dfrac{5\ \text{mL}}{325\ \text{mg}}\ \Big|\ \dfrac{65\ \text{mg}}{1\ \text{grain}}$

$\dfrac{\overset{1}{\cancel{5}}\ \cancel{\text{grain}}}{}\ \Big|\ \dfrac{5\ \text{mL}}{\underset{\underset{1}{65}}{\cancel{325}}\ \cancel{\text{mg}}}\ \Big|\ \dfrac{\cancel{65}\ \cancel{\text{mg}}}{1\ \cancel{\text{grain}}}\ \Big|\ \dfrac{1\times 5\times 1}{1\times 1}=5\ \text{mL}$

11. $\dfrac{40\ \text{mg}}{\text{m}^2}\ \Big|\ \dfrac{0.44\ \text{m}^2}{}$

$\dfrac{40\ \text{mg}}{\cancel{\text{m}^2}}\ \Big|\ \dfrac{0.44\ \cancel{\text{m}^2}}{}\ \Big|\ \dfrac{40\times 0.44}{}=17.6\ \text{mg}$

12. $\dfrac{0.1\ \text{mg}}{\text{kg}}\ \Big|\ \dfrac{1\ \text{mL}}{10\ \text{mg}}\ \Big|\ \dfrac{32\ \text{lb}}{}\ \Big|\ \dfrac{1\ \text{kg}}{2.2\ \text{lb}}$

$\dfrac{0.2\ \text{mg}}{\text{kg}}\ \Big|\ \dfrac{1\ \text{mL}}{10\ \text{mg}}\ \Big|\ \dfrac{32\ \text{lb}}{}\ \Big|\ \dfrac{1\ \text{kg}}{2.2\ \text{lb}}$

$\dfrac{0.1\ \cancel{\text{mg}}}{\cancel{\text{kg}}}\ \Big|\ \dfrac{1\ \text{mL}}{10\ \cancel{\text{mg}}}\ \Big|\ \dfrac{32\ \cancel{\text{lb}}}{}\ \Big|\ \dfrac{1\ \cancel{\text{kg}}}{2.2\ \cancel{\text{lb}}}\ \Big|\ \dfrac{0.1\times 1\times 32\times 1}{10\times 2.2}\ \Big|\ \dfrac{3.2}{22}=\dfrac{3.2}{22}=0.15\ \text{mL}$

$\dfrac{\overset{1}{\cancel{0.2}}\ \cancel{\text{mcg}}}{\cancel{\text{kg}}}\ \Big|\ \dfrac{1\ \text{mL}}{10\ \cancel{\text{mg}}}\ \Big|\ \dfrac{32\ \cancel{\text{lb}}}{}\ \Big|\ \dfrac{1\ \cancel{\text{kg}}}{\underset{11}{\cancel{2.2}}\ \cancel{\text{lb}}}\ \Big|\ \dfrac{1\times 1\times 32}{10\times 11}=\dfrac{32}{110}=0.29\ \text{mL or } 0.3\ \text{mL}$

13. $\dfrac{0.44\ \text{g}}{}\ \Big|\ \dfrac{1\ \text{mL}}{330\ \text{mg}}\ \Big|\ \dfrac{1000\ \text{mg}}{1\ \text{g}}$

$\dfrac{0.44\ \cancel{\text{g}}}{}\ \Big|\ \dfrac{1\ \text{mL}}{\cancel{330}\ \cancel{\text{mg}}}\ \Big|\ \dfrac{\cancel{1000}\ \cancel{\text{mg}}}{1\ \cancel{\text{g}}}\ \Big|\ \dfrac{0.44\times 100}{33}=\dfrac{44}{33}=1.33\ \text{mL}$

14. $\dfrac{1{,}000{,}000\ \text{units}}{}\ \Big|\ \dfrac{1\ \text{mL}}{500{,}000\ \text{units}}$

$\dfrac{\overset{2}{\cancel{1{,}000{,}000}}\ \cancel{\text{units}}}{}\ \Big|\ \dfrac{1\ \text{mL}}{\underset{1}{\cancel{500{,}000}}\ \cancel{\text{units}}}\ \Big|\ \dfrac{2\times 1}{1}=2\ \text{mL}$

15. $\dfrac{500 \text{ mL}}{6 \text{ hr}}$

$\dfrac{500 \text{ mL}}{6 \text{ hr}} \bigg| \dfrac{500}{6} = 83.3 \text{ or } 83 \text{ mL/hr}$

16. $\dfrac{1000 \text{ mL}}{16 \text{ hr}}$

$\dfrac{1000 \text{ mL}}{16 \text{ hr}} \bigg| \dfrac{1000}{16} = 62.5 \text{ or } 63 \text{ mL/hr}$

17. $\dfrac{1000 \text{ mL}}{10 \text{ hr}} \bigg| \dfrac{60 \text{ gtt}}{1 \text{ mL}} \bigg| \dfrac{1 \text{ hr}}{60 \text{ min}}$

$\dfrac{\overset{100}{\cancel{1000} \text{ mL}}}{\underset{}{\cancel{10} \text{ hr}}} \bigg| \dfrac{60 \text{ gtt}}{1 \text{ mL}} \bigg| \dfrac{1 \text{ hr}}{\underset{1}{\cancel{60} \text{ min}}} \bigg| \dfrac{100 \times 1 \times 1}{1 \times 1 \times 1} = 100 \text{ gtt/min}$

18. $\dfrac{250 \text{ mL}}{2 \text{ hr}} \bigg| \dfrac{15 \text{ gtt}}{1 \text{ mL}} \bigg| \dfrac{1 \text{ hr}}{60 \text{ min}}$

$\dfrac{250 \text{ mL}}{2 \text{ hr}} \bigg| \dfrac{\overset{1}{\cancel{15} \text{ gtt}}}{1 \text{ mL}} \bigg| \dfrac{1 \text{ hr}}{\underset{4}{\cancel{60} \text{ min}}} \bigg| \dfrac{250 \times 1 \times 1}{2 \times 1 \times 4} = \dfrac{250}{8} = 31.25 \text{ or } 31 \text{ gtt/min}$

19. $\dfrac{5 \text{ units}}{\text{hr}} \bigg| \dfrac{\overset{1}{\cancel{125} \text{ mL}}}{\underset{1}{\cancel{125} \text{ units}}} \bigg| \dfrac{5}{} = 5 \text{ mL/hr}$

20. $\dfrac{1500 \text{ units}}{\text{hr}} \bigg| \dfrac{500 \text{ mL}}{25{,}000 \text{ units}}$

$\dfrac{1500 \text{ units}}{\text{hr}} \bigg| \dfrac{\overset{1}{\cancel{500} \text{ mL}}}{\underset{50}{\cancel{25{,}000} \text{ units}}} \bigg| \dfrac{1500}{50} = 30 \text{ mL/hr}$

21. $\dfrac{30 \text{ mL}}{\text{hr}} \bigg| \dfrac{25{,}000 \text{ units}}{250 \text{ mL}}$

$\dfrac{30 \text{ mL}}{\text{hr}} \bigg| \dfrac{\overset{100}{\cancel{25{,}000} \text{ units}}}{\underset{1}{\cancel{250} \text{ mL}}} \bigg| \dfrac{30 \times 100}{} = 3000 \text{ units/hr}$

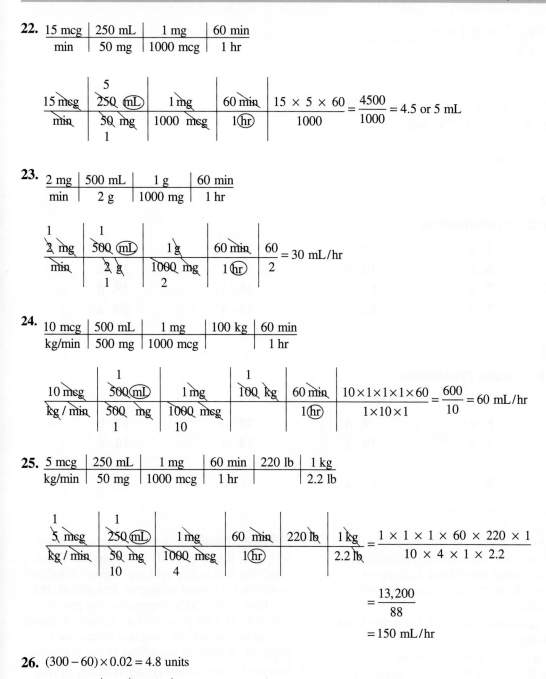

22. $\dfrac{15\ \text{mcg}}{\text{min}} \bigg| \dfrac{250\ \text{mL}}{50\ \text{mg}} \bigg| \dfrac{1\ \text{mg}}{1000\ \text{mcg}} \bigg| \dfrac{60\ \text{min}}{1\ \text{hr}}$

$$\dfrac{15\ \text{mcg}}{\text{min}} \bigg| \dfrac{\overset{5}{250}\ \text{mL}}{\underset{1}{50}\ \text{mg}} \bigg| \dfrac{1\ \text{mg}}{1000\ \text{mcg}} \bigg| \dfrac{60\ \text{min}}{1\ \text{hr}} \bigg| \dfrac{15 \times 5 \times 60}{1000} = \dfrac{4500}{1000} = 4.5\ \text{or}\ 5\ \text{mL}$$

23. $\dfrac{2\ \text{mg}}{\text{min}} \bigg| \dfrac{500\ \text{mL}}{2\ \text{g}} \bigg| \dfrac{1\ \text{g}}{1000\ \text{mg}} \bigg| \dfrac{60\ \text{min}}{1\ \text{hr}}$

$$\dfrac{\overset{1}{2}\ \text{mg}}{\text{min}} \bigg| \dfrac{\overset{1}{500}\ \text{mL}}{\underset{1}{2}\ \text{g}} \bigg| \dfrac{1\ \text{g}}{\underset{2}{1000}\ \text{mg}} \bigg| \dfrac{60\ \text{min}}{1\ \text{hr}} \bigg| \dfrac{60}{2} = 30\ \text{mL/hr}$$

24. $\dfrac{10\ \text{mcg}}{\text{kg/min}} \bigg| \dfrac{500\ \text{mL}}{500\ \text{mg}} \bigg| \dfrac{1\ \text{mg}}{1000\ \text{mcg}} \bigg| \dfrac{100\ \text{kg}}{} \bigg| \dfrac{60\ \text{min}}{1\ \text{hr}}$

$$\dfrac{10\ \text{mcg}}{\text{kg/min}} \bigg| \dfrac{\overset{1}{500}\ \text{mL}}{\underset{1}{500}\ \text{mg}} \bigg| \dfrac{1\ \text{mg}}{\underset{10}{1000}\ \text{mcg}} \bigg| \dfrac{\overset{1}{100}\ \text{kg}}{} \bigg| \dfrac{60\ \text{min}}{1\ \text{hr}} \bigg| \dfrac{10 \times 1 \times 1 \times 1 \times 60}{1 \times 10 \times 1} = \dfrac{600}{10} = 60\ \text{mL/hr}$$

25. $\dfrac{5\ \text{mcg}}{\text{kg/min}} \bigg| \dfrac{250\ \text{mL}}{50\ \text{mg}} \bigg| \dfrac{1\ \text{mg}}{1000\ \text{mcg}} \bigg| \dfrac{60\ \text{min}}{1\ \text{hr}} \bigg| \dfrac{220\ \text{lb}}{} \bigg| \dfrac{1\ \text{kg}}{2.2\ \text{lb}}$

$$\dfrac{\overset{1}{5}\ \text{mcg}}{\text{kg/min}} \bigg| \dfrac{\overset{1}{250}\ \text{mL}}{\underset{10}{50}\ \text{mg}} \bigg| \dfrac{1\ \text{mg}}{\underset{4}{1000}\ \text{mcg}} \bigg| \dfrac{60\ \text{min}}{1\ \text{hr}} \bigg| \dfrac{220\ \text{lb}}{} \bigg| \dfrac{1\ \text{kg}}{2.2\ \text{lb}} = \dfrac{1 \times 1 \times 1 \times 60 \times 220 \times 1}{10 \times 4 \times 1 \times 2.2}$$

$$= \dfrac{13{,}200}{88}$$

$$= 150\ \text{mL/hr}$$

26. $(300 - 60) \times 0.02 = 4.8\ \text{units}$

$$\dfrac{4.8\ \text{units}}{\text{hr}} \bigg| \dfrac{\overset{1}{100}\ \text{mL}}{\underset{1}{100}\ \text{units}} = 4.8\ \text{mL/hr}$$

27. $(400 - 60) \times 0.02 = 6.8\ \text{units}$

$$\dfrac{6.8\ \text{units}}{\text{hr}} \bigg| \dfrac{\overset{1}{100}\ \text{mL}}{\underset{1}{100}\ \text{units}} = 6.8\ \text{mL/hr}$$

28. $\dfrac{16\ \text{units}}{\text{kg/hr}} \bigg| \dfrac{50\ \text{kg}}{} \bigg| \dfrac{500\ \text{mL}}{\underset{50}{25000}\ \text{units}} \bigg| \dfrac{16 \times 50}{50} = 16\ \text{mL/hr}$

29. $\dfrac{60 \; \text{units}}{\text{kg}} \left| \dfrac{1 \; \text{kg}}{2.2 \; \text{lb}} \right| \dfrac{110 \; \text{lb}}{} \left| \dfrac{6600}{2.2} \right. = 3000 \; \text{units}$

30. $\dfrac{2 \; \text{units}}{\text{kg} \; / \; \text{hr}} \left| \dfrac{1 \; \text{kg}}{2.2 \; \text{lb}} \right| \dfrac{120 \; \text{lb}}{} \left| \dfrac{\overset{1}{500} \; \text{mL}}{\underset{50}{2500} \; \text{units}} \right. = \dfrac{2 \times 120}{2.2 \times 50} = 2.18 \; \text{or} \; 2.2 \; \text{mL/hr}$

$21.5 + 2.2 = 23.7 \; \text{mL/hr}$

Chapter 12

Test 1: Basic Drug Information

1. a	**5.** b	**9.** a	**13.** a	**17.** b
2. c	**6.** a	**10.** b	**14.** a	**18.** d
3. d	**7.** a	**11.** d	**15.** a	**19.** d
4. b	**8.** d	**12.** c	**16.** a	**20.** a

Chapter 13

Test 1: Administration Procedures

Part A

1. c	**5.** c	**9.** d	**13.** b	**17.** b
2. d	**6.** b	**10.** a	**14.** a	**18.** d
3. b	**7.** a	**11.** c	**15.** d	**19.** c
4. d	**8.** d	**12.** a	**16.** b	**20.** c

Part B

1. Correct. As the needle or catheter is removed, there is a possibility of bleeding at the site. In addition, the nurse should use a clamp to carry the needle or catheter to a puncture-proof container.

2. Incorrect. The nurse must wash his or her hands before leaving the room.

3. Incorrect. It is not necessary to wear gloves to prepare an IV because there is no contact at this time with the patient's blood or body fluids.

4. Correct. Standard precautions state that a mask must be worn when the patient is on strict or respiratory isolation precautions.

5. Correct. There is a potential risk of exposure to hepatitis B virus and HIV. Laboratory testing may not show the presence of the virus or antibodies to the virus.

6. Correct. Although transdermal pads are applied to intact skin, standard precaution require gloves.

7. Correct. In carrying out the vaginal douche there is a possibility of exposure to vaginal secretions.

8. Incorrect. The nurse should squeeze the finger and, after washing hands with soap and water, scrub the area with povidone–iodine (Betadine) or another accepted antiseptic. In addition, the needlestick should be reported to the proper authority and the protocol for exposure to blood should be carried out. Standard precautions apply to all patients regardless of the diagnosis.

9. Incorrect. There is always a possibility or risk when doing an invasive procedure such as an injection.

10. Incorrect. Because the patient is alert and can take the medicine cup from the nurse, hand-washing is adequate.

11. Incorrect. The CDC guidelines advise the nurse not to recap a needle, but to place it immediately in a puncture-proof container.

12. Correct. Nitroglycerin ointment is a potent vasodilator. Wearing gloves protects the nurse against the drug's effect.

13. Incorrect. The nurse's fingers may come in contact with mucous membrane in administering eye drops.

Putting It Together Answers

Chapter 6

Calculations

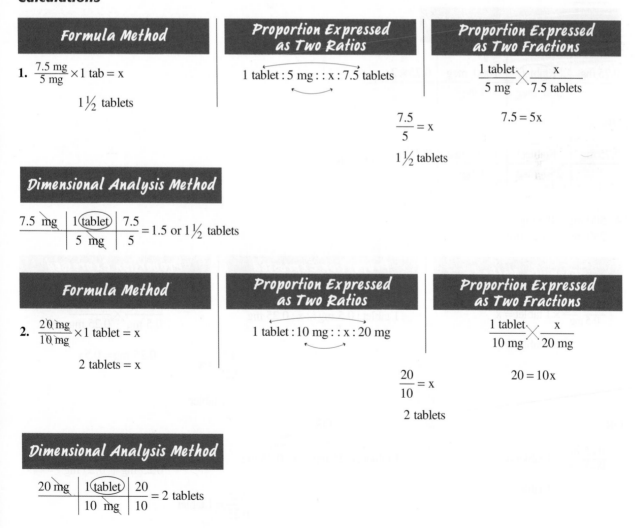

Formula Method	Proportion Expressed as Two Ratios	Proportion Expressed as Two Fractions
1. $\dfrac{7.5 \text{ mg}}{5 \text{ mg}} \times 1 \text{ tab} = x$	$1 \text{ tablet} : 5 \text{ mg} :: x : 7.5 \text{ tablets}$	$\dfrac{1 \text{ tablet}}{5 \text{ mg}} \times \dfrac{x}{7.5 \text{ tablets}}$
$1\frac{1}{2}$ tablets	$\dfrac{7.5}{5} = x$	$7.5 = 5x$
	$1\frac{1}{2}$ tablets	

Dimensional Analysis Method

$$\dfrac{7.5 \text{ mg}}{} \mid \dfrac{1 \text{ tablet}}{5 \text{ mg}} \mid \dfrac{7.5}{5} = 1.5 \text{ or } 1\frac{1}{2} \text{ tablets}$$

Formula Method	Proportion Expressed as Two Ratios	Proportion Expressed as Two Fractions
2. $\dfrac{20 \text{ mg}}{10 \text{ mg}} \times 1 \text{ tablet} = x$	$1 \text{ tablet} : 10 \text{ mg} :: x : 20 \text{ mg}$	$\dfrac{1 \text{ tablet}}{10 \text{ mg}} \times \dfrac{x}{20 \text{ mg}}$
$2 \text{ tablets} = x$	$\dfrac{20}{10} = x$	$20 = 10x$
	2 tablets	

Dimensional Analysis Method

$$\dfrac{20 \text{ mg}}{} \mid \dfrac{1 \text{ tablet}}{10 \text{ mg}} \mid \dfrac{20}{10} = 2 \text{ tablets}$$

3. 500 mcg = 0.5 mg
250 mcg = 0.25 mg

Formula Method	Proportion Expressed as Two Ratios	Proportion Expressed as Two Fractions

Formula Method

$$\frac{0.75 \text{ mg}}{0.5 \text{ mg}} \times 1 \text{ tablet} = x$$

$1\frac{1}{2}$ tablets

Proportion Expressed as Two Ratios

1 tablet : 0.5 mg : : x : 0.75 mg

Proportion Expressed as Two Fractions

$$\frac{1 \text{ tablet}}{0.5 \text{ mg}} \times \frac{x}{0.75 \text{ mg}}$$

$$0.75 \text{ mg} = 0.5x$$

$$\frac{0.75}{0.5} = x$$

$1\frac{1}{2}$ tablets

OR

$$\frac{0.75 \text{ mg}}{0.25 \text{ mg}} \times 1 \text{ tablet} = x$$

3 tablets

1 tablet : 1.25 mg : : x : 0.75 mg

$$\frac{1 \text{ tablet}}{0.25 \text{ mg}} \times \frac{x}{0.75 \text{ mg}}$$

$$0.75 \text{ mg} = 0.25x$$

$$\frac{0.75}{0.25} = x$$

3 tablets

Dimensional Analysis Method

$$\frac{0.75 \text{ mg}}{} \left| \frac{1 \text{ tablet}}{500 \text{ mcg}} \right|_{1}^{2} \frac{1000 \text{ mcg}}{1 \text{ mg}} \left| \frac{0.75 \times 2}{1} = 1.5 \right.$$

OR

$$\frac{0.75 \text{ mg}}{} \left| \frac{1 \text{ tablet}}{250 \text{ mcg}} \right|_{1}^{4} \frac{1000 \text{ mcg}}{1 \text{ mg}} \left| \frac{0.75 \times 4}{1} = 3 \text{ tablets} \right.$$

4. 500 mg = 0.5 mg
250 mcg = 0.25 mg

Formula Method	Proportion Expressed as Two Ratios	Proportion Expressed as Two Fractions

Formula Method

$$\frac{0.25 \text{ mg}}{0.5 \text{ mg}} \times 1 \text{ tablet} = x$$

$\frac{1}{2}$ tablet

Proportion Expressed as Two Ratios

1 tablet : 0.5 mg : : x : 0.25 mg

Proportion Expressed as Two Fractions

$$\frac{1 \text{ tablet}}{0.5 \text{ mg}} \times \frac{x}{0.25 \text{ mg}}$$

$$0.25 \text{ mg} = 0.5x$$

$$\frac{0.5}{0.25} = x$$

$\frac{1}{2}$ tablet

OR

$$\frac{0.25 \text{ mg}}{0.25 \text{ mg}} \times 1 \text{ tablet} = x$$

1 tablet

OR

1 tablet : 0.25 mg : : x : 0.25 mg

$$\frac{1 \text{ tablet}}{0.25 \text{ mg}} \times \frac{x}{0.25 \text{ mg}}$$

$$\frac{0.25}{0.25} = 1 \text{ tablet}$$

Dimensional Analysis Method

$$\frac{0.25\ \text{mg}}{} \left|\frac{1\ \text{tablet}}{500\ \text{mg}}\right|\frac{1000\ \text{mcg}}{1\ \text{mg}}\right| \frac{0.25 \times 2}{1} = 0.5 \text{ or } \tfrac{1}{2} \text{ tablet}$$

OR

$$\frac{0.25\ \text{mg}}{} \left|\frac{1\ \text{tablet}}{250\ \text{mcg}}\right|\frac{1000\ \text{mcg}}{1\ \text{mg}}\right| \frac{0.25 \times 4}{1} = 1 \text{ tablet}$$

5. 500 mcg = 0.5 mg
250 mcg = 0.25 mg

Formula Method	Proportion Expressed as Two Ratios	Proportion Expressed as Two Fractions

$$\frac{0.125\ \text{mg}}{0.5\ \text{mg}} \times 1 \text{ tablet} = x$$

0.25 or $\tfrac{1}{4}$ tablet = x

(may be unable to quarter the tablet)

1 tablet : 0.5 mg : : x : 0.125 mg

$$\frac{1\ \text{tablet}}{0.5\ \text{mg}} \times \frac{x}{0.125\ \text{mg}}$$

$$\frac{0.125\ \text{mg}}{0.5\ \text{mg}} = x$$

0.125 mg = 0.5x

0.25 or $\tfrac{1}{4}$ tablet

OR

$$\frac{0.125\ \text{mg}}{0.25\ \text{mg}} \times 1 \text{ tablet} = x$$

$\tfrac{1}{2}$ tablet

1 tablet : 0.25 mg : : x : 0.125 mg

$$\frac{1\ \text{tablet}}{0.25\ \text{mg}} \times \frac{x}{0.125\ \text{mg}}$$

$$\frac{0.125}{0.25} = x$$

0.125 = 0.25x

$\tfrac{1}{2}$ tablet

Dimensional Analysis Method

$$\frac{0.125\ \text{mg}}{} \left|\frac{1\ \text{tablet}}{500\ \text{mg}}\right|\frac{1000\ \text{mg}}{1\ \text{mg}}\right| \frac{0.125 \times 2}{1} = 0.25 \text{ or } \tfrac{1}{2} \text{ tablet}$$

OR

$$\frac{0.125\ \text{mg}}{} \left|\frac{1\ \text{tablet}}{250\ \text{mg}}\right|\frac{1000\ \text{mg}}{1\ \text{mg}}\right| \frac{0.125 \times 4}{1} = \tfrac{1}{2} \text{ tablet}$$

Formula Method	Proportion Expressed as Two Ratios	Proportion Expressed as Two Fractions
6. $\dfrac{15 \ \cancel{mEq}}{10 \ \cancel{mEq}} \times 750 \ mg = x$	$750 \ mg : 10 \ mEq :: x : 15 \ mEq$	$\dfrac{750 \ mg}{10 \ mEq} \diagdown \dfrac{x}{15 \ mEq}$
$1{,}125 \ mg$		$750 \times 15 = 10x$
		$\dfrac{11{,}250}{10} = x$
		$1{,}125 \ mg$

Dimensional Analysis Method

$$\frac{\overset{3}{\cancel{15}} \ \cancel{mEq}}{\underset{2}{\cancel{10}} \ \cancel{mEq}} \ \bigg| \ \frac{750 \ \boxed{mg}}{} \ \bigg| \ \frac{750 \times 3}{2} = 1{,}125 \ mg$$

Formula Method	Proportion Expressed as Two Ratios	Proportion Expressed as Two Fractions
7. $0.25 \ mg = 250 \ mcg$	$1 \ tablet : 125 \ mg :: x : 250 \ mcg$	$\dfrac{1 \ tablet}{125 \ mcg} \diagdown \dfrac{x}{250 \ mg}$
$\quad 0.5 \ mg = 500 \ mcg$		
$\dfrac{250 \ \cancel{mcg}}{125 \ \cancel{mcg}} \times 1 \ tablet = x$		$250 = 125x$
$\quad 2 \ tablets$		$\dfrac{250}{125} = 2 \ tablets$
$\dfrac{500 \ \cancel{mcg}}{125 \ \cancel{mcg}} \times 1 \ tablet = x$		
$\quad 4 \ tablets$		
	$1 \ tablet : 125 \ mg :: x : 500 \ mg$	$\dfrac{1 \ tablet}{125 \ mg} \diagdown \dfrac{x}{500 \ mg}$
		$500 = 125x$
		$\dfrac{500}{125} = x$
		$4 \ tablets$

Dimensional Analysis Method

$$\frac{0.25 \ \cancel{mg}}{} \ \bigg| \ \frac{1 \ \boxed{tablet}}{125 \ \underset{1}{\cancel{mcg}}} \ \bigg| \ \frac{\overset{8}{\cancel{1000}} \ \cancel{mcg}}{1 \ \cancel{mg}} \ \bigg| \ \frac{0.25 \times 8}{} = 2 \ tablets$$

$$\frac{0.5 \ \cancel{mg}}{} \ \bigg| \ \frac{1 \ \boxed{tablet}}{125 \ \underset{1}{\cancel{mcg}}} \ \bigg| \ \frac{\overset{8}{\cancel{1000}} \ \cancel{mcg}}{1 \ \cancel{mg}} \ \bigg| \ \frac{0.5 \times 8}{} = 4 \ tablets$$

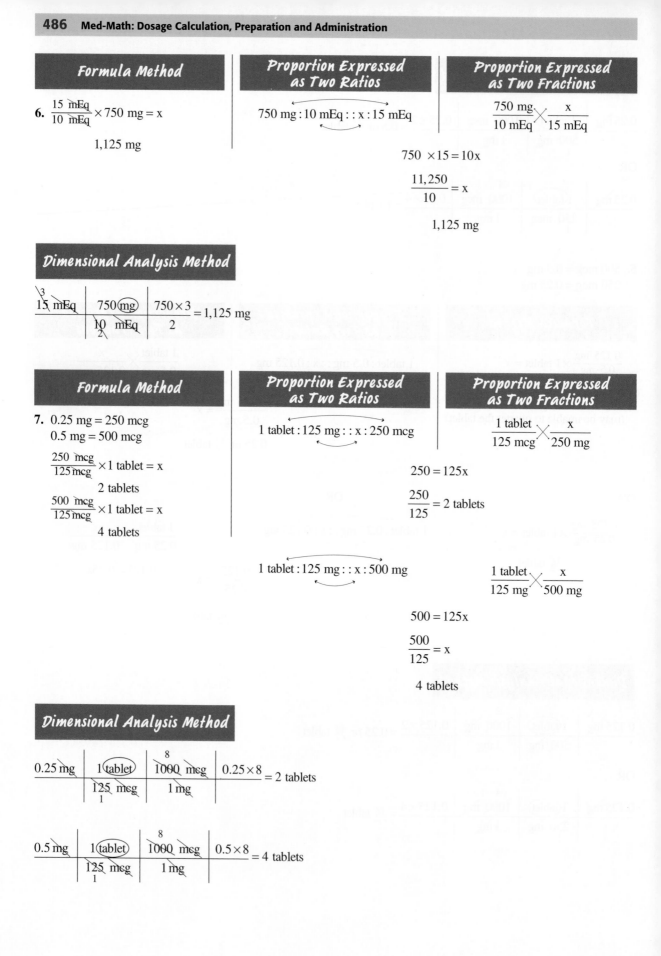

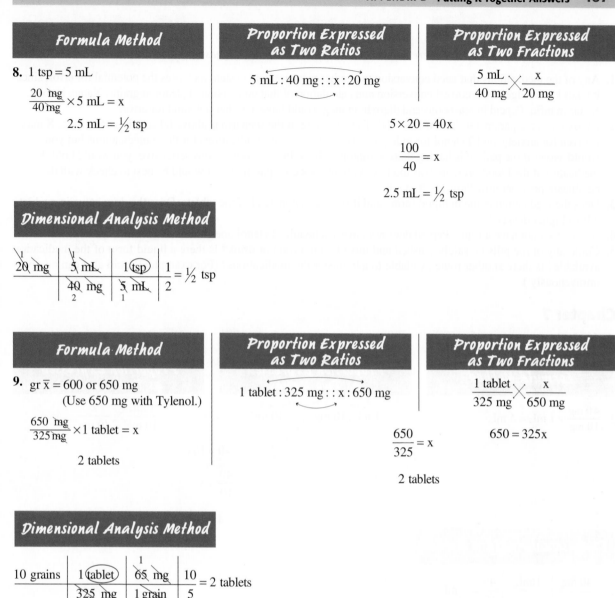

Formula Method	**Proportion Expressed as Two Ratios**	**Proportion Expressed as Two Fractions**
8. 1 tsp = 5 mL	5 mL : 40 mg : : x : 20 mg	$\dfrac{5\ mL}{40\ mg} \times \dfrac{x}{20\ mg}$
$\dfrac{20\ mg}{40\ mg} \times 5\ mL = x$		$5 \times 20 = 40x$
2.5 mL = ½ tsp		$\dfrac{100}{40} = x$
		2.5 mL = ½ tsp

Dimensional Analysis Method

$$\dfrac{20\ mg}{} \left| \dfrac{5\ mL}{40\ mg} \right| \dfrac{1\ tsp}{5\ mL} \left| \dfrac{1}{2} = \frac{1}{2}\ tsp \right.$$

Formula Method	**Proportion Expressed as Two Ratios**	**Proportion Expressed as Two Fractions**
9. gr x̄ = 600 or 650 mg (Use 650 mg with Tylenol.)	1 tablet : 325 mg : : x : 650 mg	$\dfrac{1\ tablet}{325\ mg} \times \dfrac{x}{650\ mg}$
$\dfrac{650\ mg}{325\ mg} \times 1\ tablet = x$		$650 = 325x$
2 tablets	$\dfrac{650}{325} = x$	
	2 tablets	

Dimensional Analysis Method

$$\dfrac{10\ grains}{} \left| \dfrac{1\ tablet}{325\ mg} \right| \dfrac{65\ mg}{1\ grain} \left| \dfrac{10}{5} = 2\ tablets \right.$$

Formula Method	**Proportion Expressed as Two Ratios**	**Proportion Expressed as Two Fractions**
10. 1 Gm = 1000 mg	1 tablet : 200 mg : : x : 1000 mg	$\dfrac{1\ tablet}{200\ mg} \times \dfrac{x}{1000\ mg}$
$\dfrac{1000\ mg}{200\ mg} \times 1\ tablet = x$		$1000 = 200x$
4 tablets	$\dfrac{1000}{200} = x$	
	4 tablets	

Dimensional Analysis Method

$$\dfrac{1\ Gm}{} \left| \dfrac{1\ tablet}{200\ mg} \right| \dfrac{1000\ mg}{1\ Gm} \left| \dfrac{4}{} = 4\ tablets \right.$$

Critical Thinking Questions

The "answers" are suggested and there may be other correct comments, suggestions, and answers.

1. Any of the medications that need conversion to another measurement system increases the potential for error, since it takes knowledge of the correct conversion and calculation of that conversion. Tylenol in grains, Xanax in mcg, K-dur in mEq, Pepcid in teaspoons and digoxin in mcg would have a higher potential for error.
2. Digoxin has the parameter: hold if HR < 60. The heart rate in the scenario is above 60 so it is safe to give. Xanax is given for anxiety, and Tylenol for mild pain. There are no contraindications for these medications but you would assess if the patient is having these symptoms. Since Prinivil is an antihypertensive, you would hold the medication if the blood pressure was too low-without a specific parameter, it would be best to check with the healthcare provider how "low" is "too low."
3. Does the medication come in liquid form? and if so, use that instead of the tablets. Does the drug come in a tablet with a higher dosage?
4. Xanax does not have a route. Pepcid does not have a schedule. Tylenol does not have a route.
5. Could any of the pills be safely crushed and mixed with a food or drink? Is there a liquid form of the medication available? Is there another route available to administer the medications? (For example, Pepcid also can be given intravenously.)

Chapter 7

Calculations

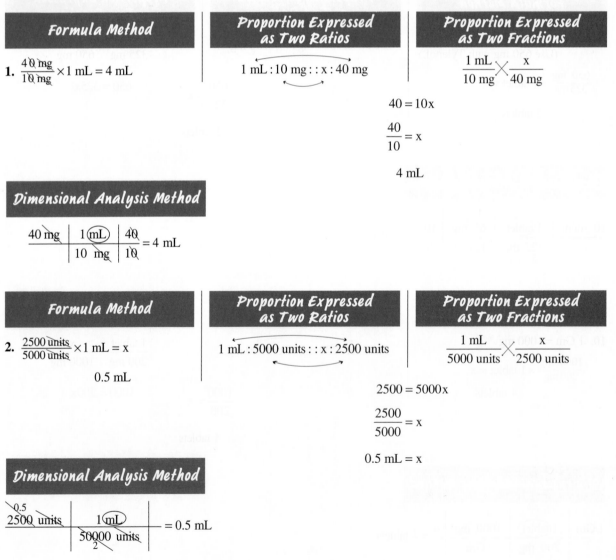

Formula Method	Proportion Expressed as Two Ratios	Proportion Expressed as Two Fractions
1. $\dfrac{40 \text{ mg}}{10 \text{ mg}} \times 1 \text{ mL} = 4 \text{ mL}$	$1 \text{ mL} : 10 \text{ mg} :: x : 40 \text{ mg}$	$\dfrac{1 \text{ mL}}{10 \text{ mg}} \times \dfrac{x}{40 \text{ mg}}$

$$40 = 10x$$

$$\frac{40}{10} = x$$

$$4 \text{ mL}$$

Dimensional Analysis Method

$$\frac{40 \text{ mg}}{} \mid \frac{1 \text{ mL}}{10 \text{ mg}} \mid \frac{40}{10} = 4 \text{ mL}$$

Formula Method	Proportion Expressed as Two Ratios	Proportion Expressed as Two Fractions
2. $\dfrac{2500 \text{ units}}{5000 \text{ units}} \times 1 \text{ mL} = x$	$1 \text{ mL} : 5000 \text{ units} :: x : 2500 \text{ units}$	$\dfrac{1 \text{ mL}}{5000 \text{ units}} \times \dfrac{x}{2500 \text{ units}}$
0.5 mL		

$$2500 = 5000x$$

$$\frac{2500}{5000} = x$$

$$0.5 \text{ mL} = x$$

Dimensional Analysis Method

$$\frac{\overset{0.5}{2500 \text{ units}}}{} \mid \frac{1 \text{ mL}}{\underset{2}{50000 \text{ units}}} = 0.5 \text{ mL}$$

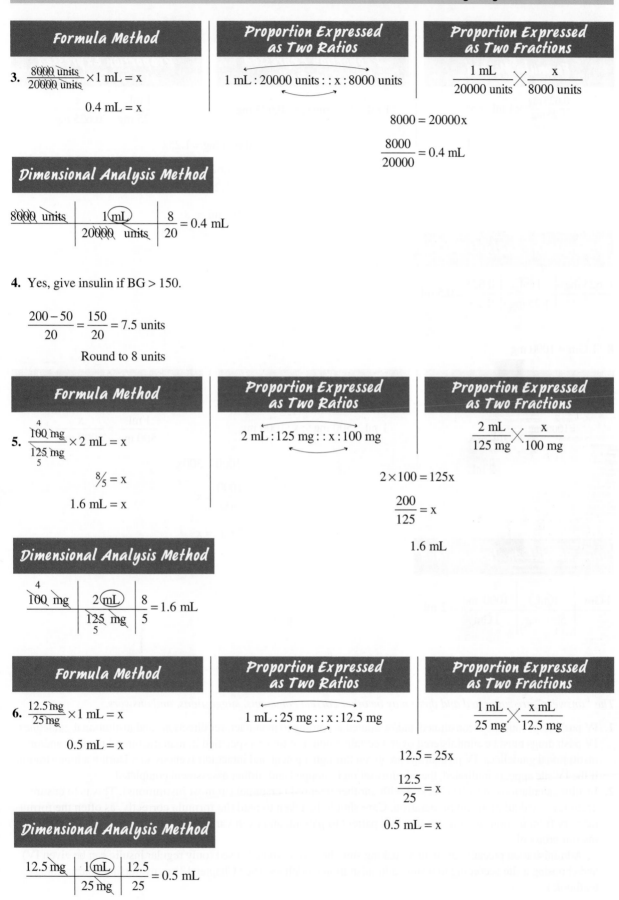

Formula Method

3. $\dfrac{8000 \text{ units}}{20000 \text{ units}} \times 1 \text{ mL} = x$

$0.4 \text{ mL} = x$

Proportion Expressed as Two Ratios

$1 \text{ mL} : 20000 \text{ units} :: x : 8000 \text{ units}$

Proportion Expressed as Two Fractions

$\dfrac{1 \text{ mL}}{20000 \text{ units}} \times \dfrac{x}{8000 \text{ units}}$

$8000 = 20000x$

$\dfrac{8000}{20000} = 0.4 \text{ mL}$

Dimensional Analysis Method

$\dfrac{8000 \text{ units}}{} \left| \dfrac{1 \text{ mL}}{20000 \text{ units}} \right| \dfrac{8}{20} = 0.4 \text{ mL}$

4. Yes, give insulin if BG > 150.

$\dfrac{200 - 50}{20} = \dfrac{150}{20} = 7.5 \text{ units}$

Round to 8 units

Formula Method

5. $\dfrac{\overset{4}{100} \text{ mg}}{\underset{5}{125} \text{ mg}} \times 2 \text{ mL} = x$

$\frac{8}{5} = x$

$1.6 \text{ mL} = x$

Proportion Expressed as Two Ratios

$2 \text{ mL} : 125 \text{ mg} :: x : 100 \text{ mg}$

Proportion Expressed as Two Fractions

$\dfrac{2 \text{ mL}}{125 \text{ mg}} \times \dfrac{x}{100 \text{ mg}}$

$2 \times 100 = 125x$

$\dfrac{200}{125} = x$

1.6 mL

Dimensional Analysis Method

$\dfrac{\overset{4}{100} \text{ mg}}{} \left| \dfrac{2 \text{ mL}}{\underset{5}{125} \text{ mg}} \right| \dfrac{8}{5} = 1.6 \text{ mL}$

Formula Method

6. $\dfrac{12.5 \text{ mg}}{25 \text{ mg}} \times 1 \text{ mL} = x$

$0.5 \text{ mL} = x$

Proportion Expressed as Two Ratios

$1 \text{ mL} : 25 \text{ mg} :: x : 12.5 \text{ mg}$

Proportion Expressed as Two Fractions

$\dfrac{1 \text{ mL}}{25 \text{ mg}} \times \dfrac{x \text{ mL}}{12.5 \text{ mg}}$

$12.5 = 25x$

$\dfrac{12.5}{25} = x$

$0.5 \text{ mL} = x$

Dimensional Analysis Method

$\dfrac{12.5 \text{ mg}}{} \left| \dfrac{1 \text{ mL}}{25 \text{ mg}} \right| \dfrac{12.5}{25} = 0.5 \text{ mL}$

7. Vasotec should be administered.

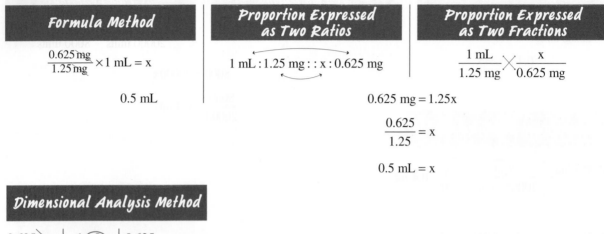

Formula Method	Proportion Expressed as Two Ratios	Proportion Expressed as Two Fractions

$$\frac{0.625\,mg}{1.25\,mg} \times 1\,mL = x$$

$$0.5\,mL$$

$$1\,mL : 1.25\,mg :: x : 0.625\,mg$$

$$\frac{1\,mL}{1.25\,mg} \times \frac{x}{0.625\,mg}$$

$$0.625\,mg = 1.25x$$

$$\frac{0.625}{1.25} = x$$

$$0.5\,mL = x$$

Dimensional Analysis Method

$$\frac{0.625\,mg}{} \mid \frac{1\,mL}{1.25\,mg} \mid \frac{0.625}{1.25} = 0.5\,mL$$

8. 1 Gm = 1000 mg

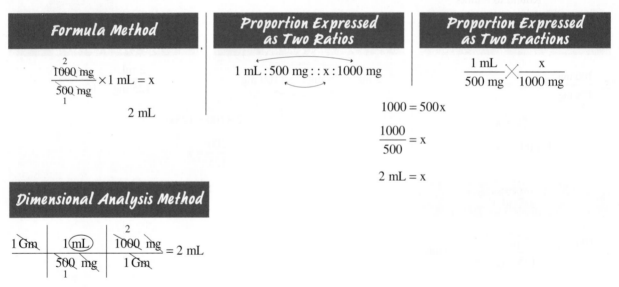

Formula Method	Proportion Expressed as Two Ratios	Proportion Expressed as Two Fractions

$$\frac{\overset{2}{1000}\,mg}{\underset{1}{500}\,mg} \times 1\,mL = x$$

$$2\,mL$$

$$1\,mL : 500\,mg :: x : 1000\,mg$$

$$\frac{1\,mL}{500\,mg} \times \frac{x}{1000\,mg}$$

$$1000 = 500x$$

$$\frac{1000}{500} = x$$

$$2\,mL = x$$

Dimensional Analysis Method

$$\frac{1\,Gm}{} \mid \frac{1\,mL}{500\,mg} \mid \frac{\overset{2}{1000}\,mg}{1\,Gm} = 2\,mL$$

Critical Thinking Questions

The "answers" are suggested and there may be other correct comments, suggestions, and answers.

1. IV push drugs must be reconstituted and/or diluted according to manufacturer directions and institutional guidelines. IV push drugs must be administered over a certain amount of time as specified in manufacturer directions and/or institutional guidelines. IV push drugs are given through a patent and intact intravenous site. During administration, if the IV site appears infiltrated, the administration is stopped and further assessment completed.

2. Insulin calculations must be checked with another licensed personnel (in most institutions). This is to ensure accuracy in calculation and preparation. Care should be taken to read the formula correctly, as often the formulas vary from institution to institution and patient to patient, and even varies with one patient depending on the insulin protocol.

Administration precautions include making sure the correct route is used (only regular insulin can be given IV) and choosing a site according to insulin administration guidelines. (See Chapter 13 or any nursing pharmacology textbook.)

3. Insulin dosages can be miscalculated as with any drug. "U" must be written as units per The Joint Commission "do not use" abbreviations as the "u" can be mistaken for a number. If the sliding scale formula changes (as it often does depending on the patient's glucose level), then care must be taken to use the new formula and calculate the new dose correctly.

4. Heparin doses can be miscalculated as with any drug. "U" must be written as units per The Joint Commission "do not use" abbreviations as the "u" can be mistaken for a number. Heparin comes in two different strengths, 10000 units in 1 mL and 1000 units in 1 mL and these are often mistaken as the vials are very similar. Many institutions require two licensed personnel to double check the heparin dose.

5. Type 2 diabetics often experience higher glucose levels and more variance of their glucose level in the hospital because it is a more stressful situation physically and emotionally, increasing the glucocorticoids in their body and therefore raising their blood glucose. This patient is also on Solu-Medrol and any exogenous steroid will raise blood glucose.

6. Phenergan should be held as it is listed under the patient's drug allergies. The patient has a history of renal cell carcinoma a nephrectomy—an assessment of renal function needs to be done. Medications that may need to be given in a lower dose would include Lasix, and Vancomycin. These two drugs may also need to be given at separate times because of the renal involvement. The PTT needs to be checked to determine the safe dose of Heparin.

Chapter 8

Calculations

1. $\dfrac{100 \text{ mL} \times \cancel{60} \text{ gtt}}{\cancel{60} \text{ min}} = 100 \text{ gtt/min}$

$\dfrac{100 \text{ mL} \times \overset{1}{\cancel{20}}}{\underset{3}{\cancel{60}} \text{ min}} = \dfrac{100}{3} = 33.33 \text{ or } 33 \text{ gtt/min}$

2. $\dfrac{100 \text{ mL} \times \overset{2}{\cancel{60}} \text{ gtt}}{\underset{1}{\cancel{30}} \text{ min}} = 200 \text{ gtt/min}$

$\dfrac{100 \text{ mL} \times \cancel{20} \text{ gtt}}{\cancel{30} \text{ min}} = \dfrac{200}{3} = 66.66 \text{ or } 67 \text{ gtt/min}$

3. $\dfrac{50 \text{ mL} \times \overset{2}{\cancel{60}} \text{ gtt}}{\underset{1}{\cancel{30}} \text{ minutes}} = 100 \text{ gtt/min}$

(guidelines: infuse 50 mL over 30 minutes if no direction is given)

$\dfrac{50 \text{ mL} \times \cancel{15} \text{ gtt}}{\underset{2}{\cancel{30}} \text{ minutes}} = \dfrac{50}{2} = 25 \text{ gtt/min}$

4. $\dfrac{1000 \text{ mL}}{40 \text{ mL}} = 25 \text{ hours}$

5. Gentamicin   100 mL (daily)   NS   40 mL/hr × 20.5 hours
    Cubicin   100 mL (daily)   (24 hours − 3.5 hours that
    Zosyn   50 mL   antibiotics are running)

$$\underline{\times\ \ 4\ \ \ }\text{(6 hours = 4 doses)}$$
$$200\ \text{mL}$$

$$40\ \text{mL/hr}$$
$$\underline{\times\ 20.5\ \text{hr}}$$
$$820\ \text{mL}$$

Total intake: 1020 mL

Critical Thinking Questions

The "answers" are suggested and there may be other correct comments, suggestions, and answers.

1. The patient complains of nausea and vomiting. The PO medications may be held and/or another route substituted (check with physician or healthcare provider for an order). Prinivil and Procardia should be held because of the low blood pressure and physician or healthcare provider notified.
2. Each antibiotic works against different organisms (note the suffixes in the names—cillin, -mycin, -micin—they are each a different category of antiinfective). The cause of the infection may not be known yet (usually dependent on the results of cultures) and so the three antibiotics together would kill most bacteria. After the cause of the infection is known, then perhaps only one antibiotic would be used.
3. 40 mL × 6 hours = 240 mL. The IV solution may not be infusing at the correct rate due to miscalculation of rate (if using gtts/min) or setting the wrong rate on the infusion pump. If the infusion is running by gravity, then the patient's position can affect the flow rate. If the patient only has one IV infusion site, then the primary fluid (NS) will be stopped when the antibiotics are infusing.
4. Yes, the dose is 20 mg. The order reads "if over 10 mg must be IVPB." Mix in 50 mL and give over 30 minutes. (If direction is not given as to amount and rate, use 50 mL as a minimum amount over 30 minutes.)

Chapter 9

Calculations

1. 30 mg in 500 mL D5W

$$\frac{30\ \text{mg}}{500\ \text{mL}} = 0.06\ \text{mg/mL}$$

$$0.06\ \text{mg} \times 1000\ \text{mcg} = 60\ \text{mcg/mL}$$

2. Dose 100 mcg/min

$$100\ \text{mcg} \times 60\ \text{min} = 6000\ \text{mcg/hr}$$

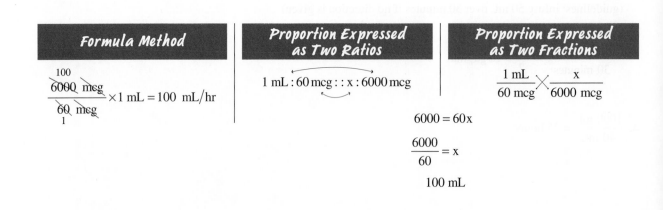

Formula Method	Proportion Expressed as Two Ratios	Proportion Expressed as Two Fractions
$$\frac{\overset{100}{\cancel{6000}\ \text{mcg}}}{\underset{1}{\cancel{60}\ \text{mcg}}} \times 1\ \text{mL} = 100\ \text{mL/hr}$$	$$1\ \text{mL} : 60\ \text{mcg} :: x : 6000\ \text{mcg}$$	$$\frac{1\ \text{mL}}{60\ \text{mcg}} \times \frac{x}{6000\ \text{mcg}}$$ $$6000 = 60x$$ $$\frac{6000}{60} = x$$ $$100\ \text{mL}$$

Dimensional Analysis Method

(combines # 1 and # 2)

$$\frac{\overset{1}{\cancel{100}\ \cancel{mcg}}}{\cancel{min}} \left| \frac{500\,\cancel{mL}}{\underset{1}{\cancel{30}\ \cancel{mg}}} \right| \frac{1\ \cancel{mg}}{\underset{10}{\cancel{1000}\ \cancel{mcg}}} \left| \frac{\overset{2}{\cancel{60}\ \cancel{min}}}{1\,\cancel{hr}} \right| \frac{500 \times 2}{10} = 100\ \text{mL/hr}$$

3. $\dfrac{4\ \text{mg}}{500\ \text{mL}} = 0.008\ \text{mg/mL}$

$0.008\ \text{mg} \times 1000\ \text{mcg} = 8\ \text{mcg/mL}$

4. Dose: $0.5\ \text{mcg/min}$

$0.5\ \text{mg} \times 60\ \text{min} = 30\ \text{mcg/hr}$

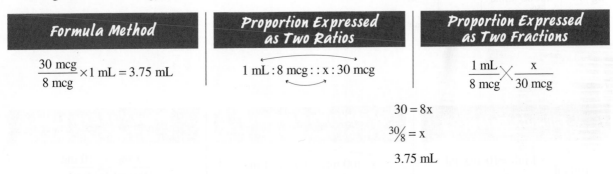

Formula Method	**Proportion Expressed as Two Ratios**	**Proportion Expressed as Two Fractions**
$\dfrac{30\ \text{mcg}}{8\ \text{mcg}} \times 1\ \text{mL} = 3.75\ \text{mL}$	$1\ \text{mL} : 8\ \text{mcg} :: x : 30\ \text{mcg}$	$\dfrac{1\ \text{mL}}{8\ \text{mcg}} \times \dfrac{x}{30\ \text{mcg}}$

$30 = 8x$

$^{30}\!/_{8} = x$

$3.75\ \text{mL}$

Dimensional Analysis Method

(combines # 1 and # 2)

$$\frac{0.5\,\cancel{mcg}}{\cancel{min}} \left| \frac{500\,\cancel{mL}}{\underset{1}{\cancel{4}\ \cancel{mg}}} \right| \frac{1\ \cancel{mg}}{\underset{2}{\cancel{1000}\ \cancel{mcg}}} \left| \frac{\overset{15}{\cancel{60}\ \cancel{min}}}{1\,\cancel{hr}} \right| \frac{0.5 \times 15}{2} = 3.75\ \text{mL} \qquad \text{Set the pump at 3.8 or 4 mL/hr}$$

5. $12\ \text{units/kg/hr}$

$12\ \text{units} \times 90\ \text{kg} = 1080\ \text{units/hr}$

6.

Formula Method	Proportion Expressed as Two Ratios	Proportion Expressed as Two Fractions

$$\frac{1080 \text{ units}}{25000 \text{ units}} \times 500 \text{ mL} = 21.6 \text{ mL/hr}$$
or 22 mL/hr

500 mL : 25000 units : : x : 1080 units

$$\frac{500 \text{ mL}}{25000 \text{ units}} \times \frac{1 \text{ mL}}{1080 \text{ units}}$$

$$500 \times 1080 = 25000x$$

$$21.6 \text{ mL/hr}$$

Dimensional Analysis Method

(combines # 5 and # 6)

$$\frac{12 \text{ units}}{\text{kg} \cdot \text{hr}} \cdot \frac{500 \text{ mL}}{25000 \text{ units}} \cdot 90 \text{ kg} \cdot \frac{12 \times 90}{50} = 21.6 \text{ mL/hr}$$ Set the pump at 21.6 or 22 mL/hr

next PTT due in 6 hours

7.

Formula Method	Proportion Expressed as Two Ratios	Proportion Expressed as Two Fractions

$$\frac{x}{100 \text{ mL}} \times 1 \text{ mL} = 10 \text{ mg/mL}$$

$$\frac{x}{100} \times 100 = 10 \times 100$$

$$x = 1000 \text{ mg}$$

x : 100 mL : : 10 mg : 1 mL

$$\frac{x \text{ mg}}{100 \text{ mL}} \times \frac{10 \text{ mg}}{1 \text{ mL}}$$

$$x = 100 \times 10$$

$$x = 1000 \text{ mg}$$

Dimensional Analysis Method

$$\frac{10 \text{ mg}}{1 \text{ mL}} \cdot 100 \text{ mL} \cdot \frac{10 \times 100}{} = 1000 \text{ mg}$$

8a. Order: 5 mcg/kg/min
5 mcg × 90 kg = 450 mcg/min

Step 1: $$\frac{1000 \text{ mg}}{100 \text{ mL}} = 10 \text{ mg in 1 mL}$$

Step 2:   10 mg × 1000 = 10000 mcg in 1 mL

Step 3:   Divide by 60 to get mcg per min
$$\frac{10000}{60} = 166.67 \text{ mcg/min}$$

Step 4:   Solve. Round to the nearest whole number.

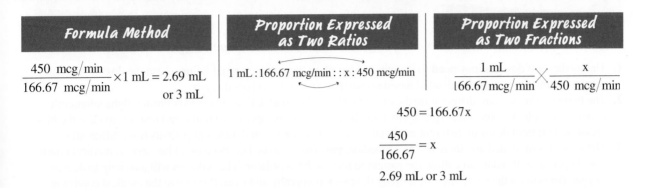

Formula Method	Proportion Expressed as Two Ratios	Proportion Expressed as Two Fractions
$\dfrac{450\ \text{mcg/min}}{166.67\ \text{mcg/min}} \times 1\ \text{mL} = 2.69\ \text{mL}$ or 3 mL	1 mL : 166.67 mcg/min : : x : 450 mcg/min	$\dfrac{1\ \text{mL}}{166.67\ \text{mcg/min}} \times \dfrac{\text{x}}{450\ \text{mcg/min}}$

$$450 = 166.67\text{x}$$

$$\frac{450}{166.67} = \text{x}$$

2.69 mL or 3 mL

Dimensional Analysis Method

(combines all steps)

$$\frac{1\ \cancel{\text{mL}}}{\underset{2}{\cancel{10}}\ \cancel{\text{mg}}} \times \frac{1\ \cancel{\text{mg}}}{1000\ \cancel{\text{mcg}}} \times \frac{\overset{1}{\cancel{5}}\ \cancel{\text{mcg}}}{\cancel{\text{kg}}\ /\ \cancel{\text{min}}} \times \frac{90\ \cancel{\text{kg}}}{} \times \frac{60\ \cancel{\text{min}}}{1\,\text{hr}} \times \frac{90 \times 60}{2 \times 1000} = \frac{5400}{2000} = 2.7\ \text{mL/hr}\ \text{or}\ 3\,\text{mL/hr}$$

Set the pump at 2.7 or 3 mL/hr.

8b. Order: 50 mcg/kg/min

50 mcg × 90 kg = 4500 mcg/min

(Steps 1–4 unchanged)

Formula Method	Proportion Expressed as Two Ratios	Proportion Expressed as Two Fractions
$\dfrac{4500\ \text{mcg/min}}{166.67\ \text{mcg/min}} \times 1\ \text{mL} = 26.99$ or 27 mL/hr	1 mL : 166.67 mcg/min : : x : 4500 mcg/min	$\dfrac{1\ \text{mL}}{166.67\ \text{mcg/min}} \times \dfrac{\text{x}}{4500\ \text{mcg/min}}$

$$4500 = 166.67\text{x}$$

$$\frac{4500}{166.67} = 26.99\ \text{or}\ 27\ \text{mL/hr}$$

Dimensional Analysis Method

(combines all steps)

$$\frac{1\ \cancel{\text{mL}}}{\underset{1}{\cancel{10}}\ \cancel{\text{mg}}} \times \frac{1\ \cancel{\text{mg}}}{1000\ \cancel{\text{mcg}}} \times \frac{\overset{5}{\cancel{50}}\ \cancel{\text{mcg}}}{\cancel{\text{kg}}\ /\ \cancel{\text{min}}} \times \frac{90\ \cancel{\text{kg}}}{} \times \frac{60\ \cancel{\text{min}}}{1\,\text{hr}} \times \frac{5 \times 90 \times 60}{1000} = \frac{27000}{1000} = 27\ \text{mL/hr}$$

Set the pump at 26.99 or 27 mL/hr.

Critical Thinking Questions

The "answers" are suggested answers and there may be other correct comments, suggestions, and answers.

1. The medication dosages may need to be adjusted based on the patient's renal failure. Also the dosages and/or administration times may be adjusted based on when the patient receives dialysis.
2. The two vasopressors are different medications and have different actions (Neo-Synephrine-alpha adrenergic agonist; Levophed-alpha adrenergic agonist and beta 1 adrenergic agonist), but the end result is to raise the blood pressure. Different doses of different medications may work better, and different patients react differently.
3. The patient is intubated and there are no immediate plans to extubate her, because of her serious medical condition. Diprivan will sedate and allow the patient to rest on the ventilator. The sedation will also help to decrease oxygen demand on the heart, thereby helping the cardiomyopathy and overall improve the medical condition.
4. A calcium channel blocker such as Nifedeipine may help atrial fibrillation but the patient is allergic to calcium channel blockers.
5. The two vasopressors may be causing the increased heart rate because of their affect on the alpha and beta receptors.
6. IV push drugs are given slowly to infuse the amount of drug concentration given over a longer time. This may be to prevent side effects, in this case, to prevent nausea.

Chapter 10

Calculations

1a. Dose: 20 mg

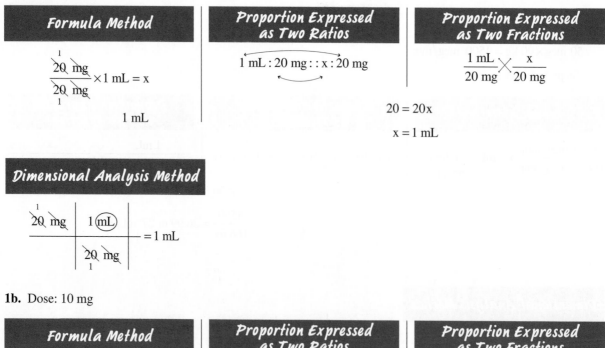

1b. Dose: 10 mg

Formula Method	Proportion Expressed as Two Ratios	Proportion Expressed as Two Fractions
$\dfrac{\overset{1}{\cancel{10}}\text{ mg}}{\underset{2}{\cancel{20}}\text{ mg}} \times 1\text{ mL} = x$ $\frac{1}{2}$ or 0.5 mL	$1\text{ mL} : 20\text{ mg} :: x : 10\text{ mg}$	$\dfrac{1\text{ mL}}{20\text{ mg}} \times \dfrac{x}{10\text{ mg}}$ $10 = 20x$ $\dfrac{10}{20} = x$ $\frac{1}{2}$ or 0.5 mL

Dimensional Analysis Method

$$\frac{\overset{1}{\cancel{10}}\ \text{mg}\ \Big|\ 1\ \textcircled{mL}\ \Big|\ 1}{\Big|\ \underset{2}{\cancel{20}}\ \text{mg}\ \Big|\ 2} = 0.5\ \text{mL}$$

2a. Dose: 400 mg

Formula Method	Proportion Expressed as Two Ratios	Proportion Expressed as Two Fractions
$\dfrac{400\ \text{mg}}{\underset{32}{\cancel{160}}\ \text{mg}} \times \overset{1}{\cancel{5}}\ \text{mL} = \dfrac{400}{32} = 12.5\ \text{mL}$	5 mL : 160 mg : : x : 400 mg	$\dfrac{5\ \text{mL}}{160\ \text{mg}} \times \dfrac{\text{x}}{400\ \text{mL}}$

$$5 \times 400 = 160\text{x}$$

$$\frac{2000}{160} = \text{x}$$

$$12.5\ \text{mL}$$

Dimensional Analysis Method

(combines both steps)

$$\frac{400\ \text{mg}\ \Big|\ \cancel{5}\ \text{mL}\ \Big|\ 1\ \textcircled{tsp}\ \Big|\ 400}{\Big|\ 160\ \text{mg}\ \Big|\ \cancel{5}\ \text{mL}\ \Big|\ 160} = 2.5\ \text{or}\ 2\tfrac{1}{2}\ \text{tsp}$$

2b. 12.5 mL = how many teaspoons
    1 tsp = 5 mL

Formula Method	Proportion Expressed as Two Ratios	Proportion Expressed as Two Fractions
$\dfrac{12.5\ \text{mL}}{5\ \text{mL}} \times 1\ \text{tsp} = 2.5\ \text{tsp}$	1 tsp : 5 mL : : x : 12.5 mL	$\dfrac{1\ \text{tsp}}{5\ \text{mL}} \times \dfrac{\text{x}}{12.5\ \text{mL}}$

$$12.5 = 5\text{x}$$

$$\frac{12.5}{5} = \text{x}$$

$$2.5\ \text{tsp}$$

3. 5 mg/kg
    $5 \times 30 = 150$ mg

Formula Method	Proportion Expressed as Two Ratios	Proportion Expressed as Two Fractions
$\dfrac{150\ \text{mg}}{\underset{20}{\cancel{100}}\ \text{mg}} \times \overset{1}{\cancel{5}}\ \text{mL} = \text{x}$ $\dfrac{150}{20} = \text{x}$ $7.5\ \text{mL}$	5 mL : 100 mg : : x : 150 mg	$\dfrac{5\ \text{mL}}{100\ \text{mg}} \times \dfrac{\text{x}}{150\ \text{mg}}$

$$5 \times 150 = 100\text{x}$$

$$\frac{750}{100} = \text{x}$$

$$7.5\ \text{mL}$$

Dimensional Analysis Method

(combines all steps)

$$\frac{5\ \cancel{mg}}{\cancel{kg}} \left| \frac{30\ \cancel{kg}}{} \right| \frac{\overset{1}{\cancel{5}}\ \cancel{(mL)}}{\underset{20}{\cancel{100}}\ \cancel{mg}} \left| \frac{5 \times 30}{20} \right. = \frac{150}{20} = 7.5\ mL$$

4. Dose: 2 Gm = 2000 mg

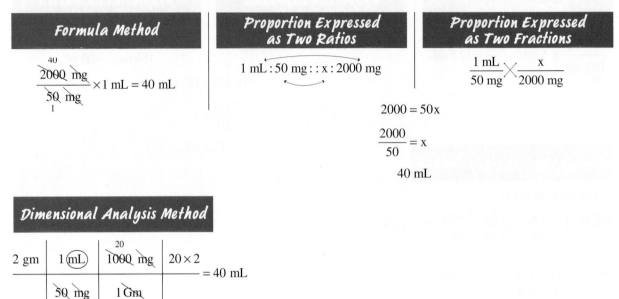

Formula Method	Proportion Expressed as Two Ratios	Proportion Expressed as Two Fractions
$\dfrac{\overset{40}{\cancel{2000}}\ \cancel{mg}}{\underset{1}{\cancel{50}}\ \cancel{mg}} \times 1\ mL = 40\ mL$	1 mL : 50 mg : : x : 2000 mg	$\dfrac{1\ mL}{50\ mg} \diagdown \dfrac{x}{2000\ mg}$

$$2000 = 50x$$
$$\frac{2000}{50} = x$$
$$40\ mL$$

Dimensional Analysis Method

$$\frac{2\ gm}{} \left| \frac{1\ \cancel{(mL)}}{\underset{1}{\cancel{50}}\ \cancel{mg}} \right| \frac{\overset{20}{\cancel{1000}}\ \cancel{mg}}{1\ \cancel{Gm}} \left| \frac{20 \times 2}{} \right. = 40\ mL$$

Infuse over 30 min. Set the pump at 80 mL/hr. The pump will deliver 40 mL in 30 minutes. Follow directions to infuse via Buterol.

5. 0.9 BSA

0.72 mg × BSA =

0.72 × 0.9 = 0.648 mg

6. Dose = 150 mg

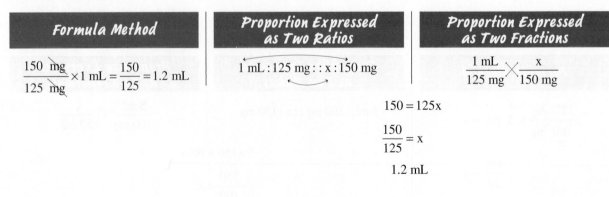

Formula Method	Proportion Expressed as Two Ratios	Proportion Expressed as Two Fractions
$\dfrac{150\ \cancel{mg}}{125\ \cancel{mg}} \times 1\ mL = \dfrac{150}{125} = 1.2\ mL$	1 mL : 125 mg : : x : 150 mg	$\dfrac{1\ mL}{125\ mg} \diagdown \dfrac{x}{150\ mg}$

$$150 = 125x$$
$$\frac{150}{125} = x$$
$$1.2\ mL$$

Dimensional Analysis Method

$$\frac{\overset{30}{\cancel{150}} \text{ mg} \quad 1 \text{ } \cancel{mL} \quad 30}{\underset{25}{\cancel{125}} \text{ mg} \quad 25} = 1.2 \text{ mL}$$

7. 1 mg/kg
$1 \times 30 = 30$ kg.

The dose is higher than the safe dose (10–25 mg). Check with the physician or healthcare provider, although the ordered dose is a correct prescribing dose.

8. 10 mL/kg/hr
$10 \times 30 = 300$ mL for 1 hour

Critical Thinking Questions

The "answers" are suggested answers and there may be other correct comments, suggestions, and answers.

1. Hold (and discontinue) the Augmentin—it contains amoxicillin and the patient is allergic to penicillin. Check with the physician or healthcare provider about giving Fortaz—sometimes the patient will have a cross-sensitivity to other antibiotics if allergic to penicillin, especially cephalosporins, which Fortaz is classified as.
2. Digoxin is ordered and there does not seem to be a medical condition that warrants the order. There may be a medical history of a cardiac condition that the nurse is unaware of. Check with the physician or healthcare provider.
3. The PO route may be difficult given the history of "flu-like" symptoms and no food and minimal drink for 28 hours. Check if any of the medications can be given via another route (need to have the physician or healthcare provider order a different route). If the patient has decreased nausea, check to see if the medications can be given in a liquid form.
4. The amount to be infused is 300 mL for one hour. Although this is a large dose of fluid for a child, the child's condition (no food and minimal drink for 48 hours) may warrant the fluid in order to prevent further dehydration. 100 mL/hr is also a higher dose, but again may be needed for the child's condition. Close monitoring of the infusion is needed.

Glossary

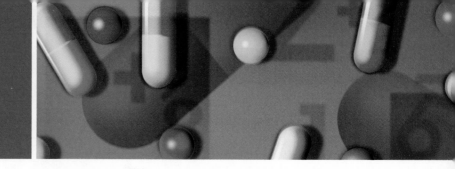

Absorption the passing of a drug in the body across tissue into the general circulation and becomes active in the body

ac before meals

ad lib as desired

Adverse effects nontherapeutic effects that may be harmful

Aerosol method of drug administration where the solid drug is delivered in a liquid spray

Agonist drug that binds with cell receptors to invoke a cellular response, usually similar to the cell's action

Allergic reaction reaction to a drug involving the body's antibody response to a perceived antigen (in this case, the medication)

Ampule (ampoule) a sealed glass container for powdered or liquid drugs

Amt amount

Analgesic drug to relieve or minimize pain

Anaphylaxis severe allergic reaction

Anaphylactic shock severe allergic reaction that results in a shock state

Antagonist drug that binds with cell receptors to block the cellular response

Antagonism the interaction between two drugs in which the combined effect is less than the sum of the effects of the drugs acting separately

Antibiotic drug that inhibits or kills bacteria, fungus or protozoans

Anticoagulant drug that inhibits formation of blood clots

Antiemetic drug that prevents vomiting and reduces nausea

Antihypertensive drug that lowers blood pressure

Antitussive drug to use to suppress coughing

Anxiolytic drugs that relieve anxiety

Apothecary system a measurement system using grains and minims, introduced into the United States from England in colonial times

AS, AD, AU left ear, right ear, both ears; JCAHO states do not use, but write out "left ear," "right ear," or "both ears" as appropriate

Autonomy self-determination. The patient/client has a right to be informed about drug therapy and to refuse it

Avoirdupois system a measurement system using ounces and pounds; used for patient weight and some drugs

Bactericidal a drug action that kills an organism

Bacteriostatic a drug action that inhibits an organism's ability to grow and reproduce

Beneficence acting in the best interests of the patient. "Doing good"

bid twice a day

Bioavailability the availability of a drug once it is absorbed and transported in the body to the site of its action

Biotransformation the conversion of an active drug to an inactive compound

Body surface area, or BSA calculation of meters squared based on height and weight, as shown in a nomogram

BP blood pressure

Bronchodilator drug that dilates the bronchioles of the lungs

Buccal the route of administration in which a drug is placed in the pouch between the teeth and cheek

C Centigrade, Celsius

Cap or Capsule a gelatin container that holds a drug in a solid or liquid form

CC or cc cubic centimeter; equal to 1 mL; JCAHO states do not use this abbreviation; use "mL"

Cardiac glycoside a drug that increases cardiac contractility and increases cardiac output. Lanoxin (digoxin) is the most common cardiac glycoside used

CDC Centers for Disease Control and Prevention

Chemical name the drug name derived from its chemical structure

Chemotherapy drug treatment of cancer

Civil law statutes concerned with the rights and duties of individuals

Clark's Rule a way to determine dosage of medications for children older than 2 years of age; based on weight

Cm centimeter

Combination drugs drugs that contain more than one active medication

Common factor a number that is a factor of two different numbers (ie, 3 is a factor of 6 and 9)

Common fraction a fraction with a whole number in the numerator and denominator (ie, 7/9)

Compliance taking a medication as prescribed or following label instructions

Concentration the amount of drug in a solution; in fraction, decimal, or percentage form

Contraindication a situation in which a drug should be avoided

Controlled drug a drug controlled by federal, state, and local law; a drug that may be lead to drug abuse or dependence

Corticosteroid hormones that help the body respond to stress; also used in immune response, anti-inflammatory. In the body, produced by the adrenal cortex

Cream a semisolid drug preparation applied externally to the skin or mucous membrane

CR controlled release

Criminal law statutes that protect the public again actions harmful to society

CSF cerebrospinal fluid

Cross tolerance becoming tolerant to one drug and then acquiring tolerance to another drug; this could be with a similar drug or a drug from a similar category or a drug with a similar classification

Cumulation or Accumulation the inability of the body to metabolize one dose of a drug before another dose is administered; cumulation leads to increased concentration of the drug in the body and possible toxicity

d day

DEA US Drug Enforcement Administration

Denominator the bottom number in a fraction

Dermal route the topical application of a drug to the skin

Diluent a liquid used to dissolve a solid, usually a powder, into a solution

Disch discharge

D/C discharge or discontinue; JCAHO states do not use; write out "discharge" or "discontinue" as appropriate

Displacement the increase in the volume of fluid added to a powder, when the powder dissolves and goes into solution

Distribution the movement of a drug through body fluids, chiefly blood, to cells

Dividend the number to be divided (eg, 40 divided by 5, 40 is the dividend)

Divisor the number by which the dividend is divided; in the previous example, 5 is the divisor

dL deciliter, 100 mL

Dose the amount of drug to be administered at one time or the total amount to be given

DR delayed release

dr dram. An apothecary measurement rarely used. One fluid dram equals approximately 4 mL

Drip or Drop factor the number of drops of an IV fluid in 1 mL; listed on the IV tubing set or package

Drip rate the number of drops of an IV solution to be infused per minute

Drop a minute (tiny) sphere of liquid

Drug a chemical agent used in the treatment, diagnosis, or prevention of disease

Dry powder inhaler (DPI) inhaler that converts a solid drug into a fine powder

Elixir a clear, aromatic, sweetened alcoholic preparation

Emulsion suspension of a fat or oil in water with the aid of an agent to reduce surface tension

Enteral refers to the small intestine

Enteral route drugs given orally or through N/G or PEG tubes

Enteric coating a layer placed over a tablet or capsule to prevent dissolution in the stomach; used to protect the drug from gastric acid or to protect the stomach from drug irritation

Enteral feedings delivery of liquid feedings through a tube

Epidural route medication is administered into the space around the dura mater of the spinal column

ER   extended release

Ethics   a system of values and morals

Excretion   the physiologic elimination of substances from the body

Expectorant   drug to increase bronchial secretions

Expiration date   a drug cannot be administered after the last day of the month stamped on the label

F   Fahrenheit

FDA   Food and Drug Administration

Fidelity   ethical principle where the nurse or health care provider keeps promises made to a patient

Film-coated tablets   compressed, powdered drugs that are smooth and easy to swallow because of their outer shell covering

First-pass effect   drugs that are administered orally that pass from the intestine to the liver and are partially metabolized before entering the circulation

Formulary   reference for pharmacists and other health care providers with lists of drugs, drug combinations, etc.

Flow rate   number of milliliters per hour of IV fluid to be infused

fl. oz.   fluid ounce; equal to 30 mL

Fluid extract or fluidextract   potent alcoholic liquid concentration of a drug

Fraction   division of one number by another

Fried's rule   a rule to calculate drug dosages for infants younger than 1 year; based on age

g   or Gm gram

G-tube   gastrostomy tube; inserted into the stomach. Can be used for drug administration and enteral feedings

Gauge   the diameter or width of a needle; the higher the gauge number, the finer the needle

Gel   an aqueous suspension of small particles of an insoluble drug in a hydrated form

Generic name   the official name of a drug as listed in the United States or other pharmacopoeia

Glucocorticoid   hormones that help the body to respond to stress. In the body manufactured by the adrenal cortex

Gram   weight of 1 mL of water at 4°C; basic unit of weight in metric system

gr   grain; approximately equal to 60 or 65 mg. an apothecary measure rarely used

gtt   drop or drops

h or hr   hour

Half-life   the time that a drug is metabolized by 50% in the body

Hepatotoxic   a drug or side effects of a drug that may affect the liver

Household system   a measurement system based on household items of measurement; uses teaspoon, tablespoon, cups

hs   hour of sleep, at bedtime; JCAHO states not to use this abbreviation; write out "at bedtime"

hypo   hypodermic syringe or injection

I & O   intake and output

IM   intramuscular

Idiosyncratic   an unexplained or unusual reaction to a drug

Improper fraction   a fraction with the numerator larger or equal to the denominator

Incompatibility   a mixture of two or more drugs that results in a harmful chemical or physical interaction

Inhalant   vapors that are inhaled via the nose, lungs, or trachea

Inhaler   a device used to spray liquid or powder in a fine mist into the lungs during inspiration

inj   injection

Interaction   either desirable or undesirable effects produced by giving two or more drugs together

IU   international unit; JCAHO states do not use, write out "international units"

Intra-articular   medication injected into the joints

Intradermal or ID   an injection given into the upper layers of the skin

Intramuscular or IM   an injection given into the muscle

Intrathecal   administration into the cerebrospinal fluid via the subarachnoid space

Intravenous or IV   medication given by injection or infusion into a vein

Isotonic   solutions that have the same osmotic pressure as physiologic body fluids

IV   intravenous

IVPB   intravenous piggyback; a medication placed in an infusion set and attached to the main line IV for delivery to the patient

JCAHO   Joint Commission on Accreditation of Healthcare Organizations; an organization responsible for safety in hospitals and other health care settings; in 2004, the JCAHO issued a list of abbreviations "not to be used" to decrease errors

J-tube a tube placed in the jejunum, can be used for drug administration and enteral feedings

Justice ethical principle that refers to all patients/clients receiving the same care and that it is the nurse's obligation to provide safe care

k or kg kilogram

lb pounds

Liter or L unit of fluid volume in the metric system; equal to one tenth of a cubic meter

Loading dose higher dose given at the initiation of drug therapy in order to build up the therapeutic effect

Lotion liquid suspension intended for external use

Lowest common denominator the smallest number that is a multiple of all denominators

Lowest terms the smallest numbers possible in the numerator and denominator of a fraction; reducing a fraction to lowest terms means the numerator and denominator cannot be reduced further

Lozenge a flat, round, or rectangular preparation held in the mouth until it dissolves

Magma a bulky suspension of an insoluble preparation in water that must be shaken before pouring

mcg microgram; previously abbreviated as µg; however, this is not an approved abbreviation by the JCAHO

MDI metered dose inhaler; an aerosol device that consists of two parts: a canister under pressure and a mouthpiece; finger pressure on the mouthpiece opens a valve that discharges one dose

Medication another word for drug. Sometimes used to a drug that has been administered

Medication Administration Record (MAR) documentation of drugs received by the patient or schedule of drugs to be received

Medication error a preventable error in medication administration, usually related to one of the six rights

Meniscus the curved surface of a liquid in a container

Metabolism the chemical biotransformation of a drug to a form that can be excreted

Meter or m a unit of length in the metric system; equals 39.27 in

Metric System a measurement system that uses meters, liters, grams; common system used

worldwide except in the United States; widely used system in dosages of drugs; based on units of 10

mg milligram

MgSO4 magnesium sulfate; JCAHO states do not use; write out "magnesium sulfate" because this abbreviation can be confused with MSO4

Military time time based on a 24-hour clock rather than the traditional 12-hour clock

Milliequivalent or mEq the number of grams of solute in a 1-mL solution; used to measure electrolytes and some medications

min minute

minim an apothecary measure, rarely used. Equals 1/60 of a dram. Also equal to one drop

Mixed number a whole number and a fraction (eg, 1 11/42)

ML or mL milliliter

mm millimeter

mo month

MS, MSO4 morphine sulfate; JCAHO states do not use; write out morphine sulfate; this abbreviation can be confused with MgSO4

Multidose large stock containers of medication

Narcotic natural or synthetic drug related to morphine; or a large classification of drugs that include hallucinogens, CNS stimulants, and illegal drugs

Nebulizer device to convert liquid drugs into a fine mist to use as an inhaled route

NDC national drug code; a number used by pharmacists to identify a drug and the packaging method

Nephrotoxic a drug or side effects of a drug that may affect the renal system

N/G tube tube inserted through the nasal opening into the stomach. Can be used for drug administration and enteral feedings.

Nomogram a tabular illustration of body surface area based on height and weight

Nonmaleficence ethical principle to not harm the patient. "Do no harm"

Nonparenteral drugs drugs administered by topical, rectal, or oral route

Nonprescription drug a drug obtained without a prescription; also called over the counter or OTC

NPO nothing by mouth

Numerator the top number in a fraction

OD right eye (suggested "do not use"—write out "right eye")

Official name a drug's official name as listed in the United States Pharmacopoeia and the National Formulary

O/G tube tube inserted through the oral cavity into the stomach. Can be used for drug administration and enteral feedings

Ointment a semisolid preparation in a petroleum or lanolin base for external use

Ophthalmic pertaining to the eye

Oral route abbreviated po; drugs given through the mouth

OS left eye (suggested "do not use"—write out "left eye")

OTC over the counter

Otic pertaining to the ear

Ototoxic a drug or side effects of the drug that may affect the ear

OU both eyes (suggested "do not use"—write out "both eyes")

oz ounce

Parenteral a general term that means administration by injection (IV, IM, or subcutaneous)

Paste a thick ointment used to protect the skin

Pastille a disklike solid that slowly dissolves in the mouth

Patch a small adhesive that releases medication over an extended period of time; applied topically

pc after meals

PEG tube a special type of gastrostomy tube, Percutaneous Endoscopic Gastrotomy. Is designed to be more permanent. Can be used for drug administration and enteral feedings.

Percentage parts per hundred, designated by a percent sign (%)

Percentage solution the solid that is dissolved in a liquid represents a percentage of the total weight of the solution; measured in grams per 100 mL solution

Pharmacodynamics the study of the chemical and physical effects of drugs in the body

Pharmacogenetics chemical and physical effects in the body to a drug related to a person's genetics

Pharmacokinetics the science of the factors that determine how much drug reaches the site of action in the body and is excreted

Pharmacology the study of the origin, nature, chemistry effects, and uses of drugs

Pharmacopoeia medical reference containing information about drugs

Pharmacotherapeutics the study of the use of drugs to treat, prevent, and diagnose diseases

Piggyback medication placed in an IV infusion set attached to the mainline IV for delivery to the patient

Placebo an inert substance used in place of a drug to determine its psychological effect and the physiologic changes caused by the psychological response

PO by mouth, oral

Potency strength of a drug at a specific concentration or dose

Powder a finely ground solid drug or mixture of drugs for internal or external use

PPN peripheral parenteral nutrition

Prefilled cartridge a small vial with a needle attached that fits into a metal or plastic holder for injection

Prefilled syringe a liquid, sterile medication that is ready to administer without further preparation

Prescription an order for medication written by an authorized prescriber

Prescription drug a drug that requires a prescription; regulated usually by state laws

Prime number a whole number only divisible by one and itself; a whole number that cannot be reduced any further (ie, 3, 5, 7)

Protocol a specific set of drug orders referring to certain physical conditions, or lab values that must be met before drug administration. Also used when titrating certain drugs, i.e. insulin and heparin.

PR per rectum

PRN when required

Product the answer in multiplication

Prolonged-release or slow-release tablet a powdered, compressed drug that disintegrates more slowly and has a longer duration of action

Proper fraction a fraction with a numerator smaller than the denominator

Proportion a set of ratios or fractions

pt patient or pint

q each, every